CLINICAL GASTROENTEROLOGY

Series Editor
George Y. Wu
University of Connecticut Health Center, Farmington, CT, USA

For further volumes:
http://www.springer.com/series/7672

Chris A. Liacouras · Jonathan E. Markowitz
Editors

Eosinophilic Esophagitis

Humana Press

Editors
Chris A. Liacouras, MD
Professor of Pediatrics
The University of Pennsylvania
School of Medicine
Co-Director
Center for Pediatric Eosinophilic Disorders
The Children's Hospital of Philadelphia
Philadelphia, PA, USA
liacouras@email.chop.edu

Jonathan E. Markowitz, MD, MSCE
Medical Director
Pediatric Gastroenterology and Nutrition
Greenville Hospital System University
Medical Center
Greenville, SC, USA
JMarkowitz@ghs.org

ISBN 978-1-60761-514-9 e-ISBN 978-1-60761-515-6
DOI 10.1007/978-1-60761-515-6
Springer New York Dordrecht Heidelberg London

Library of Congress Control Number: 2011936009

Printed on acid-free paper

Humana Press is part of Springer Science+Business Media (www.springer.com)

Preface

Eosinophilic esophagitis (EoE) is a disease that has gained increasing interest over the last decade. First appreciated in 1995, EoE is now one of the most talked about disorders among pediatric and adult gastroenterologists, allergists, and pathologists. Over the past decade, the disease has seen impressive advances with regard to the clinical recognition of patients, basic research, allergy testing, and genetic identification.

In 2007, the first consensus recommendations on EoE were published in *Gastroenterology*. Because of the significant increase in the number of publications on the subject, an update of the consensus recommendations were recently published in the *Journal of Allergy and Clinical Immunology (July 2011)*. As part of this update, a conceptual definition was generated that states, "*Eosinophilic esophagitis represents a chronic, immune/antigen mediated, esophageal disease characterized clinically by symptoms related to esophageal dysfunction and histologically by eosinophil-predominant inflammation.*" In addition, the diagnostic guideline was adjusted and now defines the disease as follows: "*EoE is a clinico-pathological disease. Clinically, EoE is characterized by symptoms related to esophageal dysfunction. Pathologically, one or more biopsies must show eosinophil predominant inflammation. With few exceptions, 15 eosinophils/hpf (peak value) is considered a minimum threshold for a diagnosis of EoE. The disease is isolated to the esophagus and other causes of esophageal eosinophilia should be excluded, specifically PPI-responsive esophageal eosinophilia. The disease should remit with treatments of dietary exclusion and/or topical corticosteroids. EoE should be diagnosed by clinicians taking into consideration all clinical and pathologic information; neither of these parameters should be interpreted in isolation.*"

The contributing authors have been selected because of their expertise not only from their clinical and research experience, but also from their long-standing interest, dedication, and efforts to increase the knowledge of EoE worldwide. They have written informative chapters providing up-to-date knowledge on both pediatric and adult manifestations of EoE. We hope that the readers will use the information presented to increase their knowledge of EoE and to aid them in the diagnosis, management, and treatment of individual patients.

As editors, we would like to thank all contributing authors for their hard work and interest in this project. Their commitment and excellence in patient care, research, and education is much appreciated and readily apparent.

Philadelphia, PA — Chris A. Liacouras
Greenville, SC — Jonathan E. Markowitz

Contents

Contributors

Seema S. Aceves, MD, PhD Division of Allergy, Immunology, Departments of Pediatrics and Medicine, University of California, Rady's Children's Hospital, San Diego, CA, USA

Steven J. Ackerman, PhD Department of Biochemistry and Molecular Genetics (M/C 669), and Sections of Hematology-Oncology and Pulmonary, Critical Care, Sleep and Allergy, The University of Illinois at Chicago College of Medicine, Chicago, IL, USA

Paola De Angelis, MD Digestive Surgery and Endoscopy Unit, Pediatric Hospital Bambino Gesú, Rome, Italy

Amindra S. Arora, MBBChir, FRCP Department of GIH, Mayo Clinic, Rochester, MN, USA

Dan Atkins, MD Professor of Pediatrics, Associate Professor of Pediatrics, Co-Director, National Jewish Health, University of Colorado Denver School of Medicine, The Children's Hospital Denver, Denver, CO, USA

Gastrointestinal Eosinophilic Diseases Program, The Children's Hospital Colorado, National Jewish Health, University of Colorado Denver School of Medicine, Aurora, CO, USA

Stephen E. Attwood, FRCS, FRCSI, MCh, BA Mod Physiol Department of Surgery, Northumbria Healthcare, Tyne + Wear, UK

Janet L. Beausoleil, MD Department of Pediatrics, Division of Allergy and Immunology, The Children's Hospital of Philadelphia, Philadelphia, PA, USA

Terri Brown-Whitehorn, MD Assistant Professor of Clinical Pediatrics, Department of Allergy and Immunology, The Children's Hospital of Philadelphia, University of Pennsylvania School of Medicine, Philadelphia, PA, USA

Matthew Bohm, DO Clinical Instructor of Medicine, Department of Medicine, Temple University Hospital, Philadelphia, PA, USA

A. Wesley Burks, MD Department of Pediatrics, Division of Allergy and Immunology, Duke University Medical Center, Durham, NC, USA

Katherine N. Cahill, MD Clinical Fellow in Allergy and Immunology, Division of Rheumatology, Immunology, and Allergy, Brigham and Women's Hospital and Harvard Medical School, Boston, MA, USA

Mirna Chehade, MD, MPH Mount Sinai center for Eosinophilic Disorders, Jaffe Food Allergy Institute, Mount Sinai School of Medicine, New York, NY, USA

Edaire Cheng, MD Department of Pediatrics, University of Texas Southwestern Medical Center, Dallas, TX, USA

Antonella Cianferoni, MD, PhD Assistant Professor of Pediatrics, Department of Allergy, The Children's Hospital of Philadelphia, Philadelphia, PA, USA

Margaret H. Collins, MD Department of Pathology, University of Cincinnati, Cincinnati Children's Hospital Medical Center, Cincinnati, OH, USA

Luigi Dall'Oglio, MD Department of Digestive Endoscopy and Surgery Unit, Bambino Gesú Children's Hospital IRCCS, Rome, Italy

Gary W. Falk, MD, MS Department of Medicine, Hospital of the University of Pennsylvania, Perelman School of Medicine, Philadelphia, PA, USA

Department of Medicine, Division of Gastroenterology, Hospital of the University of Pennsylvania, Philadelphia, PA, USA

James P. Franciosi, MD, MS, MSCE Division of Gastroenterology, Hepatology and Nutrition, Cincinnati Children's Hospital Medical Center, Cincinnati, OH, USA

Glenn T. Furuta, MD National Jewish Health, University of Colorado Denver School of Medicine, The Children's Hospital Denver, Denver, CO, USA

Gastrointestinal Eosinophilic Diseases Program, Children's Hospital Colorado, National Jewish Health, University of Colorado Denver School of Medicine, Aurora, CO, USA

Mimi Girten, BS, RD, LDN Pediatric Dietician, Department of Clinical Nutrition, The Children's Hospital of Philadelphia, Philadelphia, PA, USA

Gerald J. Gleich, MD Department of Dermatology, University of Utah Hospital, Salt Lake City, UT, USA

Elizabeth Goldberg, RN, MSN, CRNP Advance Practice Nurse, Division of Gastroenterology, Hepatology, and Nutrition, The Children's Hospital of Philadelphia, Philadelphia, PA, USA

Nirmala Gonsalves, MD Department of Medicine, Division of Gastroenterology, Northwestern University, Feinberg School of Medicine, Chicago, IL, USA

Ikuo Hirano, MD Department of Gastroenterology, Northwestern University Feinberg School of Medicine, Chicago, IL, USA

Petr Hruz, MD, PhD Department of Gastroenterology and Hepatology, University Hospital Basel, Basel, Switzerland

W. Daniel Jackson, MD Clinical Professor of Pediatrics, Department of Pediatric Gastroenterology and Nutrition, University of Utah School of Medicine, Salt Lake City, UT, USA

Amir F. Kagalwalla, MBBS Division of Gastroenterology, Hepatology, and Nutrition, Northwestern University Feinberg School of Medicine, Children's Memorial Hospital, John H. Stroger Hospital of Cook County, Chicago, IL, USA

David A. Katzka, MD Department of Medicine, Mayo Clinic, Rochester, MN, USA

Mary Klinnert, PhD Department of Pediatrics, National Jewish Health, Denver, CO, USA

Department of Psychiatry, School of Medicine, University of Colorado, Aurora, CO, USA

David A. Leiman, MD Medical Resident, Department of Medicine, Hospital of the University of Pennsylvania, Perelman School of Medicine, Philadelphia, PA, USA

Marc S. Levine, MD Professor of Radiology and Advisory Dean, Chief of Gastrointestinal Radiology, Department of Radiology, University of Pennsylvania School of Medicine, Philadelphia, PA, USA

Hospital of the University of Pennsylvania, Philadelphia, PA, USA

Chris A. Liacouras, MD Co-Director, Center for Pediatric Eosinophilic Disorders, The Children's Hospital of Philadelphia, Philadelphia, PA, USA

Professor of Pediatrics, Division of Gastroenterology, Hepatology and Nutrition, University of Pennsylvania School of Medicine, Philadelphia, PA, USA

Colleen Lukens, PhD Psychologist, Department of Child and Adolescent Psychiatry and the Behavioral Sciences, The Children's Hospital of Philadelphia, Philadelphia, PA, USA

Asim Maqbool, MD Pediatric Gastroenterology, Hepatology, and Nutrition, University of Pennsylvania School of Medicine, The Children's Hospital of Philadelphia, Philadelphia, PA, USA

Jonathan E. Markowitz, MD, MSCE Department of Pediatrics, Pediatric Gastroenterology and Nutrition, Greenville Hospital System University Medical Center, Greenville, SC, USA

Richard J. Noel, MD, PhD Division of Gastroenterology, Department of Pediatrics, Medical College of Wisconsin, Milwaukee, WI, USA

Molly O'Gorman, MD Associate Professor of Pediatrics, Department of Pediatric Gastroenterology, Hepatology, and Nutrition, Primary Children's Medical Center and University of Utah Hospital, Salt Lake City, UT, USA

Kathryn A. Peterson, MD, MSci (Epid) Assistant Professor of Medicine, Department of Gastroenterology, University of Utah Hospital, Salt Lake City, UT, USA

Philip E. Putnam, MD Division of Gastroenterology, Hepatology, and Nutrition, Cincinnati Children's Hospital Medical Center, Cincinnati, OH, USA

Cincinnati Center for Eosinophilic Disorders, Cincinnati, OH, USA

Karthik Ravi, MD GI Fellow Department of GIH, Mayo Clinic, Rochester, MN, USA

Joel E. Richter, MD, FACP, MACG Department of Medicine, Section of Gastroenterology, Temple University School of Medicine, Philadelphia, PA, USA

Sally Ritz, RD, CSP, LDN Certified Specialist in Pediatric Nutrition, Division of Gastroenterology, Hepatology, and Nutrition, Children's Memorial Hospital, Chicago, IL, USA

Marc E. Rothenberg, MD, PhD Department of Allergy and Immunology, Cincinnati Children's Hospital Medical Center, University of Cincinnati, Cincinnati, OH, USA

Hugh A. Sampson, MD Professor of Pediatrics, Dean, Translational Biomedical Sciences, Director, Jaffe Food Allergy Institute, Mount Sinai School of Medicine, New York, NY, USA

Javed Sheikh, MD Center for Eosinophilic Disorders, Beth Israel Deaconess Medical Center, Harvard Medical School, Brookline, MA, USA

Joseph D. Sherrill, PhD Department of Allergy and Immunology, Cincinnati Children's Hospital Medical Center, Cincinnati, OH, USA

Michele Shuker, MS, RD, CSP, LDN Division of Allergy and Immunology, The Children's Hospital of Philadelphia, Philadelphia, PA, USA

Scott H. Sicherer, MD Department of Pediatrics, Mount Sinai School of Medicine, Jaffe Food Allergy Institute, New York, NY, USA

Stuart Spechler, MD Chief, Department of Medicine, VA North Texas Healthcare System and the University of Texas Southwestern Medical Center, Dallas, TX, USA

Jonathan Spergel, MD, PhD Department of Pediatrics, Division of Allergy and Immunology, The Children's Hospital of Philadelphia, Philadelphia, PA, USA

Alex Straumann, MD Department of Gastroenterology, University Hospital Basel, Basel, Switzerland

Swiss EoE Research Group, Olten, Switzerland

Louanne M. Tourangeau, MD Allergy and Immunology, Department of Medicine, University of California, San Diego, CA, USA

Pooja Varshney, MD Fellow-in-Training, Department of Pediatrics, Division of Allergy and Immunology, Duke University Medical Center, Durham, NC, USA

Harland S. Winter, MD Associate Professor of Pediatrics, Department of Pediatric Gastroenterology, Harvard Medical School, MassGeneral Hospital for Children, Boston, MA, USA

Chapter 1
A History of Eosinophilic Esophagitis

Chris A. Liacouras and Jonathan E. Markowitz

Keywords Eosinophilic esophagitis • Esophageal eosiniphilia • Allergic esophagitis

Introduction

Eosinophilic esophagitis (EoE), an isolated esophageal eosinophilia associated with clinical symptoms, is a disease that has received a great deal of attention over the last 10–15 years. EoE, previously known as primary eosinophilic esophagitis, idiopathic eosinophilic esophagitis or allergic esophagitis, occurs in both children and adults. Prior to 1995, the literature contained only rare reports of individuals diagnosed with an isolated esophageal eosinophilia. However, since 1995, reports in the literature and information related to EoE have grown tremendously. This chapter focuses on the history of EoE, including initial reports of esophageal eosinophilia prior to 1995, the landmark article identifying EoE as a disorder in 1995, the growth of EoE in the literature since 1995, the development of the First International Gastrointestinal Eosinophilic Research Symposium (FIGERS) in 2006, and the creation of The International Gastrointestinal Eosinophilic Researchers (TIGERS).

C.A. Liacouras (✉)
Co-Director, Center for Pediatric Eosinophilic Disorders, The Children's Hospital of Philadelphia, 34th and Civic Center Blvd, Philadelphia, PA 19104, USA

Professor of Pediatrics, Division of Gastroenterology, Hepatology and Nutrition, University of Pennsylvania School of Medicine, Philadelphia, PA, USA
e-mail: liacouras@email.chop.edu

C.A. Liacouras and J.E. Markowitz (eds.), *Eosinophilic Esophagitis*,
Clinical Gastroenterology, DOI 10.1007/978-1-60761-515-6_1,

History of Esophagitis

Since 1970, the histologic hallmarks for reflux esophagitis have been basal zone hyperplasia, elongated papillae, and intraepithelial neutrophils [1–4]. Other nonspecific findings include dilated vascular channels in the lamina propria papillae and distended squamous or "balloon" cells. In 1982, Winter [5] reported the presence of intraepithelial eosinophils as an added criterion for the diagnosis of reflux esophagitis in children. In this study of 46 symptomatic pediatric patients and nine control subjects, the presence of esophageal eosinophils was correlated with 24-h pH probe monitoring, esophageal manometry, and other histologic features of gastroesophageal reflux, including papillary length and basal zone thickness. The presence of one of more intraepithelial eosinophils in the esophagus was established as a specific indicator of esophagitis. Abnormal esophageal acid clearance was correlated with other accepted morphologic features of esophageal injury. In addition, it was suggested that eosinophils were diagnostic of reflux esophagitis even if other accepted histologic abnormalities were absent. Although the majority of eosinophils were observed in the distal esophagus, the presence of more proximal eosinophils was associated with increasingly abnormal pH probe results. These findings were later confirmed in adults [6]. Over the years, apart from the diagnosis of reflux esophagitis, large numbers of esophageal eosinophils have been identified in children with eosinophilic gastroenteritis or allergic gastroenteritis [7], Crohn's disease and, more recently, eosinophilic esophagitis.

History of Esophageal Eosinophilia

During the last 25 years, several studies have identified patients with an isolated, severe eosinophilic esophagitis, which suggested an etiology other than acid reflux. In 1977 one of the first cases of esophageal eosinophilia was reported by Dobbins [8], involving a case of a 51-year-old male patient with asthma and allergies who developed dysphagia and substernal chest pain. Esophageal biopsies revealed a focal, marked eosinophilic infiltrate. Small bowel biopsies demonstrated villous flattening and an eosinophilia. The patient was diagnosed with eosinophilic gastroenteritis. In 1978, Landres [9] reported on the case of a patient with achalasia associated with esophageal eosinophilia who underwent esophageal myotomy that revealed eosinophilic infiltration of the muscular layer. In 1983, Matzinger [10] described an adolescent with dysphagia, food allergy, and a peripheral eosinophilia who underwent esophageal biopsy, which revealed eosinophilic infiltration of both the esophagus and stomach. In 1985, Lee [11] reported on a series of 11 patients with a severe esophageal eosinophilia, greater than 10 esophageal eosinophils per high power field (hpf), who presented with dysphagia, heartburn, vomiting, and esophageal strictures (3 of 11). However, reflux was not documented by 24-h pH probe. One patient was given steroids and clinically improved.

Between 1978 and 1990, several reports were published linking radiographic abnormalities with esophageal eosinophilia [12–14]. Clinically, patients described in these reports presented with dysphagia, heartburn, chest pain, peripheral eosinophilia, regurgitation, and vomiting. In the majority of these patients, barium radiographic studies demonstrated an esophageal stricture. While most of these patients underwent repeated esophageal dilatation, one patient was given corticosteroids, upon which, both the clinical symptoms and the esophageal stricture resolved.

In 1993, Attwood [15] reported one of the first studies comparing patients with isolated esophageal eosinophilia to patients with gastroesophageal reflux. He described 12 patients presenting with dysphagia who had more than 20 esophageal eosinophils/hpf (mean 56 eosinophils/hpf). All had visually normal esophageal mucosa and no esophageal anatomic abnormality – 11 had normal pH monitoring and seven had evidence of an allergic disorder. Only one patient had antral eosinophilia. This group was compared to another group, consisting of 90 patients with medically responsive gastroesophageal reflux (documented by an abnormal 24-h pH probe). Only 43 of these patients had esophageal eosinophils to a much lesser degree (mean 3.3 eosinophils/HPF). The author suggested that these patients represented a new clinicopathologic syndrome not previously described. Similarly, in 1995, Vitellas [16] reported on 13 male patients with idiopathic eosinophilic esophagitis and showed that the majority of these patients responded to corticosteroids. The patients' clinical symptoms included dysphagia (12 of 13), allergic manifestations (10 of 13), peripheral eosinophilia (12 of 13) and proximal esophageal strictures (10 of 13). Vitellas suggests that the identification of these patients is important because treatment with corticosteroids is much more effective than esophageal dilatation.

In 1993, Levine and Saul [17] suggested that idiopathic eosinophilic esophagitis should be considered in all patients with esophageal narrowing and a severe esophageal eosinophilia. These authors argued that the difference between the diagnosis of reflux esophagitis and idiopathic eosinophilic esophagitis depended upon the location of the eosinophilia, with the implication that, in idiopathic eosinophilic esophagitis, esophageal eosinophils were located predominantly in the proximal esophagus and that the distal esophagus was spared. In contrast, Ruchelli [18] demonstrated that a diagnosis of eosinophilic esophagitis should be considered based on the degree of esophageal eosinophilia regardless of location. Ruchelli identified 102 patients who had at least one intraepithelial esophageal eosinophil after undergoing endoscopic biopsy for symptoms of gastroesophageal reflux. Patients initially underwent upper endoscopy with distal esophageal biopsy and were subsequently treated with aggressive antireflux pharmacologic therapy. Ruchelli's results indicated that the number of esophageal eosinophils/hpf predicted patient improvement (1.1 ± 0.3 eosinophils/hpf), relapse (6.4 ± 2.4) or reflux treatment failure (24.5 ± 6.1).

Eosinophilic Gastroenteritis and Colitis

The role of the eosinophil in eosinophilic gastritis is unclear, but its presence is the unifying factor in the diagnosis. Eosinophilic granules serve in the killing of parasites and act as inflammatory mediators and chemotactic agents [19]. Tissue damage may result from the interplay between immunoglobulins, complement, eosinophils, and other inflammatory cells. Antibody-antigen complexes may be responsible for the attraction of eosinophils into the tissue of the gastrointestinal tract in association with complement activation and deposition [20]. Mast cell-associated mediators have also been shown to affect eosinophils and may play a role in the mediation of disease in eosinophilic gastroenteritis (EG). Once present in the tissue, the eosinophil may possess the ability to modulate disease in positive or negative ways. The cell may serve to control the inflammatory cascade from mast cell degranulation. Enzymes present in eosinophil granules contain enzymes that counteract the damaging substances present in mast cells. However, eosinophil granules also contain vasoactive substances such as platelet-activating factor and leukotrienes, which may contribute to the inflammatory and clinical features of the disease [21]. The relationship between eosinophils and mast cells increases the confusion in categorizing EG. Mast cells typically are thought of in allergic disease, but IgE levels in EG are not consistently elevated.

Almost 30 years ago, Moon and Kleinman classified EG into three categories: mucosal, muscular, and subserosal. Mucosal EG is the most common form and is signified by mucosal infiltration of eosinophils on biopsy or gastrointestinal edema on radiographic study [22]. Muscular EG is defined by eosinophilic infiltration of the muscular layer of the intestine and is associated with stenosis or obstruction of the gastrointestinal tract without ascites. Serosal EG is the least common form of EG and represents eosinophilic infiltration of the serosal layer associated with eosinophilic ascites. The diagnosis of EG is often missed. Biopsy results do not always coincide with the clinical picture, perhaps because of the patchy nature of the disease or the possibility of not identifying an eosinophilia with random intestinal biopsy. Mucosal EG has been reported to affect any portion of the gastrointestinal tract. In the majority of cases, the gastric antrum and small bowel are affected, resulting in nausea, vomiting, and epigastric pain. Patients with muscular EG present with symptoms of gastrointestinal obstruction or dysmotility. The muscular layer of the gastric antrum is most commonly affected and typically causes vomiting, abdominal pain, and delayed gastric emptying. Involvement of the small intestine and colon is less likely. Patients with serosal EG present with symptoms from ascites or intestinal perforation. Extraintestinal infiltration has also been described.

In contrast to other forms of EG, eosinophilic colitis or proctitis commonly represents sensitivity to cow's milk or soy protein, and symptoms abate with elimination of the offending antigen. Infants affected by this type of EG commonly lack systemic symptoms, leading to speculation that this disease may be a separate entity. In 1986, Goldman and Proujansky [7] reviewed 53 cases of allergic proctitis and gastroenteritis in children. Thirty-eight patients were identified as having symptoms and biopsy findings consistent with EG. Of the 38 patients with EG, all were found to have a mucosal eosinophilia of the gastric antrum. Seventy-nine percent also demonstrated a mucosal eosinophilia of the small intestine (duodenum), 60% had esophageal involvement, and in 52% eosinophilia was found in the gastric corpus. The majority of these patients had upper and lower gastrointestinal symptoms with multiple relapses, and many required corticosteroid therapy. In contrast, the remaining 15 patients were diagnosed with allergic proctitis. The majority of these children were aged less than 6 months and responded to dietary change without relapse. While the gastric antrum appears to be the most common location of disease, the patchy nature of the disease and the lack of full-thickness specimens on most endoscopic biopsies can lead to false negative biopsy results.

Eosinophilic Esophagitis

In 1995, Kelly [23] reported on a group of children with esophageal eosinophilia who did not respond to antireflux therapy but instead improved on an amino-acid-based formula. This study involved ten patients with histologic esophagitis who were diagnosed with reflux esophagitis and who failed pharmacologic therapy. Six patients had a persistent esophageal eosinophilia despite undergoing a Nissen fundoplication. Only one patient had a 24-h pH probe performed, which showed no evidence of reflux. These patients were subsequently placed on a strict diet consisting of an amino-acid-based formula for a median of 17 weeks. Symptomatic improvement was seen with an average of 3 weeks after the introduction of the elemental diet (resolution in eight patients, improvement in two). In addition, all ten patients demonstrated a significant improvement in esophageal eosinophilia. Subsequently, all patients reverted to previous symptoms upon reintroduction of foods. While an exact etiology was not determined, Kelly suggests an immunologic basis, either a delayed hypersensitivity or a cell-mediated hypersensitivity response, as the cause for eosinophilic esophagitis.

Liacouras confirmed the presence of EoE in 1998. He [24] identified 20 of 214 patients presenting with symptoms and histologic abnormalities suggestive of gastroesophageal reflux disease who remained symptomatic despite the use of H2-blockers, proton pump inhibitors, and prokinetic agents [25]. All of these patients had an isolated severe eosinophilic infiltration of the distal esophagus (mean of 34 ± 10 eosinophils/hpf) with normal antral/duodenal histology and minimal to no acid reflux by 24-h pH probe monitoring. Upon introduction of oral corticosteroids, 19 of 20 patients showed rapid improvement in clinical symptoms (average of 8 ± 3.5 days), and all 20 displayed histologic resolution of their esophageal eosinophilia within 1 month after being placed on corticosteroids. While corticosteroid therapy provides quick relief of symptoms and resolution of esophageal eosinophilia within 1 month, prolonged steroid therapy is not recommended. If symptoms recur soon after discontinuing steroid therapy (weeks to months), a strict elemental diet therapy should be instituted. However, if symptoms recur more than 1 year later, repeat short courses of corticosteroids are suggested.

Shortly thereafter, several other treatment regimens have been reported. One case report in 1998 demonstrated rapid clinical improvement after treatment with topical corticosteroids [25]. Patients were instructed to use inhaled corticosteroids but to immediately swallow after inhalation in order to deliver the medication to the esophagus. Histologic improvement was not determined. The mast-cell-stabilizing agent cromolyn sodium has also been tried in children with EoE. In similar fashion to its use for children with EG, oral cromolyn has been given to patients with a severe esophageal eosinophilia in conjunction with other systemic signs and symptoms of allergic disease. However, no controlled reports have been performed, and efficacy for oral cromolyn in children with EoE has not been established.

Surgical antireflux procedures were shown not to be effective in controlling patients with EoE. Liacouras [26] documented two cases of failed Nissen fundoplication in patients with symptoms suggestive of gastroesophageal reflux unresponsive to aggressive antireflux medication. In both cases, the symptoms and abnormal esophageal pathology remained after surgery. Physicians should not assume that chronic distal EoE results from acid reflux. In these cases, it is imperative that a 24-h pH probe be performed, and, if results are markedly abnormal, antireflux surgery might be considered. On the other hand, if the pH probe is normal or mildly abnormal, then the diagnosis of EoE is strongly suggested.

Liacouras [24] demonstrated that the clinical and histologic features of eosinophilic esophagitis may evolve over years. Of 20 children with eosinophilic esophagitis, five patients did not show a severe esophageal eosinophilia on initial endoscopy. Each of these patients, however, demonstrated a severe esophageal eosinophilia on repeat endoscopy after failure of anti-reflux medication. In all of these patients, esophageal histology demonstrated more than 20 eosinophils/hpf.

Initially, most of the clinical and basic research related to EoE was generated by pediatric gastroenterologists. The reason for this was likely based on the fact that pediatric gastroenterologists almost always performed mucosal biopsies regardless of the visual appearance of the gastrointestinal mucosa. Additionally, a number of children diagnosed with EoE often are fed a routine infant formula thereby allowing an easier transition to an amino-acid based formula. From 2000 to 2005, a number of pediatric gastroenterologists and allergists contributed important work to the understanding of EoE. Noel published information on the incidence of EoE [27], Rothenberg, Furuta, and Mishra contributed important information on pathophysiology [28–30], Putnam, Gupta, and Markowitz added information on the clinical manifestations [31–33] and Spergel and Aceves wrote articles on the allergic manifestations and treatment [34, 35]. Moreover, EoE became a major interest in adult patients. Straumann published the first notable work on the incidence, diagnosis and treatment of EoE [36]. In addition, Katzka reported on the clinical presentation, diagnosis, and treatment of EoE [37] while Hirano and Gonsalvas published information on dietary and medical therapy of EoE in adults [38, 39].

FIGERS

In 2005, because of the significant increase in the number of articles related to EoE appearing in the literature and the enhanced interest among clinicians, a working group of pediatric and adult physicians spanning multiple specialties was created.

The idea for this group was to develop cohesive guidelines in order to create a definition, diagnostic techniques, and therapies for individuals with EoE. The working group included pediatric and adult gastroenterologists, allergists, pathologists, and basic scientists. After a year of literature review, teleconferences and face-to-face meetings, the first international gastrointestinal eosinophilic research symposium (FIGERS) was held in October 2006 at the annual meeting held by the North American Society for Pediatric Gastroenterology, Hepatology and Nutrition (NASPGHAN). During the meeting, more than 50 specialists were invited to participate in the development of EoE guidelines. In addition, over 300 NASPGHAN members also attended the conference as observers. During the discussion of EoE, the topics included definitions, pathophysiology, incidence, epidemiology, genetics, diagnosis, endoscopic techniques, histology, allergy evaluation, therapy and future research. This conference provided invaluable information and was the framework for the EoE Consensus statement published in *Gastroenterology* in 2007 [40].

TIGERS

Following the FIGERS conference in 2007, physicians realized that a great deal of information was still unknown about many of the topics related to EoE. In addition, the literature on EoE was still rapidly growing. Thus, a subset of invited specialists formed a working group, The International Gastrointestinal Researchers (TIGERS), to not only respond to many of the unanswered questions left over from FIGERS but also to help develop future guidelines, research ideas and proposals related to EoE. Since that time, the members of TIGERS have increased worldwide knowledge of EoE in many ways. Their members created an EoE slide set used by more than 100 physicians to provide lectures and educations to clinicians all over the world. Moreover, they have helped to fund research grants to aid young scientists interested in advancing EoE knowledge, conducted research to help identify a possible genetic link in individuals with EoE, set up additional symposiums and meeting for several other international organizations, and helped to bring the study of EoE to the forefront among gastroenterologists, allergists, and pathologists worldwide.

Future

EoE has become a major focus of interest among gastroenterologists, allergists, and pathologists over the last 15 years. Initially thought of as a rare disease limited to a few children receiving gastrostomy feedings in a specific locale, we now know that the occurrence of EoE is much more common than initially thought and is increasing in frequency worldwide. From only a few published articles a year in 1997, the literature on EoE has expanded to include more than 125 published peer-reviewed articles in 2009. The names of the authors and physicians listed in this chapter have not only contributed a great deal of knowledge to the understanding of EoE but also brought EoE to the forefront of National Medical Associations such as the AAAAI, the AGA, the ASGE, and the NASPGHAN. Because of the increasing interest in EoE, further research is required in this ever-increasing population of patients and the final chapter on the history of the disease has yet to be written.

References

1. Ismail-Beigi F, Horton PF, Pope CE. Histological consequences of gastroesophageal reflux in man. Gastroenterology. 1970;58:163–74.
2. Behar J, Sheahan DC. Histologic abnormalities in reflux esophagitis. Arch Pathol Lab Med. 1975;99:387–91.
3. Seefeld U, Krejs GJ, Siebenmann RE, et al. Esophageal histology in gastroesophageal reflux. Morphometric findings in suction biopsies. Dig Dis Sci. 1977;22:956–9.
4. Johnson LF, Demeester TR, Haggitt RC. Esophageal epithelial response to gastroesophageal reflux. A quantitative study. Dig Dis Sci. 1978;23:498–502.
5. Winter HS, Madara JL, Stafford RJ. Intraepithelial eosinophils: a new diagnostic criterion for reflux esophagitis. Gastroenterology. 1982;83:818–23.
6. Brown LF, Goldman H, Antonioli DA. Intraepithelial eosiniophilis in endoscopic biopsies of adults with reflux esophagitis. Am J Surg Pathol. 1984;8:899–905.
7. Goldman H, Proujansky R. Allergic proctitis and gastroenteristis in children: clinical and mucosal biopsy features in 53 cases. Am J Surg Pathol. 1986;10:75–86.
8. Dobbins JW, Sheahan DG, Behar J. Eosinophilic gastroenteritis with esophageal involvement. Gastroenterology. 1977;72:1312–6.
9. Landres RT, Kuster GGR, Strum WB. Eosinophilic esophagitis in a patient with vigorous achalasia. Gastroenterology. 1978;74:1298–301.
10. Matzinger MA, Daneman A. Esophageal involvement in eosinophilic gastroenteritis. Pediatr Radiol. 1983;13:35–8.
11. Lee RG. Marked eosinophilia in esophageal mucosal biopsies. Am J Surg Pathol. 1985;9:475–9.
12. Teele RL, Katz AJ, Goldman H, Kettle RM. Radiographic features of eosinophilic gastroenteritis (allergic gastroenteropathy) of childhood. AJR Am J Roentgenol. 1979;132:575–80.
13. Picus D, Frank PH. Eosinophilic esophagitis. AJR Am J Roentgenol. 1981;136:1001–3.
14. Feczko PJ, Halpert RD, Zonca M. Radiologic abnormalities in eosinophilic esophagitis. Gastrointest Radiol. 1985;10:321–4.
15. Attwood SEA, Smyrk TC, Demeester TR, Jones JB. Esophageal eosinophilia with dysphagia: a district clinicopathologic syndrome. Dig Dis Sci. 1993;38:109–16.
16. Vitellas KM, Bennett WF, Bova JG, et al. Radiographic manifestations of eosinophilic gastroenteritis. Abdom Imaging. 1995;20:406–13.
17. Levine MS, Saul SH. Idophatic eosinophilic esophagitis: how common is it? Radiology. 1993;186:631–2.
18. Ruchelli E, Wenner W, Voytek T, et al. Severity of esophageal eosinophilia predicts response to conventional gastroesophageal reflux therapy. Pediatr Dev Pathol. 1999;2:15–8.
19. Wershill BK, Walker WA. The mucosal barrier, IgE-mediated gastrointestinal events, and eosinophilic gastroenteritis. Gastroenterol Clin North Am. 1990;21:387–402.
20. Cello JP. Eosinophilic gastroenteritis – a complex disease entity. Am J Med. 1979; 67:1097–104.
21. Sawaya SM, Misk RJ, Aftimos GP. Eosinophilic gastroenteritis: report of two cases and comment on the literature. Eur J Surg. 1992;158:439–41.
22. Moon A, Kleinman RE. Allergic gastroenteropathy in children. Ann Allergy Asthma Immunol. 1995;74:5–9.

23. Kelly KJ, Lazenby AJ, Rowe PC, et al. Eosinophilic esophagitis attributed to gastroesophageal reflux: improvement with an amino acid-based formula. Gastroenterology. 1995;109:1503–12.
24. Liacouras CA, Wenner WJ, Brown K, Ruchelli E. Primary eosinophilic esophagitis in children: successful treatment with oral corticosteroids. J Pediatr Gastroenterol Nutr. 1998;26:380–5.
25. Faubion Jr WA, Perrault J, Bugart LF, et al. Treatment of eosinophilic esophagitis with inhaled corticosteroids. J Pediatr Gastroenterol Nutr. 1998;27:90–3.
26. Liacouras CA. Failed Nissen fundoplication in two patients who had persistent vomiting and eosinophilic esophagitis. J Pediatr Surg. 1997;32:1504–6.
27. Noel RJ, Putnam PE, Rothenberg ME. Eosinophilic esophagitis. N Engl J Med. 2004;51(9):940–1.
28. Rothenberg ME, Mishra A, Collins MH, Putnam PE. Pathogenesis and clinical features of eosinophilic esophagitis. J Allergy Clin Immunol. 2001;108(6):891–4.
29. Furuta GT. Clinicopathologic features of esophagitis in children. Gastrointest Endosc Clin N Am. 2001;11(4):683–715.
30. Mishra A, Hogan SP, Brandt EB, Rothenberg ME. IL-5 promotes eosinophil trafficking to the esophagus. J Immunol. 2002;168(5):2464–9.
31. Noel RJ, Putnam PE, Collins MH, Assa'ad AH, Guajardo JR, Jameson SC, et al. Clinical and immunopathologic effects of swallowed fluticasone for eosinophilic esophagitis. Clin Gastroenterol Hepatol. 2004;2(7):568–75.
32. Lim JR, Gupta SK, Croffie JM, Pfefferkorn MD, Molleston JP, Corkins MR, et al. White specks in the esophageal mucosa: an endoscopic manifestation of non-reflux eosinophilic esophagitis in children. Gastrointest Endosc. 2004;59(7):835–8.
33. Markowitz JE, Spergel JM, Ruchelli E, Liacouras CA. Elemental diet is an effective treatment for eosinophilic esophagitis in children and adolescents. Am J Gastroenterol. 2003;98(4):777–82.
34. Spergel JM, Beausoleil JL, Mascarenhas M, Liacouras CA. The use of skin prick tests and patch tests to identify causative foods in eosinophilic esophagitis. J Allergy Clin Immunol. 2002;109(2):363–8.
35. Aceves SS, Dohil R, Newbury RO, Bastian JF. Topical viscous budesonide suspension for treatment of eosinophilic esophagitis. J Allergy Clin Immunol. 2005;116(3):705–6.
36. Straumann A, Spichtin HP, Grize L, Bucher KA, Beglinger C. Natural history of primary eosinophilic esophagitis: a follow-up of 30 adult patients for up to 11.5 years. Gastroenterology. 2003;125(6):1660–9.
37. Katzka DA. Eosinophilic esophagitis. Curr Treat Options Gastroenterol. 2003;6(1):49–54.
38. Stevoff C, Rao S, Parsons W, Kahrilas PJ, Hirano I. EUS and histopathologic correlates in eosinophilic esophagitis. Gastrointest Endosc. 2001;54(3):373–7.
39. Gonsalves N, Policarpio-Nicolas M, Zhang Q, Rao MS, Hirano I. Histopathologic variability and endoscopic correlates in adults with eosinophilic esophagitis. Gastrointest Endosc. 2006;64(3):313–9.
40. Furuta GT, Liacouras CA, Collins MH, Gupta SK, Justinich C, Putnam PE, et al. Eosinophilic esophagitis in children and adults: a systematic review and consensus recommendations for diagnosis and treatment. Gastroenterology. 2007;133(4):1342–63.

Chapter 2
Epidemiology, Incidence, and Prevalence of EoE in Children

Richard J. Noel

Keywords Eosinophilic esophagitis • Gastroesophageal reflux disease • Epidemiology of EoE • Demographic descriptors of EoE

Introduction

Few pediatric diseases have produced similar volumes of clinical and basic research data in as short a time as eosinophilic esophagitis (EoE). Once believed to be a rare disorder that possibly represented recalcitrant gastroesophageal reflux disease, EoE is now known to be a unique entity with a specific transcriptional signature, epidemiologic descriptors, histologic features, and treatments. This chapter delineates the epidemiology of pediatric EoE, including demographic descriptors and measures of frequency.

Esophageal Mucosal Eosinophilia in Pediatric Patients

Unlike other segments of the gastrointestinal tract, the healthy esophageal epithelium has essentially no intraepithelial eosinophils. This finding has been documented by both cadaveric studies, and retrospective review of biopsies without pathologic diagnoses [1, 2]. When Winter et al. in 1982 described intraepithelial eosinophils on esophageal biopsies that correlated with abnormal pH probe studies, the esophageal mucosal eosinophil was identified as a marker for peptic esophagitis [3].

R.J. Noel (✉)
Division of Gastroenterology, Department of Pediatrics, Medical College of Wisconsin, 9000 W. Wisconsin Avenue, Milwaukee, WI 53226, USA
e-mail: rnoel@mcw.edu

C.A. Liacouras and J.E. Markowitz (eds.), *Eosinophilic Esophagitis*, Clinical Gastroenterology, DOI 10.1007/978-1-60761-515-6_2,

The concept that esophageal mucosal eosinophilia was not solely due to peptic disease developed over time. Approximately a decade after Winter's observations, key studies by Attwood et al. [4] and Kelly et al. [5] suggested that high-grade esophageal mucosal eosinophilia may indicate a process distinct from peptic disease because the inflammation persisted despite therapies that minimized esophageal acid exposure. Ruchelli et al. later noted that the higher degree of eosinophilia appeared to distinguish EoE from peptic disease [6]. This distinction was further supported by studies that documented EoE in patients with normal pH probe results [7]. Recent studies have noted a specific transcriptional signature [8] and unique histologic features [9] that distinguish EoE from other esophageal inflammatory processes. A systematic review of the literature in 2007 led to consensus recommendations that provided a definition for EoE according to histologic and clinical criteria, including a peak eosinophil density of 15 eosinophils per 400× microscopic field in the absence of evidence of peptic disease [10].

Epidemiologic Data in Pediatric EoE

To date, two population-based studies on pediatric EoE have been published [11, 12]. Other retrospective series have provided demographic estimates from referral population from specific regions, including Western Australia and West Virginia [13, 14]. Additionally, large cohorts of referral patients are tracked at both the Cincinnati Children's Hospital Medical Center and Children's Hospital of Philadelphia [15, 16]. Other series have utilized survey results, from both patients and providers alike, to estimate demographic parameters of pediatric EoE [17, 18]. Data were also extrapolated from case series whose intent was to describe a specific treatment or feature of EoE. Notably, regardless of the study type or geographic origin, demographic descriptors of the pediatric EoE population remain consistent across the literature, and support the case that EoE is a distinct diagnostic entity.

Geographic Distribution of EoE

EoE affects children throughout the world. An internet-based patient survey tool provided data from 107 surveys that originated in multiple countries, including Canada, England, China, Israel, and the USA (32 states included) [17]. A survey of a national pathology database described 363 cases of EoE (42 pediatric) diagnosed in 26 of 34 states from which specimens were submitted [19]. A physician survey of EoE with 1,801 respondents noted cases in four regions of the USA (Northeast, Midwest, South, and West), with the highest prevalence rates in the Northeast [18]. EoE has also been reported in many European countries (Belgium, Denmark, France, Greece, Italy, the Netherlands, Spain, and Sweden), South and Central America (Argentina, Brazil, and Mexico), Japan, New Zealand, and Australia [10, 13, 20]. No cases of primary (allergic) EoE have been reported from the African continent.

Age at Diagnosis

The average age of diagnosis for pediatric EoE is between 6 and 10 years of age. The two population-based studies place the average age of diagnosis at approximately 10 years of age [11, 12]. The larger Philadelphia referral cohort has a younger age of diagnosis, estimated at 6 years of age [16]. It is likely that many children with EoE have symptoms for years before the diagnosis is made. A retrospective series of 20 patients with EoE had a mean time between onset of symptoms and diagnosis of EoE of 4.5 ± 3.5 years (mean ± standard deviation) [21]. It is therefore clear that data regarding age of diagnosis may not reflect the actual onset of disease. Furthermore, it has been well established that children with EoE may not have symptoms that parallel their esophageal inflammation [22], allowing for the occasional unexpected diagnosis of EoE made in an asymptomatic patient.

Sex Distribution

Without exception, large case series and population-based studies of EoE document a large male predominance among their cohorts or study populations (Table 2.1). The two population-based studies of pediatric EoE describe male percentages of 71 and 65.2% [11, 12]. The large Philadelphia 14-year referral cohort is 75% male [16]. Multiple studies highlighting treatments or specific clinical features of EoE going back to 1997 also have a marked male predominance with percentages ranging from 70 to 92% [23–27]. Although a male predominance is consistent in pediatric EoE, its implications as to etiology, disease course, or outcome is unknown.

Presenting Symptoms

Unlike the adult presentation of the disease where dysphagia and food impaction constitute the predominant presenting symptoms, the pediatric presentation of EoE varies dramatically across the pediatric age range (Table 2.2). Two studies, including a population-based study of Hamilton county (Cincinnati) [11] and a review of a large referral population (Philadelphia) [16] best highlight the evolution of symptoms across the pediatric age range. The youngest EoE patients present with feeding disorders characterized by feeding refusal and vomiting, sometimes associated with failure to gain weight. These youngest EoE patients may develop profound feeding aversion and require interdisciplinary care to guide feeding skill acquisition as the EoE is addressed medically [28]. Young children with feeding disorders may also be initially evaluated by otolaryngologists or speech and language pathologists who may not be aware of EoE [29]. In younger school-age children, the primary symptoms evolve to vomiting and abdominal pain. By adolescence, the disease mirrors that of adults with dysphagia and recurrent food impactions [30]. The fact that both

Table 2.1 Summary of publications with generalizable pediatric EoE epidemiologic data

	Guajardo et al. [17]	Noel et al. [11]	Cherian et al. [13]	Assa'ad [4]	Gill et al. [14]	Spergel et al. [16]	Prasad et al. [12]
Type	Patient self-report survey	Population-based	Referral population	Referral population	Referral population	Referral population	Population-based
Year	2002	2004	2006	2007	2007	2008	2009
Cases	39	103	296	89	44	620	23
Mean age (years)	8	10.5	6.58	6.2	9.0	6.2	10
% Male	82	71	66.2	78.6	63	75	65.2

Table 2.2 Publications describing presenting symptoms of pediatric EoE according to fraction and population and/or patient age

	Guajardo et al. [17]	Noel et al. [11]	Assa'ad [4]	Gill et al. [14]	Spergel [16]	Prasad et al. [12]
Cases	39	103	89	44	620	23
Presenting symptoms	%	Median age (%)	Mean age (%)	%	Median age (%)	%
Feeding disorder	NA	2 (13.6)	1 (3)	NA	2.8 (19)	NA
Vomiting	54	8.1 (26.2)	3.2 (59.5)	43	5.1 (25.4)	43.5
Abdominal pain	21	12 (26.2)	4.9 (24.7)	55	9 (14.1)	30.4
Dysphagia	36	13.4 (27.2)	4.3 (15.7)	9	11.1 (10)	60.9
Food impaction	36	16.8 (6.8)	8.8 (6.7)	NA		21.7

Data are presented according to manner in which they are reported in the publication and include population percentage alone, median age and population percentage, or mean age and population percentage

Table 2.3 Publications describing racial breakdown of pediatric EoE populations

	Assa'ad [4]	Spergel [16]
Cases	89	620
Racial breakdown		
% White	94.4	90
% AA	4.5	4
% Asian	NA	3

referral and population-based studies demonstrate similar progressions of symptoms over advancing age suggests that these features can be generalized to whole of pediatric EoE. Eventually, prospective cohort studies may be required to achieve a more precise understanding of how EoE symptoms evolve as children grow into adults.

Racial Distribution

Limited data exist regarding racial distribution of EoE (Table 2.3). The issue has been best addressed by the large Philadelphia cohort and an 8-year retrospective study from Cincinnati [15, 16]. Both studies describe a large white predominance in the population (90–94.4%), with African-American and Asians representing only 4 and 3%, respectively. This distribution differs from that of asthma in North American populations, which occurs with greater frequency in African-Americans (15.8%) vs. whites (7.3%), Asians (6%), and Latinos (3.9%) [31]. Whether these data truly reflect actual racial differences in EoE susceptibility or underreporting of minority EoE remains to be determined.

Table 2.4 Publications describing prevalence of atopic disease in populations of children with EoE

	Guajardo et al. [17]	Noel et al. [11]	Assa'ad [15]	Gill et al. [14]	Spergel [16]	Prasad et al. [12]
Cases	39	103	89	44	620	23
% Atopy, seasonal allergy, or rhinoconjunctivitis	64	57.4	NA	32	61	53.8
% Asthma	38	36.8	NA	NA	50	63.6
% Eczema	26	NA	NA	NA	21	
% Food allergic	NA	46	75	NA	NA	57.1

Association with Atopic Disease

Compared with the general population, the frequency of atopic disease is much higher in patient populations with EoE (Table 2.4). While estimates vary, demographic studies of atopic diseases in children report a prevalence of 6% for asthma, 15% for allergic rhinitis, 10% for eczema, and 3% for food allergy [32–34]. In comparison, prevalence of EoE in pediatric populations uniformly exceeded these population baselines. The Hamilton County EoE population exceeded population prevalences by 6-, 3.8-, and 15-fold for asthma, rhinitis, and food allergy, respectively [11]. The referral EoE population from Philadelphia exceeded population standards by 8.3-, 4-, and 2-fold for asthma, rhinitis, and eczema, respectively [16]. While the exact mechanism for the strong association with atopic disease is unknown, it is likely that EoE and other atopic diseases share common Th2 inflammatory mediators. Outside of animal models [35], no data exist to suggest the mechanism by which asthma (or any other atopic process) promotes EoE in children.

Airborne Allergens and Seasonal Variation in EoE

The promotion of EoE by a respiratory allergen was first demonstrated in a mouse model that developed EoE in response to intra-tracheal *Aspergillus fumigatus* sensitization that involved interleukin-5 and eotaxin [36]. Subsequent animal data propose a further connection between the respiratory tract and esophagus by demonstrating that intra-tracheal interleukin-13 deposition can produce esophageal mucosal eosinophilia suggestive of EoE [35].

A human corollary to this concept was described in a case report from 2003 that described a 21-year-old female with no detectable dietary allergen sensitivities, but multiple environmental allergies, including trees, grasses, ragweed, Aspergillus, cat, dog, and dust mite. Over a course of 4 years, she underwent five diagnostic upper endoscopies and had significant esophageal mucosal eosinophilia only in May and September during specific pollen seasons. This case supported the notion that airborne allergens, like dietary allergens, can drive EoE in sensitized individuals who swallow the allergens or cytokines from the naso-oropharynx and possibly directly activate the respiratory tract. Studies in atopic adults have also documented low-level esophageal mucosal eosinophilia during the pollen season that, alone, does not constitute EoE, but can contribute by raising the level of esophageal eosinophil recruitment [37].

The phenomenon of seasonal variation in levels of esophageal eosinophilia was described in a retrospective analysis of a referral population of 234 children with EoE [38]. In this study, the authors noted that during the winter months, they observed the lowest diagnostic frequency, as well as a trend toward lower severity of mucosal eosinophilia. Similarly in a population-based 30-year study of EoE patients in Olmstead County, MN [12], the highest frequency of diagnosis occurred in the summer/fall and the lowest in the winter months when the pollen counts were highest and lowest, respectively.

Taken together, these data strongly support a contribution, if not the core cause for EoE, from airborne allergens. However, these data do cannot establish a causal mechanism for the role of airborne allergens in human EoE to a similar degree as that of amino acid-based formulas for dietary allergens [39]. These data suggest that EoE may point to a larger "allergy epidemic" and may not be a disease limited to the gastrointestinal tract. This topic is addressed in the consensus recommendations that patients with EoE receive comprehensive evaluation and management of atopic disease [10].

Frequency Metrics

Three studies have estimated the pediatric disease prevalence at approximately 50 per 100,000 (Table 2.5) [11, 12, 18]. Compared with other well-established diseases in pediatric gastroenterology, EoE has a higher prevalence and is more likely to be encountered in general practice. At a reported yearly incidence of approximately 10 per 100,000 pediatric population, EoE occurs more frequently than other entities such as biliary atresia [40] and inflammatory bowel disease [41] that have an incidence approximating 7 per 100,000.

The Hamilton County population-based study suggested a trend toward increasing annual incidence, from 9.09 per 100,000 in 2000, to 12.81 per 100,000 in 2003 with a prevalence of approximately 43 cases per 100,000 pediatric population [11]. However, the trend for increasing incidence was not statistically significant. The data continue to be accrued in a prospective manner and will be reanalyzed in the

Table 2.5 Publications providing frequency estimates for pediatric EoE

	Noel et al. [11]	Cherian et al. [13]	Gill et al. [14]	Book [18]	Prasad et al. [12][a]
Prevalence per 100,000	43	9	NA	52	54
Incidence per 100,000	12.8	NA	7.3	NA	2.39

[a] Data include both pediatric and adult sex- and age-matched cases

future. The Olmstead County population-based study has noted increasing incidence for age and sex-matched cases describing a population prevalence of 54 cases per 100,000 (mixed adult and pediatric population) [12]. Incidence has also increased from negligible in 1976–1980 to approximately 9 per 100,000 in 2001–2005.

Despite these data, there may still be an element of recognition bias that contributes to a perception of increasing incidence. A systematic review of adult esophageal biopsy specimens between 1990 and 2005 found not significant increase in the frequency of biopsies with histologic features consistent with EoE and makes a case for increased recognition [42]. Conversely, a review of histologic specimens from children in Western Australia describes an 18-fold increase in prevalence over a similar time period, from 0.5 to 8.9 per 100,000 in 1995 and 2004, respectively [43]. In addition, the Philadelphia referral cohort data has shown a steady increase in EoE diagnosed in patients from Pennsylvania, New Jersey, and Delaware [16]. Ultimately, data from well-controlled, prospective, population samples will be required to answer this question in a definitive manner.

Environmental Theories for the Causation of EoE

While progress has been made toward explaining the molecular and immunological basis of pediatric EoE [44], changes in gene expression pattern, alone, cannot explain the rapid pace at which EoE has been established as a unique disorder. Several theories implicate environmental forces as contributors to the disease onset in the pediatric population; these have been reviewed by Bonis [45]. It must be noted that these ideas, although intriguing conjectures, have not been directly tested regarding EoE.

EoE is Part of an Allergy Epidemic in the Context of the Hygiene Hypothesis

Allergic disease (asthma, allergic rhinitis, atopic dermatitis) and autoimmune disease (type 1 diabetes, inflammatory bowel disease) both have increased in prevalence according to gradients of per capita gross national product and eradication of early life infectious disease [46]. The hygiene hypothesis suggests that as a population becomes wealthier, it becomes "cleaner" and previously common infectious diseases such as mumps, measles, hepatitis A, and tuberculosis are eradicated. As a consequence of improved hygiene, interaction between microbial proteins and Toll-like receptors does not occur, interfering with modulation of both Th1 and Th2 antigen-driven pathways [47]. Additionally, some data suggest that eradication of *Helicobacter pylori* in a population is associated with development of atopic diseases [48]. Congruent with this model is the fact that the only eosinophilic esophagitis reported from the African continent is secondary to *Gnathostoma spinigerum* infection [49].

Excesses or Deficiencies of Dietary Constituents Contribute to EoE

Studies have identified altered dietary constituents as potential contributors to atopic disease. These include decreasing intake of antioxidants in fruits and vegetables, increasing intake of ω–6 polyunsaturated fatty acids, and decreasing intake of ω–3 polyunsaturated fatty acids as potential contributors to atopy in children [50]. Dietary increases in ω–6 fatty acids result in increased production of arachidonic acid and PGE_2, promoting Th2 sensitization. Conversely, ω–3 fatty acids have inhibitory properties on cyclooxygenase, resulting in decreased production of inflammatory mediators. Decreases in the antioxidant dietary content have also been implicated in the development of atopy. Oxidant stress can induce production of inflammatory mediators that can induce Th1 cytokine production and decrease Th2 cytokine activity.

Indiscriminate Use of Acid Suppressant Medication Contributes to EoE

Acid digestion of dietary proteins interferes with binding of IgE and subsequent sensitization [51]. Theoretically, the use of proton pump inhibitors decreases the threshold for dietary protein sensitization and binding of IgE. Conversely, esophageal mucosal eosinophilia occurs as a result of acid reflux disease and can be reversed with acid-suppressant medications [52].

Disruption of the Esophageal Epithelial Barrier Contributes to EoE

Dilated intercellular spaces have been identified in adults with non-erosive reflux disease, allowing the possibility that reflux-related increased intercellular permeability may expose the esophageal mucosa to unprocessed dietary antigens [53]. Furthermore, microarray transcriptional studies from esophageal mucosal biopsies have identified overrepresented filaggrin loss-of-function mutations in a population of EoE patients when compared to healthy controls [54]. Filaggrins are components of the granular layer of the epidermis; underexpression of filaggrins has been associated with eczema and ichthyosis vulgaris. Barrier disruption may also involve the skin and allow allergic sensitization prior to the induction of oral tolerance by introduction of proteins into the diet [55, 56].

Constituents of Processed Food Contribute to EoE

Successful treatment of EoE by amino acid-based diets and some elimination diets may be interpreted as reduction in intact dietary proteins that are recognized by immune effectors. Dietary treatment may also be interpreted as a reduction in exposure to fertilizers, pesticides, antibiotics, and preservatives used in the food industry. A Dutch study reports a reduced risk in eczema in infants and toddlers who were fed diets that were 90% organic [57]. Furthermore, imazamox-related compounds have fungicidal activity and may also function as haptens with immunogenic potential when bound to larger carrier molecules [58].

Conclusion

EoE has been a dynamic disease in its short history. The fact that EoE is among the top entities listed in the differential diagnosis of adolescents with dysphagia or food impaction, or infants and toddlers with feeding disorder or vomiting with features beyond benign infantile reflux, speaks volumes for the pediatricians that have contributed to the knowledge pool since 1995. The demographic descriptors highlighted in this chapter suggest a profile for the typical patient with EoE. This patient may be a North American white male with vomiting or dysphagia, diagnosed between 6 and 10 years of age, with a personal and family history of atopic disease, including asthma, rhinitis, and food allergy. While such patients clearly exist, the profile only brings together prevalent features that are likely to exist along unrelated axes. Future research may eventually demonstrate underlying relationships between these currently disparate features. As research continues to add to the collective knowledge of pediatric EoE, our understanding of how EoE symptoms evolve in children, how specific patient factors determine long-term outcomes, and how the genetic complement of an individual and a specific population interacts with the environment to produce EoE.

References

1. Lowichik A, Weinberg AG. A quantitative evaluation of mucosal eosinophils in the pediatric gastrointestinal tract. Mod Pathol. 1996;9(2):110–4.
2. DeBrosse CW, Case JW, Putnam PE, Collins MH, Rothenberg ME. Quantity and distribution of eosinophils in the gastrointestinal tract of children. Pediatr Dev Pathol. 2006;9(3):210–8.
3. Winter HS, Madara JL, Stafford RJ, Grand RJ, Quinlan JE, Goldman H. Intraepithelial eosinophils: a new diagnostic criterion for reflux esophagitis. Gastroenterology. 1982;83(4):818–23.
4. Attwood SE, Smyrk TC, Demeester TR, Jones JB. Esophageal eosinophilia with dysphagia. A distinct clinicopathologic syndrome. Dig Dis Sci. 1993;38(1):109–16.
5. Kelly KJ, Lazenby AJ, Rowe PC, Yardley JH, Perman JA, Sampson HA. Eosinophilic esophagitis attributed to gastroesophageal reflux: improvement with an amino acid-based formula. Gastroenterology. 1995;109(5):1503–12.

6. Ruchelli E, Wenner W, Voytek T, Brown K, Liacouras C. Severity of esophageal eosinophilia predicts response to conventional gastroesophageal reflux therapy. Pediatr Dev Pathol. 1999;2(1):15–8.
7. Steiner SJ, Gupta SK, Croffie JM, Fitzgerald JF. Correlation between number of eosinophils and reflux index on same day esophageal biopsy and 24 hour esophageal pH monitoring. Am J Gastroenterol. 2004;99(5):801–5.
8. Blanchard C, Wang N, Stringer KF, et al. Eotaxin-3 and a uniquely conserved gene-expression profile in eosinophilic esophagitis. J Clin Invest. 2006;116(2):536–47.
9. Protheroe C, Woodruff SA, de Petris G, et al. A novel histologic scoring system to evaluate mucosal biopsies from patients with eosinophilic esophagitis. Clin Gastroenterol Hepatol. 2009;7(7):749–55,e711.
10. Furuta GT, Liacouras CA, Collins MH, et al. Eosinophilic esophagitis in children and adults: a systematic review and consensus recommendations for diagnosis and treatment. Gastroenterology. 2007;133(4):1342–63.
11. Noel RJ, Putnam PE, Rothenberg ME. Eosinophilic esophagitis. N Engl J Med. 2004;351(9): 940–1.
12. Prasad GA, Alexander JA, Schleck CD, et al. Epidemiology of eosinophilic esophagitis over three decades in Olmsted County, Minnesota. Clin Gastroenterol Hepatol. 2009;7(10):1055–61.
13. Cherian S, Smith NM, Forbes DA. Rapidly increasing prevalence of eosinophilic oesophagitis in Western Australia. Arch Dis Child. 2006;91(12):1000–4.
14. Gill R, Durst P, Rewalt M, Elitsur Y. Eosinophilic esophagitis disease in children from West Virginia: a review of the last decade (1995–2004). Am J Gastroenterol. 2007;102(10):2281–5.
15. Assa'ad AH, Putnam PE, Collins MH, et al. Pediatric patients with eosinophilic esophagitis: an 8-year follow-up. J Allergy Clin Immunol. 2007;119(3):731–8.
16. Spergel JM, Brown-Whitehorn TF, Beausoleil JL, et al. 14 years of eosinophilic esophagitis: clinical features and prognosis. J Pediatr Gastroenterol Nutr. 2009;48(1):30–6.
17. Guajardo JR, Plotnick LM, Fende JM, Collins MH, Putnam PE, Rothenberg ME. Eosinophil-associated gastrointestinal disorders: a world-wide-web based registry. J Pediatr. 2002;141(4):576–81.
18. Book WM. Eosinophilic gastrointestinal disorders: disease prevalence in the United States. National Harbor, MD: NASPGHAN; 2009.
19. Kapel RC, Miller JK, Torres C, Aksoy S, Lash R, Katzka DA. Eosinophilic esophagitis: a prevalent disease in the United States that affects all age groups. Gastroenterology. 2008;134(5):1316–21.
20. Cury EK, Schraibman V, Faintuch S. Eosinophilic infiltration of the esophagus: gastroesophageal reflux versus eosinophilic esophagitis in children – discussion on daily practice. J Pediatr Surg. 2004;39(2):e4–7.
21. Noel RJ, Putnam PE, Collins MH, et al. Clinical and immunopathologic effects of swallowed fluticasone for eosinophilic esophagitis. Clin Gastroenterol Hepatol. 2004;2(7):568–75.
22. Pentiuk S, Putnam PE, Collins MH, Rothenberg ME. Dissociation between symptoms and histological severity in pediatric eosinophilic esophagitis. J Pediatr Gastroenterol Nutr. 2009;48(2):152–60.
23. Gupta SK, Fitzgerald JF, Chong SK, Croffie JM, Collins MH. Vertical lines in distal esophageal mucosa (VLEM): a true endoscopic manifestation of esophagitis in children? Gastrointest Endosc. 1997;45(6):485–9.
24. Orenstein SR, Shalaby TM, Di Lorenzo C, et al. The spectrum of pediatric eosinophilic esophagitis beyond infancy: a clinical series of 30 children. Am J Gastroenterol. 2000;95(6): 1422–30.
25. Teitelbaum JE, Fox VL, Twarog FJ, et al. Eosinophilic esophagitis in children: immunopathological analysis and response to fluticasone propionate. Gastroenterology. 2002;122(5):1216–25.
26. Spergel JM, Beausoleil JL, Mascarenhas M, Liacouras CA. The use of skin prick tests and patch tests to identify causative foods in eosinophilic esophagitis. J Allergy Clin Immunol. 2002;109(2):363–8.
27. Khan S, Orenstein SR, Di Lorenzo C, et al. Eosinophilic esophagitis: strictures, impactions, dysphagia. Dig Dis Sci. 2003;48(1):22–9.

28. Pentiuk SP, Miller CK, Kaul A. Eosinophilic esophagitis in infants and toddlers. Dysphagia. 2007;22(1):44–8.
29. Smith LP, Chewaproug L, Spergel JM, Zur KB. Otolaryngologists may not be doing enough to diagnose pediatric eosinophilic esophagitis. Int J Pediatr Otorhinolaryngol. 2009;73(11):1554–7.
30. Focht DR, Kaul A. Food impaction and eosinophilic esophagitis. J Pediatr. 2005;147(4):540.
31. Simon PA, Zeng Z, Wold CM, Haddock W, Fielding JE. Prevalence of childhood asthma and associated morbidity in Los Angeles County: impacts of race/ethnicity and income. J Asthma. 2003;40(5):535–43.
32. Johnson CC, Ownby DR, Zoratti EM, Alford SH, Williams LK, Joseph CL. Environmental epidemiology of pediatric asthma and allergy. Epidemiol Rev. 2002;24(2):154–75.
33. Fennessy M, Coupland S, Popay J, Naysmith K. The epidemiology and experience of atopic eczema during childhood: a discussion paper on the implications of current knowledge for health care, public health policy and research. J Epidemiol Community Health. 2000;54(8):581–9.
34. Sampson HA. Update on food allergy. J Allergy Clin Immunol. 2004;113(5):805–19,quiz 820.
35. Mishra A, Rothenberg ME. Intratracheal IL-13 induces eosinophilic esophagitis by an IL-5, eotaxin-1, and STAT6-dependent mechanism. Gastroenterology. 2003;125(5):1419–27.
36. Mishra A, Hogan SP, Brandt EB, Rothenberg ME. An etiological role for aeroallergens and eosinophils in experimental esophagitis. J Clin Invest. 2001;107(1):83–90.
37. Onbasi K, Sin AZ, Doganavsargil B, Onder GF, Bor S, Sebik F. Eosinophil infiltration of the oesophageal mucosa in patients with pollen allergy during the season. Clin Exp Allergy. 2005;35(11):1423–31.
38. Wang FY, Gupta SK, Fitzgerald JF. Is there a seasonal variation in the incidence or intensity of allergic eosinophilic esophagitis in newly diagnosed children? J Clin Gastroenterol. 2007;41(5):451–3.
39. Markowitz JE, Spergel JM, Ruchelli E, Liacouras CA. Elemental diet is an effective treatment for eosinophilic esophagitis in children and adolescents. Am J Gastroenterol. 2003;98(4):777–82.
40. Yoon PW, Bresee JS, Olney RS, James LM, Khoury MJ. Epidemiology of biliary atresia: a population-based study. Pediatrics. 1997;99(3):376–82.
41. Kugathasan S, Judd RH, Hoffmann RG, et al. Epidemiologic and clinical characteristics of children with newly diagnosed inflammatory bowel disease in Wisconsin: a statewide population-based study. J Pediatr. 2003;143(4):525–31.
42. Vanderheyden AD, Petras RE, DeYoung BR, Mitros FA. Emerging eosinophilic (allergic) esophagitis: increased incidence or increased recognition? Arch Pathol Lab Med. 2007;131(5): 777–9.
43. Potter JW, Saeian K, Staff D, et al. Eosinophilic esophagitis in adults: an emerging problem with unique esophageal features. Gastrointest Endosc. 2004;59(3):355–61.
44. Rothenberg ME. Biology and treatment of eosinophilic esophagitis. Gastroenterology. 2009;137(4):1238–49.
45. Bonis PA. Putting the puzzle together: epidemiological and clinical clues in the etiology of eosinophilic esophagitis. Immunol Allergy Clin North Am. 2009;29(1):41–52,viii.
46. Bach JF. The effect of infections on susceptibility to autoimmune and allergic diseases. N Engl J Med. 2002;347(12):911–20.
47. Vercelli D. Mechanisms of the hygiene hypothesis–molecular and otherwise. Curr Opin Immunol. 2006;18(6):733–7.
48. Blaser MJ, Chen Y, Reibman J. Does *Helicobacter pylori* protect against asthma and allergy? Gut. 2008;57(5):561–7.
49. Muller-Stover I, Richter J, Haussinger D. Infection with *Gnathostoma spinigerum* as a cause of eosinophilic oesophagitis. Dtsch Med Wochenschr. 2004;129(38):1973–5.
50. Devereux G, Seaton A. Diet as a risk factor for atopy and asthma. J Allergy Clin Immunol. 2005;115(6):1109–17,quiz 1118.
51. Untersmayr E, Jensen-Jarolim E. The role of protein digestibility and antacids on food allergy outcomes. J Allergy Clin Immunol. 2008;121(6):1301–8,quiz 1309–1310.

52. Ngo P, Furuta GT, Antonioli DA, Fox VL. Eosinophils in the esophagus–peptic or allergic eosinophilic esophagitis? Case series of three patients with esophageal eosinophilia. Am J Gastroenterol. 2006;101(7):1666–70.
53. Orlando LA, Orlando RC. Dilated intercellular spaces as a marker of GERD. Curr Gastroenterol Rep. 2009;11(3):190–4.
54. Blanchard C, Stucke EM, Burwinkel K, et al. Coordinate interaction between IL-13 and epithelial differentiation cluster genes in eosinophilic esophagitis. J Immunol. 2010;184(7):4033–41.
55. Lack G. The concept of oral tolerance induction to foods. Nestle Nutr Workshop Ser Pediatr Program. 2007;59:63–8,discussion 68–72.
56. Lack G. Epidemiologic risks for food allergy. J Allergy Clin Immunol. 2008;121(6):1331–6.
57. Kummeling I, Thijs C, Huber M, et al. Consumption of organic foods and risk of atopic disease during the first 2 years of life in the Netherlands. Br J Nutr. 2008;99(3):598–605.
58. Gunther S, Hempel D, Dunkel M, Rother K, Preissner R. SuperHapten: a comprehensive database for small immunogenic compounds. Nucleic Acids Res. 2007;35(Database issue):D906–10.

Chapter 3
Epidemiology of Eosinophilic Esophagitis in Adults

Petr Hruz and Alex Straumann

Keywords Eosinophilic esophagitis • Esophageal eosinophilia • Epidemiology • Biopsy • Pathology • Endoscopy

Introduction

Epidemiology is derived from the Greek terms, *epi* = among; *demos* = people; and *logos* = study. It is the doctrine of factors affecting the health and the illness of populations, and serves as the foundation and logic of any interventions made in public health as well as in clinical practice. Epidemiology relies on a number of scientific disciplines, such as medicine, biology, geography, and social science.

The relevance of any given disease is primarily determined by the following three factors (1) its *epidemiological cornerstones*, in particular, its incidence and prevalence among a certain population. Incidence is defined as the number of new cases of the target disease in the population at risk within a specified time period. Prevalence is the total number of cases with the target disorder in the population at risk at a specific time point. (2) Its *natural history*, which is, *per definitionem*, the final outcome without any intervention, as well as its course as a result of therapeutic manipulation; and (3) whether a given disease has an *exemplary pathogenesis* whose understanding improves the general knowledge of basic physiologic and pathophysiologic mechanisms.

A. Straumann (✉)
Department of Gastroenterology, University Hospital Basel,
Basel, Switzerland

Swiss EoE Research Group, Roemerstrasse 7,
4600 Olten, Switzerland
e-mail: alex.straumann@hin.ch

C.A. Liacouras and J.E. Markowitz (eds.), *Eosinophilic Esophagitis*,
Clinical Gastroenterology, DOI 10.1007/978-1-60761-515-6_3,

Epidemiology is therefore one of the leading factors determining the clinical and socio-economic relevance of any disease; and thus, the knowledge of the epidemiologic parameters of a disease is crucial for identifying risk factors as well as pathogenetic mechanisms, for planning preventive measures and for determining optimal treatment approaches.

Eosinophilic esophagitis (EoE) is clinico-pathologically characterized by esophageal symptoms in combination with a dense esophageal eosinophilia, both of which are, in this disease, refractory to proton pump inhibitors [1]. It is important to bear this definition in mind when performing epidemiological studies or when analyzing the literature. To date, only limited population-based epidemiologic information on EoE is available. This is because most of the studies published have been based on retrospective analyses of pathology reports with re-examinations of biopsy specimens, or on retrospective analyses of endoscopy reports. However, it is obvious that only data from geographically confined regions subjected to longitudinal analysis provide the basis from which substantive and valid epidemiologic statements can be made.

Epidemiological Facts

Prevalence of Esophageal Eosinophilia

In the peripheral blood of healthy individuals, eosinophils are found in concentrations of up to 350 cells per mm^3 and, under physiological conditions, are additionally found in the mucosa of all areas of the digestive tract, *except the esophagus* [2, 3]. The presence of eosinophils in the esophagus is therefore commonly associated with disease. Notably, esophageal eosinophilia is not exclusively limited to EoE. In particular, eosinophilic infiltration of the distal part of the esophagus has been reported in patients having gastroesophageal reflux disease (GERD). Esophageal eosinophilia therefore requires a process of differential diagnosis and cannot, a priori, be equated with eosinophilic esophagitis [4].

In 2006, by taking endoscopic biopsies of the distal esophagus from among a random, representative sample ($n = 1{,}000$) of the adult Swedish population (mean age 54 years, 49% men), Ronkainen et al. determined the prevalence of esophageal eosinophils in the general population [5]. Eosinophilic infiltration of the esophageal epithelium was arbitrarily classified as "low grade" with 1–4 eosinophils/HPF (high power field), "possible EoE" with 5–14 eosinophils/HPF, "probable EoE" with 15 to ≤20 eosinophils/HPF, and "definite EoE" when ≥20 eosinophils/HPF were found. The prevalence of any eosinophils in the most distal parts of the esophagus was found to be 4.8% in the general population, predominantly among men (63%), with 54% of these subjects reporting reflux symptoms. This suggests that the presence of esophageal eosinophils may be more common in the general population than expected, but may also be of ambiguous clinical significance, especially as there are no data about the prevalence of eosinophils in the mid- and proximal portions of the esophagus. "Definite EoE" was found in four cases (0.4% of the general population) where three subjects reported troublesome reflux symptoms, but endoscopically, no signs of erosive esophagitis were noted (Table 3.1). Only one subject with "definite EoE" presented with asthma and dysphagia, which would suggest that this patient was suffering from clinico-pathologically defined EoE. "Probable EoE" was present in 7 and "possible EoE" in 25 subjects. In the group of "probable EoE", three subjects had reflux symptoms and two had signs of erosive esophagitis, and in the "possible EoE" group, 12 had reflux symptoms and 13 endoscopically visible erosive esophagitis, respectively. On evaluation of the two biopsy sites (taken at 2 cm above, and at, the Z-line), the presence of eosinophils was positively associated with erosive esophagitis, hiatus hernia, narrowing of the esophageal lumen and esophageal ulcer, thereby suggesting that the presence of esophageal eosinophils, especially in the distal esophageal portions, may be a manifestation of reflux disease.

Incidence and Prevalence of Eosinophilic Esophagitis

As EoE has been reported on all continents except for Africa, there seems to be a broad distribution of the disease worldwide. Several studies have addressed the increasing incidence and prevalence of EoE in the adult population during the last decades. Three of these studies that evaluated geographically confined regions will be discussed here [6–8].

Data from Australia: "Townsville County" indicator area. Townsville, located in Queensland, Australia, is a geographically isolated community of 198,000 people with a centralized gastroenterology service [6]. In a retrospective and observational study, adult residents were diagnosed with EoE after review of physician records, computerized endoscopic, and hospital records. Up to September 2002, a total of 31 patients had been diagnosed with EoE. There were no patients diagnosed with EoE between 1981 and 1994, 12 patients between 1995 and 2000, and 19 patients between January 2001 and September 2002; this indicates an increasing incidence of EoE in this geographically confined region in Australia. At the end of 2002, the prevalence of EoE was 15.6 patients per 100,000 inhabitants (Table 3.1).

Data from Europe, Switzerland: "Olten County" indicator area. The Olten County indicator area is situated in the northwestern part of Switzerland, an industrialized European country [8]. Some 90,000 inhabitants live in this geographically circumscribed area that is surrounded by a state border; for the past 50 years, most of the 35 individual communities have been urban in character. Two board-certified gastroenterologists working in closely connected referral practices in Olten City are responsible for the gastrointestinal (GI) care of this area. Both gastroenterologists work exclusively and consistently with one single pathology center. Of note, the region has

Table 3.1 Prevalence of esophageal eosinophilia and of eosinophilic esophagitis (population-based studies)

	Origin	Study design	Study period	Inclusion criteria	Prevalence (%)
Esophageal eosinophilia					
Ronkainen et al. [5]	Sweden	Prospective, random cohort	2006	≥20 Eos/HPF	0.4
Eosinophilic esophagitis					
Straumann et al. [8]	Switzerland	Prospective, longitudinal cohort	1989–ongoing	≥24 Eos/HPF + endoscopic signs + symptoms	0.013
Croese et al. [6]	Australia	Retrospective, cohort	1981–2002	≥30 Eos/HPF + endoscopic signs	0.0156
Prasad et al. [13]	USA	Retrospective, cohort	1976–2005	≥15 Eos/HPF + symptoms	0.054

experienced no relevant demographic changes and no structural changes to the medical system within the past decades. Since 1989, EoE patients with PPI-refractory esophageal symptoms, EoE-consistent endoscopic abnormalities, and a peak infiltration of the esophageal epithelium with ≥24 eosinophils/HPF are prospectively enrolled into a continuing community-based database. The diagnostic and enrolment procedures have remained almost unchanged during the past 20 years.

A recent analysis of this database suggests that the incidence and prevalence of EoE has been substantially on the rise during the last 6 years. Between 1989 and 2003, the annual incidence rate was between 0.6 and 1.3 patients per 100,000 inhabitants. Between 2004 and 2006, this rate increased to 2.7 and, during the last 3 years, on average, has reached eight newly diagnosed patients per 100,000 inhabitants per year. A similar increase has been observed for the prevalence rate, which ranged between 3 and 12 in the years 1989–2003 (Table 3.1). Thereafter, the prevalence increased from 20 in 2007, and was up to 39 per 100,000 inhabitants in 2009. Notably, the total number of esophageal gastro-duodenoscopies (EGD) performed in the region remained almost stable during this period, and the diagnostic delay (time between onset of symptoms and diagnosis of EoE) did not decrease substantially during recent years. This is suggestive that the increase in incidence and prevalence of EoE is due to neither an increased awareness of the disease by the treating physicians nor to more upper gastrointestinal tract endoscopies being performed.

Data from the USA: "Olmsted County" indicator area. Similar results are reported from Olmsted County, a geographically confined region in Minnesota (USA) which comprises about 120,000 people [7]. Sociodemographically, the community mirrors that of the US white population. County residents receive their medical care almost exclusively from two group practices. Cases were identified by an electronic search using the terms esophagitis and food bolus impaction in the Rochester Epidemiology Project database, the medical records storage system for this region. Patients having ≥15 eosinophils/HPF on endoscopy with esophageal biopsies were included in the analysis. The cumulative age- and gender-adjusted incidence rate between 1976 and 2005 was 2.39 (1.85–2.93) per 100,000 inhabitants. The prevalence of EoE in this time span was 54 per 100,000 inhabitants (Table 3.1). Analysis clearly indicated that the incidence of EoE increased over time, with a pronounced increase in the last reported 5-year period (2001–2005). The differences in the incidence and prevalence rates between Olmsted and Olten counties may be explained by the different threshold values used for the histologic diagnostic criterion in the two studies (≥15 vs. ≥24 eosinophils/HPF, respectively).

Of note, the prevalence of EoE at the end of 2002 was approximately 16 patients per 100,000 inhabitants in Townsville County, Australia; 13 in Olten County, Switzerland; and 27 in Olmsted County, USA, respectively, and, considering the methodological differences between the three studies, roughly within the same range.

Prevalence of EoE on upper endoscopy and/or esophageal biopsy specimens. Other additional information concerning the prevalence of EoE is available from studies based on analyses of pathological or endoscopic databases in non-geographically defined regions.

Between 2002 and 2005, one analysis from a US provider (Caris Diagnostics, Irving, TX) of gastrointestinal pathology services for physicians from community-based, independent endoscopy centers identified 363 cases of EoE in more than 74,000 upper endoscopies, thereby achieving a prevalence rate of approximately 0.5% per endoscopy performed [9]. A reexamination of esophageal biopsy specimens from 1992 to 2004 (pathology database at the University of Pennsylvania) showed a cumulative prevalence of 1.7% (ten cases per 584 reviewed esophageal biopsies), but clearly more cases were identified in the years 2001–2004 [10], again indicating an increasing prevalence of EoE. A prospective study performed between March and September 2007 at a tertiary US military care hospital enrolled 400 consecutive adult patients who underwent a routine upper endoscopy. Patients had EoE if ≥20 eosinophils/HPF were present in biopsy specimens. A high EoE prevalence rate of 6.5% was reported [11]. Other studies show that patients are diagnosed with EoE in 10–15% of the cases when patients are referred for an upper endoscopy due to dysphagia [12, 13], and 11% of patients with food impactions are reported to have EoE [14].Younger patients (<50 years) with dysphagia are more likely to have EoE [12, 13].

Based on these studies, we can conclude that the prevalence of adult EoE has clearly been increasing in the last years. However, still to be determined is whether this increase is based on an accumulation of EoE cases as the mortality from EoE is low, or whether it is based on an increasing incidence, as suggested by recent studies in geographically stable areas.

Demographic Profile of EoE Patients

Gender

All clinical, epidemiological, endoscopic, and pathological EoE studies concordantly demonstrate that males are much more commonly affected with EoE than females. In most studies, between 70 and 80% of all cases diagnosed are in males. Analysis of studies with detailed demographic information of adult patients showed that, on average, 76% of those affected were males, thereby suggesting a male-to-female risk ratio of 3:1 [1]. Interestingly, studies focusing on the leading EoE symptoms of dysphagia and food impaction report this striking male predominance as well [12, 14–16].

Age Distribution, Age at Diagnosis, Age at Onset, Diagnostic Delay

EoE can be found in all age groups [9]. Most studies investigating adult EoE found an average age for subjects with EoE between 34 and 42 years, which suggests that EoE is a disease of middle-aged adults [6–9, 11, 12]. Indeed, in a national US database, most EoE cases identified were in patients between 18 and 49 years of age [9].

Interestingly, age at diagnosis does not at all correlate with onset of EoE-attributed symptoms, which can be considered as onset of disease. Several studies report a substantial time lag between onset of symptoms and diagnosis (diagnostic delay) which, in some cases, can be attributed to unawareness of sentinel features at endoscopy [6]. Croese et al. describe an average diagnostic delay of 54 months (range: 0–180). Similar data are reported from the European countries of Germany and Switzerland. In Germany, the average duration between onset of symptoms and final diagnosis of EoE was 4.2 years (range: 0–44 years) [16] while in Switzerland, for patients with the main symptom of dysphagia, 4.8 years (range: 0–22 years) was required [8]. Of note, an updated analysis from the Olten County (Switzerland) database shows that the average diagnostic delay in the years 1989 to 1998 was 4.3 years ($n=10$; range: 0–17) and from 1999 to 2008, 4.8 years ($n=30$; range: 0–23) and did therefore not change significantly. Under the assumption of increased awareness by physicians for the disease in the last years, this suggests that a substantial proportion of the diagnostic delay can be attributed to the patients themselves postponing medical consultation.

Social Status and Education

Cases of EoE patients have been reported worldwide and identified in a variety of ethnic backgrounds, including Caucasian, African-American, Hispanics, and Asians. However, there are no controlled data about geographic variations of prevalence and it remains unclear whether EoE is associated with any particular ethnic or racial predilection, especially as most of the reported studies analyzed data primarily from Caucasian patients. Interestingly, a study in the USA prospectively analyzed 400 patients at a tertiary care military hospital who underwent routine upper endoscopy and demonstrated that there was no significant race difference between EoE-positive and EoE-negative patients (Caucasian EoE+60% vs. EoE−55%) [11]. In this study, African-Americans (9.3%) were slightly more frequently diagnosed with EoE than were Caucasians (7%). There were no cases of EoE diagnosed among Hispanics or Asians. However, because of this study's high overall EoE prevalence rate of 6.5% on routine upper endoscopy, these data should be interpreted with caution, especially when compared to the general population. Other studies have not reported such high EoE prevalence rates on routine endoscopy.

One case-control study from a GI and allergy cohort analyzing the sociodemographic and geographic characteristics of children with EoE in the Philadelphia area (Pennsylvania, USA) demonstrated a significant difference between EoE patients and controls in terms of predominance of Caucasian race and of male gender [17]. Other notable factors identified were that EoE patients tended to live in affluent environments, be better educated, and reside more often in suburban areas when compared to the control groups; nevertheless, after adjustment for race and gender, these differences could no longer be confirmed. These results notwithstanding, data from socioeconomic distribution are sparse and more systematic evaluations are needed to address the important questions of the contribution of environmental influences for the development of EoE.

Atopic Disease

EoE is characterized as a chronic T-helper 2-type inflammatory disorder of the esophagus [18]. The accumulation of eosinophils in the esophageal wall of EoE patients with specific patterns of cytokine expression resemble the findings in other allergic diseases [19, 20], and it has been proposed that eosinophils migrate to the esophagus in response to various ingested and/or inhaled allergens. Indeed, patients with EoE are reported to have a history of seasonal allergies in 40–50%, asthma in 30–40% and food allergies in 10–40% [6–8, 11, 12]. In a prospective evaluation, Veerappan et al. reported that the prevalence of asthma was significantly higher in the EoE-positive group than in the EoE-negative group [11]. Similarly, though not significantly different, seasonal allergies and food allergies had a higher prevalence among the EoE-positive group. A high degree of atopy was described in a case series of 23 adult EoE patients [21]. Atopic diathesis was found in 18 of the 23 patients, with allergic rhinitis being the most common, and 17 of the 23 were polysensitized to several environmental allergens. The same study identified wheat, tomato, carrot, and onion as the most commonly observed food allergens in adult EoE patients. However, despite the fact that, in children, food allergens have been identified as pathogenic factors of EoE and elemental and elimination diet often results in an improvement or even resolution of symptoms [22], this is still controversial in adults. In a small study of six adult EoE patients, known sensitization to wheat and rye did not appear to be causative as an elimination diet did not improve symptoms or endoscopic findings [22]. Though outside the scope of this chapter, these cited studies suggest that EoE in children differs in some features from EoE in adults.

Positive Family History

Studies from Australia and Switzerland report a positive family history for asthma in 35 and 43% of EoE patients, respectively, and that in 13–23%, other family members are also affected by EoE [7, 8]. Collins et al. at Cincinnati Children's Hospital Medical Center (Ohio, USA) identified 26 families with more than one person diagnosed with EoE (59 patients in total) [23]. The demographic characteristics show that the patients' mean age was 10.3 years (range: 0.25–47 years), and 69.5% were males. Cases were only found among Caucasians. Affected family members included siblings in 85%, and children and their parents in 15%. The most common complaint at diagnosis was dysphagia, reported by 68% of patients. There were considerable atopic features reported in cases of familial EE: 51% reported asthma and 73% had allergic rhinitis. More than 70% of patients had skin prick tests that were reactive either to food (76%) or aeroallergens (71%) or both (63%). The same study also focused on the clinical, pathologic, and molecular characterization (gene expression using genome-wide microarray) of familial versus sporadic EoE cases and showed that clinical manifestations, endoscopic findings, and histological abnormalities did not differ between familial and sporadic cases, thereby suggesting a common underlying pathophysiologic mechanism [24].

Symptoms

The most common presenting symptom of adult EoE is dysphagia for solids, often leading to long-lasting food impaction with the necessity of endoscopic bolus removal. Retrospective analysis of indications for upper endoscopy in EoE patients shows that the rate of dysphagia differs substantially among studies. The reasons for this are, first, the retrospective nature of data acquisition in most studies, and second, reporting of only the primary symptom vs. reporting of multiple symptoms. In most studies, dysphagia is present in 70–100% of patients with EoE [7–9, 16]. Similarly, a large variation can be observed for food impaction and/or the necessity of bolus removal, which ranges between 30 and 50% in most studies [6–8, 11, 24]. As a consequence of EoE's male predilection, it is not surprising that food impaction occurs more frequently in men [15, 24]. Interestingly, patients undergoing upper endoscopy for the diagnostic work-up of dysphagia or food impaction are reported having EoE with a prevalence of 10–15%, and an even higher risk if the age <50 years [12, 13]. Kapel et al. describe an increasing prevalence of EoE in patients having dysphagia which rose from 0.2% in 2002 to 1.9% in 2005 [9]. Finally, patients presenting with dysphagia have been observed to have a significantly higher peak eosinophil count on biopsy specimens [9]. In summary, EoE is likely a leading cause of dysphagia and food impaction.

Symptoms resembling GERD are reported in different studies ranging from 16 to 54% for EoE patients [6–9, 16]. Also, symptoms of chest pain and abdominal pain are reported in the literature. Evaluation of these symptoms is currently limited by a lack of standard symptom definition, which is again mainly due to the retrospective nature of data acquisition in most of the studies.

Relevant Questions and Outlook

Despite the fact that the data presented above are scarce and further epidemiologic investigation is needed, they raise several interesting questions and present opportunities for speculation. The following section addresses some of these aspects.

Eosinophilic Esophagitis: A Truly New or Only Newly Recognized Disease?

To answer this question, the history of EoE's recognition first has to be elucidated. Three conditions had to be present before a diagnosis of EoE was possible (1) assessment of EoE-consistent symptoms; (2) upper endoscopy; and (3) histologic examination of the esophageal tissue.

The first important condition includes recognition of symptoms indicating esophageal dysfunction. Adult patients with EoE report a typical *history* of dysphagia [1, 25–27] and in children suffering from EoE, swallowing disturbances are also present among the leading symptoms [1, 25, 28]. However, it is rare to find patients reporting EoE-consistent swallowing disturbances before the 1980s, even in larger EoE cohorts. This observation is suggestive that the onset of EoE was a rarity before 1980.

Endoscopy, as the second condition necessary for diagnosing EoE, currently represents the most important diagnostic tool for patients with symptoms of the upper GI tract, and is usually the first step in the diagnostic work-up of patients with dysphagia [29]. Upper endoscopy was widely introduced during the 1970s. Interestingly, almost 25 years passed before the initial comprehensive series of adult EoE patients were published, thereby leading to the recognition of EoE as a distinct entity [25–27]. EoE was therefore not detected by endoscopists during the first two decades of gastrointestinal endoscopy. Indeed, it is well known that EoE detection by endoscopy is often difficult [25, 30]. Nevertheless, in a substantial fraction of patients, EoE evokes spectacular abnormalities [6, 30] that lead promptly to biopsy sampling, even when the disease is unknown. It is therefore likely that gastroenterologists performing endoscopies at the beginning of the endoscopy era would have recognized – and would have taken biopsies – in at least a certain fraction of EoE patients, even despite the lower quality of the first-generation endoscopes.

The third condition, *histological examination* using hematoxylin–eosin (HE) staining, a standard method for decades, is needed to detect eosinophils in the tissue. Pathologists would have easily recognized the uncommon finding of a dense tissue eosinophilia in the esophagus. In the literature, this spectacular abnormality was first reported in 1978 as a case report and misinterpreted as vigorous achalasia [31].

Based on these considerations, one can conclude that all conditions necessary for diagnosing EoE were available since the early 1970s, but nevertheless, EoE was not observed before 1994.

To sum up, there is thus a gap of more than 20 years when EoE was not recognized. In addition, there is strong evidence that EoE-consistent symptoms did not occur before the 1980s. Regarding these timelines, it is tempting to speculate that EoE started during the last two decades of the last century, and thus provides strong evidence that EoE is truly a new disease.

Eosinophilic Esophagitis: A More-Prevalent or a More-Recognized Disease?

It is still debated whether the occurrence of adult EoE is truly increasing and the disease affects ever more individuals, or whether the diagnosis is established more frequently as a consequence of the increased awareness by health care providers. Answering this question requires population-based long-term analysis.

Unfortunately, the vast majority of studies addressing this question rely on retrospective analyses of pathology or endoscopy databases [9, 11, 32]. Data resulting from these approaches therefore represent EoE cases per esophageal biopsy or per upper endoscopy, but not EoE cases per so many inhabitants. Ronkainen et al. used a population-based, endoscopic approach to achieve robust epidemiologic data in the Swedish population [5]. However, the interpretation of this study is hampered by two facts: First, they performed an analysis based mainly on histology revealing data about the prevalence of esophageal eosinophilia, which could be different from the prevalence of EoE, and second, this cross-sectional analysis was performed at a given time point and therefore provides no information regarding changes in prevalence over time. The best evidence for a true escalation comes from Australia [6] and Switzerland [8]. As cited above, retrospective analysis by Croese et al. shows a 0 incidence of EoE in Townsville County, Australia before 1995, which increased to an annual 1.01 incidence rate with 12 cases between 1995 and 2000 (12 cases/198,000 population/6 years); and again increased to 5.48 new cases per year (19/198,000/1.75 years) by September 2002. In 1989, investigators in Switzerland created a population-based database and prospectively captured all adolescent and adult EoE patients living in the clearly defined area of Olten County. The incidence rates ranged between 0 and 8 cases per year per 100,000 inhabitants, and showed an increasing trend , whereas the cumulative prevalence increased constantly from 0 to 39 cases per 100,000 inhabitants. Furthermore, the diagnostic delay was approximately 4–5 years and remained stable throughout the entire period, indicating that the detection of EoE did not improve during these two decades.

In summary, there is strong evidence that there is a true and constant increase in the prevalence of EoE. In contrast, whether this increased prevalence is due to an increase in incidence or only due to the non-fatal character of EoE, adding ever more cases to the patient pool, is still controversial and further population-based longitudinal studies are required to confirm this assumption.

Eosinophilic Esophagitis: A Seasonal or a Perennial Disease?

This question seeks to enhance the still-limited understanding of EoE's pathogenesis. Food allergens as well as aeroallergens have been implicated as contributing factors in inducing and maintaining the eosinophilic inflammation [1, 33, 34]. Data supporting the relationship to food allergies comes predominantly from the pediatric literature [35] and indeed, several types of diets eliminating potential allergens have proven efficacious in the treatment of children with EoE [36–38]. In contrast, adults with EoE are often sensitized to aeroallergens [1, 22]. Further evidence that aeroallergens might play a crucial role in the pathogenesis of EoE was provided by a case report demonstrating a seasonal variation of EoE's activity in parallel to pollen exposure [39]. A confirmation of a seasonal dependency of EoE would be an indicator that external seasonal factors, in particular, pollen, could play a substantial role in the pathogenesis of this Th2-type inflammation.

To date, two investigators have searched for a seasonal variation of EoE's occurrence [40, 41]. Unfortunately, both studies used the time point of diagnostic endoscopy in the annual cycle as the marker of disease onset. However, it is known that there is a substantial gap between onset of symptoms (=likely onset of disease) and diagnosis. For instance, in the Swiss cohort, including more than 500 adolescent and adult EoE patients, there is a diagnostic delay of approximately 4–5 years. Therefore, in most patients, the date of endoscopy can definitely not be linked to the date of onset of disease. Conclusions regarding the influence of pollen in the pathogenesis of EoE that are drawn from endoscopic rates are thus likely to be highly speculative and most probably misleading.

Taken together, with the exception of one single case report [39], there is no solid proof that either the first onset of EoE or the course of its inflammation show a seasonal variation, or that pollen exposure could play a pathogenic role. Prospective studies using either a systematic assessment of the symptom course or of EoE's inflammatory activity in correlation to the pollen exposure are needed to answer this question.

Eosinophilic Esophagitis: An Industrialized or a Westernized Disease?

The vast majority of EoE cases and cohorts are reported from industrialized countries, such as the USA, Europe, and Australia, whereas almost no reports come from tropical areas and/or developing countries [1]. This pattern is not surprising and corresponds well with the pattern of classical allergic disorders. It might be explained by the hygiene theory which postulates that individuals who are not exposed to infections during early childhood are prone to develop allergies as adolescents or adults [42]. However, regarding the worldwide distribution of EoE, one exception is surprising: Japan is not yet infested with EoE (personal communication). This fact can neither be explained by lack of education of Japanese gastroenterologists nor by inappropriate diagnostic tools. Japanese gastroenterologists and pathologists are highly educated and best equipped with high-tech instruments. EoE must therefore be considered a westernized, but not an industrialized, disease.

Two apparent differences exist between Japan and the remaining industrialized countries: nutritional habits and genetics. While in western kitchen flavors, dairy products, potatoes and beef are familiar, the Japanese kitchen is dominated by fish and rice, and in addition, often in an uncooked form.

Conclusion

This obvious difference in nutritional habits together with the fact that, in some cases, EoE can be treated by elimination of distinct foods raises the question of whether one of the western foods could be a trigger for EoE, or in contrast, one Japanese food could exert a protective effect. However, this speculation needs further investigation and genetic factors must also be considered. In elucidating the denouement of this relatively new disease, it is important to realize that, though numerous questions remain, much progress has been made, and each new study furthers our understanding and moves us closer to alleviating the pathos of affected patients.

References

1. Furuta GT, Liacouras CA, Collins MH, et al. Eosinophilic esophagitis in children and adults: a systematic review and consensus recommendations for diagnosis and treatment. Gastroenterology. 2007;133:1342–63.
2. Kato M, Kephart GM, Talley NJ, et al. Eosinophil infiltration and degranulation in normal human tissue. Anat Rec. 1998;252:418–25.
3. Lowichik A, Weinberg AG. A quantitative evaluation of mucosal eosinophils in the pediatric gastrointestinal tract. Mod Pathol. 1996;9:110–4.
4. Ahmad M, Soetikno RM, Ahmed A. The differential diagnosis of eosinophilic esophagitis. J Clin Gastroenterol. 2000;30:242–4.
5. Ronkainen J, Talley NJ, Aro P, et al. Prevalence of oesophageal eosinophils and eosinophilic oesophagitis in adults: the population-based Kalixanda study. Gut. 2007;56:615–20.
6. Croese J, Fairley SK, Masson JW, et al. Clinical and endoscopic features of eosinophilic esophagitis in adults. Gastrointest Endosc. 2003;58:516–22.
7. Prasad GA, Alexander JA, Schleck CD, et al. Epidemiology of eosinophilic esophagitis over three decades in Olmsted County, Minnesota. Clin Gastroenterol Hepatol. 2009;7:1055–61.
8. Straumann A, Simon HU. Eosinophilic esophagitis: escalating epidemiology? J Allergy Clin Immunol. 2005;115:418–9.
9. Kapel RC, Miller JK, Torres C, et al. Eosinophilic esophagitis: a prevalent disease in the United States that affects all age groups. Gastroenterology. 2008;134:1316–21.
10. Whitney-Miller CL, Katzka D, Furth EE. Eosinophilic esophagitis: a retrospective review of esophageal biopsy specimens from 1992 to 2004 at an adult academic medical center. Am J Clin Pathol. 2009;131:788–92.
11. Veerappan GR, Perry JL, Duncan TJ, et al. Prevalence of eosinophilic esophagitis in an adult population undergoing upper endoscopy: a prospective study. Clin Gastroenterol Hepatol. 2009;7:420–6,e421–422.
12. Mackenzie SH, Go M, Chadwick B, et al. Eosinophilic oesophagitis in patients presenting with dysphagia – a prospective analysis. Aliment Pharmacol Ther. 2008;28:1140–6.
13. Prasad GA, Talley NJ, Romero Y, et al. Prevalence and predictive factors of eosinophilic esophagitis in patients presenting with dysphagia: a prospective study. Am J Gastroenterol. 2007;102:2627–32.
14. Byrne KR, Panagiotakis PH, Hilden K, et al. Retrospective analysis of esophageal food impaction: differences in etiology by age and gender. Dig Dis Sci. 2007;52:717–21.
15. Desai TK, Stecevic V, Chang CH, et al. Association of eosinophilic inflammation with esophageal food impaction in adults. Gastrointest Endosc. 2005;61:795–801.
16. Muller S, Puhl S, Vieth M, et al. Analysis of symptoms and endoscopic findings in 117 patients with histological diagnoses of eosinophilic esophagitis. Endoscopy. 2007;39:339–44.

17. Franciosi JP, Tam V, Liacouras CA, et al. A case-control study of sociodemographic and geographic characteristics of 335 children with eosinophilic esophagitis. Clin Gastroenterol Hepatol. 2009;7:415–9.
18. Straumann A, Bauer M, Fischer B, et al. Idiopathic eosinophilic esophagitis is associated with a T(H)2-type allergic inflammatory response. J Allergy Clin Immunol. 2001;108:954–61.
19. Akdis CA, Akdis M, Simon D, et al. T cells and T cell-derived cytokines as pathogenic factors in the nonallergic form of atopic dermatitis. J Invest Dermatol. 1999;113:628–34.
20. Bousquet J, Vignola AM, Demoly P. Links between rhinitis and asthma. Allergy. 2003;58:691–706.
21. Roy-Ghanta S, Larosa DF, Katzka DA. Atopic characteristics of adult patients with eosinophilic esophagitis. Clin Gastroenterol Hepatol. 2008;6:531–5.
22. Simon D, Straumann A, Wenk A, et al. Eosinophilic esophagitis in adults – no clinical relevance of wheat and rye sensitizations. Allergy. 2006;61:1480–3.
23. Collins MH, Blanchard C, Abonia JP, et al. Clinical, pathologic, and molecular characterization of familial eosinophilic esophagitis compared with sporadic cases. Clin Gastroenterol Hepatol. 2008;6:621–9.
24. Kerlin P, Jones D, Remedios M, et al. Prevalence of eosinophilic esophagitis in adults with food bolus obstruction of the esophagus. J Clin Gastroenterol. 2007;41:356–61.
25. Attwood SE, Smyrk TC, Demeester TR, et al. Esophageal eosinophilia with dysphagia. A distinct clinicopathologic syndrome. Dig Dis Sci. 1993;38:109–16.
26. Straumann A, Spichtin HP, Bernoulli R, et al. Idiopathic eosinophilic esophagitis: a frequently overlooked disease with typical clinical aspects and discrete endoscopic findings. Schweiz Med Wochenschr. 1994;124:1419–29.
27. Vitellas KM, Bennett WF, Bova JG, et al. Idiopathic eosinophilic esophagitis. Radiology. 1993;186:789–93.
28. Liacouras CA, Spergel JM, Ruchelli E, et al. Eosinophilic esophagitis: a 10-year experience in 381 children. Clin Gastroenterol Hepatol. 2005;3:1198–206.
29. Varadarajulu S, Eloubeidi MA, Patel RS, et al. The yield and the predictors of esophageal pathology when upper endoscopy is used for the initial evaluation of dysphagia. Gastrointest Endosc. 2005;61:804–8.
30. Straumann A, Spichtin HP, Bucher KA, et al. Eosinophilic esophagitis: red on microscopy, white on endoscopy. Digestion. 2004;70:109–16.
31. Landres RT, Kuster GG, Strum WB. Eosinophilic esophagitis in a patient with vigorous achalasia. Gastroenterology. 1978;74:1298–301.
32. Vanderheyden AD, Petras RE, DeYoung BR, et al. Emerging eosinophilic (allergic) esophagitis: increased incidence or increased recognition? Arch Pathol Lab Med. 2007;131:777–9.
33. Arora AS, Yamazaki K. Eosinophilic esophagitis: asthma of the esophagus? Clin Gastroenterol Hepatol. 2004;2:523–30.
34. Rothenberg ME, Mishra A, Collins MH, et al. Pathogenesis and clinical features of eosinophilic esophagitis. J Allergy Clin Immunol. 2001;108:891–4.
35. Spergel JM, Beausoleil JL, Mascarenhas M, et al. The use of skin prick tests and patch tests to identify causative foods in eosinophilic esophagitis. J Allergy Clin Immunol. 2002;109:363–8.
36. Kagalwalla AF, Sentongo TA, Ritz S, et al. Effect of six-food elimination diet on clinical and histologic outcomes in eosinophilic esophagitis. Clin Gastroenterol Hepatol. 2006;4:1097–102.
37. Kelly KJ, Lazenby AJ, Rowe PC, et al. Eosinophilic esophagitis attributed to gastroesophageal reflux: improvement with an amino acid-based formula. Gastroenterology. 1995;109:1503–12.
38. Orenstein SR, Shalaby TM, Di Lorenzo C, et al. The spectrum of pediatric eosinophilic esophagitis beyond infancy: a clinical series of 30 children. Am J Gastroenterol. 2000;95:1422–30.
39. Fogg MI, Ruchelli E, Spergel JM. Pollen and eosinophilic esophagitis. J Allergy Clin Immunol. 2003;112:796–7.
40. Almansa C, Krishna M, Buchner AM, et al. Seasonal distribution in newly diagnosed cases of eosinophilic esophagitis in adults. Am J Gastroenterol. 2009;104:828–33.
41. Wang FY, Gupta SK, Fitzgerald JF. Is there a seasonal variation in the incidence or intensity of allergic eosinophilic esophagitis in newly diagnosed children? J Clin Gastroenterol. 2007;41:451–3.
42. Braun-Fahrlander C, Riedler J, Herz U, et al. Environmental exposure to endotoxin and its relation to asthma in school-age children. N Engl J Med. 2002;347:869–77.

Chapter 4
Eosinophil Biology in the Pathogenesis of Eosinophilic Disorders

Steven J. Ackerman

Keywords Eosinophil • Biology • Differentiation • Migration • Recruitment • Activation • Secretion

Introduction

In the 100+ years following the identification of the eosinophilic leukocyte by Paul Ehrlich in 1879, a significant number of diseases and syndromes characterized by blood or tissue eosinophilia were identified. However, specific functional roles for the eosinophil in host defense and innate immunity, allergic and related inflammatory responses, tissue injury, repair, remodeling, and fibrosis have only been delineated in the past ~30 years [1–3]. These studies served to characterize many of the unique biologic characteristics of blood and activated tissue eosinophils, their preformed granule proteins, and inducible lipid, oxidative, and cytokine products, focusing initially on the eosinophil's pro-inflammatory and cytotoxic potential in the pathogenesis of allergic, parasitic, and a variety of idiopathic eosinophil-associated syndromes [4]. Recognition of the eosinophil as an effector cell in asthma pathogenesis fueled the initial surge in interest in this granulocyte [5], and the "epidemics" of eosinophil myalgia syndrome related to ingestion of tainted L-tryptophan [6], and more recent identification and increasing prevalence of eosinophilic esophagitis (EoE) have markedly increased clinical and public awareness and interest in the eosinophil [7].

S.J. Ackerman (✉)
Department of Biochemistry and Molecular Genetics (M/C 669), and Sections of Hematology-Oncology and Pulmonary, Critical Care, Sleep and Allergy, The University of Illinois at Chicago College of Medicine, Molecular Biology Research Building, Rm. 2074, 900S. Ashland Avenue, Chicago, IL 60607, USA
e-mail: sackerma@uic.edu

C.A. Liacouras and J.E. Markowitz (eds.), *Eosinophilic Esophagitis*,
Clinical Gastroenterology, DOI 10.1007/978-1-60761-515-6_4,

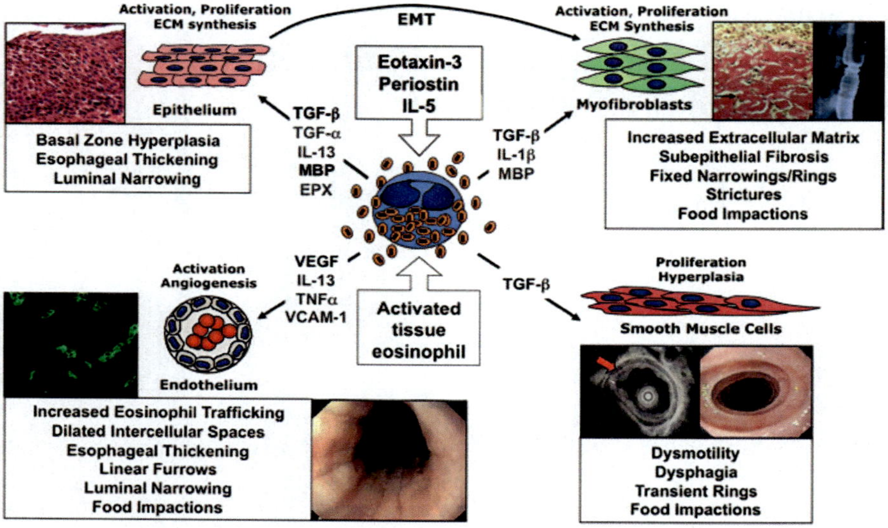

Fig. 4.1 Role of the eosinophil in the pathogenesis of EoE: relationships to clinical, endoscopic and histologic pathologies. Eosinophil activation during recruitment to the esophagus occurs in response to eotaxin-3, periostin, IL-5 and interactions with vascular endothelium, epithelium, and fibroblasts, leading to their expression of fibrogenic factors such as TGF-β. Eosinophil-expressed TGF-β and granule proteins (MBP, EPX) induce epithelial basal zone hyperplasia, contributing to esophageal thickening and luminal narrowing. Eosinophil-derived TGF-β induces fibroblast activation, with transdifferentiation to myofibroblasts and consequent over-production of ECM leading to subepithelial fibrosis, fixed narrowings/rings, strictures, and food impactions. Alternatively, TGF-β expressed by eosinophils or MBP/EPX damaged epithelium itself may induce epithelial to mesenchymal (myofibroblast) transition (EMT) contributing to subepithelial fibrosis [85]. Eosinophil-expressed TGF-β may induce smooth muscle cell hypertrophy/hyperplasia leading to thickening of the esophageal muscularis propria, contributing to dysmotility, dysphagia, transient rings, and non-stricture food impactions. Eosinophil expression of VEGF likely supports increased angiogenic responses of vascular endothelium with VCAM-1 activation by IL-13 and TNF-α, contributing to increased eosinophil trafficking, dilated intercellular spaces, esophageal thickening, furrowing, luminal narrowing, and non-stricture food impactions. (Updated and reproduced in color with permission from [80] Aceves SS, Ackerman SJ. Immunol Allergy Clin N Am. 2009;29:197–211)

The current paradigm, that eosinophils subserve pro-inflammatory and tissue-damaging roles in the pathogenesis of eosinophil-associated diseases and hypereosinophilic syndromes such as EoE (Fig. 4.1), is supported by a growing number of definitive mouse model and human studies. A pivotal role for the eosinophil in the development of tissue remodeling and fibrosis, in part through their elaboration of remodeling and fibrogenic growth factors, is now widely accepted [8–10]. Studies using IL-5 knockout mice and two strains of eosinophil-deficient mice strongly support the concept that eosinophils contribute to the pathology of airway remodeling and subepithelial fibrosis in asthma [11, 12] and are required for T cell polarization for Th2 responses in the lung in response to allergen challenge [13], and recent clinical trials using anti-IL-5 antibody (Mepolizumab™) to ablate eosinophils in the bone marrow, blood and tissues of patient with "eosinophilic", but not neutrophilic, asthma, showed efficacy in reversing aspects of eosinophil-mediated tissue damage, remodeling and fibrosis in allergic diseases such as asthma [14, 15], eosinophilic esophagitis (EoE) [16], and the hypereosinophilic syndrome (HES) [17]. This chapter will review basic aspects of eosinophil cellular, molecular, and immunobiology that are pertinent to understanding their inflammatory and pathologic activities, the mechanisms that regulate eosinophil development and eosinophilia in the bone marrow, blood, and tissues, and their relationships to the pathogenesis of eosinophil-mediated allergic disorders such as EoE.

Eosinophil Morphology and Mediators of Inflammation

Eosinophils contain a number of distinct membrane-bound granules produced during their differentiation from IL-5R+ eosinophil progenitors (EoP) in the bone marrow. These include: (1) uniformly electron dense primary granules present mainly in eosinophil promyelocytes; (2) secondary (specific) granules containing the hallmark electron dense crystalloid core and less dense granule matrix (>95% of granules in mature eosinophils); and (3) small granules, sites of hydrolytic enzymes such as acid phosphatase and arylsulfatase, that may be functionally analogous to cellular lysosomes. The secondary granule is the major storage site for the eosinophil's cationic proteins, which confer the eosinophil's unique affinity for acidic fluorone dyes such as eosin, the basis for Paul Ehrlich's discovery, and naming of the eosinophil in 1879. As well, eosinophils contain non-membrane-bound lipid-rich organelles called lipid bodies [18], the numbers of which increase in activated eosinophils, both in vitro and at sites of tissue inflammatory reactions [19]. Lipid bodies incorporate fatty acids such as arachidonate and likely serve as intracellular depots for their storage and metabolism, including the formation of leukotrienes, since they contain all of the required eicosanoid-forming enzymes (5-lipoxygenase, leukotriene C4 synthase, cyclooxygenase) [20]. These organelles, along with vesiculotubular "sombrero" structures and small vesicles involved in transport and secretion during eosinophil activation [21], represent the major storage sites for the eosinophil's preformed cytotoxic and inflammatory proteins.

The Granule Cationic Proteins

Initial studies of the biochemistry, biologic activities and tissue localization of the cationic enzymes and non-enzymatic proteins isolated from the eosinophil secondary granule provided the first clues to this granulocyte's role in the pathogenesis of inflammation and tissue damage in eosinophil-associated diseases [4]. As well, immunohistochemical detection of eosinophil-specific granule constituents in tissue biopsies provided evidence for the participation of the eosinophil in diseases not normally associated with blood or tissue eosinophilia, e.g., certain skin diseases such as atopic dermatitis [22]. These studies provided compelling evidence supporting a pathologic effector role for eosinophils in the induction of tissue and end-stage organ damage [23]. These cationic granule proteins include the two major basic proteins (MBP-1, MBP-2), eosinophil peroxidase (EPX), and the eosinophil's ribonucleases, eosinophil-derived neurotoxin (EDN, RNase2) and eosinophil cationic protein (ECP, RNase3).

Studies of the mechanisms by which the eosinophil granule cationic proteins are secreted or released into tissues have shown that they can be independently (selectively) secreted, depending on the type and strength of the activating stimulus, through a number of different secretory pathways ranging from classical granule fusion and exocytosis (e.g., in the killing parasitic helminths), piecemeal degranulation (a vesicular transport process from secondary granules in the absence of exocytosis), and cytolytic degranulation (the release of intact, membrane-bound, and secretory-competent secondary granules directly into the tissue upon eosinophil apoptosis/cell death) [24, 25].

In addition to secretion of their preformed granule cationic proteins, eosinophils have the capacity to express potent toxic reactive oxygen species (ROS) [26], eicosanoids (e.g. prostaglandins, leukotrienes, lipoxins) and other inflammatory lipid mediators [18] (see below), and importantly, a significant number of hematopoietic and inflammatory cytokines key to the normal and pathophysiologic roles of the eosinophil [27, 28].

Cytokines and Growth Factors

In addition to their granule proteins, eosinophils are also a considerable source of both preformed (stored) and newly synthesized cytokines, chemokines and growth factors, including Th1 and Th2 type cytokines, that can participate in linking innate and adaptive immune responses, regulation of Th2 responses, leukocyte chemotaxis, tissue remodeling and fibrosis, and cell growth and survival, including the eosinophil's own survival through expression of GM-CSF (Table 4.1) [27, 29]. Although T cells and other lymphocytes generally express greater amounts of these cytokines at sites of allergic tissue inflammatory responses, the ability of the eosinophil to both synthesize and store these cytokines in their cytoplasmic granules, and to secrete them from both the intact cell and from cell-free secondary granules in the tissue [25], suggests eosinophils may provide both a more rapid and highly focused release of these immune regulators at sites of allergic inflammation [27, 29].

Eosinophils are classically associated with the development of Th2-polarized allergic and anti-parasite host immune responses and are recruited into immune environments rich in Th2 cytokines, particularly IL-4, IL-5, and IL-13. IL-5, the eosinophilopoietin, regulates the development of blood and tissue eosinophilia through its multiple actions on eosinophil progenitor (EoP) cell expansion and

Table 4.1 Eosinophils express and secrete multiple stored and newly synthesized interleukins, chemokines, and growth factors upon priming and activation

Interleukins
IL-1 (α and β), IL-2, IL-3, IL-4, IL-5, IL-6, IL-9, IL-10, IL-11, IL-12, IL-13, IL-16, IL-17
Chemokines
Epithelial cell-derived neutrophil activating peptide (CXCL5), eotaxin (CCL11), growth-related oncogene (CXCL1), interleukine-8 (CXCL8), IFN-γ inducible protein (CXCL10), IFN-inducible T-cell alpha chemoattractant (CXCL11), macrophage inflammatory protein 1alpha (MIP1α), monocyte chemoattractant protein 1 (CCL3), monokine induced by IFN-γ (CXCL9), MCP-3 (CCL7), MCP-4 (CCL13), RANTES (CCL5)
Growth factors
Heparin-binding epidermal growth factor-like binding protein (HB-EGF-LBP), nerve growth factor (NGF), platelet-derived growth factor (PDGF-BB), transforming growth factor-alpha (TGF-α), transforming growth factor-beta (TGF-β)
Autocrine survival factors
Granulocyte-macrophage colony-stimulating factor (GM-CSF)
Other immune regulators
Interferon-gamma (IFN-γ), tumor necrosis factor alpha (TNF-α)

Modified with permission from: Fillon S, Ackerman SJ, Furuta GT. Eosinophils. In: Charles N. Serhan, Peter Ward and Derek Gilroy, editors. Fundamentals of Inflammation, Chapter 7. Cambridge: Cambridge University Press; 2010. pp. 86–95.

terminal differentiation in the bone marrow, eosinophil recruitment, priming, and activation in tissue inflammatory sites, and can also prolong eosinophil survival in response to allergic stimuli [30, 31]. However, activated eosinophils express their own GM-CSF, which signals in an autocrine manner to prevent apoptosis [32], thus significantly prolonging their tissue survival, e.g. in the lung in asthma [32, 33], and likely in the GI tract in eosinophil-associated GI diseases such as EoE. Notably, treatment of asthma [34] or EoE [35] patients with anti-IL-5 antibody (Mepolizumab) only depletes ~50% of lung or esophageal eosinophils, likely due to their autocrine GM-CSF-mediated long-term survival in these tissues.

Although IL-5 is the only lineage-specific eosinophilopoietin, basal levels of eosinophil differentiation occurs in the bone marrow in the absence of IL-5, i.e., in IL-5 and IL-5R knockout mice, but these mice do not develop blood or tissue eosinophilia in response to allergic or parasitic challenges. This suggests IL-5's primary role is the rapid expansion of the eosinophil lineage for the development of blood and tissue eosinophilia. Consistent with this is the finding that IL-5 upregulates eosinophil progenitor cell expression of the transmembrane isoform of its receptor (specifically the IL-5-binding α chain of the heterodimeric IL-5R) and downregulates the soluble "decoy" isoform of the α-chain [36]. Numerous studies of IL-5 in experimental mouse asthma models using gain-of-function transgenic lung-specific over-expression and loss of function IL-5 knockouts and anti-IL-5 neutralizing antibodies, have confirmed its role in allergic responses, particularly in amplifying blood and tissue eosinophilia. For example, transgenic over-expression of IL-5 either systemically or in an organ-specific manner in the mouse is sufficient to induce eosinophilia [37–40], while antibody neutralization or gene knockout of IL-5 blocks multiple aspects of the asthmatic response [41, 42], including suppression of pulmonary eosinophilia in response to allergen sensitization/inhalation challenge, airways hyperreactivity [43], and airways remodeling in terms of goblet cell mucus metaplasia, subepithelial fibrosis and airway smooth muscle hyperplasia [44]. Likewise, eosinophil trafficking to the allergen sensitized and challenged lung is significantly reduced in IL-5 deficient (knockout) mice and those treated with anti-IL-5 neutralizing antibodies [41, 42, 44]. Importantly, clinical studies show that anti-IL-5 antibody (Mepolizumab) in asthmatics fully depletes their bone marrow and blood eosinophils, significantly reduces pulmonary eosinophils by >50% [15, 34, 45], and shows efficacy in reducing sputum eosinophils and asthma exacerbations [46], and improving airway function and reducing steroid use [47], both in patients with clearly defined refractory, steroid-dependent eosinophilic asthma.

Eosinophils can express a number of cytokines normally associated with Th2 T cells such as IL-4 and IL-13, which can activate human vascular endothelial and respiratory epithelial cells to produce eosinophil chemotactic cytokines (chemokines) [48], thus amplifying eosinophil recruitment to the tissues. Both IL-4 and IL-13, produced in greater quantities by Th2 T cells than eosinophils, also recruits and activates IgE-producing B lymphocytes and enhances IgE-mediated allergic responses [49]. Unlike IL-4, IL-13 has a distinct role in allergic inflammation, acting as a primary regulator of allergen-induced airway inflammation and goblet cell mucus metaplasia in asthma [50] and eosinophilic esophageal inflammation and remodeling in EoE [51–54]. Although both IL-4 and IL-13 induce the expression of eotaxins by epithelial cells in a STAT6-dependent manner [55], IL-13 alone expressed by T cells or eosinophils themselves in asthma, EoE and other eosinophil-associated inflammatory diseases [51, 56], may participate as an important eosinophil chemoattractant [31].

Of interest, eosinophils also produce a number of cytokines associated with Th1 immune responses including IL-2, IL-6, IL-12, TNF-α and IFN-γ, suggesting they share some functional activities with Th1 T cells [57–59]. Of note, Th1 cells are recruited by CXCL9 (a monokine induced by IFN-γ) and CXCL10 (IFN-γ-inducible protein-10) [60]. IL-6 has been shown to inhibit Th1 and increase Th2 differentiation of eosinophils through induction of naïve T cell IL-4 production [61]. In some Th1 models of inflammation, eosinophil-derived IFN-γ is increased [29]. In addition, TNF-α is essential for eosinophil-derived IFN-γ-induced secretion of Th1 chemokines [59].

Eosinophils also secrete a number the major chemoattractants (chemokines) involved in their own recruitment into tissues including the eotaxins and RANTES, suggesting eosinophils may amplify or perpetuate their recruitment to sites of allergic inflammatory responses, even after the initiating stimulus is no longer present, i.e., mast cell or epithelial cell activation. The eotaxins (1, 2 and 3) in particular, principally secreted by both activated epithelial cells and T cells, are the most highly selective of the chemokines involved in eosinophil tissue recruitment identified to date. Eosinophils selectively express CCR3 on their plasma membrane, the cognate receptor for the eotaxins. In contrast, RANTES is less eosinophil-selective and induces both eosinophil and neutrophil granulocyte influx, whereas the chemokine MIP-1α, also expressed by eosinophils, is primarily involved in the trafficking of neutrophils [62].

Eosinophils also participate in other biological processes, not the least of which is regulation of the immune microenvironment in the lung and other tissues [3, 13, 63], including their recently identified requirement for the development of Th2-mediated allergic responses and recruitment of effector T cells into the lung in experimental allergic asthma models [13], indicating an important role in bridging innate and adaptive immune responses in allergic airway inflammation [2, 3]. Eosinophil-deficient (named "PHIL") mice have significantly blunted Th2 cytokine responses in the airways and fail to recruit Th2 effector T cells into the lung during allergic inflammation [11, 13]. As well, IL-4-deficient mice have reduced allograft transplant-associated eosinophilia, and impaired development of Th2 inflammation at sites of allograft transplants in these mice, suggesting eosinophils may regulate immune responses leading to transplant rejection [64]. Moreover, IL-4 and IL-13 are strongly associated with tumor cell death in several types of cancer [65], and tumor cells engineered to over-express IL-4, but not IL-5, induce tumors that undergo eosinophil-mediated regression in a murine cancer model [66–68]. Of note, IL-4 therapy of cancer patients in a Phase I clinical trial was shown to induce mild eosinophilia, systemic and tissue (skin) eosinophil activation and degranulation, increased levels of MBP1 (both systemically and extracellular in the skin), and significantly enhanced eosinophil survival due to IL-5, GM-CSF and IL-3, suggesting an association between IL-4 and eosinophil-induced pathologies in certain human cancers and allergic responses [69]. Of interest, almost all human and murine tumors become infiltrated by eosinophils at some point in their growth [3, 70], with the presence of eosinophils being either a positive or negative prognostic factor, depending on the type of cancer [3, 70].

Finally, eosinophils are a very rich source of TGF-β [71–76], comprise the major TGF-β expressing cell population in the airways in human asthma [73, 77] and experimental mouse asthma models [44], and in the esophagus in EoE [71, 78], and are clinically and experimentally associated with multiple aspects of tissue remodeling (e.g. epithelial cell hyperplasia, smooth muscle hyperplasia, angiogenesis) and fibrosis [10, 79] (fibroblast activation, transdifferentiation into myofibroblasts and increased deposition of extracellular matrix) in many eosinophil-associated allergic diseases and hypereosinophilic syndromes including asthma [8, 9, 78] and EoE [71, 80] (reviewed in greater detail below). Recent studies have implicated the eosinophil in the development of subepithelial fibrosis through the induction of epithelial mesenchymal transition (EMT) in the airway epithelial cells in asthma [81–84] and in the esophagus in EoE [85].

Lipid Mediators Expressed By Eosinophils

Eosinophils express all of the required lipoxygenase and cyclooxygenase enzymes involved in the generation of a variety of potent lipid mediators of inflammation derived from arachidonic acid, and when appropriately activated they synthesize and secrete lipid mediators including cysteinyl leukotrienes (mainly LTC_4), prostaglandins (mainly PGE_2), and platelet-activating factor (PAF). These eosinophil-derived eicosanoids can increase leukocyte trafficking and adhesion to endothelial cells, induce airway smooth muscle contraction, increase vascular permeability and mucus secretion, and are considered one of the pro-inflammatory functions of the eosinophil [1], particularly in late-phase allergic reactions. In contrast, eosinophil-derived arachidonate-derived lipid mediators are also likely to participate in the resolution of allergic inflammation. For example, airway challenge with allergen in a mouse asthma model has recently been shown to initiate airway biosynthesis of functionally significant amounts of lipoxin A_4 and increase its receptor expression. Notably, a stable analog of Lipoxin A_4 has been shown to block the development of airway hyperresponsiveness, diminish airway inflammation, and decrease overall leukocyte recruitment and its consequent expression of Th2 cytokines (IL-5, IL-13), eotaxins, prostanoids, and cysteinyl leukotrienes (i.e. LTC_4) in the airways [45]. As well, lipoxin A_4 analogues have been found to block the development of allergic pleural eosinophil effusions and inhibit the early edema and neutrophil recruitment seen in allergic responses [86]. These lipoxin A_4 mediated responses were found to be independent of mast cell degranulation and included inhibition of the generation and activities of IL-5, eotaxin and platelet activating factor [86]. Finally, eosinophils themselves express receptors for the cysteinyl leukotrienes (CysLT1R and CysLT2R), prostaglandins (PGD2 type 2 receptor), and PAF [87–89], consistent with the induction of eosinophil recruitment by leukotrienes (LTB4, D4, E4), PAF, and 5-oxo-6,8,11,14-eicosatetraenoic acid, suggesting a role for these chemoattractant lipids in the tissue recruitment of eosinophils to sites of allergic reactions [86, 90, 91].

Monitoring of Eosinophil Activity in Disease

Increased appreciation of the importance of both the numbers and functional status of tissue eosinophils, as well as important functional differences between circulating blood eosinophils and those recruited into tissues and exposed to cytokines and other factors in the tissue microenvironment [92], led to the development and increasingly more routine use of approaches to monitor eosinophil activation in situ. Tissue biopsies are routinely employed for both the clinical diagnosis and experimental evaluation of eosinophil activity in diseases involving the skin [22, 93, 94], lungs [95–97], lymph nodes [98], heart [99], and other tissues such as the esophagus in EoE [100], contributing significantly to current appreciation of the eosinophil's roles in disease pathogenesis, particularly tissue remodeling and fibrosis [78, 80]. The difficulties, tediousness, and sampling errors inherent in accurately quantifying the numbers and functional status of eosinophils in tissue biopsies, even using antibodies that recognize eosinophil-specific cell surface activation markers or secretion of the granule cationic proteins with quantitative morphometric assessments, still makes routine clinicopathologic evaluation of tissue eosinophils by these methods somewhat impractical clinically. Alternatives such as analysis of eosinophil-specific biomarkers in tissue secretions from affected organs, e.g., bronchoalveolar lavage or induced sputum, have met with some success in the clinical and experimental evaluation of eosinophil participation in diseases such as asthma [101], and more recently using biopsy tissue sections in EoE [100]. In addition to routine histochemical enumeration of eosinophils by H&E staining, and immunohistochemical localization of cell-associated and secreted eosinophil granule cationic proteins such as eosinophil peroxidase (EPX) [100] and eosinophil-derived neurotoxin (EDN) [102], two additional methods were previously used to monitor eosinophil activation, secretion, and participation in the pathogenesis of allergic disease. These included identification of activated eosinophils (erroneously) by staining with a monoclonal anti-ECP antibody EG2 that recognized a secreted, deglycosylated form of the protein (no longer available) [103–105], and measurement of the eosinophil granule cationic protein biomarkers including MBP, ECP, and EDN by radioimmunoassay [106–108], and more recently by commercially available ELISAs (for EDN, ECP) in various body fluids including serum, plasma, urine, sputum, nasal lavage, and BAL fluid [109]. Under well-controlled sampling conditions, measurements of these eosinophil granule biomarkers is an excellent indicator of eosinophil secretory activity in vivo and eosinophil involvement in a variety of allergic, parasitic, inflammatory, and skin diseases [93], some not normally associated with blood or tissue eosinophilia [110]. Such measurements likely reflect in vivo secretion in tissues or secretory activity of eosinophils in the fluid sampled [109], or both, and have provided compelling evidence for relationships between eosinophil secretory activity, pathogenesis, and disease severity [111–113].

Eosinophil Development and Trafficking

Eosinophilopoiesis in the Bone Marrow

Eosinophils develop from a recently re-defined population of lineage-committed stem cell-derived CD34+/IL-5Rα+ eosinophil progenitors (EoP) in the bone marrow [114], principally in response to T cell-derived cytokines that include eosinophil lineage-specific IL-5, as well as IL-3 and GM-CSF. These cytokines regulate eosinophil differentiation and function at a number of levels including: (1) EoP proliferation and terminal differentiation, (2) priming, activation and/or survival of eosinophils in blood and tissues, and (3) recruitment of eosinophils into allergic reactions. Activated Th2 polarized T-cells are a primary source for these eosinophil-active cytokines in allergic and parasitic diseases, and hypereosinophilic syndromes, e.g., HES. However, other leukocytes including mast cells, macrophages, and natural killer cells, and endothelial cells and stromal cells such as fibroblasts are also producers of these factors. Thus, IL-5, principally from activated Th2 T cells [115] and mast cells [116, 117] regulates the development of blood and tissue eosinophilia in vivo [118–120]. While IL-3 and GM-CSF are multipotent cytokines with activities on many other blood cell lineages, IL-5 is eosinophil-selective and plays a crucial role in driving committed EoP cell proliferation, terminal differentiation, and post-mitotic activation in the development of eosinophilia [121]. IL-5 is maximally active on the IL-5R+ EoP pool that is initially expanded by IL-3 and GM-CSF [121]. Although IL-5 is necessary and sufficient for the development of eosinophilia [121, 122], eosinophil differentiation itself, at least in the mouse, does not require IL-5 [123]. IL-5-mediated upregulated expression of the IL-5 receptor (IL-5R) on the EoP is a prerequisite for IL-5-induced eosinophil terminal differentiation and development of eosinophilia, and IL-5 over-expression underlies many eosinophil-associated diseases and hypereosinophilic syndromes such as HES [124–126]. IL-5-overexpressing transgenic mice develop profound eosinophilias [37, 127], further evidence that IL-5 is key in promoting both the production and activities of eosinophils. Conversely, IL-5-deficient (gene knockout) mice [123, 128] do not develop significant blood or tissue eosinophilia, airways hyperresponsiveness to cholinergics, and airways remodeling in murine allergic asthma models [128], nor do they develop blood or tissue eosinophilia in response to infection with helminth parasites [123]. The finding that IL-5-deficient mice still generate basal numbers of bone marrow eosinophils fits the current paradigm that basal blood cell development: (1) occurs independently of the lineage-specific cytokines (i.e., EPO, G-CSF, M-CSF and IL-5), and (2) is regulated at the level of gene transcription through combinatorial networks of transcription factors acting to resolve lineage promiscuous gene expression patterns in early uncommitted hematopoietic progenitors [129–131].

Transcriptional Regulation of Eosinophil Lineage Commitment and Differentiation

Avian, mouse, and human studies have shown that only a handful of transcription factors and their functional interactions are key to specifying eosinophil lineage-commitment and terminal differentiation [132]. The combinatorial activities of GATA-1, C/EBPα, and PU.1 are required, with GATA-1 the pivotal player that determines if granulocyte-macrophage progenitors will differentiate to the eosinophil (GATA-1 required), or neutrophil and macrophage lineages (absence of GATA-1). As well, a GATA-1 co-activator called FOG-1 (friend of GATA-1) that is required for erythroid differentiation, functions instead as a co-repressor of GATA-1 in the eosinophil lineage [133], and must be downregulated for eosinophil differentiation [134]. Thus, eosinophil development is deficient in GATA-1 knockout mice [135], and transgenic deletion of a high affinity double GATA site in the murine GATA-1 promoter itself blocks eosinophil development [136]. Notably, similar high-affinity double GATA sites are present in the promoters of a number of hallmark eosinophil-specific genes including MBP1, EPX, CLC/Gal-10, IL-5Rα [137], and the eotaxin receptor, CCR3 [138]. The current consensus for the combinatorial transcription factor "code" that specifies the eosinophil relative to the other hematopoietic lineages is outlined in Fig. 4.2. Regulation of both the levels and time of expression of these transcription factors are required to generate eosinophils, such that commitment and terminal differentiation of eosinophils from EoP

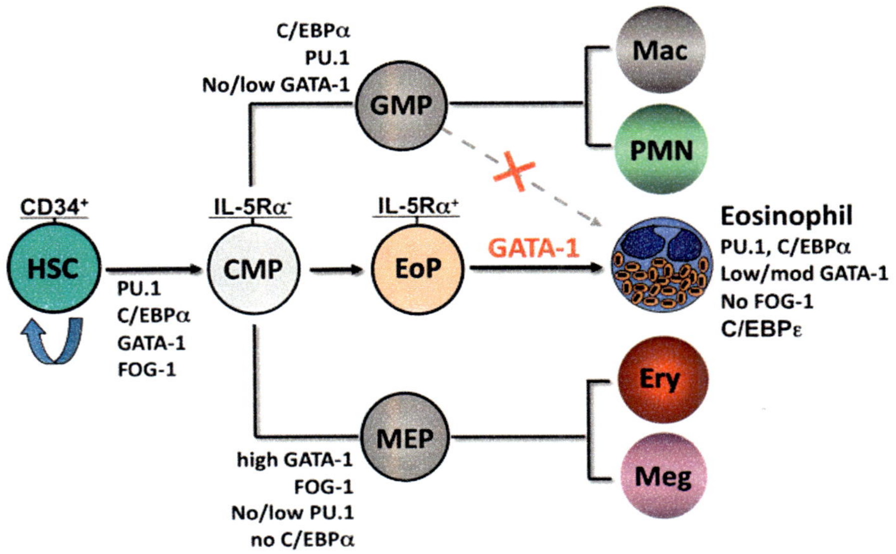

Fig. 4.2 Combinatorial transcription factor "codes" that specify eosinophil lineage commitment and terminal differentiation. GATA-1 is both necessary and sufficient to drive eosinophil development, and C/EBPε is required for eosinophil terminal differentiation. Eosinophils have recently been shown to develop from a distinct CD34+/IL-5Rα+ eosinophil progenitor (EoP) derived from the common myeloid progenitor (CMP) pool and not from the granulocyte-macrophage progenitor (GMP) as previously thought [114]. C/EBPα, CCAAT enhancer-binding protein α: *Ery* erythrocyte; *FOG-1* friend of GATA-1; *GMP* granulocyte-macrophage progenitors; *HSC* CD34+ hematopoietic stem cells; *Mac* macrophage; *Meg* megakaryocyte; *MEP* megakaryocyte/erythroid progenitors; *PMN* polymorphonuclear leukocyte; *PU.1* ets factor (identical to Spi-1 oncogene). (Modified and updated with permission from: McNagny K, Graf T. Making eosinophils through subtle shifts in transcription factor expression. J Exp Med. 2002;195(11):F43–47)

requires coordinated expression of C-EBPα, PU.1, a moderate level of GATA-1, and absence of FOG-1 [132]. As well, C/EBPε expressed mainly during the promyelocyte to myelocyte transition, is required for eosinophil development; studies of C/EBPε knockout mice showed that eosinophil (and neutrophil) differentiation requires C/EBPε, since these mice lack terminally differentiated and functionally mature eosinophils and neutrophils [139, 140]. Similarly, patients with specific granule deficiency (SGD) have a mutation in their C/EBPε gene that leads to a failure of both neutrophil and eosinophil differentiation, with failed expression of important secondary granule protein genes in both granulocytes [141]. Greater understanding of the complex combinatorial and functional interactions of transcription factors that regulate eosinophil lineage commitment, differentiation, and gene expression may lead to novel targets for ablating eosinophil development in general, or selectively knocking down eosinophil expression of key inflammatory mediators, e.g., the granule cationic proteins or eotaxin receptor CCR3, as novel therapeutic approaches to treating eosinophil-mediated allergic diseases such as EoE.

Eosinophilopoiesis and Eosinophil Extravasation

Studies with anti-IL-5 antibody in both mouse and human subjects show clearly that IL-5 is crucial for the generation of both allergic and idiopathic eosinophilias [142, 143], a key initiating step involving EoP surface expression of the high-affinity IL-5 receptor (CD125/CD131) [144]. Up to this point, eosinophils and basophils share a common differentiation pathway, the remnants of which persist even in the mature cells; blood eosinophils express low levels of the α chain of the high affinity IgE receptor (FcεRI) [145, 146], while basophils express low levels of MBP1 [147], Charcot-Leyden crystal protein/Galectin-10 (CLC/Gal-10) [148], EDN, ECP, and EPX [149]. Both cells in the peripheral blood express the eotaxin receptor CCR3 [150]. Another shared differentiation marker is Siglec-8 (Siglec-F in the mouse [151, 152]), expressed more highly on blood eosinophils than bone marrow eosinophils, and at higher levels than basophils [153, 154].

IL-5-deficient mice have very few bone marrow, tissue, and circulating eosinophils [123], while the opposite is true for IL-5-overexpressing transgenic mice [37, 127]. The precise signals that regulate eosinophil egress from the bone marrow are incompletely understood; besides a role for IL-5 itself [155], eotaxin-1 (CCL11), and perhaps other CCR3 ligands participate in this process [156]. As well, blocking antibodies to β2 integrins have been shown to prevent IL-5-mediated eosinophil release from the bone marrow, whereas blocking α4 integrins enhances their release. The mechanism for this is still unclear, but both IL-5 and CCR3 agonists have been reported to alter integrin function in a manner that aids cellular detachment from various counter-ligands [157–159]. Allergen sensitization and challenge murine asthma models also suggest that the extravasation of eosinophils from the bone marrow is partly T cell dependent [160].

Eosinophil Mobilization, Trafficking, Survival, and Death at Sites of Tissue Inflammation

In healthy individuals, following bone marrow extravasation, eosinophils reside for only a short time in the peripheral circulation before transit into extravascular sites, preferentially in tissues and organs exposed to the external environment, mainly submucous membranes and loose connective tissue of the skin, gastrointestinal and genital tracts, and the lungs [161]. In eosinophil-associated diseases, both the acute and chronic recruitment of eosinophils into tissue inflammatory sites occurs principally in response to components of classical IgE-mediated early and late phase immediate hypersensitivity reactions, but also in response to a number of non-allergic immunologically mediated inflammatory reactions and in idiopathic hypereosinophilic syndromes (see below). As well, diurnal variations in blood eosinophil levels are well documented, with the lowest number of intravascular eosinophils early in the morning and highest number late at night, mirroring the circadian rhythms in adrenal corticosteroid levels in the blood [162]. Likewise, diurnal variations also occur in the mobilization, recruitment, and activation of eosinophils in tissues in diseases such as nocturnal asthma [97, 163].

The mechanisms by which eosinophils are selectively recruited in large numbers relative to other leukocytes in inflammatory reactions are fairly well understood; [31] their mobilization from the vasculature, as for other leukocytes, involves rolling and adherence to vascular endothelium via L-selectin, followed by interactions with intercellular adhesion molecule-1 (ICAM-1) through CD18/CD11a,b-dependent mechanisms, and migration in response to eosinophil-specific chemoattractants, particularly the eotaxins. Adherence via CD18-independent mechanisms involves binding to cytokine-activated endothelial cells via either E-selectin (also known as endothelial leukocyte adhesion molecule-1 (ELAM)), or vascular cell adhesion molecule-1 (VCAM). Selective recruitment of eosinophils also involves adhesion to VCAM via the β1 integrin very late activation antigen-4 (VLA-4), expressed by eosinophils but not neutrophils [164]. The selective recruitment of eosinophils into tissue inflammatory sites likely involves both these complex interactions with the adhesion pathways and chemotactic gradients of eotaxin-1 (CCL11), eotaxin-2 (CCL24), or eotaxin-3 (CCL26), depending on the tissue (e.g. eotaxin-3 in the esophagus in EoE). The eotaxins, the most potent and eosinophil-selective chemokines identified to date, bind, and signal through the CCR3 receptor expressed selectively on eosinophils [165–167]. Other less potent eosinophil chemoattractants include complement fragment C5a, platelet activating factor (PAF), and the eosinophil-active cytokines (IL-3, IL-5, GM-CSF) that prime eosinophils for enhanced migratory responses to these agents. Other more potent eosinophil chemoattractants (active in the 10^{-12} to 10^{-11} M range, ~1,000-fold more active than PAF and C5a), include the sulfidopeptide leukotrienes [168], IL-2, the CD8+ T-cell-derived lymphocyte chemoattractant factor (LCF) that uses CD4 expressed by activated eosinophils as its receptor [169], and the chemokine RANTES (CCL5), which is chemotactic for certain T-cell subsets and monocytes, but not for neutrophils; [170] its production by CD4+ T-cells in cutaneous and pulmonary allergen-induced late-phase reactions may contribute to the eosinophil recruitment in these responses.

Two interrelated mechanisms that regulate the tissue accumulation of eosinophils are linked to eosinophil-associated pathophysiology [171]. First, IL-5 plays a critical role in expanding and terminally differentiating the EoP pools in the bone marrow in response to peripheral allergic or other tissue inflammatory stimuli. Th2 cytokines such as IL-4 and IL-13 operate within tissues to regulate eosinophil transmigration from the vascular bed, a process that exclusively promotes tissue accumulation of eosinophils over other leukocytes, likely by activating the eosinophil-specific endothelial adhesion pathways noted above, and by regulating the production of IL-5 and eotaxin expression in the target tissue. As well, IL-4 and IL-13 act as potent inducers of the eotaxins [171]. Thus, IL-5 and the eotaxins cooperate locally to selectively promote eosinophilia, the former working both systemically and within the tissues to promote the local chemoattractant signals provided by the latter. The regulation of IL-5 and eotaxin levels within tissues by cytokines that include IL-4 and IL-13, allows Th2 cells to coordinate both tissue and blood

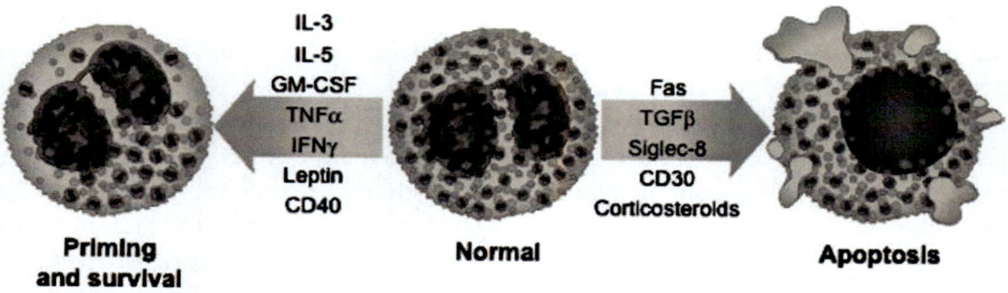

Fig. 4.3 Factors that may influence eosinophil life or death decisions at sites of tissue inflammation. Stimuli that are known to promote eosinophil priming and survival are indicated, and are contrasted with those that facilitate eosinophil apoptosis (programmed cell death). Also shown are some of the phenotypic characteristics that accompany the primed state of the eosinophil compared to those seen in eosinophils undergoing apoptosis. *GM-CSF* granulocyte-macrophage colony-stimulating factor; *IL* interleukin; *IFNγ* interferon-γ; *TGFβ* transforming growth factor-β; *TNFα* tumor necrosis factor-α. (Reproduced with permission from: Ackerman SJ, Bochner BS. Mechanisms of eosinophilia in the pathogenesis of hypereosinophilic disorders. Immunol Allergy Clin N Am. 2007;27:357–375; Art by Jacqueline Schaffer)

eosinophilia. These observations highlight the importance of targeting both IL-5 and the eotaxin/CCR3 signaling systems to effectively block eosinophil-associated inflammation and tissue pathology [171–173].

Diseases associated with peripheral blood eosinophilia, e.g., the hypereosinophilic syndrome (HES), are frequently associated with elevated serum levels of IL-5 and/or GM-CSF, [174–177] and administration of IL-5 or GM-CSF in humans results in a rapid and sustained peripheral blood eosinophilia [178, 179]. Eosinophils normally persist in the peripheral circulation for approximately 18–24 h before migrating into extravascular tissue sites, but their transit time in the circulation may be extended under conditions that induce peripheral blood eosinophilia. Although the bone marrow is the largest reservoir of eosinophil progenitors (EoP) and differentiating cells, their predominant destination in the healthy individual is the gastrointestinal tract; homing to the GI tract occurs in response to constitutive expression of eotaxin-1 (CCL11) by gut epithelial cells [180]. Once eosinophils migrate into extravascular tissue sites, they do not appear to re-circulate through the blood, although animal model studies suggest that eosinophils implanted into the lungs can traffic to regional lymph nodes where they may participate in antigen presentation [181]. Eosinophil survival in tissues is dependent on autocrine or local production of anti-apoptotic cytokines such as IL-5 and GM-CSF; other locally produced survival factors may include IL-3, TNF-α, IFN-γ, leptin [182], engagement of CD40 [183] and others [1] (Fig. 4.3). In the right tissue microenvironment, studies indicate that eosinophils and their precursors may be capable of surviving for several days [184–186] to months, even after administration of anti-IL-5 antibody that depletes both bone marrow and peripheral blood eosinophils [34, 35]. Of interest, eosinophils obtained by BAL of asthmatic subjects or after lung subsegmental bronchoprovocation with allergen, show prolonged survival ex vivo for 24–48 h in the absence of exogenous survival cytokines, whereas their peripheral blood counterparts do not [187, 188], consistent with either in vivo exposure to these cytokines in the inflamed airways, or induction of autocrine expression of GM-CSF by the eosinophil [32]. Eosinophil interactions with specific tissue matrix proteins, particularly fibronectin and laminin, may also be important in inducing their autocrine GM-CSF-driven prolonged survival within tissues [189, 190]. Eosinophils in the tissues that do not encounter the necessary survival factors undergo rapid apoptosis and phagocytic clearance. As well, there are pathways that selectively induce eosinophil apoptosis. For example, corticosteroids rapidly decrease the numbers of both circulating and tissue eosinophils, although the mechanisms responsible for this are complex and poorly understood, likely involving a combination of decreased release from the bone marrow, decreased circulation time, redistribution to other organs such as spleen or inhibited expression of survival cytokines and chemokines [191–195]. Other pro-apoptotic stimuli for eosinophils include lidocaine [196], TGF-β [197], Siglec-8/Siglec-F [198, 199], Fas (CD95) [200] and CD30 [201]. Other drugs used to reduce eosinophil numbers in hypereosinophilic syndromes include hydroxyurea, which causes a global inhibition of hematopoiesis, and IFN-α that reduces the numbers of circulating eosinophils [202]. Tyrosine kinase inhibitors, particularly imatinib mesylate (Gleevec), have profound effects on eosinophil numbers in a subset of individuals with HES who have a chromosome 4 deletion mutation that generates a fusion between the FIP1L1 and PDGFRα genes, resulting in a chronic eosinophil leukemia due to the constitutively active tyrosine kinase [203].

Eosinophil Activation and Functions

Activation of Eosinophil Secretion and Degranulation

Eosinophil participation in the pathogenesis of tissue inflammation, damage, remodeling and fibrosis in allergic diseases such as EoE requires more than their selective recruitment, i.e. to the esophagus. The activation state of the recruited eosinophil, and importantly, its exposure to components of the inflammatory tissue microenvironment, is equally important in determining its varied contributions to tissue pathology. For example, strains of IL-5 transgenic mice that express IL-5 systemically typically have profound blood, organ, and tissue eosinophilia, but in the absence of additional secretory signals, show little if any eosinophil-mediated tissue pathology and remain relatively healthy [37, 126]. The required secondary signals include cross-linking of surface immunoglobulin receptors, particularly for IgA and to a lesser extent for IgG [168], as well as exposure to activating rather than priming levels of a number of cytokines, chemokines, complement and lipid mediators for which they express receptors including IL-5 itself, the eotaxins, IL-4, the cysteinyl leukotrienes, complement fragments (C3a, C5a), neuropeptides, and others [30, 204]. Notably missing from this list is IgE, for which there is now ample evidence that mouse eosinophils do not express the high affinity IgE receptor (FcεRI), and human eosinophils, which express very low if any functional FcεRI on their surface, lack the β chain of the receptor, making direct activation of eosinophils highly unlikely [205–207]. Eosinophil activation by many of the above-mentioned agonists induces eosinophil piecemeal degranulation with selective secretion of the granule cationic proteins (ECP, EDN, EPX and MBP1) depending on the stimulus, the generation of reactive oxygen species directed extracellularly (ROS, e.g. superoxide,) and lipid mediators including cysteinyl leukotriene LTC_4 and PAF. Activated eosinophils also generate and secrete a wide range of cytokines and chemokines including IL-1β and TGF-β, two of the major mediators of eosinophil-induced tissue remodeling and fibrosis seen in many eosinophil-associated diseases [10, 75, 208, 209].

The quantities of cytokines and chemokines released by activated eosinophils in vitro and at sites of allergic tissue inflammation in vivo can vary widely compared to other leukocytes; [27, 30] of these, GM-CSF is one of those produced in greatest amounts [168], and as discussed previously, functions as an autocrine anti-apoptotic signal that prolongs eosinophil survival at sites of tissue inflammation. As well, eosinophil exposure to low levels of IL-5 and the eotaxins primes them for increased secretory and oxidative responses to other physiologically relevant stimuli including IL-5 itself, sIgA, IFN-γ and others that induce the secretion of the granule proteins (ECP, EDN, EPX, MBP1) and eosinophil-elaborated cytokines (RANTES, IL-4) via the process of piecemeal degranulation (PMD) [210, 211], a unique mechanism that allows for their selective mobilization through vesicular transport to the plasma membrane into the extracellular space [212, 213]. In contrast, granule fusion and classical exocytosis are rarely observed in eosinophils at sites of tissue inflammation [214], but are frequently seen in eosinophil-mediated killing of larval helminth parasites such as schistosomula of *Schistosoma mansoni*.

Once secreted, the eosinophil's granule proteins have varied pro-inflammatory activities that have been extensively defined in both in vitro and in vivo studies; these include plasma membrane, cell, and tissue-damaging cytotoxicities [215, 216]. They can also selectively activate other inflammatory cells such as basophils and mast cells to release vasoactive mediators such as histamine [217], and induce an oxidative burst in neutrophils [218]. Of note, MBP1 is a potent antagonist of inhibitory M2 muscarinic receptors in vitro and in the airways in Guinea pig allergic asthma models [219], and it potently enhances the ability of TGF-β primed fibroblasts to express and secrete members of the pro-inflammatory and pro-fibrotic IL-6 family of cytokines including IL-6 and IL-11 [220]. Thus, eosinophils come fully armed with pre-formed mediators of inflammation, tissue damage, remodeling, and fibrogenesis that are secreted at sites of eosinophilic inflammation in eosinophil-associated allergic diseases such as asthma and hypereosinophilic syndromes such as EoE, and have the capacity when appropriately primed and activated to synthesize and secrete cytokines, chemokines, and lipid mediators of inflammation in the process of their recruitment from the bone marrow and peripheral circulation into tissues in response to allergic (e.g. mast cell, basophil) and other inflammatory and/or Th2 T-cell stimuli.

Pathogenesis of Tissue and End Organ Damage in Eosinophilic Diseases

Based on current understanding of eosinophil functions in hypereosinophilic conditions, sustained eosinophilia, regardless of its origin (i.e., reactive, clonal, allergic or idiopathic), has the capacity to lead to end organ damage. The multiple manifestations of eosinophil-associated end organ damage are considerable [221], but not all cases of sustained blood or tissue hypereosinophilia lead to end organ damage. For example, patients with hypereosinophilic syndromes such as eosinophilic pneumonia and episodic angioedema with eosinophilia [222] characteristically fail to develop the cardiac damage and endomyocardial fibrosis associated with untreated eosinophilia in patients with the HES. As noted above, IL-5 transgenic mice, which develop extremely high numbers of peripheral blood eosinophils, do not develop significant tissue or end organ damage, indicating that other factors are required for tissue-specific eosinophil recruitment, activation, and damage [37, 126]. Likewise, other factors may be necessary to induce eosinophilic end organ tissue damage, such as secretion of eosinophil-active inflammatory or hematopoietic cytokines (e.g., GM-CSF), genetic predisposition, clonal T-cell dysfunction, T-cell polarization to a Th2 rather than Th1 phenotype, or in situ production of cytokines that enhance eosinophil long-term tissue survival and activation by blocking eosinophil apoptosis. A number of the eosinophil granule cationic proteins are capable of inducing thrombotic events [223], endothelial and endocardial damage [99], and neurotoxicity (the ribonucleases EDN and ECP) [224, 225]. MBP and ECP are potent cellular toxins capable of damaging normal host cells and tissues in a manner reminiscent of end-organ tissue damage associated with chronic tissue eosinophilia [168]. As well, upon priming and activation, the eosinophil has the capacity to undergo a potent respiratory burst, generating ROS that can directly, or in association with the enzymatic activities of EPX, induce significant oxidant-mediated tissue damage [226–228].

Eosinophil Induction and Regulation of Tissue Remodeling and Fibrosis

One of the most experimentally and clinically well-defined roles of the eosinophil is as an inducer of tissue remodeling and fibrosis, for which the paradigms developed for other eosinophil-mediated diseases provide insights into the pathogenesis and clinical manifestations of EoE (Fig. 4.1). Tissue remodeling in Th2-mediated and other eosinophil-associated diseases was first characterized in the hypereosinophilic syndrome (HES) and asthma; [9, 11, 63, 99] in HES, eosinophil recruitment, activation, and secretion (degranulation) in the heart leads to significant patient morbidity and mortality due to the development of endomyocardial fibrosis and associated cardiac failure [99, 208]. Asthma, another Th2/eosinophil-associated disease, is characterized by significant airway remodeling consisting of goblet cell metaplasia with hyperproduction of mucous, smooth muscle hyperplasia and hypertrophy, subepithelial fibrosis, and increased angiogenesis; [9] these structural changes contribute to the clinical manifestations of bronchial hyperreactivity, airway edema, mucous plugging, and subsequent narrowing of the airway lumen. In a subset of patients, this airways obstruction becomes irreversible. Although the pathogenic role of the eosinophil in HES is relatively clear, its role in asthma is still being resolved [13, 63]. Mouse models of asthma support a significant contribution of the eosinophil to airway pathology and remodeling. Of note, double transgenic mice expressing both airway eotaxin-2 and systemic IL-5 have severe human asthma-like pathologies including subepithelial collagen deposition that is essentially eliminated if the animals are crossed to eosinophil-deficient mice [11, 40]. In this regard, the best human "experiment" for the effects of eosinophil deficiency is treatment of patients with tissue eosinophilia with neutralizing anti-IL-5 antibodies to remove the principal eosinophilopoietic stimulus. For example, asthmatic patients treated with monoclonal anti-IL-5 antibody (Mepolizumab™) showed decreased amounts of subepithelial extracellular matrix proteins in the airways including tenascin, pro-collagen III, and lumican [15]. Similar studies testing the efficacy of anti-IL-5 antibodies for treatment of pediatric [16] and adult EoE [35] should provide further insights into the roles of the eosinophil in the various aspects of tissue remodeling and fibrosis that contribute to the pathogenesis of EoE [229, 230] (Fig. 4.1) and other EGIDs.

Pathogenic Mechanisms of Eosinophil-Mediated Tissue Fibrosis

Eosinophils are considered a major inducer of tissue remodeling and fibrosis [209] in a variety of eosinophil-associated allergic diseases and hypereosinophilic syndromes including asthma [8, 73], eosinophil myalgia syndrome [231], eosinophilic endomyocardial fibrosis [208], idiopathic pulmonary fibrosis [232], scleroderma [231], and most recently EoE [229, 230]. Eosinophils are implicated in fibrogenesis through these clinical disease associations, their elaboration of fibrogenic growth factors such as TGF-β [74, 233], PDGF-BB [234], IL-1β [10] and their secretion of the granule proteins MBP1 [220] and EPX [235]. The association of degranulating eosinophils and granule protein deposition in tissues with pathological fibrosis is a recurrent finding in a broad group of eosinophilic diseases including EoE [100, 102, 236], and eosinophils are one of the major TGF-β producing cells in the esophagus in pediatric EoE [71] and in the lungs of asthmatics [73].

Both human and animal model studies provide compelling evidence for eosinophils as effectors of tissue remodeling and fibrosis. As noted above, reduction in bronchial eosinophils by only ~55% in asthmatics treated with anti-IL-5 antibody (Mepolizumab™) was sufficient to decrease the expression of ECM proteins in the reticular basement membrane [15], and anti-IL-5 similarly decreased both eosinophils and deposition of ECM proteins in the skin of atopic subjects in allergen-induced late-phase reactions [14]. Direct evidence for eosinophil induction of remodeling and fibrosis comes from studies in eosinophil-deficient mice, demonstrating their essential role in the development of airway remodeling, including mucus (goblet) cell metaplasia, smooth muscle cell hyperplasia, and subepithelial fibrosis [11, 12, 44].

A number of growth factors and cytokines expressed by the eosinophil [27] are implicated in tissue remodeling and fibrosis, TGF-β being the most potently fibrogenic and well studied. TGF-β regulates the expression of the pro-fibrogenic cytokine IL-6, the myofibroblast marker α-smooth muscle actin (α-SMA) and other ECM proteins such as the collagens, and its expression is correlated with bronchial airway fibrosis and asthma severity [237], and its over-expression in the lung in rodent animal models induces pulmonary fibrosis [233]. Eosinophil-fibroblast interactions have been implicated in the generation of subepithelial fibrosis and airway remodeling characteristic of human asthma in murine allergic asthma models [238, 239], but mechanistic assessments of eosinophil-fibroblast interactions that induce tissue fibrosis are still relatively limited. Eosinophil granule MBP1 synergizes with TGF-β or IL-1β primed lung fibroblasts to induce significant increases in gene transcription and secretion of the IL-6 family of inflammatory and fibrogenic cytokines, including IL-6 and IL-11 [220], and TGF-β-induced fibroblast secretion of IL-6 is implicated in the overproduction of collagens, tissue inhibitor of metalloproteinases (TIMPs), and glycosaminoglycans in fibrogenesis [240, 241]. Eosinophil-lung fibroblast co-culture in the presence of IL-5 induces fibroblasts to trans-differentiate into myofibroblasts with increased expression of α-SMA and ECM proteins [79]. Similarly, eosinophils may indirectly impact fibroblast phenotype and fibrogenesis through activation of the epithelial-mesenchymal trophic unit [242], e.g., through secretion of MBP and EPX (Fig. 4.1) [235]. Alternatively, eosinophils may induce fibrogenesis through TGF-β induction of the epithelial to mesenchymal transition (EMT), as recently shown to occur in the lung in asthma [243] and most recently by the authors laboratory in the esophagus in EoE [85].

Subepithelial fibrosis, a component of airway remodeling in asthma, is initiated by insults that include Th2-mediated allergic responses; eosinophils recruited into the airways are thought to drive the differentiation of airway fibroblasts to myofibroblasts as characterized by the expression of myofibroblast-specific markers such as α-SMA, the deposition of ECM proteins such as collagens, fibronectin, and other ECM constituents such as tenascin and lumican [9, 15, 242]. Correlations between pulmonary expression of eotaxin-1, expression of eotaxin-1 receptor (CCR3), TGF-β_1, and pulmonary fibrosis have been reported in a bleomycin mouse model, further supporting this general mechanism [244]. In contrast, studies of eosinophil-mediated tissue remodeling and fibrosis in EoE have been limited to date, principally due to the difficulties inherent in obtaining biopsies containing sufficient esophageal lamina propria below the stiffened hyperplastic epithelium. For this reason, evidence for progressive remodeling and fibrosis of the esophagus has been derived principally from endoscopic and radiologic features of the disease [245]. However, several recent studies by Aceves and colleagues show that esophageal biopsies from pediatric EoE patients have increased subepithelial fibrosis, expression of TGF-β_1 by eosinophils, and activation of TGF-β SMAD-mediated signaling pathways compared with GERD and normal subjects [71]. Beyond these reports, the mechanisms regulating esophageal remodeling and fibrosis in chronic

EoE have not been systematically studied to define the changes in epithelial cell and fibroblast phenotype, the role of eosinophil-fibroblast interactions, or the contributions of EMT to this process. Genome-wide expression profiling studies of EoE esophageal biopsies identified eotaxin-3 as the principal mediator of eosinophil recruitment to the esopahgus [246], but interestingly did not identify many genes involved in tissue remodeling and fibrosis. However, one of these genes, periostin, is expressed predominantly in collagen-rich fibrous connective tissues subject to mechanical stresses and in wound healing, and was reported to participate in the subepithelial fibrosis in asthma, downstream of the IL-4 and IL-13 signals [247]. Primary esophageal fibroblasts release periostin when cultured with IL-13 and TGF-β [248], and the periostin localized mainly in vascular papillae (projections of subepithelial lamina propria into the epithelium) in the esophagus, may contribute to eosinophil recruitment by increasing their adhesion to fibronectin [248]. Thus, eosinophil-derived TGF-β, by inducing fibroblast expression of periostin, could provide an esophageal eosinophil inflammation amplification loop, and its consequent induction of the esophageal remodeling and fibrosis seen in EoE.

Summary

The eosinophil is clearly a multifunctional granulocyte that participates in both the pathogenesis and pathophysiology of allergic diseases in terms of both the initiation and propagation of allergic and related inflammatory responses, including roles in tissue damage, repair and remodeling. However, there is still much to be determined in terms of the cell biology, immunobiology, and effector roles of the eosinophil in these processes, particularly the eosinophil's newly recognized role as a regulator of tissue microenvironments into which it is recruited, whether homeostatically in health or in disease pathogenesis [2, 3]. While some aspects of eosinophil biology and functions reviewed in this chapter are by no means certain, i.e., they are based on murine and other animal model studies, the eosinophil's presence at mucosal surfaces in the gastrointestinal tract in healthy individuals suggests a sentry role in host innate immunity. Their abnormal presence in large numbers in the esophagus in EoE supports a role for the eosinophil in the pathogenesis of the profound esophageal tissue remodeling and fibrosis characteristic of this disease (Fig. 4.1).

Acknowledgment Dr. Ackerman was supported in part by NIH grant R21AI079925, a Translational Research Award from the American Gastroenterology Association (AGA), the Campaign Urging Research on Eosinophilic Diseases (CURED), the Thrasher Research Foundation, and the American Partnership for Eosinophilic Diseases (APFED).

References

1. Rothenberg ME, Hogan SP. The eosinophil. Annu Rev Immunol. 2006;24:147–74.
2. Lee JJ, Jacobsen EA, McGarry MP, Schleimer RP, Lee NA. Eosinophils in health and disease: the LIAR hypothesis. Clin Exp Allergy. Apr 2010;40(4):563–75.

3. Jacobsen EA, Taranova AG, Lee NA, Lee JJ. Eosinophils: singularly destructive effector cells or purveyors of immunoregulation? J Allergy Clin Immunol. Jun 2007;119(6):1313–20.
4. Gleich GJ, Adolphson CR, Leiferman KM. The biology of the eosinophilic leukocyte. Annu Rev Med. 1993;44:85–101.
5. Frigas E, Gleich GJ. The eosinophil and the pathophysiology of asthma. J Allergy Clin Immunol. 1986;77(4):527–37.
6. Belongia EA, Mayeno AN, Osterholm MT. The eosinophilia-myalgia syndrome and tryptophan. Annu Rev Nutr. 1992;12:235–56.
7. Furuta GT, Liacouras CA, Collins MH, et al. Eosinophilic esophagitis in children and adults: a systematic review and consensus recommendations for diagnosis and treatment. Gastroenterology. Oct 2007;133(4):1342–63.
8. Kay AB. The role of eosinophils in the pathogenesis of asthma. Trends Mol Med. Apr 2005;11(4):148–52.
9. Kay AB, Phipps S, Robinson DS. A role for eosinophils in airway remodelling in asthma. Trends Immunol. Sep 2004;25(9):477–82.
10. Gomes I, Mathur SK, Espenshade BM, Mori Y, Varga J, Ackerman SJ. Eosinophil-fibroblast interactions induce fibroblast IL-6 secretion and extracellular matrix gene expression: implications in fibrogenesis. J Allergy Clin Immunol. Oct 2005;116(4):796–804.
11. Lee JJ, Dimina D, Macias MP, et al. Defining a link with asthma in mice congenitally deficient in eosinophils. Science. 2004;305(5691):1773–6.
12. Humbles AA, Lloyd CM, McMillan SJ, et al. A critical role for eosinophils in allergic airways remodeling. Science. 2004;305(5691):1776–9.
13. Jacobsen EA, Ochkur SI, Pero RS, et al. Allergic pulmonary inflammation in mice is dependent on eosinophil-induced recruitment of effector T cells. J Exp Med. 2008; 205(3):699–710.
14. Phipps S, Flood-Page P, Menzies-Gow A, Ong YE, Kay AB. Intravenous anti-IL-5 monoclonal antibody reduces eosinophils and tenascin deposition in allergen-challenged human atopic skin. J Invest Dermatol. Jun 2004;122(6):1406–12.
15. Flood-Page P, Menzies-Gow A, Phipps S, et al. Anti-IL-5 treatment reduces deposition of ECM proteins in the bronchial subepithelial basement membrane of mild atopic asthmatics. J Clin Invest. Oct 2003;112(7):1029–36.
16. Stein ML, Collins MH, Villanueva JM, et al. Anti-IL-5 (mepolizumab) therapy for eosinophilic esophagitis. J Allergy Clin Immunol. Dec 2006;118(6):1312–9.
17. Rothenberg ME, Klion AD, Roufosse FE, et al. Treatment of patients with the hypereosinophilic syndrome with mepolizumab. N Engl J Med. 2008;358(12):1215–28.
18. Weller PF. Lipid, peptide and cytokine mediators elaborated by eosinophils. In: Smith H, Cook RM, editors. Immunopharmacology of eosinophils. London: Academic; 1993. p. 25–42.
19. Weller PF, Monahan-Earley RA, Dvorak HF, Dvorak AM. Cytoplasmic lipid bodies of human eosinophils. Subcellular isolation and analysis of arachidonate incorporation. Am J Pathol. 1991;138(1):141–8.
20. Bozza PT, Yu W, Penrose JF, Morgan ES, Dvorak AM, Weller PF. Eosinophil lipid bodies: specific, inducible intracellular sites for enhanced eicosanoid formation. J Exp Med. 1997;186(6):909–20.
21. Melo RC, Spencer LA, Perez SA, Ghiran I, Dvorak AM, Weller PF. Human eosinophils secrete preformed, granule-stored interleukin-4 through distinct vesicular compartments. Traffic. Nov 2005;6(11):1047–57.
22. Leiferman KM. A current perspective on the role of eosinophils in dermatologic diseases. J Am Acad Dermatol. 1991;24(6 Pt 2):1101–12.
23. Ackerman SJ. Characterization and functions of eosinophil granule proteins. In: Makino S, Fukuda T, editors. Eosinophils: biological and clinical aspects. Boca Raton: CRC Press; 1993. p. 33–74.
24. Moqbel R, Lacy P. New concepts in effector functions of eosinophil cytokines. Clin Exp Allergy. Dec 2000;30(12):1667–71.
25. Neves JS, Perez SA, Spencer LA, et al. Eosinophil granules function extracellularly as receptor-mediated secretory organelles. Proc Natl Acad Sci USA. 2008;105(47):18478–83.

26. Weiss SJ, Test ST, Eckmann CM, Roos D, Regiani S. Brominating oxidants generated by human eosinophils. Science. 1986;234(4773):200–3.
27. Lacy P, Moqbel R. Eosinophil cytokines. Chem Immunol. 2000;76:134–55.
28. Lacy P, Moqbel R. Immune effector functions of eosinophils in allergic airway inflammation. Curr Opin Allergy Clin Immunol. Feb 2001;1(1):79–84.
29. Spencer LA, Szela CT, Perez SA, et al. Human eosinophils constitutively express multiple Th1, Th2, and immunoregulatory cytokines that are secreted rapidly and differentially. J Leukoc Biol. Jan 2009;85(1):117–23.
30. Hogan SP, Rosenberg HF, Moqbel R, et al. Eosinophils: biological properties and role in health and disease. Clin Exp Allergy. May 2008;38(5):709–50.
31. Rosenberg HF, Phipps S, Foster PS. Eosinophil trafficking in allergy and asthma. J Allergy Clin Immunol. 2007;119(6):1303–10. quiz 1311–1302.
32. Esnault S, Malter JS. GM-CSF regulation in eosinophils. Arch Immunol Ther Exp (Warsz). 2002;50(2):121–30.
33. Esnault S, Fang Y, Kelly EA, et al. Circadian changes in granulocyte-macrophage colony-stimulating factor message in circulating eosinophils. Ann Allergy Asthma Immunol. Jan 2007;98(1):75–82.
34. Flood-Page PT, Menzies-Gow AN, Kay AB, Robinson DS. Eosinophil's role remains uncertain as anti-interleukin-5 only partially depletes numbers in asthmatic airway. Am J Respir Crit Care Med. 2003;167(2):199–204.
35. Straumann A, Conus S, Grzonka P, et al. Anti-interleukin-5 antibody treatment (mepolizumab) in active eosinophilic oesophagitis: a randomised, placebo-controlled, double-blind trial. Gut. Jan 2010;59(1):21–30.
36. Tavernier J, Van der Heyden J, Verhee A, et al. Interleukin 5 regulates the isoform expression of its own receptor alpha-subunit. Blood. 2000;95(5):1600–7.
37. Dent LA, Strath M, Mellor AL, Sanderson CJ. Eosinophilia in transgenic mice expressing interleukin-5. J Exp Med. 1990;172(5):1425–31.
38. Lee JJ, McGarry MP, Farmer SC, et al. Interleukin-5 expression in the lung epithelium of transgenic mice leads to pulmonary changes pathognomonic of asthma. J Exp Med. 1997;185(12): 2143–56.
39. Crosby JR, Shen HH, Borchers MT, et al. Ectopic expression of IL-5 identifies an additional CD4(+) T cell mechanism of airway eosinophil recruitment. Am J Physiol Lung Cell Mol Physiol. Jan 2002;282(1):L99–108.
40. Ochkur SI, Jacobsen EA, Protheroe CA, et al. Coexpression of IL-5 and eotaxin-2 in mice creates an eosinophil-dependent model of respiratory inflammation with characteristics of severe asthma. J Immunol. 2007;178(12):7879–89.
41. Mauser PJ, Pitman A, Witt A, et al. Inhibitory effect of the TRFK-5 anti-IL-5 antibody in a guinea pig model of asthma. Am Rev Respir Dis. 1993;148(6 Pt 1):1623–7.
42. Trifilieff A, Fujitani Y, Coyle AJ, Kopf M, Bertrand C. IL-5 deficiency abolishes aspects of airway remodelling in a murine model of lung inflammation. Clin Exp Allergy. Jun 2001;31(6):934–42.
43. Hamelmann E, Oshiba A, Loader J, et al. Antiinterleukin-5 antibody prevents airway hyperresponsiveness in a murine model of airway sensitization. Am J Respir Crit Care Med. 1997;155(3):819–25.
44. Cho JY, Miller M, Baek KJ, et al. Inhibition of airway remodeling in IL-5-deficient mice. J Clin Invest. Feb 2004;113(4):551–60.
45. Menzies-Gow A, Flood-Page P, Sehmi R, et al. Anti-IL-5 (mepolizumab) therapy induces bone marrow eosinophil maturational arrest and decreases eosinophil progenitors in the bronchial mucosa of atopic asthmatics. J Allergy Clin Immunol. 2003;111(4):714–9.
46. Haldar P, Brightling CE, Hargadon B, et al. Mepolizumab and exacerbations of refractory eosinophilic asthma. N Engl J Med. 2009;360(10):973–84.
47. Nair P, Pizzichini MM, Kjarsgaard M, et al. Mepolizumab for prednisone-dependent asthma with sputum eosinophilia. N Engl J Med. 2009;360(10):985–93.
48. Terada N, Hamano N, Nomura T, et al. Interleukin-13 and tumour necrosis factor-alpha synergistically induce eotaxin production in human nasal fibroblasts. Clin Exp Allergy. Mar 2000;30(3):348–55.

49. LaPorte SL, Juo ZS, Vaclavikova J, et al. Molecular and structural basis of cytokine receptor pleiotropy in the interleukin-4/13 system. Cell. 2008;132(2):259–72.
50. Wills-Karp M. Interleukin-13 in asthma pathogenesis. Immunol Rev. Dec 2004;202:175–90.
51. Straumann A, Kristl J, Conus S, et al. Cytokine expression in healthy and inflamed mucosa: probing the role of eosinophils in the digestive tract. Inflamm Bowel Dis. Aug 2005;11(8): 720–6.
52. Blanchard C, Mingler MK, Vicario M, et al. IL-13 involvement in eosinophilic esophagitis: transcriptome analysis and reversibility with glucocorticoids. J Allergy Clin Immunol. Dec 2007;120(6):1292–300.
53. Mishra A, Rothenberg ME. Intratracheal IL-13 induces eosinophilic esophagitis by an IL-5, eotaxin-1, and STAT6-dependent mechanism. Gastroenterology. Nov 2003;125(5):1419–27.
54. Zuo L, Mingler M, Blanchard C, Finkelman FD, Fulkerson PC, Rothenberg ME. IL-13 transgene induced experimental eosinophilic esophagitis is associated with increased esophageal circumference and extensive angiogenesis. J Allergy Clin Immunol. 2008;121(2):S72.
55. Zimmermann N, Hershey GK, Foster PS, Rothenberg ME. Chemokines in asthma: cooperative interaction between chemokines and IL-13. J Allergy Clin Immunol. Feb 2003;111(2): 227–42.
56. Schmid-Grendelmeier P, Altznauer F, Fischer B, et al. Eosinophils express functional IL-13 in eosinophilic inflammatory diseases. J Immunol. 2002;169(2):1021–7.
57. Kita H. The eosinophil: a cytokine-producing cell? J Allergy Clin Immunol. Apr 1996;97(4): 889–92.
58. Straumann A, Simon HU. The physiological and pathophysiological roles of eosinophils in the gastrointestinal tract. Allergy. Jan 2004;59(1):15–25.
59. Liu LY, Bates ME, Jarjour NN, Busse WW, Bertics PJ, Kelly EA. Generation of Th1 and Th2 chemokines by human eosinophils: evidence for a critical role of TNF-alpha. J Immunol. 2007;179(7):4840–8.
60. Bisset LR, Schmid-Grendelmeier P. Chemokines and their receptors in the pathogenesis of allergic asthma: progress and perspective. Curr Opin Pulm Med. Jan 2005;11(1):35–42.
61. Rincon M, Anguita J, Nakamura T, Fikrig E, Flavell RA. Interleukin (IL)-6 directs the differentiation of IL-4-producing CD4+ T cells. J Exp Med. 1997;185(3):461–9.
62. Ottonello L, Montecucco F, Bertolotto M, et al. CCL3 (MIP-1alpha) induces in vitro migration of GM-CSF-primed human neutrophils via CCR5-dependent activation of ERK 1/2. Cell Signal. Mar 2005;17(3):355–63.
63. Jacobsen EA, Ochkur SI, Lee NA, Lee JJ. Eosinophils and asthma. Curr Allergy Asthma Rep. Apr 2007;7(1):18–26.
64. Surquin M, Le Moine A, Flamand V, et al. Skin graft rejection elicited by beta 2-microglobulin as a minor transplantation antigen involves multiple effector pathways: role of Fas-Fas ligand interactions and Th2-dependent graft eosinophil infiltrates. J Immunol. 2002;169(1):500–6.
65. Debinski W, Obiri NI, Pastan I, Puri RK. A novel chimeric protein composed of interleukin 13 and Pseudomonas exotoxin is highly cytotoxic to human carcinoma cells expressing receptors for interleukin 13 and interleukin 4. J Biol Chem. 1995;270(28):16775–80.
66. Tepper RI, Pattengale PK, Leder P. Murine interleukin-4 displays potent anti-tumor activity in vivo. Cell. 1989;57(3):503–12.
67. Tepper RI, Coffman RL, Leder P. An eosinophil-dependent mechanism for the antitumor effect of interleukin-4. Science. 1992;257(5069):548–51.
68. Tepper RI, Mule JJ. Experimental and clinical studies of cytokine gene-modified tumor cells. Hum Gene Ther. 1994;5(2):153–64.
69. Sosman JA, Bartemes K, Offord KP, et al. Evidence for eosinophil activation in cancer patients receiving recombinant interleukin-4: effects of interleukin-4 alone and following interleukin-2 administration. Clin Cancer Res. 1995;1(8):805–12.
70. Cormier SA, Taranova AG, Bedient C, et al. Pivotal advance: eosinophil infiltration of solid tumors is an early and persistent inflammatory host response. J Leukoc Biol. Jun 2006;79(6):1131–9.
71. Aceves SS, Newbury RO, Dohil R, Bastian JF, Broide DH. Esophageal remodeling in pediatric eosinophilic esophagitis. J Allergy Clin Immunol. Jan 2007;119(1):206–12.

72. Elovic AE, Ohyama H, Sauty A, et al. IL-4-dependent regulation of TGF-alpha and TGF-beta1 expression in human eosinophils. J Immunol. 1998;160(12):6121–7.
73. Minshall EM, Leung DY, Martin RJ, et al. Eosinophil-associated TGF-beta1 mRNA expression and airways fibrosis in bronchial asthma. Am J Respir Cell Mol Biol. 1997;17(3): 326–33.
74. Ohno I, Nitta Y, Yamauchi K, et al. Transforming growth factor beta 1 (TGF beta 1) gene expression by eosinophils in asthmatic airway inflammation. Am J Respir Cell Mol Biol. 1996;15(3):404–9.
75. Levi-Schaffer F, Garbuzenko E, Rubin A, et al. Human eosinophils regulate human lung- and skin-derived fibroblast properties in vitro: a role for transforming growth factor beta (TGF-beta). Proc Natl Acad Sci USA. 1999;96(17):9660–5.
76. Ohno I, Lea RG, Flanders KC, et al. Eosinophils in chronically inflamed human upper airway tissues express transforming growth factor 1 gene (TGF·1). J Clin Invest. 1992;89:1662–8.
77. Broide DH. Immunologic and inflammatory mechanisms that drive asthma progression to remodeling. J Allergy Clin Immunol. 2008;121(3):560–70. quiz 571–562.
78. Aceves SS, Broide DH. Airway fibrosis and angiogenesis due to eosinophil trafficking in chronic asthma. Curr Mol Med. Aug 2008;8(5):350–8.
79. Phipps S, Ying S, Wangoo A, Ong YE, Levi-Schaffer F, Kay AB. The relationship between allergen-induced tissue eosinophilia and markers of repair and remodeling in human atopic skin. J Immunol. 2002;169(8):4604–12.
80. Aceves SS, Ackerman SJ. Relationships between eosinophilic inflammation, tissue remodeling, and fibrosis in eosinophilic esophagitis. Immunol Allergy Clin North Am. 2009;29(1): 197–211.
81. Doerner AM, Zuraw BL. TGF-beta1 induced epithelial to mesenchymal transition (EMT) in human bronchial epithelial cells is enhanced by IL-1beta but not abrogated by corticosteroids. Respir Res. 2009;10:100.
82. Hackett TL, Warner SM, Stefanowicz D, et al. Induction of epithelial-mesenchymal transition in primary airway epithelial cells from patients with asthma by transforming growth factor-beta1. Am J Respir Crit Care Med. 2009;180(2):122–33.
83. Zhang M, Zhang Z, Pan HY, Wang DX, Deng ZT, Ye XL. TGF-beta1 induces human bronchial epithelial cell-to-mesenchymal transition in vitro. Lung. 2009;187(3):187–94.
84. Holgate ST, Holloway J, Wilson S, Bucchieri F, Puddicombe S, Davies DE. Epithelial-mesenchymal communication in the pathogenesis of chronic asthma. Proc Am Thorac Soc. 2004;1(2):93–8.
85. Akhtar N, Woodruff SA, Mukkada V, et al. Identification of epithelial mesenchymal transition in eosinophilic esophagitis and its relationship to esophageal remodeling and fibrosis. Gastroenterology. 2010;138 Suppl 1:S-172.
86. Bandeira-Melo C, Bozza PT, Diaz BL, et al. Cutting edge: lipoxin (LX) A4 and aspirin-triggered 15-epi-LXA4 block allergen-induced eosinophil trafficking. J Immunol. 2000;164(5): 2267–71.
87. Wang H, Tan X, Chang H, Huang W, Gonzalez-Crussi F, Hsueh W. Platelet-activating factor receptor mRNA is localized in eosinophils and epithelial cells in rat small intestine: regulation by dexamethasone and gut flora. Immunology. Jul 1999;97(3):447–54.
88. Fujii M, Tanaka H, Abe S. Interferon-gamma up-regulates expression of cysteinyl leukotriene type 2 receptors on eosinophils in asthmatic patients. Chest. Nov 2005;128(5):3148–55.
89. Zinchuk O, Fukushima A, Zinchuk V, Fukata K, Ueno H. Direct action of platelet activating factor (PAF) induces eosinophil accumulation and enhances expression of PAF receptors in conjunctivitis. Mol Vis. 2005;11:114–23.
90. Ohshima N, Nagase H, Koshino T, et al. A functional study on CysLT(1) receptors in human eosinophils. Int Arch Allergy Immunol. Sep 2002;129(1):67–75.
91. Powell WS, Chung D, Gravel S. 5-Oxo-6,8,11,14-eicosatetraenoic acid is a potent stimulator of human eosinophil migration. J Immunol. 1995;154(8):4123–32.
92. Sedgwick JB, Calhoun WJ, Vrtis RF, Bates ME, McAllister PK, Busse WW. Comparison of airway and blood eosinophil function after in vivo antigen challenge. J Immunol. 1992;149(11):3710–8.

93. Ackerman SJ, Kephart GM, Francis H, Awadzi K, Gleich GJ, Ottesen EA. Eosinophil degranulation. An immunologic determinant in the pathogenesis of the Mazzotti reaction in human onchocerciasis. J Immunol. 1990;144(10):3961–9.
94. Leiferman KM, Ackerman SJ, Sampson HA, Haugen HS, Venencie PY, Gleich GJ. Dermal deposition of eosinophil-granule major basic protein in atopic dermatitis. Comparison with onchocerciasis. N Engl J Med. 1985;313(5):282–5.
95. Filley WV, Holley KE, Kephart GM, Gleich GJ. Identification by immunofluorescence of eosinophil granule major basic protein in lung tissues of patients with bronchial asthma. Lancet. 1982;2(8288):11–6.
96. Gleich GJ, Motojima S, Frigas E, Kephart GM, Fujisawa T, Kravis LP. The eosinophilic leukocyte and the pathology of fatal bronchial asthma: evidence for pathologic heterogeneity. J Allergy Clin Immunol. 1987;80(3 Pt 2):412–5.
97. Kraft M, Djukanovic R, Torvik J, et al. Evaluation of airway inflammation by endobronchial and transbronchial biopsy in nocturnal and nonnocturnal asthma. Chest. 1995;107(3 Suppl):162S.
98. Samoszuk MK, Nathwani BN, Lukes RJ. Extensive deposition of eosinophil peroxidase in Hodgkin's and non-Hodgkin's lymphomas. Am J Pathol. Dec 1986;125(3):426–9.
99. Tai PC, Ackerman SJ, Spry CJ, Dunnette S, Olsen EG, Gleich GJ. Deposits of eosinophil granule proteins in cardiac tissues of patients with eosinophilic endomyocardial disease. Lancet. 1987;1(8534):643–7.
100. Protheroe C, Woodruff SA, de Petris G, et al. A novel histologic scoring system to evaluate mucosal biopsies from patients with eosinophilic esophagitis. Clin Gastroenterol Hepatol. 2009;7(7):749–55. e711.
101. Pizzichini E, Pizzichini MM, Efthimiadis A, et al. Indices of airway inflammation in induced sputum: reproducibility and validity of cell and fluid-phase measurements. Am J Respir Crit Care Med. 1996;154(2 Pt 1):308–17.
102. Kephart GM, Alexander JA, Arora AS, et al. Marked deposition of eosinophil-derived neurotoxin in adult patients with eosinophilic esophagitis. Am J Gastroenterol. Feb 2010;105(2): 298–307.
103. Rosenberg HF, Tiffany HL. Characterization of the eosinophil granule proteins recognized by the activation-specific antibody EG2. J Leukoc Biol. 1994;56(4):502–6.
104. Moqbel R, Barkans J, Bradley BL, Durham SR, Kay AB. Application of monoclonal antibodies against major basic protein (BMK-13) and eosinophil cationic protein (EG1 and EG2) for quantifying eosinophils in bronchial biopsies from atopic asthma. Clin Exp Allergy. 1992;22(2):265–73.
105. Tai PC, Spry CJ, Peterson C, Venge P, Olsson I. Monoclonal antibodies distinguish between storage and secreted forms of eosinophil cationic protein. Nature. 1984;309(5964):182–4.
106. Bascom R, Pipkorn U, Proud D, et al. Major basic protein and eosinophil-derived neurotoxin concentrations in nasal-lavage fluid after antigen challenge: effect of systemic corticosteroids and relationship to eosinophil influx. J Allergy Clin Immunol. 1989;84(3):338–46.
107. Wassom DL, Loegering DA, Solley GO, Moore SB, Schooley RT, Fauci A. Elevated serum levels of the eosinophil granule major basic protein in patients with eosinophilia. J Clin Invest. 1981;67(3):651–61.
108. Peterson CG, Enander I, Nystrand J, Anderson AS, Nilsson L, Venge P. Radioimmunoassay of human eosinophil cationic protein (ECP) by an improved method. Establishment of normal levels in serum and turnover in vivo. Clin Exp Allergy. 1991;21(5):561–7.
109. Venge P. The eosinophil granulocyte in allergic inflammation. Pediatr Allergy Immunol. 1993;4(4 Suppl):19–24.
110. Wassom DL, Loegering DA, Solley GO, et al. Elevated serum levels of the eosinophil granule major basic protein in patients with eosinophilia. J Clin Invest. 1981;67(3):651–61.
111. Gundel RH, Gerritsen ME, Gleich GJ, Wegner CD. Repeated antigen inhalation results in a prolonged airway eosinophilia and airway hyperresponsiveness in primates. J Appl Physiol. 1990;68(2):779–86.
112. Wardlaw AJ, Dunnette S, Gleich GJ, Collins JV, Kay AB. Eosinophils and mast cells in bronchoalveolar lavage in subjects with mild asthma. Relationship to bronchial hyperreactivity. Am Rev Respir Dis. 1988;137(1):62–9.

113. Kapp A. The role of eosinophils in the pathogenesis of atopic dermatitis – eosinophil granule proteins as markers of disease activity. Allergy. 1993;48:1–5.
114. Mori Y, Iwasaki H, Kohno K, et al. Identification of the human eosinophil lineage-committed progenitor: revision of phenotypic definition of the human common myeloid progenitor. J Exp Med. 2009;206(1):183–93.
115. Takatsu K, Tominaga A, Harada N, et al. T cell-replacing factor (TRF)/interleukin 5 (IL-5): molecular and functional properties. Immunol Rev. 1988;102:107–35.
116. Plaut M, Pierce JH, Watson CJ, Hanley-Hyde J, Nordan RP, Paul WE. Mast cell lines produce lymphokines in response to cross-linkage of Fc epsilon RI or to calcium ionophores. Nature. 1989;339(6219):64–7.
117. Galli SJ, Gordon JR, Wershil BK, Elovic A, Wong DT, Weller PF. Mast cell and eosinophil cytokines in allergy and inflammation. In: Kay AB, Gleich GJ, editors. Eosinophils in allergy and inflammation, vol. 2. New York: Marcel Dekker; 1994. p. 255–80.
118. Palacios R, Karasuyama H, Rolink A. Ly1+ PRO-B lymphocyte clones. Phenotype, growth requirements and differentiation in vitro and in vivo. EMBO J. 1987;6(12):3687–93.
119. Takatsu K, Yamaguchi N, Hitoshi Y, Sonoda E, Mita S, Tominaga A. Signal transduction through interleukin-5 receptors. Cold Spring Harb Symp Quant Biol. 1989;2:745–51.
120. Yamaguchi Y, Suda T, Suda J, et al. Purified interleukin 5 supports the terminal differentiation and proliferation of murine eosinophilic precursors. J Exp Med. 1988;167(1):43–56.
121. Sanderson CJ. Eosinophil differentiation factor (interleukin-5). Immunol Ser. 1990;49: 231–56.
122. Sanderson CJ. Control of eosinophilia. Int Arch Allergy Appl Immunol. 1991;94(1–4):122–6.
123. Kopf M, Brombacher F, Hodgkin PD, et al. IL-5-deficient mice have a developmental defect in CD5+ B-1 cells and lack eosinophilia, but have normal antibody and cytotoxic T cell responses. Immunity. 1996;4:15–24.
124. Owen WF, Rothenberg ME, Petersen J, et al. Interleukin 5 and phenotypically altered eosinophils in the blood of patients with the idiopathic hypereosinophilic syndrome. J Exp Med. 1989;170(1):343–8.
125. Owen Jr W, Petersen J, Sheff DM, et al. Hypodense eosinophils and interleukin 5 activity in the blood of patients with the eosinophilia-myalgia syndrome. Proc Natl Acad Sci USA. 1990;87(21):8647–51.
126. Sanderson CJ. Interleukin-5, eosinophils, and disease. Blood. 1992;79(12):3101–9.
127. Tominaga A, Takaki S, Koyama N, et al. Transgenic mice expressing a B cell growth and differentiation factor gene (interleukin 5) develop eosinophilia and autoantibody production. J Exp Med. 1991;173(2):429–37.
128. Foster PS, Hogan SP, Ramsay AJ, Matthaei KI, Young IG. Interleukin 5 deficiency abolishes airways eosinophilia, airways hyperreactivity, and lung damage in mouse asthma model. J Exp Med. 1996;183:195–201.
129. Cantor AB, Orkin SH. Hematopoietic development: a balancing act. Curr Opin Genet Dev. Oct 2001;11(5):513–9.
130. Miyamoto T, Akashi K. Lineage promiscuous expression of transcription factors in normal hematopoiesis. Int J Hematol. Jun 2005;81(5):361–7.
131. Akashi K. Lineage promiscuity and plasticity in hematopoietic development. Ann N Y Acad Sci. Jun 2005;1044:125–31.
132. McNagny K, Graf T. Making eosinophils through subtle shifts in transcription factor expression. J Exp Med. 2002;195(11):F43–7.
133. Yamaguchi Y, Nishio H, Kishi K, Ackerman SJ, Suda T. C/EBPbeta and GATA-1 synergistically regulate activity of the eosinophil granule major basic protein promoter: implication for C/EBPbeta activity in eosinophil gene expression. Blood. 1999;94(4):1429–39.
134. Querfurth E, Schuster M, Kulessa H, et al. Antagonism between C/EBPbeta and FOG in eosinophil lineage commitment of multipotent hematopoietic progenitors. Genes Dev. 2000;14(19):2515–25.
135. Hirasawa R, Shimizu R, Takahashi S, et al. Essential and instructive roles of GATA factors in eosinophil development. J Exp Med. 2002;195(11):1379–86.

136. Yu C, Cantor AB, Yang H, et al. Targeted deletion of a high-affinity GATA-binding site in the GATA-1 promoter leads to selective loss of the eosinophil lineage in vivo. J Exp Med. 2002;195(11):1387–95.
137. Du J, Stankiewicz MJ, Liu Y, et al. Novel combinatorial interactions of GATA-1, PU.1, and C/EBPepsilon isoforms regulate transcription of the gene encoding eosinophil granule major basic protein. J Biol Chem. 2002;277(45):43481–94.
138. Zimmermann N, Colyer JL, Koch LE, Rothenberg ME. Analysis of the CCR3 promoter reveals a regulatory region in exon 1 that binds GATA-1. BMC Immunol. 2005;6(1):7.
139. Yamanaka R, Barlow C, Lekstrom-Himes J, et al. Impaired granulopoiesis, myelodysplasia, and early lethality in CCAAT/enhancer binding protein epsilon-deficient mice. Proc Natl Acad Sci USA. 1997;94(24):13187–92.
140. Yamanaka R, Lekstrom-Himes J, Barlow C, Wynshaw-Boris A, Xanthopoulos KG. CCAAT/enhancer binding proteins are critical components of the transcriptional regulation of hematopoiesis (Review). Int J Mol Med. 1998;1(1):213–21.
141. Rosenberg HF, Gallin JI. Neutrophil-specific granule deficiency includes eosinophils. Blood. 1993;82(1):268–73.
142. Klion AD, Law MA, Noel P, Kim YJ, Haverty TP, Nutman TB. Safety and efficacy of the monoclonal anti-interleukin-5 antibody SCH55700 in the treatment of patients with hypereosinophilic syndrome. Blood. 2004;103(8):2939–41.
143. Menzies-Gow A, Flood-Page P, Sehmi R, et al. Anti-IL-5 (mepolizumab) therapy induces bone marrow eosinophil maturational arrest and decreases eosinophil progenitors in the bronchial mucosa of atopic asthmatics. J Allergy Clin Immunol. Apr 2003;111(4):714–9.
144. Clutterbuck EJ, Hirst EMA, Sanderson CJ. Human interleukin-5 (IL-5) regulates the production of eosinophils in human bone marrow cultures: comparison and interaction with IL-1, IL-3, IL-6, and GMCSF. Blood. 1989;73:1504–12.
145. Seminario M-C, Saini SS, MacGlashan Jr DW, Bochner BS. Intracellular expression and release of FcεRIα (epsilon) (alpha) by human eosinophils. J Immunol. 1999;162: 6893–900.
146. Smith SJ, Ying S, Meng Q, et al. Blood eosinophils from atopic donors express messenger RNA for the alpha, beta, and gamma subunits of the high-affinity IgE receptor (Fc epsilon RI) and intracellular, but not cell surface, alpha subunit protein. J Allergy Clin Immunol. 2000;105(2 Pt 1):309–17.
147. Ackerman SJ, Kephart GM, Habermann TM, Greipp PR, Gleich GJ. Localization of eosinophil granule major basic protein in human basophils. J Exp Med. 1983;158:946–61.
148. Ackerman SJ, Weil GJ, Gleich GJ. Formation of Charcot-Leyden crystals by human basophils. J Exp Med. 1982;155(6):1597–609.
149. Abu-Ghazaleh RI, Dunnette SL, Loegering DA, et al. Eosinophil granule proteins in peripheral blood granulocytes. J Leukoc Biol. Dec 1992;52(6):611–8.
150. Bochner BS, Schleimer RP. Mast cells, basophils, and eosinophils: distinct but overlapping pathways for recruitment. Immunol Rev. Feb 2001;179:5–15.
151. Aizawa H, Zimmermann N, Carrigan PE, Lee JJ, Rothenberg ME, Bochner BS. Molecular analysis of human Siglec-8 orthologs relevant to mouse eosinophils: identification of mouse orthologs of Siglec-5 (mSiglec-F) and Siglec-10 (mSiglec-G). Genomics. Nov 2003;82(5):521–30.
152. Zhang JQ, Biedermann B, Nitschke L, Crocker PR. The murine inhibitory receptor mSiglec-E is expressed broadly on cells of the innate immune system whereas mSiglec-F is restricted to eosinophils. Eur J Immunol. Apr 2004;34(4):1175–84.
153. Kikly KK, Bochner BS, Freeman S, et al. Identification of SAF-2, a novel siglec expressed on eosinophils, mast cells and basophils. J Allergy Clin Immunol. 2000;105:1093–100.
154. Voehringer D, van Rooijen N, Locksley RM. Eosinophils develop in distinct stages and are recruited to peripheral sites by alternatively activated macrophages. J Leukoc Biol. 2007;81(6):1434–44.
155. Palframan RT, Collins PD, Severs NJ, Rothery S, Williams TJ, Rankin SM. Mechanisms of acute eosinophil mobilization from the bone marrow stimulated by interleukin 5: the role of specific adhesion molecules and phosphatidylinositol 3-kinase. J Exp Med. 1998;188(9):1621–32.

156. Palframan RT, Collins PD, Williams TJ, Rankin SM. Eotaxin induces a rapid release of eosinophils and their progenitors from the bone marrow. Blood. 1998;91(7):2240–8.
157. Werfel S, Yednock T, Matsumoto K, Sterbinsky SA, Schleimer RP, Bochner BS. Functional regulation of β(beta)1 integrins and human eosinophils by divalent cations and cytokines. Am J Respir Cell Mol Biol. 1996;14:45–52.
158. Weber C, Kitayama J, Springer TA. Differential regulation of β1 (beta)and β2(beta) integrin avidity by chemoattractants in eosinophils. Proc Natl Acad Sci USA. 1996;93:10939–44.
159. Tachimoto H, Burdick M, Hudson SA, Kikuchi M, Konstantopoulous K, Bochner BS. CCR3-active chemokines promote rapid detachment of eosinophils from VCAM-1 in vitro. J Immunol. 2000;165:2748–54.
160. Minshall EM, Schleimer R, Cameron L, et al. Interleukin-5 expression in the bone marrow of sensitized Balb/c mice after allergen challenge. Am J Respir Crit Care Med. Sep 1998;158(3):951–7.
161. Rytomaa T. Organ distribution and histochemical properties of eosinophil granulocytes in the rat. Acta Pathol Microbiol Scand. 1960;50 Suppl 140:1.
162. Winkel P, Statland BE, Saunders AM, Osborn H, Kupperman H. Within-day physiologic variation of leukocyte types in healthy subjects as assayed by two automated leukocyte differential analyzers. Am J Clin Pathol. May 1981;75(5):693–700.
163. Martin RJ, Cicutto LC, Smith HR, Ballard RD, Szefler SJ. Airways inflammation in nocturnal asthma. Am Rev Respir Dis. 1991;143(2):351–7.
164. Schleimer RP, Sterbinsky SA, Kaiser J, et al. IL-4 induces adherence of human eosinophils and basophils but not neutrophils to endothelium. Association with expression of VCAM-1. J Immunol. 1992;148(4):1086–92.
165. Rothenberg ME, MacLean JA, Pearlman E, Luster AD, Leder P. Targeted disruption of the chemokine eotaxin partially reduces antigen-induced tissue eosinophilia. J Exp Med. 1997;185(4):785–90.
166. Daugherty BL, Siciliano SJ, DeMartino JA, Malkowitz L, Sirotina A, Springer MS. Cloning, expression, and characterization of the human eosinophil eotaxin receptor. J Exp Med. 1996;183(5):2349–54.
167. Rothenberg ME, Ownbey R, Mehlhop PD, et al. Eotaxin triggers eosinophil-selective chemotaxis and calcium flux via a distinct receptor and induces pulmonary eosinophilia in the presence of interleukin 5 in mice. Mol Med. 1996;2(3):334–48.
168. Kita H, Adolphson CR, Gleich GJ. Biology of eosinophils. In: Adkinson Jr NF, Yunginger JW, Busse WW, Bochner BS, Holgate ST, Simons FER, editors. Allergy principles and practice. 6th ed. Philadelphia: Mosby; 2003. p. 305–32.
169. Weller PF. Intercellular interactions in the recruitment and functions of human eosinophils. Ann N Y Acad Sci. 1992;664:116–25.
170. Kameyoshi Y, Dorschner A, Mallet AI, Christophers E, Schroder JM. Cytokine RANTES released by thrombin-stimulated platelets is a potent attractant for human eosinophils. J Exp Med. 1992;176(2):587–92.
171. Foster PS, Mould AW, Yang M, et al. Elemental signals regulating eosinophil accumulation in the lung. Immunol Rev. Feb 2001;179:173–81.
172. Foster PS, Hogan SP, Yang M, et al. Interleukin-5 and eosinophils as therapeutic targets for asthma. Trends Mol Med. 2002;8(4):162–7.
173. Foster PS, Martinez-Moczygemba M, Huston DP, Corry DB. Interleukins-4, -5, and -13: emerging therapeutic targets in allergic disease. Pharmacol Ther. Jun 2002;94(3):253–64.
174. Bochner BS, Friedman B, Krishnaswami G, Schleimer RP, Lichtenstein LM, Kroegel C. Episodic eosinophilia-myalgia-like syndrome in a patient without L-tryptophan use: association with eosinophil activation and increased serum levels of granulocyte-macrophage colony-stimulating factor. J Allergy Clin Immunol. Oct 1991;88(4):629–36.
175. Butterfield JH, Leiferman KM, Abrams J, et al. Elevated serum levels of interleukin-5 in patients with the syndrome of episodic angioedema and eosinophilia. Blood. 1992;79(3):688–92.
176. Fang J, Viksman MY, Ebisawa M, Bochner BS. Increased circulating levels of interleukin-5 in a case of steroid-resistant hypereosinophilic syndrome with ileal involvement. J Allergy Clin Immunol. 1994;94:129–31.

177. Simon HU, Plotz SG, Dummer R, Blaser K. Abnormal clones of T cells producing interleukin-5 in idiopathic eosinophilia. N Engl J Med. 1999;341(15):1112–20.
178. Groopman JE, Mitsuyasu RT, DeLeo MJ, Oette DH, Golde DW. Effect of recombinant human granulocyte-macrophage colony-stimulating factor on myelopoiesis in the acquired immunodeficiency syndrome. N Engl J Med. 1987;317:593–8.
179. Shi HZ, Xiao CQ, Zhong D, et al. Effect of inhaled interleukin-5 on airway hyperreactivity and eosinophilia in asthmatics. Am J Respir Crit Care Med. 1998;157(1):204–9.
180. Mishra A, Hogan SP, Lee JJ, Foster PS, Rothenberg ME. Fundamental signals that regulate eosinophil homing to the gastrointestinal tract. J Clin Invest. 1999;103(12):1719–27.
181. Shi HZ, Humbles A, Gerard C, Jin Z, Weller PF. Lymph node trafficking and antigen presentation by endobronchial eosinophils. J Clin Invest. 2000;105(7):945–53.
182. Conus S, Bruno A, Simon HU. Leptin is an eosinophil survival factor. J Allergy Clin Immunol. Dec 2005;116(6):1228–34.
183. Bureau F, Seumois G, Jaspar F, et al. CD40 Engagement enhances eosinophil survival through induction of cellular inhibitor of apoptosis protein 2 expression: possible involvement in allergic inflammation. J Allergy Clin Immunol. 2002;110:443–9.
184. Simon HU, Yousefi S, Schranz C, Schapowal A, Bachert C, Blaser K. Direct demonstration of delayed eosinophil apoptosis as a mechanism causing tissue eosinophilia. J Immunol. 1997;158(8):3902–8.
185. Cameron L, Christodoulopoulos P, Lavigne F, et al. Evidence for local eosinophil differentiation within allergic nasal mucosa: inhibition with soluble IL-5 receptor. J Immunol. 2000;164(3):1538–45.
186. Denburg JA, Keith PK. Systemic aspects of chronic rhinosinusitis. Immunol Allergy Clin North Am. Feb 2004;24(1):87–102.
187. Broide DH, Lotz M, Cuomo AJ, Coburn DA, Federman EC, Wasserman SI. Cytokines in symptomatic asthma airways. J Allergy Clin Immunol. 1992;89(5):958–67.
188. Kroegel C, Liu MC, Hubbard WM, Lichtenstein LM, Bochner BS. Blood and bronchoalveolar eosinophils in allergic subjects following segmental antigen challenge: surface phenotype, density heterogeneity, and prostanoid production. J Allergy Clin Immunol. 1994;93:725–34.
189. Anwar ARF, Moqbel R, Walsh GM, Kay AB, Wardlaw AJ. Adhesion to fibronectin prolongs eosinophil survival. J Exp Med. 1993;177(3):839–43.
190. Georas SN, McIntyre BW, Ebisawa M, Bednarczyk J, Schleimer RP, Bochner BS. Expression of a functional laminin receptor (α6β1,(alpha and beta) VLA-6) on human eosinophils. Blood. 1993;82:2872–9.
191. Gleich GJ, Hunt LW, Bochner BS, Schleimer RP. Glucocorticoid effects on human eosinophils. In: Schleimer RP, Busse WW, O'Byrne P, editors. Inhaled glucocorticoids in asthma: mechanisms and clinical actions. New York: Marcel Dekker, Inc.; 1996. p. 279–308.
192. Stellato C, Matsukura S, Fal A, et al. Differential regulation of epithelial-derived C-C chemokine expression by IL-4 and the glucocorticoid budesonide. J Immunol. 1999;163(10):5624–32.
193. Druilhe A, Letuve S, Pretolani M. Glucocorticoid-induced apoptosis in human eosinophils: mechanisms of action. Apoptosis. Oct 2003;8(5):481–95.
194. Fan J, Heller NM, Gorospe M, Atasoy U, Stellato C. The role of post-transcriptional regulation in chemokine gene expression in inflammation and allergy. Eur Respir J. Nov 2005;26(5): 933–47.
195. Simon HU. Molecules involved in the regulation of eosinophil apoptosis. Chem Immunol Allergy. 2006;91:49–58.
196. Okada S, Hagan JB, Kato M, et al. Lidocaine and its analogues inhibit IL-5-mediated survival and activation of human eosinophils. J Immunol. 1998;160(8):4010–7.
197. Alam R, Forsythe P, Stafford S, Fukuda Y. Transforming growth factor beta abrogates the effects of hematopoietins on eosinophils and induces their apoptosis. J Exp Med. 1994;179(3):1041–5.
198. Nutku E, Aizawa H, Hudson SA, Bochner BS. Ligation of Siglec-8: a selective mechanism for induction of human eosinophil apoptosis. Blood. 2003;101(12):5014–20.
199. Zhang M, Angata T, Cho JY, Miller M, Broide DH, Varki A. Defining the in vivo function of Siglec-F, a CD33-related Siglec expressed on mouse eosinophils. Blood. 2007;109:4280–7.

200. Matsumoto K, Schleimer RP, Saito H, Iikura Y, Bochner BS. Induction of apoptosis in human eosinophils by anti-fas antibody treatment in vitro. Blood. 1995;86:1437–43.
201. Matsumoto K, Terakawa M, Miura K, Fukuda S, Nakajima T, Saito H. Extremely rapid and intense induction of apoptosis in human eosinophils by anti-CD30 antibody treatment in vitro. J Immunol. 2004;172(4):2186–93.
202. Klion AD, Bochner BS, Gleich GJ, et al. Approaches to the treatment of hypereosinophilic syndromes: a workshop summary report. J Allergy Clin Immunol. 2006;117:1292–302.
203. Cools J, DeAngelo DJ, Gotlib J, et al. A tyrosine kinase created by fusion of the PDGFRA and FIP1L1 genes as a therapeutic target of imatinib in idiopathic hypereosinophilic syndrome. N Engl J Med. 2003;348(13):1201–14.
204. Abu-Ghazaleh RI, Kita H, Gleich GJ. Eosinophil activation and function in health and disease. Immunol Ser. 1992;57:137–67.
205. Kita H, Kaneko M, Bartemes KR, et al. Does IgE bind to and activate eosinophils from patients with allergy? J Immunol. 1999;162:6901–11.
206. Sihra BS, Kon OM, Grant JA, Kay AB. Expression of high-affinity IgE receptors (FcεRI) on peripheral blood basophils, monocytes, and eosinophils in atopic and nonatopic subjects: relationship to total serum IgE concentrations. J Allergy Clin Immunol. 1997;99(5): 699–706.
207. Kayaba H, Dombrowicz D, Woerly G, Papin JP, Loiseau S, Capron M. Human eosinophils and human high affinity IgE receptor transgenic mouse eosinophils express low levels of high affinity IgE receptor, but release IL-10 upon receptor activation. J Immunol. 2001;167(2):995–1003.
208. Spry CJ. The pathogenesis of endomyocardial fibrosis: the role of the eosinophil. Springer Semin Immunopathol. 1989;11(4):471–7.
209. Gharaee-Kermani M, Phan SH. The role of eosinophils in pulmonary fibrosis (Review). Int J Mol Med. 1998;1(1):43–53.
210. Melo RC, Perez SA, Spencer LA, Dvorak AM, Weller PF. Intragranular vesiculotubular compartments are involved in piecemeal degranulation by activated human eosinophils. Traffic. Oct 2005;6(10):866–79.
211. Dvorak AM, Ackerman SJ, Furitsu T, Estrella P, Letourneau L, Ishizaka T. Mature eosinophils stimulated to develop in human-cord blood mononuclear cell cultures supplemented with recombinant human interleukin-5. II. Vesicular transport of specific granule matrix peroxidase, a mechanism for effecting piecemeal degranulation. Am J Pathol. 1992;140(4):795–807.
212. Moqbel R, Lacy P. Exocytotic events in eosinophils and mast cells. Clin Exp Allergy. Aug 1999;29(8):1017–22.
213. Logan MR, Odemuyiwa SO, Moqbel R. Understanding exocytosis in immune and inflammatory cells: the molecular basis of mediator secretion. J Allergy Clin Immunol. May 2003;111(5):923–32.
214. Dvorak AM, Ackerman SJ, Weller PF. Subcellular morphology and biochemistry of eosinophils. In: Harris JR, editor. Blood cell biochemistry: megakaryocytes, platelets, macrophages and eosinophils, vol. 2. London: Plenum Publishing Corporation; 1990. p. 237–344.
215. Martin LB, Kita H, Leiferman KM, Gleich GJ. Eosinophils in allergy: role in disease, degranulation, and cytokines. Int Arch Allergy Immunol. Mar 1996;109(3):207–15.
216. Gleich GJ. Mechanisms of eosinophil-associated inflammation. J Allergy Clin Immunol. Apr 2000;105(4):651–63.
217. Thomas LL, Page SM. Inflammatory cell activation by eosinophil granule proteins. Chem Immunol. 2000;76:99–117.
218. Moy JN, Gleich GJ, Thomas LL. Noncytotoxic activation of neutrophils by eosinophil granule major basic protein. Effect on superoxide anion generation and lysosomal enzyme release. J Immunol. 1990;145(8):2626–32.
219. Jacoby DB, Costello RM, Fryer AD. Eosinophil recruitment to the airway nerves. J Allergy Clin Immunol. Feb 2001;107(2):211–8.
220. Rochester CL, Ackerman SJ, Zheng T, Elias JA. Eosinophil-fibroblast interactions. Granule major basic protein interacts with IL-1 and transforming growth factor-beta in the stimulation of lung fibroblast IL-6-type cytokine production. J Immunol. 1996;156(11):4449–56.

221. Ackerman SJ, Butterfield JH. Eosinophilia, eosinophil-associated diseases, chronic eosinophil leukemia, and the hypereosinophilic syndromes. In: Hoffman R, Benz Jr EJ, Shattil SJ, et al., editors. Hematology, basic principles and practice. 5th ed. Philadelphia: Churchill Livingstone/ Elsevier Inc.; 2008. p. 1167–86.
222. Gleich GJ, Schroeter AL, Marcoux JP, Sachs MI, O'Connell EJ, Kohler PF. Episodic angioedema associated with eosinophilia. N Engl J Med. 1984;310(25):1621–6.
223. Rohrbach MS, Wheatley CL, Slifman NR, Gleich GJ. Activation of platelets by eosinophil granule proteins. J Exp Med. 1990;172(4):1271–4.
224. Rosenberg HF, Ackerman SJ, Tenen DG. Human eosinophil cationic protein. Molecular cloning of a cytotoxin and helminthotoxin with ribonuclease activity. J Exp Med. 1989;170(1):163–76.
225. Rosenberg HF, Tenen DG, Ackerman SJ. Molecular cloning of the human eosinophil-derived neurotoxin: a member of the ribonuclease gene family. Proc Natl Acad Sci USA. 1989;86(12):4460–4.
226. Slungaard A, Mahoney Jr J. Bromide-dependent toxicity of eosinophil peroxidase for endothelium and isolated working rat hearts: a model for eosinophilic endocarditis. J Exp Med. 1991;173(1):117–26.
227. Slungaard A, Mahoney Jr J. Thiocyanate is the major substrate for eosinophil peroxidase in physiologic fluids. Implications for cytotoxicity. J Biol Chem. 1991;266(8):4903–10.
228. Slungaard A, Vercellotti GM, Walker G, Nelson RD, Jacob HS. Tumor necrosis factor alpha/ cachectin stimulates eosinophil oxidant production and toxicity towards human endothelium. J Exp Med. 1990;171(6):2025–41.
229. Rothenberg ME. Eosinophilic gastrointestinal disorders (EGID). J Allergy Clin Immunol. 2004;113(1):11–28. quiz 29.
230. Fox VL, Nurko S, Teitelbaum JE, Badizadegan K, Furuta GT. High-resolution EUS in children with eosinophilic "allergic" esophagitis. Gastrointest Endosc. Jan 2003;57(1):30–6.
231. Varga J, Kahari VM. Eosinophilia-myalgia syndrome, eosinophilic fasciitis, and related fibrosing disorders. Curr Opin Rheumatol. 1997;9(6):562–70.
232. Gharaee-Kermani M, Phan SH. Molecular mechanisms of and possible treatment strategies for idiopathic pulmonary fibrosis. Curr Pharm Des. 2005;11(30):3943–71.
233. Gauldie J, Sime PJ, Xing Z, Marr B, Tremblay GM. Transforming growth factor-beta gene transfer to the lung induces myofibroblast presence and pulmonary fibrosis. Curr Top Pathol. 1999;93:35–45.
234. Ohno I, Nitta Y, Yamauchi K, et al. Eosinophils as a potential source of platelet-derived growth factor B-chain (PDGF-B) in nasal polyposis and bronchial asthma. Am J Respir Cell Mol Biol. Dec 1995;13(6):639–47.
235. Pegorier S, Wagner LA, Gleich GJ, Pretolani M. Eosinophil-derived cationic proteins activate the synthesis of remodeling factors by airway epithelial cells. J Immunol. 2006;177(7): 4861–9.
236. Liacouras CA, Bonis P, Putnam PE, et al. Summary of the first international gastrointestinal research sypmosium. J Pediatr Gastroenterol Nutr. 2007;45(3):370–91.
237. Minshall EM, Cameron L, Lavigne F, et al. Eotaxin mRNA and protein expression in chronic sinusitis and allergen-induced nasal responses in seasonal allergic rhinitis. Am J Respir Cell Mol Biol. 1997;17(6):683–90.
238. Hoshino M, Nakamura Y, Sim J, Shimojo J, Isogai S. Bronchial subepithelial fibrosis and expression of matrix metalloproteinase-9 in asthmatic airway inflammation. J Allergy Clin Immunol. 1998;102(5):783–8.
239. Hoshino M, Nakamura Y, Sim JJ. Expression of growth factors and remodelling of the airway wall in bronchial asthma. Thorax. 1998;53(1):21–7.
240. Varga J, Jimenez SA. Modulation of collagen gene expression: its relation to fibrosis in systemic sclerosis and other disorders. Ann Intern Med. 1995;122:60–2.
241. Eickelberg O, Pansky A, Mussmann R, et al. Transforming growth factor-beta1 induces interleukin-6 expression via activating protein-1 consisting of JunD homodimers in primary human lung fibroblasts. J Biol Chem. 1999;274(18):12933–8.

242. Phipps S, Benyahia F, Ou TT, Barkans J, Robinson DS, Kay AB. Acute allergen-induced airway remodeling in atopic asthma. Am J Respir Cell Mol Biol. Dec 2004;31(6):626–32.
243. Kim KK, Kugler MC, Wolters PJ, et al. Alveolar epithelial cell mesenchymal transition develops in vivo during pulmonary fibrosis and is regulated by the extracellular matrix. Proc Natl Acad Sci USA. 2006;103(35):13180–5.
244. Huaux F, Gharaee-Kermani M, Liu T, et al. Role of Eotaxin-1 (CCL11) and CC chemokine receptor 3 (CCR3) in bleomycin-induced lung injury and fibrosis. Am J Pathol. Dec 2005;167(6):1485–96.
245. Straumann A, Spichtin HP, Grize L, Bucher KA, Beglinger C, Simon HU. Natural history of primary eosinophilic esophagitis: a follow-up of 30 adult patients for up to 11.5 years. Gastroenterology. Dec 2003;125(6):1660–9.
246. Blanchard C, Wang N, Stringer KF, et al. Eotaxin-3 and a uniquely conserved gene-expression profile in eosinophilic esophagitis. J Clin Invest. Feb 2006;116(2):536–47.
247. Takayama G, Arima K, Kanaji T, et al. Periostin: a novel component of subepithelial fibrosis of bronchial asthma downstream of IL-4 and IL-13 signals. J Allergy Clin Immunol. Jul 2006;118(1):98–104.
248. Blanchard C, Mingler MK, McBride M, et al. Periostin facilitates eosinophil tissue infiltration in allergic lung and esophageal responses. Mucosal Immunol. 2008;1(4):289–96.

Chapter 5
Role of Lymphocytes and Mast Cells in Eosinophilic Esophagitis

Mirna Chehade and Hugh A. Sampson

Keywords Eosinophilic esophagitis • Esophageal mucosa • Food antigens • Aeroallergens • Lymphocytes • Mast cells • Eosinophils

Introduction

Eosinophilic esophagitis (EoE) is a chronic inflammatory disease of the esophagus characterized by significant eosinophilic infiltration of the esophageal mucosa. Although the exact pathogenesis of EoE remains unclear, an immunological reaction to foods and possibly to aeroallergens has been implicated based on several short-term clinical trials consisting of dietary eliminations with resultant disease remission [1–4] and observations of seasonal variability in disease severity [5, 6]. The immunological reaction to dietary and environmental antigens is thought to consist of a mix of IgE-mediated and non-IgE-mediated, i.e., cell-mediated, allergic reactions [1, 3]. Histopathologically, similar to allergic diseases in other organs, various inflammatory cells are found in increased numbers in the esophagus, including lymphocytes, mast cells, and eosinophils, the latter serving as the diagnostic hallmark for the disease [7]. In this chapter, we summarize data demonstrating increased numbers of lymphocytes and mast cells in the esophagus of EoE patients. We also discuss evidence for the role of lymphocytes in EoE, focusing on the allergic phenotype of some of these cells. Since the role of mast cells in EoE has not been well studied, we speculate on the potential role of these cells in the pathogenesis of EoE.

M. Chehade (✉)
Mount Sinai Center for Eosinophilic Disorders, Jaffe Food Allergy Institute,
Mount Sinai School of Medicine, One Gustave L. Levy Place,
Box 1198, New York, NY 10029, USA
e-mail: mirna.chehade@mssm.edu

C.A. Liacouras and J.E. Markowitz (eds.), *Eosinophilic Esophagitis*,
Clinical Gastroenterology, DOI 10.1007/978-1-60761-515-6_5,

The Esophagus Is an Immunological Organ

Until recently, most studies of the esophagus focused on its physical properties as a conduit of food. Its role as an immunological organ did not emerge until diseases such as EoE were studied.

The normal esophagus is a highly distensible muscular tube that extends from the epiglottis in the pharynx at the level of the C6 vertebra, to the gastroesophageal junction at the level of the T11 or T12 vertebra [8]. The wall of the esophagus consists of a mucosa, submucosa, muscularis propria, and adventitia, reflecting the general structural organization of the gastrointestinal tract, except for the lack of a serosal coat [8].

The esophageal mucosa is composed of three parts: a non-keratinizing stratified squamous epithelial layer, lamina propria, and muscularis mucosa. The epithelial layer has mature squamous cells overlying basal cells that have great proliferative potential. The basal cell zone occupies 10–15% of the epithelial layer thickness. Various immune cells including dendritic cells, lymphocytes, and mast cells are present in the deeper portion of the epithelial layer [7, 9, 10]. Eosinophils are normally absent in the esophageal epithelium [7, 11]. The lamina propria is situated between the epithelial layer and the muscularis mucosa, and consists of loose areolar connective tissue, vascular structures, and leukocytes. The muscularis mucosa consists of longitudinally oriented smooth muscle bundles.

Deep to the mucosa is the submucosa, consisting of loose connective tissue containing blood vessels, a rich network of lymphatics, leukocytes, occasional lymphoid follicles, nerve fibers, and submucosal glands that secrete mucin-containing fluid to lubricate the esophagus. The muscularis propria consists of an inner circular coat and an outer longitudinal coat of smooth muscle with an intervening myenteric plexus.

The combination of esophageal peristalsis, presence of a lower esophagogastric junction sphincter, squamous epithelial barrier, salivary and submucosal gland products, and immune cells in the esophagus contributes to esophageal defense against injury.

Lymphocytes and Mast Cells Are Present in the Normal Esophagus

In the normal esophageal epithelium of healthy individuals, rare lymphocytes are present [7, 12, 13], historically referred to as squiggle cells by histopathologists, due to their irregular nuclear contours as they tightly intermingle with epithelial cells, as seen by microscopic examination of hematoxylin and eosin-stained sections of the esophageal epithelium [13]. These squiggle cells were shown to be T lymphocytes [12, 13]. In the esophageal epithelial layer, CD8 positive T lymphocytes are more predominant than CD4 positive cells [7, 9]; whereas CD4 T lymphocytes are the predominant ones in the normal esophageal lamina propria [9]. B lymphocytes on the other hand, while absent in the esophageal epithelium of healthy individuals [7], are present in the subepithelial lamina propria along with the CD4 positive T cells [9].

Mast cells are present in the mucosa and submucosa of the esophagus of healthy individuals [10]. Subtyping of mast cells (MC_T or MC_{TC}) in the esophagus has not been done.

In EoE, studies characterizing lymphocytes and mast cells in the esophagus of patients with the disease are limited by the depth of endoscopically obtained biopsies. Most biopsies are limited to the epithelial layer of the mucosa, and very few are deep enough to include a portion of the subepithelial lamina propria. Both lymphocytes and mast cells were found to be increased in number in the esophageal epithelium of patients with EoE [7, 10].

Lymphocytes Are Increased in Number in the EoE Esophagus

T lymphocytes were found to be increased in the esophageal epithelium of patients with EoE compared to that of healthy controls, demonstrated by immunohistochemical staining of esophageal biopsies for the T-lymphocyte marker CD3 [7, 14, 15]. T cells tended to be distributed in the deeper layers of the epithelium, being denser closer to the regenerative epithelial basal cell layer [7]. Both T cell subsets, CD4 and CD8 cells, are present, with a maintenance of CD8 predominance over CD4 cells [7, 14]. Since all histopathological studies are limited to the esophageal epithelium, it is not known whether this predominance is also true in the deeper, subepithelial layers of the esophagus in EoE. The overall number of T lymphocytes in the deeper layers of the EoE esophagus is also not known.

B lymphocytes were shown to infiltrate the esophageal epithelium of EoE patients, as demonstrated by immunohistochemical staining for the B-cell marker CD20, albeit in small numbers [7, 16]. Their number in the deeper esophageal layers in EoE patients has not been studied.

Lymphocytes May Play a Role in the Induction of EoE

A possible role for lymphocytes in the induction of disease in EoE is available based on studies of a murine model of allergen-induced esophageal eosinophilia developed by Mishra et al. [17], though the eosinophilia in the mouse model is mostly concentrated in the deeper esophageal layers including the lamina propria rather than the esophageal epithelium as seen in patients with EoE. In their mouse model, intranasal instillation of Aspergillus fumigatus as an antigen resulted in pulmonary and esophageal eosinophilia. Lymphocytes were found to be increased in the esophagus of Aspergillus-treated mice compared to saline-treated mice [18]. Both B and T lymphocytes were detected in the mucosal and submucosal regions of the esophagus. Specifically, a twofold increase in B cells and a four- to fivefold increase in

CD4 and CD8 T cells were found. When mice lacking B and T cells (RAG-1 gene-deficient) were intranasally challenged with Aspergillus antigen in the same fashion, no esophageal eosinophilic infiltration was found, indicating an important role for lymphocytes in EoE induction. When the authors performed the same experiments using B-cell-deficient mice (IgH6) and T-cell-deficient mice (Foxn1), they were able to demonstrate that T cells, rather than B cells, were important in the induction of esophageal eosinophilia. Within T-cell populations, CD4 rather than CD8 cells were shown to be important: CD4-deficient mice were moderately protected from the induction of EoE, while CD8α-deficient mice developed EoE in the regular fashion.

In humans, the role of T lymphocytes, especially CD4 cells, in the induction of EoE is less clear. Both CD4 and CD8 subsets of T lymphocytes have been found to decrease in number in the esophageal epithelium of patients with EoE following successful treatment with topical corticosteroids [7, 14]. Various descriptive studies point to a T-helper type 2 (Th2) adaptive immunity in EoE, detailed later in this chapter. The role of Th2 cytokines in the induction of EoE was demonstrated in mice by intratracheal delivery of the Th2 cytokine IL-13, which resulted in dose-dependent esophageal eosinophilia via an IL-5 and STAT6-dependent mechanism [19]. These results implicate Th2 cells as playing a crucial role in EoE pathogenesis in humans.

B-lymphocyte function in human EoE has not been examined. B lymphocytes are known to be capable of holding antigens on their surface for recognition by specific T lymphocytes along with MHC class II molecules [20]. A potential role for B lymphocytes in EoE was recently highlighted by Vicario et al. [16], who established that the esophageal mucosa in EoE was a site of initiation and development of humoral responses and local IgE production. Increased B lymphocytes and expression of molecular immunoglobulin machinery in the esophagus of children with EoE was found, regardless of the patients' atopic status. These results point to a possible local IgE-mediated response to foods and could provide a possible explanation as to the clinical response to food eliminations despite the absence of food sensitizations by skin tests in some patients with EoE [21].

No studies have addressed the presence or the role of regulatory T cells in EoE, important in oral tolerance to foods, and their secreted cytokines such as TGF-β. Co-existence of Th1 predominant diseases such as celiac disease and the Th2 disease EoE [22, 23] points to a possible global disturbance in regulatory cell function in EoE, and warrants further investigation.

T Lymphocytes in Patients with EoE Carry an Allergic Phenotype

Short-term clinical trials, mostly in children with EoE, have established a link between common food allergens and the induction of EoE, pointing toward an allergic, Th2 type of immune response [1, 3, 4]. In addition, the cytokine milieu of the esophagus and peripheral blood of patients with EoE was found to be consistent with a Th2 phenotype.

In the peripheral circulation, Bullock et al. [24] examined cytokine expression by peripheral blood mononuclear cells (PBMCs) and found that children with active EoE had an increased percentage of CD4 cells expressing the Th2 cytokine IL-5 compared to non-atopic controls. This percentage was lower in EoE patients in remission than in patients with active disease. Straumann et al. [15] measured cytokine secretion by PBMCs of EoE patients in response to in vitro stimulation with phytohemagglutinin, a polyclonal T-cell stimulant. Increased release of the Th2 cytokine IL-13 was found in 40% of the patients studied. Yamazaki et al. [25] found similar results with specific allergen stimulants. PBMCs from 15 adult patients with EoE were incubated in vitro with food allergen extracts and aeroallergen extracts. Food extracts consisted of milk, egg, soy, wheat, and peanut. Compared to healthy controls, PBMCs from EoE patients secreted significantly more of the Th2 cytokines IL-5 and/or IL-13 in response to various allergens, even in the absence of clear-cut sensitization to the allergens when serum levels of allergen-specific IgE were measured. Results from these studies are limited by the fact that many EoE patients studied had concomitant allergic diseases that may have contributed to the Th2 response. A study comparing EoE patients to allergic controls is needed to confirm these findings.

Increased levels of the Th2 cytokines IL-5 and IL-13 were found in the esophagus of patients with EoE compared to that of controls [15, 26, 27]. IL-13 likely plays an important role in the pathogenesis of EoE. When stimulated with IL-13 in vitro, esophageal epithelial cells were shown to produce high levels of eotaxin-3 [27], a highly induced chemokine in EoE shown to regulate eosinophil responses in vitro [28] and to correlate with the severity of esophageal eosinophilia in children with EoE [29]. One major limitation in all these esophageal cytokine studies is the lack of identification of the specific inflammatory cells producing these Th2 cytokines. Therefore, the contribution of lymphocytes to the production of Th2 cytokines is not yet known, especially given that other immune cells are capable of secreting these cytokines. For example, esophageal intraepithelial eosinophils of patients with EoE were found to express IL-4 and IL-13 by immunohistochemical staining of esophageal biopsies [30]. Studies addressing the specific contribution of esophageal lymphocytes into the production of Th2 cytokines in the esophagus, especially in response to specific dietary allergens, need to be performed.

Mast Cells Are Increased in Number in the EoE Esophagus

Various studies have demonstrated an increase in mast cell number in the esophageal epithelium of patients with EoE compared to that of healthy individuals (three- to sevenfold increase) [10, 29]. Mast cells were mostly located in the deeper layers of the epithelium, close to the basal epithelial regenerative layer and to other immune cells such as dendritic cells and lymphocytes [31]. The number of esophageal intraepithelial mast cells was found to correlate with that of intraepithelial eosinophils [10, 29], and was found to decrease significantly following successful EoE therapy [7].

Possible Mechanisms of Mast Cell Activation in EoE

Several studies have demonstrated that mast cells exist in an activated state in the esophageal epithelium of some patients with EoE, as evidenced by mast cell degranulation and release of tryptase into the esophageal mucosa, seen upon immunohistochemical staining of esophageal tissue for tryptase [31]. Other evidence of mast cell activation was also provided by electron microscopic examination of esophageal mast cells in EoE, demonstrating features of degranulation [32]. Using microarray analysis of esophageal tissue from EoE patients and controls, several mast cell genes were found to be induced in EoE (sixfold increase for tryptase, twofold increase for chymase, and 20-fold increase for carboxipeptidase A3) [29].

The mechanism of activation of mast cells in EoE has not been determined. In allergic diseases such as EoE, one would expect food-specific IgE cross-linking on the mast cell surface via the high affinity IgE receptor (FcεRI) to be the predominant mechanism. However, many patients with EoE do not demonstrate evidence of clear-cut food sensitization, as measured by elevated serum food-specific IgE levels or positive prick skin tests to foods [21]. Although absence of systemic sensitization does not rule out a local response restricted to esophageal tissue, Vicario et al. found esophageal mast cells that are not bearing IgE on their surface in some children with EoE [16]. A higher percentage of esophageal mast cells bearing IgE was found in children with EoE who have concomitant atopy (asthma, allergic rhinitis, or eczema) than in non-atopic EoE children. Therefore, other mechanisms for mast cell activation besides cross-linking of IgE on the cell surface may exist in EoE.

Alternative pathways for mast cell activation that are independent of IgE include stem cell factor, complement fragments, neuropeptides, and eosinophil-derived proteins, none of which have been investigated in EoE [33–35]. The eosinophil-derived granular proteins, major basic protein, and eosinophil cationic protein, are of particular interest since they have been shown to be increased in the esophageal epithelium of EoE patients and were found to be particularly prevalent in the extracellular space following eosinophilic degranulation [10], allowing potential activation of mast cells.

Possible Role of Mast Cells in the Pathogenesis of EoE

The role that mast cells play in the pathogenesis of EoE has not been studied. When activated, mast cells are known to release a variety of mediators, either stored in their preformed granules, or synthesized following activation (Table 5.1) [34]. As a result, mast cells may have an effect on several immune and non-immune cells in EoE, hence contributing to its pathogenesis.

Table 5.1 Molecules released by mast cells upon activation [34]

Class of product	Examples	Biological effects
Enzyme	Tryptase, chymase, and carboxypeptidase	Remodel connective tissue matrix
Toxic mediator	Histamine and heparin	Increase vascular permeability Cause smooth muscle contraction
Cytokine	IL-4 and IL-13	Stimulate and amplify Th2 response
	IL-3, IL-5, and GM-CSF	Promote eosinophil production and activation
	TNF-α	Promotes inflammation and stimulates cytokine production by many cell types
Chemokine	MIP-1α	Attracts monocytes, macrophages, and neutrophils
Lipid mediator	Leukotrienes C4, D4, and E4	Cause smooth muscle contraction Increase vascular permeability Stimulate mucus secretion
	Platelet-activating factor	Attracts leukocytes Amplifies production of lipid mediators Activates neutrophils, eosinophils, and platelets

Cross talk between mast cells and eosinophils may be an important contributor to the pathogenesis of EoE in humans. Activated intestinal mast cells were shown to be a potent source of IL-5 in patients with intestinal inflammatory diseases [36], a cytokine important in eosinophilic recruitment. Tryptase was also shown to stimulate the selective release of interleukin-8 [37], a cytokine that participates in eosinophilic migration [38]. Using mast cell-depleted mice, Das et al. [39] also demonstrated a role for mast cells in eotaxin-induced eosinophil accumulation after allergen sensitization. Therefore, cross talk between mast cells and eosinophils may be a two-way phenomenon, possibly contributing to the pathogenesis of EoE.

Upon activation, mast cells are also capable of releasing Th2 cytokines such as IL-4, IL-5, and IL-13 [34], and therefore may be contributing to the Th2 phenotype present in EoE [15, 26, 27]. Furthermore, through secretion of the cytokine TNF-α, mast cells are capable of coordinating and driving a Th2 immune response to antigens through maturation and Th2 skewing of dendritic cells [40]. Dendritic cells are found in the esophagus mostly concentrated in the deeper layers of the esophageal epithelium, close to other immune cells including mast cells [9].

Mast cells may also participate in the pathogenesis of EoE through their effect on non-immune cells. Mast cell components such as histamine and leukotrienes are known to have the capacity to cause smooth muscle contraction [34]. Therefore, they may hypothetically play an important role in muscular disturbances found in some patients with EoE [41].

Similar to eosinophils, mast cells also are capable of secreting TGF-β [33], a cytokine implicated in esophageal subepithelial fibrosis in EoE [42]. However, esophageal fibrosis in EoE was found to be associated with activated esophageal eosinophils, but not activated esophageal mast cells in a pediatric study [10].

Despite the potential role for mast cells in EoE, the use of leukotriene receptor antagonists in therapy has shown limited response. When used at high doses in adult patients with EoE, the leukotriene receptor antagonist montelukast resulted in clinical response in some patients, but no histological remission of the disease [43]. Furthermore, leukotriene levels were not found to be increased in the esophageal mucosa of children with EoE [44]. Studies are needed to elucidate the exact role of mast cells in the pathogenesis of EoE and the stage at which they play a role in the disease, so that therapeutic trials can be tailored accordingly.

Conclusion

In conclusion, several immune cells orchestrate disease pathogenesis in EoE, among which lymphocytes and mast cells likely play an important role. Lymphocytes, especially T cells, are increased in the EoE esophagus, and the esophageal milieu is compatible with an allergic Th2 phenotype. However, the contribution of lymphocytes into this Th2 milieu is still unclear. Mast cells are also increased in the EoE esophagus, but their exact role in the disease pathogenesis is still unclear. Figure 5.1 summarizes the proposed role that these cells may play in EoE. Further translational studies are needed to clarify the role for these two important immune cells, to allow future tailored biological therapies for EoE.

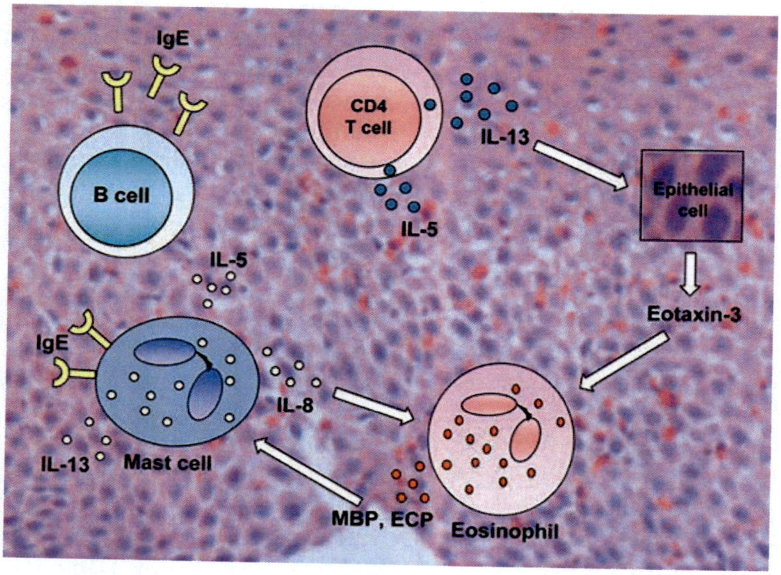

Fig. 5.1 Proposed role potentially played by lymphocytes and mast cells in eosinophilic esophagitis

References

1. Kelly KJ, Lazenby AJ, Rowe PC, Yardley JH, Perman JA, Sampson HA. Eosinophilic esophagitis attributed to gastroesophageal reflux: improvement with an amino acid-based formula. Gastroenterology. 1995;109:1503–12.
2. Markowitz JE, Spergel JM, Ruchelli E, Liacouras CA. Elemental diet is an effective treatment for eosinophilic esophagitis in children and adolescents. Am J Gastroenterol. 2003;98:777–82.
3. Spergel JM, Beausoleil JL, Mascarenhas M, Liacouras CA. The use of skin prick tests and patch tests to identify causative foods in eosinophilic esophagitis. J Allergy Clin Immunol. 2002;109:363–8.
4. Kagalwalla AF, Sentongo TA, Ritz S, Hess T, Nelson SP, Emerick KM, et al. Effect of six-food elimination diet on clinical and histologic outcomes in eosinophilic esophagitis. Clin Gastroenterol Hepatol. 2006;4:1097–102.
5. Fogg MI, Ruchelli E, Spergel JM. Pollen and eosinophilic esophagitis. J Allergy Clin Immunol. 2003;112:796–7.
6. Wang FY, Gupta SK, Fitzgerald JF. Is there a seasonal variation in the incidence or intensity of allergic eosinophilic esophagitis in newly diagnosed children? J Clin Gastroenterol. 2007;41:451–3.
7. Lucendo AJ, Navarro M, Comas C, Pascual JM, Burgos E, Santamaria L, et al. Immunophenotypic characterization and quantification of the epithelial inflammatory infiltrate in eosinophilic esophagitis through stereology: an analysis of the cellular mechanisms of the disease and the immunologic capacity of the esophagus. Am J Surg Pathol. 2007;31:598–606.
8. Liu C, Crawford JM. The gastrointestinal tract. In: Kumar V, Abbas AK, Fausto N, editors. Robbins and cotran pathologic basis of disease. 7th ed. Philadelphia, PA: Elsevier; 2005. p. 797–875.
9. Geboes K, De Wolf-Peeters C, Rutgeerts P, Janssens J, Vantrappen G, Desmet V. Lymphocytes and Langerhans cells in the human oesophageal epithelium. Virchows Arch A Pathol Anat Histopathol. 1983;401:45–55.
10. Chehade M, Sampson HA, Morotti RA, Magid MS. Esophageal subepithelial fibrosis in children with eosinophilic esophagitis. J Pediatr Gastroenterol Nutr. 2007;45:319–28.
11. Winter HS, Madara JL, Stafford RJ, Grand RJ, Quinlan JE, Goldman H. Intraepithelial eosinophils: a new diagnostic criterion for reflux esophagitis. Gastroenterology. 1982;83:818–23.
12. Mangano MM, Antonioli DA, Schnitt SJ, Wang HH. Nature and significance of cells with irregular nuclear contours in esophageal mucosal biopsies. Mod Pathol. 1992;5:191–6.
13. Cucchiara S, D'Armiento F, Alfieri E, Insabato L, Minella R, De Magistris TM, et al. Intraepithelial cells with irregular nuclear contours as a marker of esophagitis in children with gastroesophageal reflux disease. Dig Dis Sci. 1995;40:2305–11.
14. Teitelbaum JE, Fox VL, Twarog FJ, Nurko S, Antonioli D, Gleich G, et al. Eosinophilic esophagitis in children: immunopathological analysis and response to fluticasone propionate. Gastroenterology. 2002;122:1216–25.
15. Straumann A, Bauer M, Fischer B, Blaser K, Simon HU. Idiopathic eosinophilic esophagitis is associated with a T(H)2-type allergic inflammatory response. J Allergy Clin Immunol. 2001;108:954–61.
16. Vicario M, Blanchard C, Stringer KF, Collins MH, Mingler MK, Ahrens A, et al. Local B cells and IgE production in the oesophageal mucosa in eosinophilic oesophagitis. Gut. 2010;59:12–20.
17. Mishra A, Hogan SP, Brandt EB, Rothenberg ME. An etiological role for aeroallergens and eosinophils in experimental esophagitis. J Clin Invest. 2001;107:83–90.
18. Mishra A, Schlotman J, Wang M, Rothenberg ME. Critical role for adaptive T cell immunity in experimental eosinophilic esophagitis in mice. J Leukoc Biol. 2007;81:916–24.
19. Mishra A, Rothenberg ME. Intratracheal IL-13 induces eosinophilic esophagitis by an IL-5, eotaxin-1, and STAT6-dependent mechanism. Gastroenterology. 2003;125:1419–27.

20. Pierce SK, Morris JF, Grusby MJ, Kaumaya P, van Buskirk A, Srinivasan M, et al. Antigen-presenting function of B lymphocytes. Immunol Rev. 1988;106:149–80.
21. Furuta GT, Liacouras CA, Collins MH, Gupta SK, Justinich C, Putnam PE, et al. Eosinophilic esophagitis in children and adults: a systematic review and consensus recommendations for diagnosis and treatment. Gastroenterology. 2007;133:1342–63.
22. Verzegnassi F, Bua J, De Angelis P, Dall'oglio L, Di Leo G, Ventura A. Eosinophilic oesophagitis and coeliac disease: is it just a casual association? Gut. 2007;56:1029–30.
23. Quaglietta L, Coccorullo P, Miele E, Pascarella F, Troncone R, Staiano A. Eosinophilic oesophagitis and coeliac disease: is there an association? Aliment Pharmacol Ther. 2007;26:487–93.
24. Bullock JZ, Villanueva JM, Blanchard C, Filipovich AH, Putnam PE, Collins MH, et al. Interplay of adaptive th2 immunity with eotaxin-3/c-C chemokine receptor 3 in eosinophilic esophagitis. J Pediatr Gastroenterol Nutr. 2007;45:22–31.
25. Yamazaki K, Murray JA, Arora AS, Alexander JA, Smyrk TC, Butterfield JH, et al. Allergen-specific in vitro cytokine production in adult patients with eosinophilic esophagitis. Dig Dis Sci. 2006;51:1934–41.
26. Gupta SK, Fitzgerald JF, Kondratyuk T, HogenEsch H. Cytokine expression in normal and inflamed esophageal mucosa: a study into the pathogenesis of allergic eosinophilic esophagitis. J Pediatr Gastroenterol Nutr. 2006;42:22–6.
27. Blanchard C, Mingler MK, Vicario M, Abonia JP, Wu YY, Lu TX, et al. IL-13 involvement in eosinophilic esophagitis: transcriptome analysis and reversibility with glucocorticoids. J Allergy Clin Immunol. 2007;120:1292–300.
28. Kitaura M, Suzuki N, Imai T, Takagi S, Suzuki R, Nakajima T, et al. Molecular cloning of a novel human CC chemokine (Eotaxin-3) that is a functional ligand of CC chemokine receptor 3. J Biol Chem. 1999;274:27975–80.
29. Blanchard C, Wang N, Stringer KF, Mishra A, Fulkerson PC, Abonia JP, et al. Eotaxin-3 and a uniquely conserved gene-expression profile in eosinophilic esophagitis. J Clin Invest. 2006;116:536–47.
30. Straumann A, Kristl J, Conus S, Vassina E, Spichtin HP, Beglinger C, et al. Cytokine expression in healthy and inflamed mucosa: probing the role of eosinophils in the digestive tract. Inflamm Bowel Dis. 2005;11:720–6.
31. Chehade M, Castro R, Magid M, Benkov K, Birnbaum A, Pittman N, et al. Tryptase is a potential diagnostic marker for eosinophilic esophagitis and eosinophilic gastroenteritis with esophageal involvement. J Pediatr Gastroenterol Nutr. 2002;35:A105.
32. Kirsch R, Bokhary R, Marcon MA, Cutz E. Activated mucosal mast cells differentiate eosinophilic (allergic) esophagitis from gastroesophageal reflux disease. J Pediatr Gastroenterol Nutr. 2007;44:20–6.
33. Metz M, Grimbaldeston MA, Nakae S, Piliponsky AM, Tsai M, Galli SJ. Mast cells in the promotion and limitation of chronic inflammation. Immunol Rev. 2007;217:304–28.
34. Janeway CA, Travers P, Walport M, Shlomchik M. Immunobiology; the immune system in health and disease. 5th ed. New York, NY: Garland Publishing; 2001. p. 471–500.
35. Piliponsky AM, Gleich GJ, Nagler A, Bar I, Levi-Schaffer F. Non-IgE-dependent activation of human lung- and cord blood-derived mast cells is induced by eosinophil major basic protein and modulated by the membrane form of stem cell factor. Blood. 2003;101:1898–904.
36. Lorentz A, Schwengberg S, Mierke C, Manns MP, Bischoff SC. Human intestinal mast cells produce IL-5 in vitro upon IgE receptor cross-linking and in vivo in the course of intestinal inflammatory disease. Eur J Immunol. 1999;29:1496–503.
37. Compton SJ, Cairns JA, Holgate ST, Walls AF. The role of mast cell tryptase in regulating endothelial cell proliferation, cytokine release, and adhesion molecule expression: tryptase induces expression of mRNA for IL-1 beta and IL-8 and stimulates the selective release of IL-8 from human umbilical vein endothelial cells. J Immunol. 1998;161:1939–46.
38. Oliveira SH, Faccioli LH, Cunha FQ, Ferreira SH. Participation of interleukin-5 and interleukin-8 in the eosinophil migration induced by a large volume of saline. Int Arch Allergy Immunol. 1996;111:244–52.

39. Das AM, Flower RJ, Perretti M. Resident mast cells are important for eotaxin-induced eosinophil accumulation in vivo. J Leukoc Biol. 1998;64:156–62.
40. Hofmann AM, Abraham SN. New roles for mast cells in modulating allergic reactions and immunity against pathogens. Curr Opin Immunol. 2009;21:679–86.
41. Lucendo AJ, Castillo P, Martin-Chavarri S, Carrion G, Pajares R, Pascual JM, et al. Manometric findings in adult eosinophilic oesophagitis: a study of 12 cases. Eur J Gastroenterol Hepatol. 2007;19:417–24.
42. Aceves SS, Newbury RO, Dohil R, Bastian JF, Broide DH. Esophageal remodeling in pediatric eosinophilic esophagitis. J Allergy Clin Immunol. 2007;119:206–12.
43. Attwood SE, Lewis CJ, Bronder CS, Morris CD, Armstrong GR, Whittam J. Eosinophilic oesophagitis: a novel treatment using Montelukast. Gut. 2003;52:181–5.
44. Gupta SK, Peters-Golden M, Fitzgerald JF, Croffie JM, Pfefferkorn MD, Molleston JP, et al. Cysteinyl leukotriene levels in esophageal mucosal biopsies of children with eosinophilic inflammation: are they all the same? Am J Gastroenterol. 2006;101:1125–8.

Chapter 6
Esophageal Remodeling in Eosinophilic Esophagitis

Louanne M. Tourangeau and Seema S. Aceves

Keywords Squamous epithelium • Esophageal epithelium • Lamina propria • Muscularis mucosa • Submucosa • Muscularis propria • Epithelial eosinophilia

Introduction

The normal esophagus is composed of layers from the lumen to the adventitia. The non-keratinized stratified squamous epithelium abuts the lumen while the subepithelial regions contain the underlying lamina propria, muscularis mucosa, submucosa, and muscularis propria [1]. The esophageal epithelium contains regenerative cells in the basal zone, which usually comprises 15% of the total epithelial height, and projections of lamina propria, known as the vascular papillae, that extend to approximately one third of the thickness of the squamous epithelium [2]. In the normal esophagus, the LP comprises non-fibrotic, reticular collagen filaments and the epithelium is devoid of eosinophilic infiltration. Therefore, epithelial eosinophilia indicates a pathologic condition [3] (Fig. 6.1).

S.S. Aceves (✉)
Division of Allergy, Immunology, Departments of Pediatrics and Medicine, University of California, Rady's Children's Hospital, San Diego, CA, USA
e-mail: saceves@ucsd.edu; saceves@rcshd.org

C.A. Liacouras and J.E. Markowitz (eds.), *Eosinophilic Esophagitis*, Clinical Gastroenterology, DOI 10.1007/978-1-60761-515-6_6,

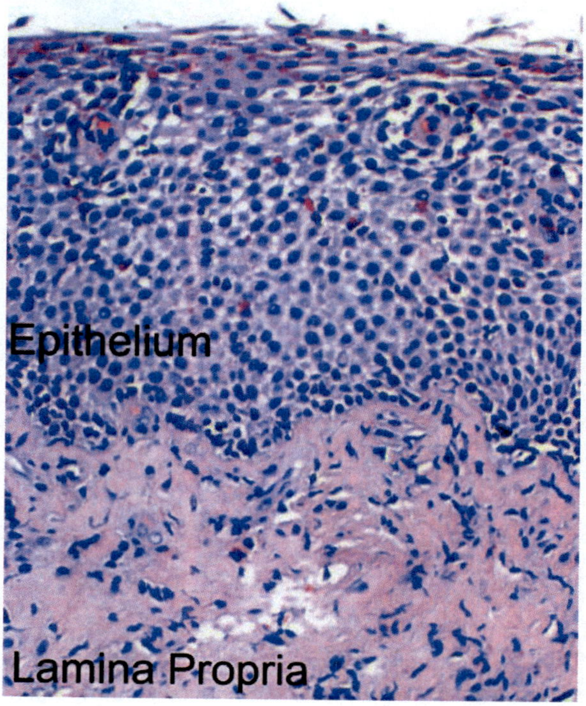

Fig. 6.1 Esophageal pathology in eosinophilic esophagitis. A representative image of a biopsy from an EoE patient demonstrates basal zone hyperplasia and epithelial eosinophil accumulation. The lamina propria demonstrates significant fibrosis with increased collagen density

Esophageal Fibrosis and Remodeling in EoE

Although Eosinophilic Esophagitis (EoE) is a clinicopathological diagnosis with typical endoscopic features such as esophageal pallor, linear furrowing, white plaques, and esophageal strictures as well as characteristic clinical symptoms such as dysphagia, abdominal pain, and poor appetite, ultimately, the diagnosis of EoE relies on the histologic finding of ≥15 eosinophils per high power field despite acid blockade [4]. It should be mentioned that there are several additional disease states that can be accompanied by esophageal eosinophilic infiltration which have not been systematically assessed for associated fibrosis. These include gastroesophageal reflux disease, the hypereosinophilic syndrome, eosinophilic gastroenteritis, inflammatory bowel disease, collagen vascular diseases, and drug reactions [3] (Fig. 6.1).

Subepithelial fibrosis was first noted to be a feature of EoE in adult patients [11]. Histologically, fibrosis can be defined as an increase in the total collagen deposition in the subepithelium [5] and reflects an important component of a more global process referred to as "tissue remodeling". In essence, remodeling is a response of tissue regeneration and repair to injurious and inflammatory states. Tissue remodeling as

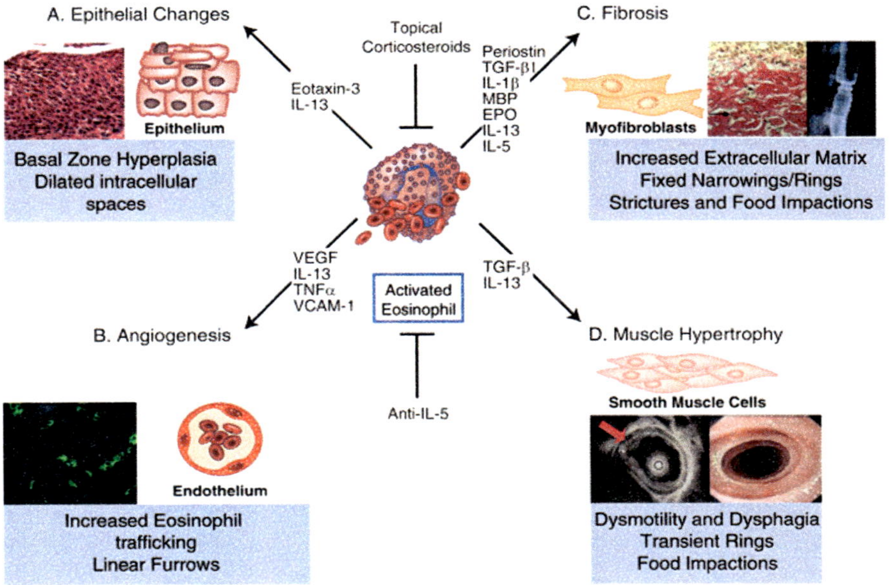

Fig. 6.2 Eosinophil activation and remodeling in EoE: (**a**) Epithelial changes due to epithelial cells in the esophagus increasing eotaxin-3 transcription in a STAT6-dependent manner when stimulated with IL-13 resulting in BZH and intracellular edema. (**b**) Eosinophil expression of vascular endothelial growth factor (VEGF) with vascular cell adhesion molecule-1 activation (VCAM-1) by IL-13 and TNF-α (alpha) increased eosinophil trafficking leads to structural changes including non-stricture food impactions. (**c**) Eosinophil-derived TGF-β induces myofibroblasts which increases the EC matrix leading to fibrosis, rings, strictures, and food impactions. Additional factors likely contributing to fibrosis include periostin, IL-1-β, MBP, EPO, IL-13, and IL-5. (**d**) Activated eosinophils express TGF-β which may induce smooth muscle hypertrophy and dysfunction leading to muscularis propria thickening which can contribute to the development of rings, food impactions, dysmotility, and dysphagia. (*Adapted from* Aceves SS, Ackerman SA. Relationships between eosinophilic inflammation, tissue remodeling, and fibrosis in eosinophilic esophagitis. Immunol Allergy Clin N Am. 2009;29:199; Fox VL, et al. High resolution EUS in children with eosinophilic "allergic" esophagitis. Gastro Endo. 2003;57:31, 33; Aceves SS, Newbury RO, Dohil R, et al. Esophageal remodeling in pediatric eosinophilic esophagitis. J Allergy Clin Immunol. 2007;119:210; with permission.)

a result of Th2 and eosinophilic disease was initially described in the hypereosinophilic syndrome and in asthma [6–9]. Asthmatic airway remodeling has a number of histologic features and has been well characterized to include epithelial cell metaplasia to a mucous-producing phenotype, subepithelial fibrosis, angiogenesis, and smooth muscle hypertrophy and hyperplasia. While animal models have been pivotal in understanding the mechanisms of asthmatic airway remodeling, the true clinical consequences and natural history of human airway remodeling remain enigmatic, especially in children, due to adequate surrogate asthma disease markers such as wheeze, cough, and airway obstruction on pulmonary function testing.

These surrogate markers obviate the need for repeated tissue procurement. As such, the correlations between a patient's clinical state and his/her tissue state are difficult to determine. In contrast, EoE is currently a disease without an adequate serologic or surrogate marker of activity. As such, patients with EoE require repeated tissue biopsy in order to follow their clinical course. This lends investigators the opportunity to study eosinophil-associated tissue remodeling over time and in response to therapy. Importantly, it also will allow us to understand the presence and clinical effects of eosinophil-associated tissue remodeling in young children. In addition, the relevance of remodeling to severe EoE complications such as stricture formation can be evaluated. Indeed, EoE studies have begun to provide a new model for understanding the mechanisms and clinical implications of tissue remodeling in children and adults.

Although first noted in adult patients, esophageal fibrosis also occurs in children with EoE [10, 11]. In 2007, two pediatric studies documented lamina propria fibrosis in pediatric EoE patients. Aceves et al. demonstrated that pediatric patients with long-standing or stricture-associated EoE had significantly more fibrosis than pediatric patients with a histologically normal esophagus or patients with reflux esophagitis [12]. Chehade and colleagues retrospectively reviewed biopsies of EoE patients and found that 57% had subepithelial fibrosis [13]. Notably, of fibrotic patients, 42% had dysphagia and 80% had food impactions. Dysphagia was not part of the EoE symptom complex in the absence of fibrosis and fibrosis appeared to precede the development of dysphagia. Additionally, fibrosis was not significantly linked to peripheral eosinophil counts, duration of symptoms, or the presence of food or environmental allergies. Endoscopically, all patients with concentric rings had both fibrosis and dysphagia [13]. However, further studies done by our group have demonstrated that fibrosis is not isolated to patients with dysphagia, strictures, or concentric rings and can occur even in children as young as 24 months [14]. As such, fibrosis appears to be an integral part of EoE pathogenesis that can begin early in life.

Potential Mechanisms of Esophageal Fibrosis in EoE

Pro-fibrotic Factors

Transforming Growth Factor beta-1 (TGFβ1)

In order to assess potential pro-fibrotic molecules that could contribute to esophageal remodeling in pediatric EoE, we analyzed the expression of transforming growth factor-beta-1 (TGFβ1) and its signaling molecule phosphorylated Smad2/3 (pSmad2/3). TGFβ1 binds to its receptor complex TGFβ RI/RII, resulting in a signal transduction cascade that phosphorylates the Smad transcription factor complex, allowing nuclear translocation and transcriptional activation of pro-fibrotic target genes. Pediatric EoE patients have increased numbers of TGFβ1-positive cells in the lamina propria compared with subjects with gastroesophageal reflux disease (GERD) or patients with a histologically normal esophagus [12]. Consistent with activation of the TGFβ1 signaling pathway, there are increased numbers of nuclear pSmad2/3 positive cells in the lamina propria of EoE patients as compared with GERD or normal patients. Messenger RNA for TGFβ1 is also increased in EoE patients as compared with controls [15]. In vitro studies have suggested the clinical consequences of elevated TGFβ1 in EoE. Using EoE fibroblasts, Blanchard et al. demonstrated that TGFβ1 can increase the production of the extracellular matrix protein, periostin [16]. Importantly, human esophageal eosinophils produce TGFβ1, directly implicating the eosinophil in EoE remodeling.

Interleukin-5

IL-5 is an essential eosinophilopoetic factor that can be sufficient for increasing eosinophil trafficking into the esophagus. IL-5 overexpression using a mini-osmotic pump or T cell transgene results in significant esophageal eosinophil accumulation. In addition, animal models of EoE have demonstrated that intranasal *Aspergillus fumigatus* induces EoE concurrent with pulmonary eosinophilia in Aspergillus challenged mice as compared with naïve mice. In this model system, Aspergillus causes significantly increased collagen accumulation in the lamina propria of allergen-challenged animals. In addition to subepithelial fibrosis, the thickened muscularis mucosa also demonstrates increased collagen deposition in the stromal papillae between the smooth muscle bundles. As such, this animal model reflects multiple components of both esophageal and airway remodeling including fibrosis, muscular hypertrophy, and basal cell proliferation [15].

In addition to fibrosis, Mishra et al. demonstrated further features of esophageal remodeling in allergen-challenged mice. Specifically, transcript levels of TGFβ1 and the mucin MUC5AC gene were increased in allergen-induced EoE as compared with control mice. Interestingly, MUC5AC mRNA levels were also significantly increased in EoE human subjects compared with healthy controls. The role of IL-5 and eosinophils (see below) was shown to be critical in murine EoE-associated esophageal remodeling. IL-5-deficient mice did not show a significant increase in collagen deposition in the lamina propria, stromal papillae, or muscularis mucosa following allergen stimulation. The lamina propria collagen thickness was 21.2 ± 2.2 μm in the allergen-challenged wild type mouse versus 5.2 ± 1.0 μm in the IL-5 gene-deficient mouse. Additionally, the histologic finding of basal zone hyperplasia was significantly lower in the IL-5 knockout mice as compared with allergen-challenged wild type mice [15].

Demonstrating potential sufficiency of IL-5 to induce esophageal remodeling, CD2-IL-5 transgenic mice demonstrate worsened esophageal remodeling with a thickened epithelium, expansion of connective tissue, and collagen accumulation in the lamina propria and the stromal papillae than their wild type counterparts. Interplay of eosinophil chemokines with IL-5 was suggested by the fact that eotaxin-1-deficient CD2-IL-5 double transgenic mice were relatively protected from esophageal remodeling [15]. Interestingly, systemic over-expression of IL-5 did not induce esophageal remodeling, leading to the conclusion that the *local* effects of IL-5 are necessary to induce esophageal remodeling. It is interesting to note that IL-5 and eotaxins can synergize to activate eosinophils and, as such, the induction of eosinophil degranulation may be pivotal to the remodeling process.

Interleukin-13

Murine models have demonstrated that pulmonary expression of IL-13 is sufficient for inducing significant airway fibrosis. Studies have shown that IL-13 mRNA levels are significantly higher in biopsy specimens from EoE pediatric patients when compared with normal controls [17]. Additionally, cultured EoE epithelial cells increase eotaxin-3 transcription in a STAT6-dependent (signal transducer activation transcription-6) manner when stimulated with IL-13 [17, 18]. Interestingly, IL-13 also induces the expression of periostin, which causes increase in eosinophil adherence to the extracellular matrix and subsequent eosinophil accumulation in target tissues, potentially providing a positive feedback loop for esophageal eosinophil trafficking.

Recently, Zuo and colleagues utilized murine models to assess the ability of increased airway IL-13 to induce EoE in the esophagus [19]. Transgenic (CC10-iIL-13) mice, with IL-13 overexpression in the lung, demonstrated increased esophageal IL-13, accumulation of eosinophil and collagen with fibrosis, angiogenesis, and increased overall esophageal circumference. Tissue remodeling appeared to be independent of eosinophils, and IL-13-induced esophageal eosinophilia appeared to be dependent on eotaxin-1 but not on eotaxin-2. Furthermore, an IL-13Rα2 (alpha) deletion caused a significant increase in IL-13 induced fibrosis. These results suggest that tissue remodeling may be largely independent of eosinophils and that IL-13 may be sufficient to induce esophageal fibrosis in vivo. As such, the fibrotic process may be inhibited by IL-13Rα2, which may function as a potential future therapeutic target.

Inflammatory Cells

Eosinophils have long been considered a key cellular component of tissue fibrosis [20] and have been implicated in a variety of diseases as a major effector cell causing fibrogenesis through their production of and interactions with fibrogenic growth factors, such as TGFβ1 [21, 22], PDGF-BB [23], IL-1β [24] and through their granule products such as MBP [25] and eosinophil peroxidase [26]. Eosinophil degranulation has been implicated in several disease states, including EoE. Indeed eosinophil granules alone can respond to IL-5 and function as cell-independent organelles [27].

We initially demonstrated that human esophageal eosinophils in EoE could express TGFβ1 [12]. Definitive proof of the importance of the eosinophil in EoE-associated tissue remodeling comes from Mishra and colleagues who demonstrated that animals lacking eosinophils due to the mutation delta double GATA are protected from EoE-associated fibrosis [15].

Recent data demonstrate that tryptase-positive mast cells in EoE also produce TGFβ1 [29, 30]. Aceves et al. explored the role of mast cells in esophageal smooth muscle, the functional role of mast cell TGF-β1 expression in contractility of human esophageal smooth muscle cells in vitro, and the effect of topical steroid therapy on tryptase-positive mast cells and chymase-positive mast cells. EoE subjects had significantly higher numbers of tryptase-positive mast cells (median of 261 cells/mm^2 in EoE versus median of 85 cells/mm^2 in controls; $p=0.002$) and TGF-β1-positive cells in the smooth muscle as compared to normal controls ($p=0.005$). Interestingly, the tryptase-positive mast cells expressed TGF-β1 which enhanced the contraction of primary human esophageal smooth muscle cells in vitro. While topical budesonide significantly decreased epithelial tryptase-positive mast cells, lamina propria tryptase- and chymase-positive mast cells remained a relatively static population and did not differ between EoE and control subjects. Additionally, they demonstrated the novel finding that in patients with EoE, the absolute number of mast cells in the smooth muscle is significantly greater than the number of eosinophils. As a result, they propose a possible link between the mast cell numbers and the smooth muscle contractility in patients with EoE similar to that seen in asthmatic subjects. As such, mast cells may also participate largely in the fibrotic process during EoE pathogenesis. Studies using mast cell-deficient mice in experimental EoE have not yet been reported.

Structural Cells of the Esophagus

Epithelium

During inflammation or injurious conditions of the esophagus such as acid reflux or EoE, the esophageal layers can be uniformly involved in structural changes. For example, in both reflux and eosinophilic esophagitis, the basal zone can become hyperplastic. In EoE, an active proliferation of the basal cells leads to significant basal zone hyperplasia. Not uncommonly, the basal zone occupies >75% of the total epithelial height in EoE [11]. In addition, the lamina propria papillae elongate and intercellular edema occurs within the esophageal epithelium during EoE [2]. Indeed, basal zone hyperplasia can be considered an epithelial feature of esophageal tissue remodeling. Studies of esophageal tissue from EoE patients have shown increased epithelial expression of eotaxin-3 as the principal mediator of eosinophil recruitment [31].

Fibroblasts

Esophageal fibroblasts have been shown to produce periostin when cultured with TGFβ1 or IL-13; but, their numbers, function, and phenotype as well as their role in disease progression to fibrosis requires further study. A recent abstract demonstrated the potential for epithelial-mesenchymal transformation in EoE, the severity of which correlated with the degree of eosinophilia, TGFβ1 expression, and fibrosis [28].

One of the identified genes in genome-wide expression profiling studies of EoE esophageal tissue was periostin. Studies have shown that primary esophageal fibroblasts release periostin when stimulated with IL-13 and TGFβ [16]. As such, periostin expression in the vascular papillae and lamina propria could increase eosinophil trafficking by allowing eosinophil adhesion to fibronectin [16].

Vascular Changes in Remodeling

Esophageal remodeling, like airway remodeling, is associated with increased vascular density. In 2007, our group reported increased numbers of esophageal blood vessels using the endothelial marker vonWillebrand factor in EoE patients as compared with GERD and normal control patients [12]. Furthermore, EoE patients had increased numbers of blood vessels expressing the activation molecule Vascular Cell Adhesion Molecule (VCAM)-1 as compared with GERD patients and normal controls [12]. It is interesting to postulate that Th2 cytokines such as IL-4 and IL-13 could increase vascular expression of VCAM-1 in EoE, thereby allowing eosinophil and inflammatory cell trafficking via the VCAM-1 ligand, Very Late Antigen (VLA)-4.

Clinical Implications of Esophageal Fibrosis and Response to Therapies

Correlation of Remodeling with Symptoms and Endoscopy

A recently published prospective study demonstrated that features of esophageal remodeling correlated with typical symptoms and endoscopic features in pediatric EoE patients [32]. Specifically, lamina propria fibrosis and inflammation correlates with dysphagia while epithelial inflammation, basal zone hyperplasia, and dilated intracellular spaces correlate with dysphagia + anorexia/early satiety [32]. Endoscopic features also correlate with histological remodeling features. While epithelial changes correlated with white plaques and lichenification/linear furrows, subepithelial fibrosis was associated specifically with lichenification and linear furrows. Interestingly, in our cohort of patients, only the symptoms of dysphagia and anorexia/early satiety were capable of identifying EoE patients from those with reflux esophagitis and remodeling features correlated only with these EoE symptoms [32].

Natural History

The most significant complication of EoE is esophageal stricture formation and it is likely that fibrosis plays an important role in the esophageal narrowing leading to strictures. We have reported that patients who are non-responders to therapy have persistent esophageal remodeling, sometimes with progression of fibrosis [14]. However, the predisposing factors for a more fibrotic EoE phenotype and the predictors for progression to strictures needs to be clarified. The long-term natural history of esophageal fibrosis in EoE patients has not been fully elucidated, but unlike other disease states where repeated tissue procurement is not required as a routine part of clinical care, EoE offers a new ability to answer these important questions.

Effects of Therapeutic Interventions on EoE Associated Esophageal Remodeling

Corticosteroids

The question of whether therapeutic interventions can reduce esophageal remodeling is beginning to be elucidated. Our group recently demonstrated that esophageal remodeling improved following topical corticosteroid use in the subset of patients who responded to therapy [14]. Patients were defined as "responders" (≤7 epithelial eosinophils per hpf following budesonide therapy) and "non-responders" (>20 epithelial eosinophils per hpf following budesonide therapy). Following therapy with oral viscous budesonide for at least 3 months, responders had a significant decrease in the degree of lamina propria fibrosis whereas the non-responders had unchanged fibrosis following treatment with budesonide.

In addition, potential mediators of fibrosis including TGFβ1 and its signaling pathway transcription factor, pSmad2/3, were decreased in the lamina propria of responder patients but not in non-responders following budesonide therapy. The mean number of TGFβ1 positive cells prior to therapy was not significantly different between responders (mean = 84 TGFβ1 positive cells/hpf) and non-responders (mean = 109 TGFβ1 positive cells/hpf). After 3 months of therapy with swallowed budesonide, the responders had significant decreases in the numbers of TGFβ1 positive cells per high power field (hpf) as compared with the non-responders (See Table 6.1) [14].

To assess the effects of steroid therapy on the downstream pathway from $TGF\beta_1$, pSmad2/3 positive cells were examined before and after therapy. Similar numbers of pSmad2/3 positive cells were found before initiation of therapy. After oral viscous budesonide use, the mean number of pSmad2/3 positive cells in responders decreased to 86; non-responders continued to have a mean of 119 pSmad2/3 positive cells per hpf. Similarly, responders demonstrated a decrease in VCAM-1 positive vessels

Table 6.1 Patient data tabulated before and after treatment with oral viscous budesonide

	Responders	Non-responders
Epithelial score	Before tx: 2.2 After tx: 0.2	Before tx: 2.5 After tx: 2.3
LP eosinophils per hpf	Before tx: 12.5 After tx: 1.8	Before tx: 13 After tx: 32
LP fibrosis score	Before tx: 1.6 After tx: 0.67	Before tx: 2.3 After tx: 2.9
$TGF\beta_1$ positive cells per hpf	Before tx: 84 After tx: 35	Before tx: 109 After tx: 97
pSmad2/3 positive cells	Before tx: 152 After tx: 86	Before tx: 156 After tx: 119
VCAM-1 positive vessels per hpf	Before tx: 19 After tx: 13	Before tx: 21 After tx: 20
Dilated Intercellular Spaces	Before tx: 0.55 After tx: 0	Before tx: 0.71 After tx: 0.70

The epithelial score was generated by adding the BZH severity score (graded as 1 to 3 with 1 = 21–50%, 2 = 51–75%, and 3 = >75%) to the Epithelial Desquamation score (graded as 0 = absent, 1 = present). Epithelial edema was determined as dilated intercellular spaces and based on the presence = 1 or absence = 0 of this finding. The LP fibrosis score was assessed using an H&E stain and was graded from 0 to 3 based on the thickness of collagen bundles and the number of fibroblasts present [14]

and epithelial edema following therapy. The non-responders did not have a significant change. It is important to note that the responders and non-responders had similar severity prior to therapy in all aspects of remodeling including fibrosis, TGFβ1, pSmad2/3, and VCAM-1.

As such, it appears that topical corticosteroids are capable of inducing remission and/or improvements in esophageal remodeling in those patients who have decreased esophageal epithelial eosinophil numbers following corticosteroid therapy. However, the dynamic nature of these changes and the potential progression to strictures in non-responder patients remains to be understood.

Anti-IL5

A humanized monoclonal anti-IL5 antibody initially showed promise as a potential treatment option for EoE patients. In one small open-label study, it was demonstrated that anti-IL5 (mepolizumab) therapy was associated with improvement in EoE-associated strictures, esophageal narrowing, basal zone hyperplasia, and eosinophilic inflammation [33]. In contrast, a placebo-controlled adult EoE study showed that mepolizumab monotherapy reduced the average numbers of eosinophils in the esophageal tissue of patients with severe EoE by approximately 55%, but did not effectively reduce patients' clinical symptom scores [34]. In addition to decreases in esophageal eosinophils, Straumann and colleagues reported decreased expression of TGFβ1 following anti-IL-5 as well as decreased expression of tenascin C, a basement membrane protein. Further studies are needed to see if anti-IL-5 reduces subepithelial changes of fibrosis and vascularity. Two recently completed pediatric trials of anti-IL-5 in EoE will help to determine the answers to these questions in children.

Esophageal Dilation

A recent study Schoepfer et al. investigated the effectiveness, safety, and impact of esophageal dilation with or without additive anti-eosinophilic medication on underlying inflammation and fibrosis in EoE patients. They found that esophageal dilation was effective for dysphagia, with a median duration of symptom relief of 15 months with dilation alone and 17 months in the cohort with dilation plus anti-eosinophilic medication [35]. Of note, they did not find a difference in eosinophilic infiltration or total eosinophilic load following dilation. Furthermore, they did not identify any significant difference in basal cell hyperplasia, spongiosis, or papillary elongation pre- versus post-dilation. Schoepfer and colleagues found an increase in submucosal fibrosis with disease duration [35]. In summary, they concluded that dilation is effective at decreasing dysphagia symptoms in the short-term but does not have any effect on the underlying fibrotic changes or on eosinophilic infiltration. Additionally, it is effective for dealing with strictures but does not affect the evolution of fibrosis or EoE itself and thus does not offer a solution to the underlying driving pathology of EoE.

Potential Future Targets to Decrease Esophageal Fibrosis in EoE

Aceves and Ackerman have speculated on different therapies both in the context of additive medications to IL-5 therapy or perhaps as lone therapy. These include blocking eosinophil recruitment through possible antagonism of eotaxin-3 or the eotaxin-3 receptor, CCR3, on eosinophils [5]. As mentioned previously, recent evidence from murine models of EoE show that IL-4, IL-5, IL-13, and STAT-6 signaling are important in the development of experimental EoE and that blockade of these abrogates esophageal eosinophilia [36]. As a result, these cytokines and their signaling pathways may be queried as potential targets for therapy.

IL-13

As noted above, IL-13 has been described as an increasingly important cytokine in the underlying pathology of EoE and esophageal epithelial cells are known to express the IL-13 receptor [18,37]. Blanchard et al. recently reported dysregulation of the epidermal differentiation complex gene (EDC) expression in EoE. The authors examined the effects of IL-13 on EDC gene expression and the presence of gene variants in the EDC gene filaggrin in human subjects with EoE. They concluded that the primary defect in epithelial responses in subjects with EoE is not intrinsic to the epithelium but is more likely secondary to the effects of IL-13, as a regulator of EDC genes [38]. Therefore, agents that interfere with IL-13 could prove to be highly effective for patients with EoE and, if IL-13 is capable of recapitulating remodeling EoE features as it does in asthma, it could possibly aid in the prevention of esophageal fibrosis.

Eotaxin-3 and CCR3 Blockade

Eotaxin-3 has been shown to be the single-most dysregulated gene in esophageal tissue in patients with EoE and an eotaxin-3 gene SNP has been associated with increased susceptibility to EoE [31]. This idea was supported through the use of a murine model where a genetic deletion in the eotaxin-3 receptor, CC chemokine receptor 3 (CCR3), protected mice from developing EoE [31]. Interestingly, IL-4 and IL-13 induce expression of eotaxins [17]. As a result, eotaxin-3 and its receptor CCR3 remain promising potential targets for future therapeutic options.

TGFβ1

Elevated levels of TGFβ1 have been demonstrated in adult and pediatric EoE. Functional consequences of TGFβ1 in EoE include increased expression of pro-fibrotic and pro-eosinophil genes such as periostin [16]. We have demonstrated that a single nucleotide polymorphism in the TGFβ1 gene is associated with therapeutic response in EoE patients [14]. As such, TGFβ1 may serve as a therapeutic target in EoE, especially in patients who are prone to a more fibrotic disease phenotype.

Summary

Overall, the long-term effects of subepithelial esophageal fibrosis in EoE have yet to be fully understood. There is a great deal of promise in terms of the effectiveness of topical esophageal corticosteroid therapy in reversal of fibrotic change in patients who respond to steroid therapy in terms of eosinophil decreases in the epithelium. However, treatment options for the steroid-non-responsive patients still needs to be studied and potential therapies identified. In addition, the genetic predisposition to a fibrotic, stricture-associated variant of EoE requires further investigation.

Acknowledgements The authors thank Dr. Robert Newbury for EE image. Author support from the Women in Allergy Junior Faculty Development Grant and NIH/NIAID R01AI092135 (SSA) and NIHT32 AI training grant to UCSD (LMT).(SSA) and NIH T32 Training grant (LT)

References

1. Odze RD. Pathology of eosinophilic esophagitis: what the clinician needs to know. Am J Gastroenterol. 2009;104(2):485–90.
2. DeNardi FG, Riddell RH. The normal esophagus. Am J Surg Pathol. 1991;15(3):296–309.
3. Bhattacharya B et al. Increased expression of eotaxin-3 distinguishes between eosinophilic esophagitis and gastroesophageal reflux disease. Hum Pathol. 2007;38(12):1744–53.
4. Furuta GT, Straumann A. Review article: the pathogenesis and management of eosinophilic oesophagitis. Aliment Pharmacol Ther. 2006;24(2):173–82.
5. Aceves SS, Ackerman SJ. Relationships between eosinophilic inflammation, tissue remodeling, and fibrosis in eosinophilic esophagitis. Immunol Allergy Clin North Am. 2009;29(1): 197–211. xiii-xiv.
6. Jacobsen EA et al. Eosinophils and asthma. Curr Allergy Asthma Rep. 2007;7(1):18–26.
7. Kay AB, Phipps S, Robinson DS. A role for eosinophils in airway remodelling in asthma. Trends Immunol. 2004;25(9):477–82.
8. Lee JJ et al. Defining a link with asthma in mice congenitally deficient in eosinophils. Science. 2004;305(5691):1773–6.
9. Tai PC et al. Deposits of eosinophil granule proteins in cardiac tissues of patients with eosinophilic endomyocardial disease. Lancet. 1987;1(8534):643–7.
10. Straumann A et al. Natural history of primary eosinophilic esophagitis: a follow-up of 30 adult patients for up to 11.5 years. Gastroenterology. 2003;125(6):1660–9.
11. Parfitt JR et al. Eosinophilic esophagitis in adults: distinguishing features from gastroesophageal reflux disease: a study of 41 patients. Mod Pathol. 2006;19(1):90–6.
12. Aceves SS et al. Esophageal remodeling in pediatric eosinophilic esophagitis. J Allergy Clin Immunol. 2007;119(1):206–12.
13. Chehade M et al. Esophageal subepithelial fibrosis in children with eosinophilic esophagitis. J Pediatr Gastroenterol Nutr. 2007;45(3):319–28.
14. Aceves SS et al. Resolution of remodeling in eosinophilic esophagitis correlates with epithelial response to topical corticosteroids. Allergy. 2010;65(1):109–16.
15. Mishra A et al. Esophageal remodeling develops as a consequence of tissue specific IL-5-induced eosinophilia. Gastroenterology. 2008;134(1):204–14.
16. Blanchard C et al. Periostin facilitates eosinophil tissue infiltration in allergic lung and esophageal responses. Mucosal Immunol. 2008;1(4):289–96.
17. Mishra A, Rothenberg ME. Intratracheal IL-13 induces eosinophilic esophagitis by an IL-5, eotaxin-1, and STAT6-dependent mechanism. Gastroenterology. 2003;125(5):1419–27.
18. Blanchard C et al. IL-13 involvement in eosinophilic esophagitis: transcriptome analysis and reversibility with glucocorticoids. J Allergy Clin Immunol. 2007;120(6):1292–300.
19. Zuo L et al. IL-13 induces esophageal remodeling and gene expression by an eosinophil-independent, IL-13Ra2-inhibited pathway. J Immunol. 2010;184(1):660–9.
20. Gharaee-Kermani M, Phan SH. The role of eosinophils in pulmonary fibrosis (Review). Int J Mol Med. 1998;1(1):43–53.
21. Gauldie J et al. Transforming growth factor-beta gene transfer to the lung induces myofibroblast presence and pulmonary fibrosis. Curr Top Pathol. 1999;93:35–45.
22. Ohno I et al. Transforming growth factor beta 1 (TGF beta 1) gene expression by eosinophils in asthmatic airway inflammation. Am J Respir Cell Mol Biol. 1996;15(3):404–9.
23. Ohno I et al. Eosinophils as a potential source of platelet-derived growth factor B-chain (PDGF-B) in nasal polyposis and bronchial asthma. Am J Respir Cell Mol Biol. 1995;13(6):639–47.

24. Gomes I et al. Eosinophil-fibroblast interactions induce fibroblast IL-6 secretion and extracellular matrix gene expression: implications in fibrogenesis. J Allergy Clin Immunol. 2005;116(4):796–804.
25. Rochester CL et al. Eosinophil-fibroblast interactions. Granule major basic protein interacts with IL-1 and transforming growth factor-beta in the stimulation of lung fibroblast IL-6-type cytokine production. J Immunol. 1996;156(11):4449–56.
26. Pegorier S et al. Eosinophil-derived cationic proteins activate the synthesis of remodeling factors by airway epithelial cells. J Immunol. 2006;177(7):4861–9.
27. Neves JS, Radke AL, Weller PF. Cysteinyl leukotrienes acting via granule membrane-expressed receptors elicit secretion from within cell-free human eosinophil granules. J Allergy Clin Immunol. 2010;125(2):477–82.
28. Akhtar N et al. Epithelial mesenchymal transition in eosinophilic esophagitis: identification and contributions to esophageal remodeling and fibrosis. J Allergy Clin Immunol. 2010;125(2 Suppl 1):161.
29. Aceves SS et al. Mast cells infiltrate the esophageal smooth muscle in patients with eosinophilic esophagitis, express TGF-b1, and increase esophageal smooth muscle contraction. J Allergy Clin Immunol. 2010;126(6):1198–204.
30. Abonia JP, Franciosi JP, Rothenberg ME. TGF-b1: mediator of a feedback loop in eosinophilic esophagitis – or should we really say mastocytic esophagitis? J Allergy Clin Immunol. 2010;126(6):1205–7.
31. Blanchard C et al. Eotaxin-3 and a uniquely conserved gene-expression profile in eosinophilic esophagitis. J Clin Invest. 2006;116(2):536–47.
32. Aceves SS, Newbury R, Dohil MA, Bastian JF, Dohil R. A symptom scoring tool for identifying pediatric patients with eosinophilic esophagitis and correlating symptoms with inflammation. Ann Allergy Asthma Immunol. 2009;103(5):401–6.
33. Stein ML et al. Anti-IL-5 (mepolizumab) therapy for eosinophilic esophagitis. J Allergy Clin Immunol. 2006;118(6):1312–9.
34. Straumann A et al. Anti-interleukin-5 antibody treatment (mepolizumab) in active eosinophilic esophagitis: a randomised, placebo-controlled, double-blind trial. Gut. 2010;59:21–30.
35. Schoepfer AM et al. Esophageal dilation in eosinophilic esophagitis: effectiveness, safety, and impact on the underlying inflammation. Am J Gastroenterol. 2009;105(5):1062–70.
36. Rothenberg ME, Hogan SP. The eosinophil. Annu Rev Immunol. 2006;24:147–74.
37. Kagami S, Saeki H, Komine M. Interleukin-4 and interleukin-13 enhance CCL26 production in a human keratinocyte cell line, HaCaT cells. Clin Exp Immunol. 2005;141:459–66.
38. Blanchard C et al. Coordinate interaction between IL-13 and epithelial differentiation cluster genes in eosinophilic esophagitis. J Immunol. 2010;184(7):4033–41.

Chapter 7
The Genetic Basis of Eosinophilic Esophagitis*

Joseph D. Sherrill and Marc E. Rothenberg

Keywords Eosinophilic esophagitis • Genetic influences • Gene regulatory networks • Polygenic disorder • DNA

Introduction

The epidemiology of eosinophilic esophagitis (EoE), a chronic inflammatory condition of the esophagus, indicates a worldwide increase in disease prevalence over the last 10 years with a disease bias among certain demographic populations [1, 2]. Retrospective studies have shown the prevalence of EoE is almost three times higher in males and is primarily restricted to Caucasians [3, 4]. The disease risk among siblings of EoE patients is estimated to be 40 times higher [5] than the risk of asthma, a more widely prevalent disease with a well-accepted genetic component. These factors suggest that EoE is a polygenic disorder with a heritable genetic basis. Snapshots of whole-genome expression patterns from patient-derived biopsies and genome-wide polymorphism mapping of patient DNA have provided great insight at the molecular level into the genetic influences contributing to EoE. In this chapter, we will highlight seminal studies that have identified critical gene regulatory networks that are operational in EoE and discuss genetic polymorphisms associated with disease susceptibility.

* This work was supported in part by NIH U19 AI070235, NIH R01 DK076893, the PHS Grant P30 DK0789392, Department of Defense, Food Allergy Project, the Buckeye Foundation, the Campaign Urging Research for Eosinophilic Disorders (CURED) Foundation, and the Dana Foundation Human Immunology Consortium. J.D.S. was supported by a T32 NIH training grant (HL091805).

M.E. Rothenberg (✉)
Department of Allergy and Immunology, Cincinnati Children's Hospital Medical Center, University of Cincinnati, MLC 7028, 3333 Burnett Avenue, Cincinnati, OH 45229, USA
e-mail: Rothenberg@cchmc.org

C.A. Liacouras and J.E. Markowitz (eds.), *Eosinophilic Esophagitis*,
Clinical Gastroenterology, DOI 10.1007/978-1-60761-515-6_7,

The EoE Transcriptome

Gene expression profiling of diseased tissue describes in accurate detail the global changes in gene expression that may serve as key molecular markers in disease. Work by Blanchard, et al. used such an approach to analyze whole-genome expression patterns from patient esophageal biopsies and defined a characteristic gene signature that differentiates EoE from normal individuals [6]. The expression levels of 574 genes (230 downregulated and 344 upregulated transcripts) were significantly altered in EoE, representing approximately 1% of transcripts in the human genome. This molecular profile was independent of patient gender, age, and atopic history and correlated with esophageal eosinophil levels. There was also a high level of conservation among sporadic and familial EoE cases [7]. Moreover, there was a clear distinction in gene expression not only between EoE patients and normal controls but also between EoE and non-EoE chronic esophagitis patients [6], indicating the presence of a unique EoE "transcriptome". Interestingly, the EoE transcriptome is dynamic in nature as evidenced by the reversibility of a large majority of the dysregulated genes (98%) in patients responsive to swallowed glucocorticoid therapy, a mechanism that is mediated in part by FK506-binding protein 5 [8]. However, there exists a subset of dysregulated genes including cadherin-like 26, uroplakin 1B, periostin, and desmoglein 1 [9] that are resistant to glucocorticoids, suggesting alternative mechanisms of transcriptional regulation or potential disease-associated mutations affecting glucocorticoid-responsive elements.

A prominent source for the gene transcriptional changes in EoE is the non-immune cells of the esophagus, namely esophageal epithelial cells. Global expression analysis of cultured primary esophageal epithelial cells stimulated with IL-13 recapitulated the transcript profile observed in EoE patient biopsies to a high degree (Spearman $p < 0.0001$) [9]. As expected, many of the non-overlapping genes between the two model systems were immune cell-specific, reflecting the presence of these cell types within the biopsy tissue itself. Taken together, these seminal studies suggest that a large number of gene networks, many of which are sensitive to IL-13, operate synergistically in a conserved and disease-specific manner to contribute to EoE pathogenesis.

The most highly dysregulated gene in the esophagus of EoE patients is the eosinophil chemoattractant eotaxin-3 (CCL26), which was overexpressed 53-fold in EoE esophageal biopsies compared to normal esophageal biopsies. Eotaxin-3 belongs to the eotaxin family of CC chemokines (eotaxins 1–3) that stimulate eosinophil migration through binding to the G protein-coupled receptor CCR3 and activation of downstream signaling pathways. Notably, eotaxins 1 and 2 were not differentially regulated at the transcript level, indicating a specific contribution of eotaxin-3 in the disease [6]. Moreover, the level of eotaxin-3 gene expression correlated with the number of infiltrating eosinophils and mast cells [6]. Eotaxin-3 was also the most highly upregulated gene in cultured esophageal epithelial cells, with IL-13 inducing 279-fold expression compared to untreated cells [9]. Immunofluorescence and in situ hybridization studies on esophageal biopsies localized eotaxin-3 expression within esophageal epithelial cells [6]. In vivo models have further supported the essential role of eotaxin-3 in EoE; for example, CCR3-deficient mice are protected from esophageal eosinophilia following intranasal allergen challenge in a mouse model of experimental EoE [6].

In addition to enhanced expression of eosinophil-associated genes such as eoatxin-3, molecular markers of other key cell lineages involved in EoE have also been established. As previously noted, multiple immune cell types can be found within the esophagus of EoE patients. For instance, the presence of mast cells within the lamina propria and epithelium of the esophagus in addition to eosinophils is a distinguishing feature of EoE that separates the disease from chronic esophagitis [10]. Within the EoE transcriptome, increases in expression levels of mast cell-specific genes including carboxypeptidase A3, high-affinity IgE receptor (FceRI), and mast cell tryptase-α (sigma) were also observed (13-, 4-, and 6-fold, respectively) [6]. Correlated with the increased esophageal mast cell numbers is an increase in resident B cell populations, particularly within the epithelium and vascular papillae; likewise, a similar increase was observed in B cell-specific transcripts involved in class switch recombination and IgE production [11].

The esophageal epithelium is at the forefront of EoE pathogenesis at both the tissue and molecular levels. Many of the pathological features of the esophagus that are associated with EoE indicate gross defects in cell adherence, cell proliferation, and extracellular matrix deposition. Further histological analyses of EoE patient esophageal biopsies have shown intercellular edema and acanthylosis [12], marked basal epithelial hyperplasia, and fibrotic lamina propria [13]. Meanwhile, the effect of IL-13 on esophageal epithelial cell gene expression, including the dramatic induction of eotaxin-3 expression, strikingly mimics the gene expression pattern observed in vivo. Thus, it is not surprising that a vast number of dysregulated genes in EoE regulate critical processes that control epithelial structure and promote tissue remodeling. Spanning a 1.6 Mbp interval on 1q21 is a cluster of genes that regulate terminal differentiation and formation of the cornified envelope of the epithelium termed the epidermal differentiation complex (EDC) [14]. Interestingly, the expression levels of many of the EDC genes including filaggrin and several small proline-rich repeat (SPRR) family members (2C, 2D, and 3) are downregulated in EoE, also implicating a role for the EDC in the diseased state of the esophageal epithelium [15]. The mechanism(s) of downregulation are partially dependent on IL-13, as IL-13 treatment directly dampens transcript levels of filaggrin, involucrin, and SPRR genes in vitro [15]. Loss of filaggrin expression and subsequent defects in epidermal barrier function have been demonstrated in atopic dermatitis [16, 17], which frequently co-occurs with EoE. However, no significant difference in filaggrin expression was observed between atopic and non-atopic EoE patients [15], suggesting an alternative function for filaggrin in regulating the epithelial structure within the human esophagus.

Thus far, the functions of EDC genes have been studied primarily in the context of the epidermis; as a result, little is known about how these genes contribute to the normal architecture of the esophageal epithelium. The epithelium of the human esophagus is comparatively simpler in terms of structure than the epidermis, being composed of stratified squamous epithelial cells and lacking a cornified layer. Despite these histological differences, one hypothesis is that the EDC genes preserve the integrity of the esophageal barrier in a similar fashion as the epidermis and that loss of this function through decreased EDC gene expression could underlie the esophageal tissue fragility that is associated with EoE [18]. Alternatively, esophageal barrier dysfunction could augment exposure to food antigens and contribute to the subsequent development of food allergies that is frequent in EoE patients [19, 20].

Increased expression of additional, non-EDC genes that govern tissue remodeling has also been identified in EoE. Studies of cardiac development and remodeling have described periostin as a cell adhesion molecule that regulates extracellular matrix deposition [21, 22]. Surprisingly, periostin is induced dramatically by 47-fold in the esophagus of EoE patients [6] with periostin protein localized in the lamina propria [23]. TGF-β, which has been shown to be expressed by eosinophils and mast cells in EoE patient biopsies [24, 25], induced a dramatic upregulation of periostin expression in primary esophageal fibroblasts, indicating a potential mechanism for the tissue fibrosis observed in EoE [23]. A functional role for periostin in EoE was evidenced both in vitro and in vivo as exogenous periostin was shown to directly enhance eosinophil adhesion, and periostin-null mice were protected from lung and esophageal eosinophilia following intranasal allergen challenge, respectively [23]. Periostin has also been shown to enhance cross-linking of collagen fibrils by upregulating the cleavage of mature, active lysyl oxidase [26]. Interestingly, a lysyl oxidase family member, lysyl oxidase-like 4 (LOXL4) is induced ninefold in IL-13-treated primary esophageal epithelial cells [9], suggesting a coordinate interaction between two highly upregulated genes (periostin and LOXL4) to synergistically promote esophageal tissue remodeling in EoE.

In summary, the identification of an EoE transcriptome has yielded a global view of the unique changes in gene expression associated with the disease. It has become evident that there exist two broad classifications of dysregulated transcripts, one specific to the infiltrating immune cells within the esophageal biopsies and the other from the affected esophageal epithelium. However, these genes do not act individually to promote disease, but rather act in concert with one another as demonstrated by the effects of IL-13 and TGF-β (beta) on eotaxin-3 and periostin expression, respectively. Thus, while a number of critical genes involved in the development and pathogenesis of EoE have been identified, much work remains in defining the interactions between larger gene networks that can cooperatively affect disease severity.

Genetic Risk Variants in EE

The high rate of EoE within families indicates that genetic heritability plays a predisposing role in disease susceptibility. Approaches commonly employed to identify single nucleotide polymorphisms (SNP)s linked with disease risk typically fall into two categories: the candidate gene approach, which focuses on SNPs in genes known to be potentially involved in a particular disease (based on pathophysiology), and the genome-wide approach, which screens in an unbiased manner for all SNPs across the genome that associate with disease. The availability of the EoE transcriptome paved the way for the identification of the first EoE risk variant in the eotaxin-3 gene [6]. The eotaxin-3 SNP rs2302009 resides in the 3′ untranslated region of the gene with the minor G allele having a frequency of approximately 22% in the Caucasian population. However, the G allele was significantly overrepresented in EE patients (32% compared to 22% in controls) with an associated $p = 0.007$ and odds ratio = 1.63 [6]. The association was further confirmed in a separate family-based model of disease risk allele transmission in which the minor G allele was transmitted more frequently than the T allele ($p = 0.005$, odds ratio = 2.13) from heterozygous parents to an affected offspring [6].

Mutations in a second EoE candidate gene, filaggrin, were screened for by restriction fragment length polymorphism mapping in 329 EoE patients and 157 normal controls [15]. Multiple studies have shown variants of filaggrin are associated with increased susceptibility to atopic dermatitis [27]. One rare filaggrin polymorphism in particular, 2282del4 (rs61816761), results in a null frameshift mutation and was not only identified as a risk variant for atopic dermatitis [28] but also occurred in 3% (20 out of 329) of EoE patients. This association was significant ($p = 0.018$) when compared to 157 normal controls (minor allele frequency = 0.6%) with an odds ratio = 4.89. The combined frequency of 2282del4 and another filaggrin SNP, R501X, which encodes a nonsense mutation, was also significantly associated with EoE ($p = 0.036$, odds ratio = 2.38) compared to normal controls. The results from these candidate gene approaches collectively demonstrate that polymorphisms in two EoE signature genes, eotaxin-3 and filaggrin, confer disease susceptibility. Moreover, the fact that both eotaxin-3 and filaggrin are derived from the esophageal epithelium further underscores the significance of this tissue in disease pathogenesis.

With the progress toward completing the human haplotype map [29] and the advent of SNP genotyping chips capable of genotyping greater than 10^6 SNPs across the human genome, many common variants have been identified as risk variants for multiple heritable human diseases. This genome-wide association approach was used to identify EoE risk variants by interrogating 550,000 SNPs in two independent EoE patient populations ($n_{total} = 351$) and two independent control populations ($n_{total} = 3{,}104$) [30]. Surprisingly, in both case-control cohorts a single EoE susceptibility locus on 5q22.1 was uncovered (Fig. 7.1) in which 11 SNPs resided within a single haplotype block spanning the thymic stromal lymphopoietin (TSLP) and WD-repeat domain 36 (WDR36) genes. TSLP is an epithelial-derived, IL-7-like cytokine shown to act on multiple immune cell types to regulate mucosal immune responses [31], whereas WDR36 is co-regulated with IL-2 expression in activated T cells [32] and is a susceptibility gene for primary open-angle glaucoma [33]. Interestingly, this same chromosome locus was linked with peripheral blood eosinophilia [34], suggesting a role for either TSLP or WDR36 in promoting eosinophilia.

The strongest associated EoE risk variant from the 5q22 block was the SNP rs3806932 located in the upstream region of TSLP, reaching genome-wide significance

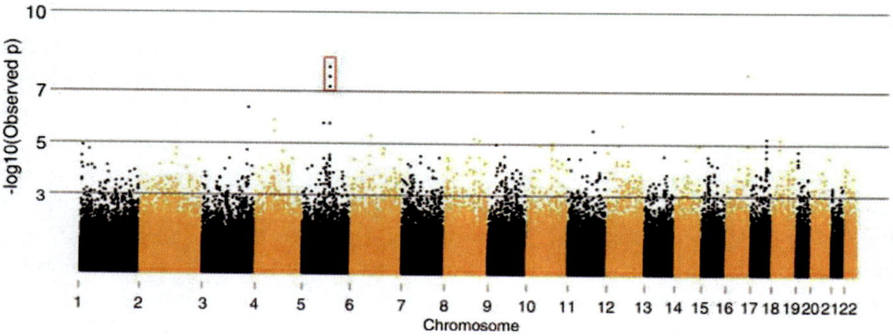

Fig. 7.1 An EoE susceptibility locus on 5q22. A Manhattan plot of the meta-analysis from the two case-control cohorts genotyped in the EoE genome-wide association study is shown. Represented by *dots* are the individual SNPs plotted by chromosomal base pair location and their associated −log10 *p* values. *Highlighted* are the significantly associated SNPs in the 5q22 locus covering the genes encoding TSLP and WDR36. Figure adapted from Rothenberg, et al. Nat Genetics 2010; 42:289–91. Used with permission

with a combined $p = 3.19 \times 10^{-9}$ across the two case-control cohorts and an odds ratio of ~0.6 [30]. Expression analysis from esophageal biopsies showed that TSLP, but not WDR36, mRNA levels were in increased in EoE. Notably, a genotype effect on TSLP expression was observed where EoE patients homozygous for the protective G allele for rs3806932 had significantly lower levels of expression compared to the other genotypes. The dramatic effects of TSLP on dendritic cells [35], B and T lymphocytes, mast cells [36, 37], and eosinophils [38] toward a Th2 phenotype have implicated TSLP as a key initiator of allergic diseases. A role for TSLP in asthma has also been demonstrated by increased TSLP expression in human asthmatic lung lavage fluid [39], asthma-like phenotypes in lung-specific TSLP transgenic mice [40], and the association of TSLP with asthma susceptibility [41, 42]. However, inclusion of patient asthma status had no effect on the association between TSLP variants and EoE, which is particularly remarkable given the high prevalence of asthma in the two EoE patient populations (20–40%) [30]. Further phenotypic analysis using allergic and non-allergic control cohorts demonstrated that the strength of the TSLP SNP association with EoE was independent of allergic status [43]. In this study, an additional association between EoE and a coding SNP (rs36133495, Ala to Val) in the TSLP receptor, which is encoded in a pseudoautosomal region on the X and Y chromosomes, was identified within male EoE patients, suggesting a potential mechanism for the increased male predilection of EoE [43].

The association of polymorphisms in eotaxin-3 and filaggrin and the identification of 5q22 as a susceptibility locus for EE have begun to uncover the role of genetic variation in EoE (Table 7.1). However, much work remains to determine the true causal variants and their effects on gene expression, mRNA stability, and protein translation. In particular, the common frequency of SNPs in the 5q22 haplotype block within the general population suggests that the EoE-associated SNPs are not

Table 7.1 Genetic studies identifying EoE risk variants

Reference	Gene (chromosome)	Study design	SNP	Associated *p*	Odds ratio	Significance
Blanchard et al. [15]	Eotaxin-3 (7q11)	Candidate gene (117 cases, 225 controls) (67 trios)	rs2302009	0.007[a]	1.63[a]	Identifies the first EoE risk variant in the most highly induced EoE transcriptome gene
Rothenberg et al. [30]	TSLP/WDR36 (5q22)	Genome-wide association (351 cases, 3,104 controls)	rs3806932	3.19×10^{-9}[b]	0.54–0.73[c]	Links EoE to genetic susceptibility locus for blood eosinophilia and gene region of Th2 regulating cytokine TSLP; finding replicated in an independent case-control cohort
Blanchard et al. [15]	Filaggrin (1q21)	Candidate gene (329 cases, 157 controls)	rs61816761	0.018	4.89	Associates a rare null mutation in an EDC gene with EoE; mutation previously linked to enhanced atopic dermatitis susceptibility
Sherrill et al. [43]	TSLP (5q22) TSLP receptor (Xp22;Yp11)	Candidate gene (170 cases, 466 controls) (199 male cases, 78 male controls)	rs10062929 rs36133495	3.16×10^{-6}[b] 0.039	0.36–0.45[c] 2.05	Determines the TSLP association is independent of allergic status and validates TSLP as an EoE susceptibility gene. Associates a coding SNP in the TSLP receptor with male EoE patients

[a] *p* value and odds ratio reported for case-control analysis
[b] Fisher's combined *p* value from meta-analysis of all study case-control cohorts
[c] Odds ratio range from all study case-control analyses

causal, but most likely co-segregate with one or more causal variant(s). Moreover, the fact that the identified polymorphisms are present only in a percentage of EoE patients indicates that additional EoE risk variants exist.

Conclusion

Our current understanding of the genetic basis of EoE is that a complex set of esophageal epithelial and immune cell-derived genes involving eotaxin-3, TSLP, and filaggrin, impacted by variation at the single nucleotide level, synergize to create a primed inflammatory environment within the esophagus that is manifested in EoE (Fig. 7.2).

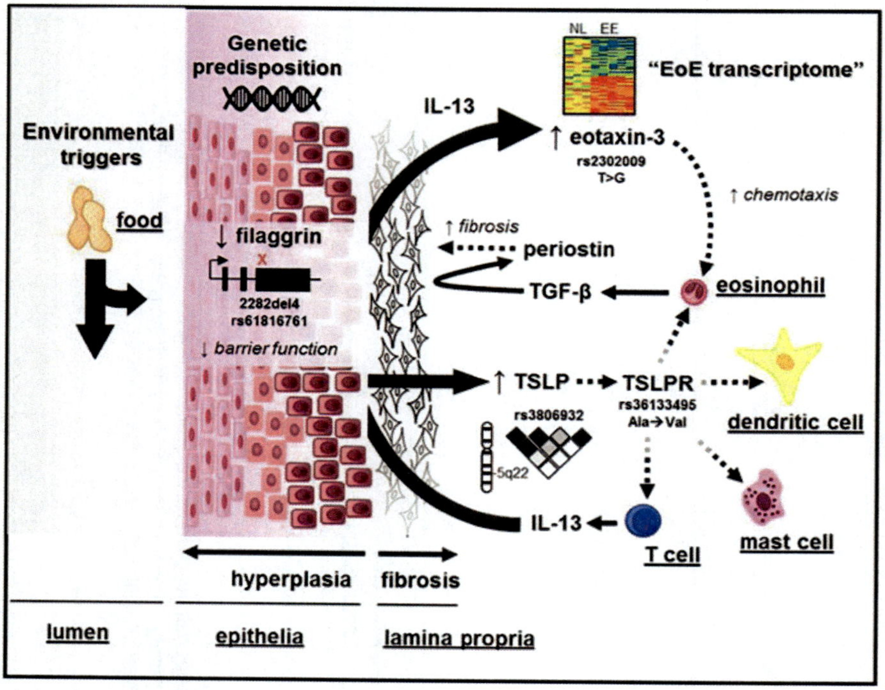

Fig. 7.2 Genetic regulation of the esophageal environment in EoE. The EoE transcriptome, an integrated network of esophageal epithelial- and immune cell-derived gene products that is regulated by IL-13 and/or impacted by genetic polymorphisms, mediates the pathophysiological changes of the esophagus in EoE

References

1. Rothenberg ME. Biology and treatment of eosinophilic esophagitis. Gastroenterology. Oct 2009;137(4):1238–49.
2. Franciosi JP, Tam V, Liacouras CA, Spergel JM. A case-control study of sociodemographic and geographic characteristics of 335 children with eosinophilic esophagitis. Clin Gastroenterol Hepatol. Apr 2009;7(4):415–9.
3. Spergel JM, Brown-Whitehorn TF, Beausoleil JL, et al. 14 years of eosinophilic esophagitis: clinical features and prognosis. J Pediatr Gastroenterol Nutr. Jan 2009;48(1):30–6.
4. Noel RJ, Putnam PE, Rothenberg ME. Eosinophilic esophagitis. N Engl J Med. Aug 2004;351(9):940–1.
5. Blanchard C, Wang N, Rothenberg ME. Eosinophilic esophagitis: pathogenesis, genetics, and therapy. J Allergy Clin Immunol. Nov 2006;118(5):1054–9.
6. Blanchard C, Wang N, Stringer KF, et al. Eotaxin-3 and a uniquely conserved gene-expression profile in eosinophilic esophagitis. J Clin Invest. Feb 2006;116(2):536–47.
7. Collins MH, Blanchard C, Abonia JP, et al. Clinical, pathologic, and molecular characterization of familial eosinophilic esophagitis compared with sporadic cases. Clin Gastroenterol Hepatol. Jun 2008;6(6):621–9.
8. Caldwell JM, Blanchard C, Collins MH, et al. Glucocorticoid-regulated genes in eosinophilic esophagitis: a role for FKBP51. J Allergy Clin Immunol. Apr 2010;125(4):879–88. e878.
9. Blanchard C, Mingler MK, Vicario M, et al. IL-13 involvement in eosinophilic esophagitis: transcriptome analysis and reversibility with glucocorticoids. J Allergy Clin Immunol. Dec 2007;120(6):1292–300.
10. Abonia JP, Blanchard C, Buckmeier BB, et al. Involvement of mast cells in eosinophilic esophagitis. J Allergy Clin Immunol. Jul 2010;126(1):140–9.
11. Vicario M, Blanchard C, Stringer KF, et al. Local B cells and IgE production in the esophageal mucosa in eosinophilic esophagitis. Gut. Jan 2010;59(1):12–20.
12. Parfitt JR, Gregor JC, Suskin NG, Jawa HA, Driman DK. Eosinophilic esophagitis in adults: distinguishing features from gastroesophageal reflux disease: a study of 41 patients. Mod Pathol. Jan 2006;19(1):90–6.
13. Furuta GT, Liacouras CA, Collins MH, et al. Eosinophilic esophagitis in children and adults: a systematic review and consensus recommendations for diagnosis and treatment. Gastroenterology. Oct 2007;133(4):1342–63.
14. South AP, Cabral A, Ives JH, et al. Human epidermal differentiation complex in a single 2.5 Mbp long continuum of overlapping DNA cloned in bacteria integrating physical and transcript maps. J Invest Dermatol. Jun 1999;112(6):910–8.
15. Blanchard C, Stucke EM, Burwinkel K, et al. Coordinate interaction between IL-13 and epithelial differentiation cluster genes in eosinophilic esophagitis. J Immunol. Apr 2010;184(7):4033–41.
16. Fallon PG, Sasaki T, Sandilands A, et al. A homozygous frameshift mutation in the mouse Flg gene facilitates enhanced percutaneous allergen priming. Nat Genet. May 2009;41(5):602–8.
17. O'Regan GM, Sandilands A, McLean WH, Irvine AD. Filaggrin in atopic dermatitis. J Allergy Clin Immunol. Sep 2009;124(3 Suppl 2):R2–6.
18. Jacobs Jr JW, Spechler SJ. A systematic review of the risk of perforation during esophageal dilation for patients with eosinophilic esophagitis. Dig Dis Sci. Jun 2010;55(6):1512–5.
19. Assa'ad AH, Putnam PE, Collins MH, et al. Pediatric patients with eosinophilic esophagitis: an 8-year follow-up. J Allergy Clin Immunol. Mar 2007;119(3):731–8.
20. Spergel JM. Eosinophilic esophagitis in adults and children: evidence for a food allergy component in many patients. Curr Opin Allergy Clin Immunol. Jun 2007;7(3):274–8.
21. Conway SJ, Molkentin JD. Periostin as a heterofunctional regulator of cardiac development and disease. Curr Genomics. Dec 2008;9(8):548–55.
22. Snider P, Hinton RB, Moreno-Rodriguez RA, et al. Periostin is required for maturation and extracellular matrix stabilization of noncardiomyocyte lineages of the heart. Circ Res. Apr 2008;102(7):752–60.

23. Blanchard C, Mingler MK, McBride M, et al. Periostin facilitates eosinophil tissue infiltration in allergic lung and esophageal responses. Mucosal Immunol. Jul 2008;1(4):289–96.
24. Aceves SS, Newbury RO, Dohil R, Bastian JF, Broide DH. Esophageal remodeling in pediatric eosinophilic esophagitis. J Allergy Clin Immunol. Jan 2007;119(1):206–12.
25. Aceves SS, et al. JACI. Dec 2010;126(6):1198–204.
26. Maruhashi T, Kii I, Saito M, Kudo A. Interaction between periostin and BMP-1 promotes proteolytic activation of lysyl oxidase. J Biol Chem. Apr 2010;285(17):13294–303.
27. Barnes KC. An update on the genetics of atopic dermatitis: scratching the surface in 2009. J Allergy Clin Immunol. Jan 2010;125(1):16–29. e1–11; quiz 30–11.
28. Palmer CN, Irvine AD, Terron-Kwiatkowski A, et al. Common loss-of-function variants of the epidermal barrier protein filaggrin are a major predisposing factor for atopic dermatitis. Nat Genet. Apr 2006;38(4):441–6.
29. International HapMap Consortium. The International HapMap Project. Nature. Dec 2003;426(6968):789–96.
30. Rothenberg ME, Spergel JM, Sherrill JD, et al. Common variants at 5q22 associate with pediatric eosinophilic esophagitis. Nat Genet. Apr 2010;42(4):289–91.
31. Ziegler SF, Artis D. Sensing the outside world: TSLP regulates barrier immunity. Nat Immunol. Apr 2010;11(4):289–93.
32. Mao M, Biery MC, Kobayashi SV, et al. T lymphocyte activation gene identification by coregulated expression on DNA microarrays. Genomics. Jun 2004;83(6):989–99.
33. Monemi S, Spaeth G, DaSilva A, et al. Identification of a novel adult-onset primary open-angle glaucoma (POAG) gene on 5q22.1. Hum Mol Genet. Mar 2005;14(6):725–33.
34. Gudbjartsson DF, Bjornsdottir US, Halapi E, et al. Sequence variants affecting eosinophil numbers associate with asthma and myocardial infarction. Nat Genet. Mar 2009;41(3):342–7.
35. Soumelis V, Reche PA, Kanzler H, et al. Human epithelial cells trigger dendritic cell mediated allergic inflammation by producing TSLP. Nat Immunol. Jul 2002;3(7):673–80.
36. Allakhverdi Z, Comeau MR, Jessup HK, et al. Thymic stromal lymphopoietin is released by human epithelial cells in response to microbes, trauma, or inflammation and potently activates mast cells. J Exp Med. Feb 2007;204(2):253–8.
37. Okayama Y, Okumura S, Sagara H, et al. FcepsilonRI-mediated thymic stromal lymphopoietin production by interleukin-4-primed human mast cells. Eur Respir J. Aug 2009;34(2):425–35.
38. Wong CK, Hu S, Cheung PF, Lam CW. TSLP induces chemotactic and pro-survival effects in eosinophils: implications in allergic inflammation. Am J Respir Cell Mol Biol. Sep 2010;43(3):305–15.
39. Ying S, O'Connor B, Ratoff J, et al. Expression and cellular provenance of thymic stromal lymphopoietin and chemokines in patients with severe asthma and chronic obstructive pulmonary disease. J Immunol. Aug 2008;181(4):2790–8.
40. Zhou B, Comeau MR, De Smedt T, et al. Thymic stromal lymphopoietin as a key initiator of allergic airway inflammation in mice. Nat Immunol. Oct 2005;6(10):1047–53.
41. He JQ, Hallstrand TS, Knight D, et al. A thymic stromal lymphopoietin gene variant is associated with asthma and airway hyperresponsiveness. J Allergy Clin Immunol. Aug 2009;124(2):222–9.
42. Harada M, Hirota T, Jodo AI, et al. Functional analysis of the thymic stromal lymphopoietin variants in human bronchial epithelial cells. Am J Respir Cell Mol Biol. Mar 2009;40(3):368–74.
43. Sherrill JD, Gao PS, Stucke EM, et al. Variants of thymic stromal lymphopoietin and its receptor associate with eosinophilic esophagitis. J Allergy Clin Immunol. Jul 2010;126(1):160–5.

Chapter 8
Relationships Between Eosinophilic Esophagitis and Eosinophilic Gastroenteritis

Dan Atkins and Glenn T. Furuta

Keywords Eosinophilic esophagitis • Eosinophilic gastroenteritis • Mucosal eosinophilia • Eosinophilic gastrointestinal diseases

Introduction

Over the last two decades, an increased recognition of gastrointestinal mucosal eosinophilia has heightened awareness and stimulated discussion regarding a number of often confusing but clinically relevant questions. What constitutes pathological mucosal eosinophilia? What are pathophysiolgical mechanisms leading to this response? What diseases are characterized by mucosal eosinophilia? What treatments resolve mucosal eosinophilia and its associated symptoms? This chapter will focus on describing the differences between and similarities shared by a narrow group of diseases referred to as eosinophilic gastrointestinal diseases or EGIDs. EGIDs are a group of gastrointestinal diseases characterized by a wide range of abdominal symptoms that occur in association with intestinal eosinophilia, when other causes of eosinophilia have been ruled out [1, 2]. Traditional descriptions of these diseases categorized them by histological groupings (mucosal, muscular, serosal) whereas more recent classifications have subdivided EGIDs by the primary organ affected [eosinophilic esophagitis, eosinophilic gastritis (EG), eosinophilic gastroenteritis (EGE) and eosinophilic colitis (EC)] [2, 3].

G.T. Furuta (✉)
National Jewish Health, University of Colorado Denver School of Medicine,
The Children's Hospital Denver, Denver, CO, USA

Gastrointestinal Eosinophilic Diseases Program, Children's Hospital Colorado,
National Jewish Health, University of Colorado Denver School of Medicine,
13123 East 16th Ave. B290, Aurora, CO 80016, USA
e-mail: glenn.furuta@childrenscolorado.org

C.A. Liacouras and J.E. Markowitz (eds.), *Eosinophilic Esophagitis*,
Clinical Gastroenterology, DOI 10.1007/978-1-60761-515-6_8,

Historical Perspective

Kaijser first described eosinophilic gastroenteritis in 1937 in the German surgical literature as a heterogeneous group of diseases characterized by abdominal symptoms and intestinal eosinophilia [4]. In 1970, Klein published a case series of seven patients with eosinophilic gastroenteritis and divided them into different subtypes according to where the eosinophilia was predominant, i.e., mucosal, muscular and serosal disease [3]. This categorization provides a useful clinical paradigm that correlates with disease presentation: i.e. mucosal disease presents with diarrhea or bleeding, muscular involvement often manifests with symptoms of obstruction and serosal disease with ascites. The publication of two studies that spanned 57 years and included 99 patients provided the greatest insights into the clinical features and natural history of eosinophilic gastroenteritis [5, 6]. In 1990, Tally et al. published their experiences with 40 adults with eosinophilic gastroenteritis who were seen from 1950 to 1987 [5]. According to the Klein criteria, patients were categorized into mucosal disease (23), muscular disease (12) and subserosal disease (5) phenotypes. In 2010, the same group published their experience with 59 patients seen from 1987 to 2007 with an observed shift to predominantly mucosal disease (52) compared to muscular disease (3) and subserosal disease (4) [6]. While the clinical experience documents that EG is a rare disease with only three patients per year seen in a large tertiary care center (out of four million patients total), these studies document a rise from approximately one patient per year from 1950 to 1987 to three patients per year from 1897 to 2007. No complications were identified in these patients although the long-term follow-up period was short. Thus, over the past 7 decades, a diverse set of patients has been described with idiopathic gastrointestinal eosinophilia and a variety of distinct and perhaps changing phenotypes.

Concurrent with these reports, findings in another group of patients were leading to the definition of another disorder involving mucosal eosinophilia in another part of the GI tract. The first report surfaced in 1978, when an adult patient with achalasia and esophageal eosinophilia was described [7]. Over the course of the next 15 years a series of case reports described esophageal rings and strictures as the radiological hallmarks of eosinophilic esophagitis or EoE [8, 9]. In 1993 and 1994, two articles described 22 adults with isolated esophageal eosinophilia and dysphagia [10, 11]. These early reports provided clear clinical descriptions of adults with dysphagia accompanied by endoscopic findings of esophageal rings, furrows and exudates were accompanied by esophageal eosinophilia. In 1995, ten children were described with symptoms of GERD recalcitrant to medical and, in some cases surgical management, with esophageal eosinophilia, who responded to an elemental formula [12]. Together, these reports set the stage for the coming decades during which the clinicopathological features of a new esophageal inflammatory disease, EoE, would be recognized and refined. The acronym of EoE will be used in this chapter because the original acronym of EE is often confused with *erosive esophagitis* by gastroenterologists.

In summary, EGIDs have become increasingly recognized as a group of diseases that present with a variety of abdominal complaints that share a unifying histological feature, intestinal eosinophilia. Though linked by the presence of an eosinophilic infiltrate, EoE, EG, EGE and EC, also share distinct clinical phenotypes that are important to recognize.

Gastrointestinal Mucosal Eosinophils

Enumeration of Eosinophils

While the normal presence of eosinophils in the mucosae of the stomach, intestine and colon is well recognized, the exact numbers that distinguish physiological from pathological eosinophilic infiltration is uncertain. Two studies, one from Dallas, Texas and another from Cincinnati, Ohio, have addressed this in small numbers of children [13, 14]. These studies compared the numbers of eosinophils along the entire length of the gastrointestinal tract yielding two strikingly similar findings. First, eosinophils increase in numbers within the mucosae along the length of the gastrointestinal tract. Second, the greatest numbers of eosinophils are present in the distal small bowel and cecum. The reasons for this pattern of eosinophil distribution are unclear but speculations include various environmental factors (dietary patterns and climate), host factors (age, gender) and/or the specific microenvironmental conditions of each intestinal organ that may be dictated by exposure to various food particles, enzymes and/or microbiota.

Metrics used to distinguish "physiological" from "pathological" numbers of eosinophils in routine practice and research studies are quite varied and include: eosinophil number (presence of one/both nuclear lobes in conjunction with eosin-stained granules), degranulation, size of a high power field (HPF), number of HPFs counted, mucosal location of the eosinophils (epithelia, lamina propria etc.) and number of biopsies examined [15–19]. Other associated morphological features such as presence of other inflammatory cells that might aid in defining chronicity of the inflammation may also be helpful. In a busy clinical practice, routine scrutiny, this level of detail may not be possible, but it is often critical in isolated cases in which eosinophils predominate. For example, "reactive eosinophilia" may actually represent a normal host response rather than a pathological finding. As the clinical need increases and research progresses, these features and others will need to be examined in greater detail and, in some circumstances, validated. Other studies to document mucosal inflammation such as contrast radiography, capsule visualization, CAT and MRI scans, push enteroscopy and others await further definition and validation. Interpretations of histological patterns is of paramount importance only when taking into consideration the clinical context in which they were obtained.

Esophageal Eosinophilia

In comparison to other areas of the GI tract, the histological interpretation of esophageal eosinophilia is reasonably straightforward. Since eosinophils are not found in the healthy esophagus, the presence of eosinophils usually indicates a pathological process. The predominant causes of esophageal eosinophilia are gastroesophageal reflux disease and eosinophilic esophagitis. Symptomatic individuals with >15 eosinophils/HPF in whom other etiologies have been excluded and who respond to anti-allergic treatments including dietary exclusions and steroids, have eosinophilic esophagitis [20]. The diagnostic decision point of 15 eos/HPF was agreed upon after vigorous debate among a group of pediatric and adult gastroenterologists, pathologists and allergists during the First International Gastrointestinal Eosinophil Research Symposium in 2006 [21]. The basis for this choice was founded on clinical experiences of those involved as well as the current published literature. This threshold was intentionally set on the low end with the proviso that all other causes of esophageal eosinophilia had been excluded. Continuing scrutiny will likely lead to a revision of this criterion as more data emerges and clinical experience increases.

Eosinophilia of the Stomach, Small Intestine and Colon

In contrast, interpretation of mucosal eosinophilia in GI organs distal to the esophagus is complex requiring astute judgement and careful consideration of whether the finding is related to a pathological process or represents an appropriate response to an exogenous insult. Because of the current lack of clarity in diagnostic criteria for these EGIDs, the finding of mucosal eosinophilia has sometimes led to the over diagnosis of EGIDs in patients who may in fact have functional abdominal pain or inflammatory bowel diseases.

Pathophysiological Mechanisms Associated with Mucosal Eosinophilia

When considering the mechanisms that result in eosinophil migration to the intestinal mucosa, it is critical to consider the regulation of this process in at least four separate locations [22]. The bone marrow is the site of differentiation, maturation and proliferation of progenitor cells into eosinophils. The vascular endothelium regulates the selective transport of eosinophils to mucosal sites. When stimulated, a variety of cells in the intestinal mucosae release chemotactic factors, forming gradients that beckon eosinophils to their terminal locations. Finally, resident and recruited cells in the mucosae stimulate newly arrived eosinophils in a regulated fashion to synthesize and release biologically active products including granule proteins, cytokines, arachidonic acid mediators and reactive oxygen species. To date, the extent of the consequences of these eosinophil products in the gastrointestinal tract are unknown, but correlations with findings in other organs can be speculated. For instance, studies of the murine lung associate the presence of activated eosinophils with increased smooth muscle contraction, diminished epithelial permeability, goblet cell hyperplasia and tissue remodelling.

Esophageal Eosinophilia

Murine models of esophageal eosinophilia have been developed that, similar to the human condition, rely on chronic exposure of the esophageal mucosa to an exogenous immunogen [23–26]. Murine systems utilized the ubiquitous aeroallergen, *Aspergillus fumigates* and more recently extracts from, cockroach/dust mites to stimulate esophageal eosinophilia. To determine which eosinophil-associated chemokines control this response, experiments were performed using IL-5 and eotaxin-1 null mice. In contrast to the robust esophageal eosinophilia observed in wild type mice, IL-5 null mice were significantly protected from eosinophilia [24]. Additional studies showed that eotaxin-1 was sufficient, but not necessary for esophageal eosinophilia. Translational studies support a role for IL-5 in this response. Mucosal biopsies from adults with EoE have provided immunohistochemical evidence of increased IL-5 [27].

On the basis of these findings, several therapeutic trials have been performed using IL-5 as a therapeutic target. In the first two case series, a dramatic reduction in eosinophilia, symptomatology, mucosal eosinophilia and in once case, resolution of esophageal stenosis was reported [28, 29]. Since then a blinded study of 11 adults showed that intravenous anti-IL5 infusions lead to a significant decrease in esophageal eosinophils and remodelling mediators and a slight, but not significant, reduction in dysphagia [30]. This lack of symptom reduction is likely due to redundant pathways promoting eosinophilia and the lack of scoring systems that adequately measure symptoms. In fact, basic and translational studies support roles for a number of other mediators including IL-13, eotaxin-3 and thymic stromal lymphopoeitin in the pathogenesis of EoE [31–33].

Although eosinophils remain the hallmark of EoE, their exact functional role in this disorder remains uncertain. Functional studies have shown that EoE patients exhibit increased sensitivity to intraluminal noxious stimuli and have altered motility with increased isolated contractions but do not demonstrate increased acid or non-acid reflux [34–37]. Murine research and translational studies in humans support a role for eosinophils in esophageal remodelling and fibrosis [38–42]. Studies remain technologically encumbered by the fact that tissue sampling is limited to the superficial mucosa and that esophageal functional assessments are invasive, uncomfortable, time-consuming and expensive. Overcoming these hurdles will allow further understanding of eosinophil functions in esophagitis.

Eosinophilia of the Stomach, Small Intestine and Colon

In contrast to the above studies, less is known about the pathogenesis of eosinophilia in gastrointestinal organs beyond the esophagus. Most studies have focused on the clinical and histological descriptions of EG, EGE and EC, but several basic studies have shed light on mechanisms of eosinophil participation in GI inflammation. Using murine models, eotaxin-1 has been shown to be the key mediator for eosinophil accumulation in the gastric mucosa [43–45]. Following sensitization and challenge to ovalbumin, wild type mice developed eosinophilic gastritis and gastric dysmotility. When the same protocol was administered to eotaxin-1 deficient mice, eosinophilia was diminished to the level observed in unchallenged control mice. Translational studies have shown that the immune milieu of the mucosa affected by eosinophilia is skewed towards a Th2 phenotype [46].

Several studies have identified a key role for eosinophils in colitis. Following induction of chemically induced colitis with dextran sodium sulfate (DSS), the colonic mucosae of mice develop increased mucosal eosinophilia [47–49]. When DSS is administered to mice deficient in eosinophils, colitis is diminished as evidenced by disease activity indices and histological parameters. In vitro studies determined that eosinophils can participate in loss of epithelial barrier function and induction of proinflammatory cytokine release from mast cells [50–53].

Whether these studies are truly reflective of the pathophysiology of EGIDs remains to be determined. Goals of future studies will be to account for the genetic predisposition toward a Th2/eosinophilic response, altered development of oral tolerance, mechanisms governing an altered epithelial barrier predisposing to sensitization upon exposure, impact of microbial populations/microbial sensing in different GI mucosal microenvironments on the development of eosinophilic inflammation and the role of exogenous/swallowed food, chemicals and medications on the epithelia and mucosa.

Clinical Implications of Mucosal Eosinophilia

Whereas the previous section identified different potential pathophysiological mechanisms for mucosal eosinophilia, it is important to consider the clinical ramifications of this finding in different parts of the GI tract and their potential impact on therapeutic interventions.

Differences Between EoE and Other EGIDs

Clinical presentations. EoE occurs with an estimated prevalence of 1–4 in 10,000, has a male predominance and typically presents with GERD-like symptoms in the young and food impaction/dysphagia in adolescents and adults [20]. The esophagus affected by EoE typically appears abnormal as manifested by edema and exudates in children and evidence of remodelling in adults. Bleeding is rare and the mucosa often feels "rubbery" during procurement of mucosal biopsies [54]. In contrast, limited data suggest that other EGIDs occur much less frequently than EoE, do not show gender predilection, and present with bleeding, diarrhea, or abdominal pain [1]. Epithelial exudates as seen on endoscopy in patients with EoE is rare. The typical endoscopic findings in EGIDs include mucosal friability, ulceration and polyp formation with some mucosal surfaces appearing normal.

Complications. Some patients with EoE develop strictures that are localized or occasionally involve long segments of the esophagus. In addition, the esophageal mucosa can become "fragile" and disrupt longitudinally, sometimes merely in response to passage of the endoscope [55]. Ulceration is rarely seen in children with EoE. In contrast, strictures or narrowings are not commonly reported in other EGIDs. Symptoms of partial obstruction are typically related to muscular involvement but fibrosis is not a typical finding. It is difficult to know whether this problem is fully recognized in other EGIDs because of the limitations of endoscopic analysis; push enteroscopy and capsule endoscopy may allow for better characterization of EGIDs in the future.

Similarities Between EoE and EGID

Mucosal eosinophilia does not typically "spread". To date, clinical experiences suggest that esophageal eosinophilia usually remains stable over time and does not spread proximally towards the mouth or distally to the stomach, small intestine or colon. Nonetheless, EGIDs can be patchy diseases that can be missed by random mucosal biopsies. It is important to remember that typical mucosal pinch biopsies, obtained at the time of an endoscopy, are limited to sampling 3 mm of the mucosal surface. In the esophagus, this size biopsy represents 0.01% of the total esophageal surface area and much less in the rest of the GI tract. If a patient with EoE begins developing lower intestinal symptoms such as diarrhea or blood in the stool, studies to identify the etiologic causes should be obtained. Depending on symptom severity, this may be limited to simple stool studies or lactose breath tests, or, alternatively, require colonoscopy and capsule endoscopy to determine if other causes exist. In contrast, if dysphagia develops in someone with eosinophilic colitis, EoE may be present and a barium esophagram and upper endoscopy may be necessary.

No obvious trend toward malignancy. Malignant potential does not appear to be increased in any EGID. Case reports describe adults with Barrets esophagus, myofibroblastic esophageal malignancy and leiomyomatosis in association with esophageal eosinophilia [56–58]. Whether these represent chance occurrences or true relationships with EoE is not yet certain [59]. EGIDs themselves have not been associated with other gastrointestinal or extraintestinal malignancies but mucosal eosinophilia in itself has been associated with malignancies or their associated treatments. Prior to assigning a diagnosis of EGIDs, malignancy or a drug effect should be considered and/or ruled out in the appropriate clinical setting.

Feeding/eating dysfunction. An emerging body of literature implicates EGIDs in the development of feeding dysfunction in children [60–65]. Whether this represents a non-specific occurrence that occurs with any gastrointestinal inflammatory disease or is unique to EGIDs remains to be determined. Nonetheless, when children exhibit significant evidence of feeding dysfunction, especially if they have atopic diseases, EGIDs, as well as other GI diseases such as gastroesophageal reflux disease (GERD) or food allergy, should be considered as a potential underlying cause. In adults, eating problems may manifest themselves as coping behaviors. A patient may deny problems with swallowing or eating, but, in fact, may have developed strategies that permit the ingestion of foods that allow for the avoidance of symptoms. For instance, chewing food for long periods, swallowing food with a glass of water or cutting foods into small pieces may have developed over time.

Therapeutic Implications of Mucosal Eosinophilia

The majority of patients with EGIDs, regardless of the type, respond to treatment with corticosteroids. However, the vehicle used to administer the corticosteroid may vary.

Systemic administration of corticosteroids provides therapeutic benefit in most patients with EGIDs. Alternatively, topical steroids have successfully reduced clinicopathological features of EoE, despite the fact that the exact distribution and pharmacokinetics remain unknown. Some patients do not respond to steroid preparations for a number of reasons including a lack of corticosteroid receptors, non-adherence, inadequate delivery to the target mucosa site or improper administration technique and inadequate dosing.

A large body of data underscores the clinical impact of dietary exclusions in the treatment of EoE and some EGIDs. Clinical experiences suggest that the more proximal the eosinophilia in the gastrointestinal tract, the more likely that a nutritional approach involving dietary elimination will be effective.

Summary

Eosinophilic gastrointestinal diseases (eosinophilic esophagitis, eosinophilic gastritis, eosinophilic gastroenteritis and eosinophilic colitis) represent a broad category of diseases with different clinicopathological features and likely different pathogenetic mechanisms. EoE appears to be increasing in incidence while other EGIDs remain rare. Though both are characterized by increased eosinophils in the gastrointestinal tissues and associated with allergic diseases, increasing evidence suggests that there may be different mechanisms responsible for this histological finding depending on the organ involved. Over the course of the next decades, phenotypic patterns of EGIDs will continue to be identified by observant health care providers. Identifying the specific mechanisms governing these phenotypes will reveal a number of novel molecular pathways. Identification of these pathways and their associated biomarkers, will allow for targeted treatments, monitoring protocols and prevention strategies.

References

1. Fleischer DM, Atkins D. Evaluation of the patient with suspected eosinophilic gastrointestinal disease. Immunol Allergy Clin North Am. 2009;29:53–63. ix.
2. Rothenberg ME. Eosinophilic gastrointestinal disorders (EGID). J Allergy Clin Immunol. 2004;113:11–28. quiz 29.
3. Klein NC, Hargrove RL, Sleisenger MH, Jeffries GH. Eosinophilic gastroenteritis. Medicine (Baltimore). 1970;49:299–319.
4. Kaijser R. Zur Kenntnis der allergischen affecktionen des verdauungsekanals vom standpunkt des chirurgen aus. Arch Klin Chir. 1937;188:36–64.
5. Talley NJ, Shorter RG, Phillips SF, Zinsmeister AR. Eosinophilic gastroenteritis: a clinicopathological study of patients with disease of the mucosa, muscle layer, and subserosal tissues. Gut. 1990;31:54–8.
6. Chang JY, Choung RS, Lee RM, Locke III GR, Schleck CD, Zinsmeister AR, et al. A shift in the clinical spectrum of eosinophilic gastroenteritis toward the mucosal disease type. Clin Gastroenterol Hepatol. 2010;8:669–75. quiz e88.
7. Landres RT, Kuster GG, Strum WB. Eosinophilic esophagitis in a patient with vigorous achalasia. Gastroenterology. 1978;74:1298–301.
8. Picus D, Frank PH. Eosinophilic esophagitis. AJR Am J Roentgenol. 1981;136:1001–3.
9. Vitellas KM, Bennett WF, Bova JG, Johnston JC, Caldwell JH, Mayle JE. Idiopathic eosinophilic esophagitis. Radiology. 1993;186:789–93.
10. Attwood S, Smyrk T, Demeester T, Jones J. Esophageal eosinophilia with dysphagia. A distinct clinicopathologic syndrome. Dig Dis Sci. 1993;38:109–16.
11. Straumann A, Spichtin HP, Bernoulli R, Loosli J, Vogtlin J. Idiopathic eosinophilic esophagitis: a frequently overlooked disease with typical clinical aspects and discrete endoscopic findings. Schweiz Med Wochenschr. 1994;124:1419–29.
12. Kelly KJ, Lazenby AJ, Rowe PC, Yardley JH, Perman JA, Sampson HA. Eosinophilic esophagitis attributed to gastroesophageal reflux: improvement with an amino acid-based formula. Gastroenterology. 1995;109:1503–12.
13. DeBrosse CW, Case JW, Putnam PE, Collins MH, Rothenberg ME. Quantity and distribution of eosinophils in the gastrointestinal tract of children. Pediatr Dev Pathol. 2006;9:210–8.
14. Lowichik A, Weinberg A. A quantitative evaluation of mucosal eosinophils in the pediatric gastrointestinal tract. Mod Pathol. 1996;9(2):110–4.
15. Collins MH. Histopathology associated with eosinophilic gastrointestinal diseases. Immunol Allergy Clin North Am. 2009;29:109–17. x-xi.
16. Dellon ES, Aderoju A, Woosley JT, Sandler RS, Shaheen NJ. Variability in diagnostic criteria for eosinophilic esophagitis: a systematic review. Am J Gastroenterol. 2007;102(10):2300–13.
17. Mueller S, Aigner T, Neureiter D, Stolte M. Eosinophil infiltration and degranulation in oesophageal mucosa from adult patients with eosinophilic oesophagitis: a retrospective and comparative study on pathological biopsy. J Clin Pathol. 2006;59:1175–80.
18. Mueller S, Neureiter D, Aigner T, Stolte M. Comparison of histological parameters for the diagnosis of eosinophilic oesophagitis versus gastro-oesophageal reflux disease on oesophageal biopsy material. Histopathology. 2008;53:676–84.

19. Odze RD. Pathology of eosinophilic esophagitis: what the clinician needs to know. Am J Gastroenterol. 2009;104:485–90.
20. Furuta GT, Liacouras CA, Collins MH, Gupta SK, Justinich C, Putnam PE, et al. Eosinophilic esophagitis in children and adults: a systematic review and consensus recommendations for diagnosis and treatment. Gastroenterology. 2007;133:1342–63.
21. Liacouras C, Bonis PA, Putnam PE, Straumann A, Ruchelli E, Gupta SK, et al. Summary of First International Gastrointestinal Eosinophil Research Symposium. J Pediatr Gastroenterol Nutr. 2007;45:370–91.
22. Rothenberg ME, Hogan SP. The eosinophil. Annu Rev Immunol. 2006;24:147–74.
23. Akei HS, Mishra A, Blanchard C, Rothenberg ME. Epicutaneous antigen exposure primes for experimental eosinophilic esophagitis in mice. Gastroenterology. 2005;129:985–94.
24. Mishra A, Hogan SP, Brandt EB, Rothenberg ME. IL-5 promotes eosinophil trafficking to the esophagus. J Immunol. 2002;168:2464–9.
25. Mishra A, Rothenberg ME. Intratracheal IL-13 induces eosinophilic esophagitis by an IL-5, eotaxin-1, and STAT6-dependent mechanism. Gastroenterology. 2003;125:1419–27.
26. Rayapudi M, Mavi P, Zhu X, Pandey AK, Abonia JP, Rothenberg ME, et al. Indoor insect allergens are potent inducers of experimental eosinophilic esophagitis in mice. J Leukoc Biol. 2010;88:337–46.
27. Straumann A, Bauer M, Fischer B, Blaser K, Simon HU. Idiopathic eosinophilic esophagitis is associated with a T(H)2-type allergic inflammatory response. J Allergy Clin Immunol. 2001;108:954–61.
28. Garrett JK, Jameson SC, Thomson B, Collins MH, Wagoner LE, Freese DK, et al. Anti-interleukin-5 (mepolizumab) therapy for hypereosinophilic syndromes. J Allergy Clin Immunol. 2004;113:115–9.
29. Stein ML, Collins MH, Villanueva JM, Kushner JP, Putnam PE, Buckmeier BK, et al. Anti-IL-5 (mepolizumab) therapy for eosinophilic esophagitis. J Allergy Clin Immunol. 2006;118:1312–9.
30. Straumann A, Conus S, Grzonka P, Kita H, Kephart G, Bussmann C, et al. Anti-interleukin-5 antibody treatment (mepolizumab) in active eosinophilic oesophagitis: a randomised, placebo-controlled, double-blind trial. Gut. 2010;59:21–30.
31. Zuo L, Fulkerson PC, Finkelman FD, Mingler M, Fischetti CA, Blanchard C, et al. IL-13 induces esophageal remodeling and gene expression by an eosinophil-independent, IL-13R alpha2-inhibited pathway. J Immunol. 2010;185:660–9.
32. Rothenberg ME, Spergel JM, Sherrill JD, Annaiah K, Martin LJ, Cianferoni A, et al. Common variants at 5q22 associate with pediatric eosinophilic esophagitis. Nat Genet. 2010;42:289–91.
33. Blanchard C, Wang N, Stringer KF, Mishra A, Fulkerson PC, Abonia JP, et al. Eotaxin-3 and a uniquely conserved gene-expression profile in eosinophilic esophagitis. J Clin Invest. 2006;116:536–47.
34. Krarup AL, Villadsen GE, Mejlgaard E, Olesen SS, Drewes AM, Funch-Jensen P. Acid hypersensitivity in patients with eosinophilic oesophagitis. Scand J Gastroenterol. 2010;45:273–81.
35. Lucendo AJ, Arias A, Perez-Martinez I, Lopez-Vazquez A, Ontanon-Rodriguez J, Gonzalez-Castillo S, et al. Adult patients with eosinophilic esophagitis do not show an increased frequency of the HLA-DQ2/DQ8 genotypes predisposing to celiac disease. Dig Dis Sci. 2011;56(4):1107–11.
36. Nurko S, Rosen R, Furuta GT. Esophageal dysmotility in children with eosinophilic esophagitis: a study using prolonged esophageal manometry. Am J Gastroenterol. 2009;104(12):3050–7.
37. Rosen R, Furuta G, Fritz J, Donovan K, Nurko S. Role of acid and nonacid reflux in children with eosinophilic esophagitis compared with patients with gastroesophageal reflux and control patients. J Pediatr Gastroenterol Nutr. 2008;46:520–3.
38. Mishra A, Wang M, Pemmaraju VR, Collins MH, Fulkerson PC, Abonia JP, et al. Esophageal remodeling develops as a consequence of tissue specific IL-5-induced eosinophilia. Gastroenterology. 2008;134:204–14.
39. Chehade M, Sampson HA, Morotti RA, Magid MS. Esophageal subepithelial fibrosis in children with eosinophilic esophagitis. J Pediatr Gastroenterol Nutr. 2007;45:319–28.

40. Abu-Sultaneh SM, Durst P, Maynard V, Elitsur Y. Fluticasone and food allergen elimination reverse sub-epithelial fibrosis in children with eosinophilic esophagitis. Dig Dis Sci. 2011;56(1):97–102.
41. Aceves SS, Newbury RO, Chen D, Mueller J, Dohil R, Hoffman H, et al. Resolution of remodeling in eosinophilic esophagitis correlates with epithelial response to topical corticosteroids. Allergy. 2010;65:109–16.
42. Dohil R, Newbury R, Fox L, Bastian J, Aceves S. Oral viscous budesonide is effective in children with eosinophilic esophagitis in a randomized, placebo-controlled trial. Gastroenterology. 2010;139:418–29.
43. Hogan S, Mishra A, Brandt E, Royalty M, Pope S, Zimmerman N, et al. A pathological function for eotaxin and eosinophils in eosinophilic gastrointestinal inflammation. Nat Immunol. 2001;2:353–60.
44. Hogan SP, Foster PS, Rothenberg ME. Experimental analysis of eosinophil-associated gastrointestinal diseases. Curr Opin Allergy Clin Immunol. 2002;2:239–48.
45. Hogan SP, Mishra A, Brandt EB, Foster PS, Rothenberg ME. A critical role for eotaxin in experimental oral antigen-induced eosinophilic gastrointestinal allergy. Proc Natl Acad Sci USA. 2000;97:6681–6.
46. Schmid-Grendelmeier P, Altznauer F, Fischer B, Bizer C, Straumann A, Menz G, et al. Eosinophils express functional IL-13 in eosinophilic inflammatory diseases. J Immunol. 2002;169:1021–7.
47. Forbes E, Murase T, Yang M, Matthaei KI, Lee JJ, Lee NA, et al. Immunopathogenesis of experimental ulcerative colitis is mediated by eosinophil peroxidase. J Immunol. 2004;172:5664–75.
48. Brandt EB, Zimmermann N, Muntel EE, Yamada Y, Pope SM, Mishra A, et al. The alpha4b-beta7-integrin is dynamically expressed on murine eosinophils and involved in eosinophil trafficking to the intestine. Clin Exp Allergy. 2006;36:543–53.
49. Forbes E, Hulett M, Ahrens R, Wagner N, Smart V, Matthaei KI, et al. ICAM-1-dependent pathways regulate colonic eosinophilic inflammation. J Leukoc Biol. 2006;80:330–41.
50. Furuta GT, Ackerman SJ, Lu L, Williams RE, Wershil BK. Stem cell factor influences mast cell mediator release in response to eosinophil-derived granule major basic protein. Blood. 1998;92:1055–61.
51. Furuta GT, Nieuwenhuis EE, Karhausen J, Gleich G, Blumberg RS, Lee JJ, et al. Eosinophils alter colonic epithelial barrier function: role for major basic protein. Am J Physiol Gastrointest Liver Physiol. 2005;289:G890–7.
52. Michail S, Abernathy F. A new model for studying eosinophil migration across cultured intestinal epithelial monolayers. J Pediatr Gastroenterol Nutr. 2004;39:56–63.
53. Michail S, Mezoff E, Abernathy F. Role of selectins in the intestinal epithelial migration of eosinophils. Pediatr Res. 2005;58:644–7.
54. Fox VL. Eosinophilic esophagitis: endoscopic findings. Gastrointest Endosc Clin N Am. 2008;18:45–57. viii.
55. Straumann A, Rossi L, Simon HU, Heer P, Spichtin HP, Beglinger C. Fragility of the esophageal mucosa: a pathognomonic endoscopic sign of primary eosinophilic esophagitis? Gastrointest Endosc. 2003;57:407–12.
56. Francalanci P, De Angelis P, Minnei F, Diomedi Camassei F, Torroni F, Dall'Oglio L, et al. Eosinophilic esophagitis and Barrett's esophagus: an occasional association or an overlap disease? Esophageal "double trouble" in two children. Digestion. 2008;77:16–9.
57. Wolfsen HC, Hemminger LL, Achem SR. Eosinophilic esophagitis and Barrett's esophagus with dysplasia. Clin Gastroenterol Hepatol. 2007;5:A18.
58. Morris CD, Wilkinson J, Fox D, Armstrong GR, Attwood SE. Diffuse esophageal leiomyomatosis with localized dense eosinophilic infiltration. Dis Esophagus. 2002;15:85–7.
59. Mukkada V, Atkins D, Furuta GT. Uncertain association of Barrett's esophagus with eosinophilic esophagitis. Clin Gastroenterol Hepatol. 2008;6:832. author reply 832–3.
60. Chelimsky G, Czinn SJ. Techniques for the evaluation of dyspepsia in children. J Clin Gastroenterol. 2001;33:11–3.

61. Duca AP, Dantas RO, Rodrigues AA, Sawamura R. Evaluation of swallowing in children with vomiting after feeding. Dysphagia. 2008;23:177–82.
62. Haas AM, Maune NC. Clinical presentation of feeding dysfunction in children with eosinophilic gastrointestinal disease. Immunol Allergy Clin North Am. 2009;29:65–75. ix.
63. Mukkada VA, Haas A, Maune NC, Capocelli KE, Henry M, Gilman N, et al. Feeding dysfunction in children with eosinophilic gastrointestinal diseases. Pediatrics. 2010;126(3):e672–7.
64. Pentiuk SP, Miller CK, Kaul A. Eosinophilic esophagitis in infants and toddlers. Dysphagia. 2007;22:44–8.
65. Spergel JM, Brown-Whitehorn TF, Beausoleil JL, Franciosi J, Shuker M, Verma R, et al. 14 years of eosinophilic esophagitis: clinical features and prognosis. J Pediatr Gastroenterol Nutr. 2009;48:30–6.

Chapter 9
Clinical Manifestations of Eosinophilic Esophagitis in Children

Philip E. Putnam

Keywords Eosinophilic esophagitis • Dietary antigens • Dysphagia • Eosinophil inflammation • Esophageal dilation • Lamina propria fibrosis

Introduction

Eosinophilic esophagitis (EoE) is a condition that affects nearly all ages. The histological features are unmistakable, but the clinical features are nonspecific and vary among individuals as well as across age ranges. The clinical manifestations are explored and placed into context for the evaluating physician.

EoE is a chronic disease with rare spontaneous remission, but it is manageable such that symptoms and inflammation can be kept at bay with consistent, effective therapy for most individuals. Patients and their physicians need to understand that the process of establishing the diagnosis and maintaining control over the inflammation are intertwined and require attention over many years.

EoE typically develops as a manifestation of adverse reaction to food antigens, although there is a clear subset of patients whose esophagitis does not respond to any degree of dietary elimination, up to and including an elemental diet with an amino acid-based formula. For reasons that have not been fully elucidated, EoE occurs mainly in males, many of whom have other manifestations of atopy, such as chronic rhinitis, eczema, asthma, or food allergies.

P.E. Putnam (✉)
Division of Gastroenterology, Hepatology, and Nutrition,
Cincinnati Children's Hospital Medical Center,
3333 Burnet Ave, ML 2010, Cincinnati, OH 45229, USA

Cincinnati Center for Eosinophilic Disorders,
3333 Burnet Ave, ML 2010, Cincinnati, OH 45229, USA
e-mail: phil.putnam@cchmc.org

C.A. Liacouras and J.E. Markowitz (eds.), *Eosinophilic Esophagitis*,
Clinical Gastroenterology, DOI 10.1007/978-1-60761-515-6_9,

Some of the overt manifestations of the esophagitis may be difficult to separate from those of the atopy (e.g., sore throat). To further complicate the evaluation of children who have EoE as a manifestation of food allergy, it is common for a child or caregiver to alter the diet or environment in response to consistent or perceived exposure-related symptoms. For example, vomiting generated consistently by exposure to a particular food often results in elimination of that antigen before any evaluation has been undertaken. If the diagnosis is EoE, ongoing symptoms despite the withdrawal of that antigen will drive additional investigation, and the existing eosinophilic inflammation will most likely be a response to at least one other dietary antigen to which there is insufficient immediate response to recognize the association.

The challenge for the evaluating physician is to understand that symptoms may have been affected by direct or empiric therapeutic maneuvers. To complicate the evaluation, symptoms vary by age, and the age at onset of symptoms and the age at presentation can be quite disparate. Therefore, the physician must be cognizant of the stage in the condition that the evaluation is taking place. Some symptoms may have come and gone, others may have progressed, and some may have been managed by prior attempts at therapy.

The physician's role is made more difficult by the information from recent studies that have determined that there is little predictable correlation between symptoms and the degree of histologic esophagitis [1]. One cannot assume that the absence of symptoms is a reflection of the absence of inflammation, and some symptoms may persist despite the resolution of histologic esophagitis.

The goal of therapy for EoE is control over symptoms and resolution of esophagitis [2]. The disparity between symptoms and the degree of esophagitis creates a dilemma for the treating physician. If significant injury to the esophageal wall occurs as a consequence of chronic inflammation, and if the inflammation is present without symptoms, the inflammation must be controlled even in the absence of symptoms. Lamina propria fibrosis, seen in children and adults who have EoE, has been seen to improve with therapy, such that prevention of permanent injury should be possible with well-maintained treatment [3]. Progressive fibrosis consequent to inadequate control over the inflammation responds, if temporarily, to esophageal dilatation, but dilatation should not be necessary with effective treatment [4, 5]. To summarize, assessment of both symptoms and histology is required to direct treatment and assure consistent control over the inflammatory process.

Symptoms

Esophageal inflammation of any sort has the potential to cause chest pain, odynophagia, or dysphagia. Associated symptoms, such as nausea, vomiting, effortless regurgitation, early satiety, poorly localized abdominal pain, and anorexia, are less specific reflections of esophageal pathology that have been reported by children who have EoE. Individuals who have EoE can present with any combination of these [6–10].

Case series have reported that symptoms from EoE vary by age in a fashion that is not universal, but common enough to warrant comment [11]. Age may also interfere symptom reporting. The evaluation of young children is necessarily affected by interpretation and reporting by an observer (the parent or caregiver) rather than the patient, so there is always some element of uncertainty as to the sophistication and precision of the report, particularly when the outward manifestation of esophagitis is nonspecific (e.g., poor feeding).

Infants and toddlers are more likely to present with difficulty feeding, manifest as gagging, choking, food refusal, and perhaps vomiting. Early school age children tend to present with vomiting or abdominal pain, whereas overt dysphagia is most common in adolescents and adults. These generalizations have held up quite well across several case series, but there are individuals whose symptoms are different from those more commonly reported by their age cohort.

Dysphagia

The term "dysphagia" has been diluted somewhat in pediatric practice in recent years, being used more broadly to indicate feeding problems rather than being strictly applied to disordered swallowing. The term does not distinguish well between disorders of oropharyngeal swallowing and pure esophageal problems. Feeding disorders may well include overt dysphagia, but infants or toddlers who are developmentally unable to describe accurately those abnormal sensations and perceptions that interfere with their ability to feed successfully may be labeled as having dysphagia despite the absence of overt esophageal pathology. Physical and psychological interference with feeding develop as a consequence of a multitude of disorders in children, including EoE [12]. Feeding disorders are one of the more common presentations in toddlers who have EoE, but the lack of history from the affected child precludes an understanding of exactly why. Extrapolating from the descriptions from older children, one may speculate that toddlers have pain, nausea, or the perception of food going down slowly that result in symptoms, such as food refusal or aversion, gagging or retching.

Intermittent or persistent dysphagia, which is the most common symptom from EoE in adults, tends to appear in late childhood or early adolescence. Although possible at younger ages, it is often the primary complaint in adolescents. It is not unusual for an adolescent to present with a food impaction that requires urgent admission for endoscopic removal of the bolus [13]. Those individuals, who have complete esophageal obstruction complain of something being stuck (usually meat), are unable to swallow their saliva and have no overt respiratory compromise. They are easily recognized in the Emergency Department – carrying a vessel of some sort containing their clear saliva, which they must expectorate instead of swallow. The esophageal lumen is full of liquid above the impaction, such that any further attempt to swallow would be unsuccessful and lead to spillage into the airway, causing coughing and choking. Those with near complete obstruction are able to successfully swallow enough saliva, such that they do not need the container, but they are nevertheless unable to swallow a bolus of anything else and are acutely aware of something being stuck.

Endoscopy with biopsies at the time of food bolus retrieval is both immediately therapeutic and diagnostic, with biopsies setting into motion the process of explaining the dysphagia and treating the underlying disorder to prevent future impactions. It is good practice to biopsy the esophagus remote from the position of the bolus, in any child or adult with a food impaction [14]. Even a nonfood foreign body, such as a coin, may fail to pass through an inflamed esophagus, so an exam of the esophagus apart from the foreign body is important to make the diagnosis when the opportunity presents itself.

Food bolus impactions in those who have EoE generally occur in the absence of overt luminal narrowing by either stricture or small caliber esophagus. Manometric abnormalities are nonspecific, but the efficiency of peristalsis must be sufficiently diminished to preclude normal food bolus transit [15].

As a symptom, dysphagia from EoE may be of any degree, and it may be intermittent, persistent, or progressive. Older individuals with chronic dysphagia tend to do a remarkable job of adapting to the limitation in swallowing by eating slowly, drinking extra fluids to encourage passage through the esophagus, and by avoiding the food textures and consistencies that are most problematic for them (e.g., meat and thick breads). Many children deny or underreport their dysphagia, having gained sufficient compensatory skill to avoid the symptom without recognizing exactly why they eat the way they do.

Pain is not a significant feature of a dysphagia, but when present should suggest a diagnosis other than EoE, even if the patient also has the perception of impaired esophageal transit. Pill-induced esophagitis and viral esophagitis (usually herpetic) may produce remarkable ulceration of the esophageal mucosa that is very painful. It creates the perception of altered passage of the food bolus, creating dysphagia along with odynophagia. However, when compared to primary dysphagia, the individual who has pill-induced esophagitis is more likely to be bothered by odynophagia and reluctant to attempt to eat because of the pain. The history is usually very suggestive of pill-induced esophagitis, as the patient reports taking medications, such as tetracycline or oral contraceptives without sufficient fluid, and may recall the dose that seemed not to proceed normally down the esophagus.

Dysphagia is not unique to EoE. Progressive dysphagia for solids and liquids associated with regurgitating undigested food, night cough, weight loss and/or recurrent pneumonia are features of achalasia. Achalasia should be apparent on barium esophagography and confirmed by manometric study of the esophagus. The dysphagia of achalasia is qualitatively different from that of EoE and develops insidiously. Because the esophagus becomes progressively dilated due to the distal functional obstruction in well-developed achalasia, it functions like a reservoir, retaining food and liquid that are then available to be regurgitated and potentially aspirated. Common comorbidities of EoE, including food allergy, asthma, eczema, and chronic rhinitis are not expected in achalasia.

In addition to achalasia, the differential diagnosis of dysphagia in a child is relatively limited, and includes foreign body in the esophagus, esophagitis or peptic strictures due to poorly controlled gastroesophageal reflux disease (GERD), Schtazki ring, and extrinsic vascular compression of the esophagus (i.e., by an aberrant subclavian artery). Congenital esophageal strictures do occur, but are rare. Anastomotic strictures after tracheoesophageal fistula (TEF) repair are not unusual. Children who have had a TEF repaired often have dysphagia due to the intrinsic dysmotility of the congenitally abnormal esophagus, even in the absence of overt luminal narrowing at the anastomotic site. Importantly, we and others have diagnosed EoE in children who have VATER syndrome or other condition in which a TEF was the primary anatomic abnormality [16].

Evaluation of Dysphagia

For the physician, dysphagia requires considerable thought and aggressive diagnostic evaluation. The history is crucial to gain an understanding of severity and chronicity. The causes of dysphagia for liquids are different from the causes of dysphagia for solids, so the evaluation is necessarily different depending on the consistency that is mishandled. EoE should only cause dysphagia for solids; therefore, if dysphagia for liquids is the presenting concern, an alternative diagnostic strategy is employed. Warning signs, such as weight loss due to inadequate intake, demand urgent evaluation and effective treatment. It may be difficult to extract the entire picture from an adolescent who is reluctant to admit to having a problem but the family will be well acquainted with the mealtime disruption generated by the dysphagia.

There are no set rules for the evaluation of dysphagia for solids. Videofluoroscopic evaluation of swallowing assesses bolus handling from lips to upper esophagus, but may not include a thorough investigation of the length of the esophagus. Modified barium esophagogram can assess the bolus passage of different consistencies through the esophagus, and is a good method for detecting stenotic areas that impede solid food bolus passage. It may suggest dysmotility if the bolus does not progress normally to the stomach despite normal caliber.

Contrast radiography to document the anatomy and gross function of the esophagus is often performed first to generate a "road map" of the esophagus. The presence, location, and caliber of a stricture should be evident on esophagogram, as should achalasia.

Additional tests available to evaluate the esophagus include esophageal manometry and endoscopy. A tissue diagnosis obtained at endoscopy is essential when an inflammatory disorder is responsible for dysphagia. For mild, intermittent dysphagia that lacks the clinical features of a stricture, endoscopy alone may be sufficient to establish a diagnosis, avoiding the radiation exposure of the contrast studies. Manometric evaluation may be required to confirm the diagnosis of achalasia or other condition that affects esophageal peristalsis in the absence of inflammation, but is not indicated in the routine evaluation of EoE.

Isolated dysphagia for liquids is rarely, if ever, a feature of EoE, but when present in a child who has EoE should promote an aggressive search for other pathology, such as a laryngeal cleft or Chiari malformation (or other posterior fossa or brainstem lesion). Those conditions have been discovered in children who also have EoE. They impact the pharyngeal phase of swallowing and cause choking on liquids. The most direct means for detection of these anomalies include brain MRI with attention to the posterior fossa, and direct laryngoscopy for the cleft.

Pain

Although EoE can create rather striking inflammation endoscopically and histologically, odynophagia is not characteristic of it. Complaints of epigastric or periumbilical abdominal pain may seem illogical as a manifestation of esophagitis, but these complaints are common in children, if vague and nonspecific.

Heartburn and chest pain (sometimes substernal and severe) are associated with EoE, but seldom are sole presenting concerns. Intermittent or chronic sore throat, with the child clearly indicating a pharyngeal rather then intrathoracic source of discomfort is more common in the author's experience.

Pain associated with EoE correlates poorly with the number of eosinophils/hpf on biopsy, does not necessarily improve with treatment on the one hand and may be completely absent despite rather remarkable inflammation on the other [1].

School aged children may present with abdominal pain as the most bothersome manifestation of EoE, and sometimes have symptoms, such as dysphagia, that provide a clinical clue that esophageal pathology may be at fault. One should be particularly concerned for the possibility of EoE in a male who has abdominal pain associated with asthma, eczema, or food allergies.

Vomiting

Vomiting is a very distressing symptom to children and their families, and arguably gets attention earlier than less troublesome concerns. Although the effortless regurgitation of reflux in infancy is common and inconsequential most of the time, overt retching and vomiting is seldom normal. Delayed evaluation and diagnosis remains a dogged complaint from families of babies who vomit but are brushed off by medical providers if weight gain is adequate. The implication that vomiting is acceptable as long as weight gain continues is absurd.

Nonbilious, nonbloody emesis has a very long differential diagnosis that includes EoE. GI physicians typically depend on the history, pattern, and associated symptoms in making an initial assessment as to the etiology of vomiting. Warning signs, such as weight loss, hematemesis, or bilious emesis warrant aggressive evaluation.

Initial study by upper GI series is useful to broadly evaluate for serious conditions that need urgent attention (e.g., pyloric stenosis or malrotation). When anatomic concerns have been allayed, further evaluation for infectious, inflammatory, toxic, metabolic, and nongastrointestinal causes for vomiting is undertaken, with the history and physical directing the order and priority of testing.

Perhaps the most common features of the vomiting associated with EoE is the development of the symptom in the second half of the first year of life when solid foods are introduced to the diet. Often erroneously attributed to reflux, this vomiting is true vomiting, not the effortless regurgitation that characterizes GERD, which usually has already peaked by 6 months of age [17]. On rare occasions, it may be consistently and obviously attributable to the ingestion of a particular food antigen, in which case food has been taken from the diet before presentation to the gastroenterologist or allergist. Chronic, intermittent vomiting not associated with a particular antigen is more often the complaint.

Other Symptoms

Some children are found to have eosinophilic esophageal inflammation during evaluation for symptoms that are clearly not of esophageal origin, such as diarrhea. Diarrhea can be a manifestation of eosinophilic inflammation in the small intestine or colon, and individuals with eosinophilic gastroenteritis may well have esophageal involvement. Children who have other inflammatory bowel disorders, including gluten-sensitive enteropathy (celiac disease) or Crohn's disease can have eosinophil-predominant esophageal inflammation that meets the criteria for EoE histologically [18]. However, it is not appropriate to make a clinical diagnosis of EoE when there is a clear diagnosis of another condition such as Crohn's that could account for the histologic changes. Similarly, the presence of systemic symptoms, such as fever or weight loss, should promote evaluation for a disease process other than EoE.

Children have been diagnosed with EoE after presenting with airway complaints. A good example is recurrent croup, with no symptoms between episodes of croup. It is difficult to conceive of a pathogenetic mechanism that might underlie the development of episodic airway symptoms from esophageal pathology in the absence of clinically significant GERD, but such individuals have been identified. Longitudinal studies to determine the impact of treatment for the EoE on the frequency or severity of the croup have not been reported.

Other respiratory symptoms are common in children with EoE. Chronic rhinitis and reactive airways are the predominant complaints. Presentation to the otorhinolaryngologist with a complaint of hoarseness or adenotonsillar hypertrophy is also possible [18, 19]. It is conceivable that these associated conditions are not primary manifestations of the esophageal inflammation, but rather concurrent manifestations of immune dysregulation or atopy. Irrespective of the mechanism, symptoms, or mode of presentation, active management of the esophagitis is important.

Associated Conditions

EoE does occur in children who have other medical conditions. It has been diagnosed in children who have Down syndrome, Pfeiffer syndrome, VATER syndrome, [syndrome including vertebral defects (V), anal atresia (A), TEF with esophageal atresia (TE), and radial or renal dysplasia (R)], and CHARGE syndrome (association of coloboma of the eye; heart anomaly; atresia, choanal; retardation of mental and somatic development; microphallus; ear abnormalities and/or deafnesscolobomas, heart defect, renal anomaly). There is no evidence to date to suggest or support any sort of common pathogenetic mechanism. The author has observed EoE in children who have other neurological and neurodevelopmental conditions, including cerebral palsy, seizures, autism spectrum, attention deficit disorder, as well as structural brain conditions, such as Chiari malformation. Once again, the association is loose without suggestion of any cause-effect relationship, but the loose association still demands that EoE be included in the differential of gastrointestinal symptoms in these children.

The Impact of Chronic Disease

As noted above, evaluation of the child with EoE might be initiated at one of many points in the course of the illness. Some children who have EoE have had a protracted or more severe course prior to evaluation and may have signs of poorly controlled disease, such as inadequate weight gain, nutritional deficiencies, poor feeding skills, or poor behavior, and limited social skills surrounding meals and feeding. It is arguable that some of these symptoms are primary manifestations of disease, whereas others develop as a consequence chronic illness, difficult therapy, or limited exposure to expected feeding opportunity at critical times during development.

One of the duties of the examining physician is to understand the impact of the condition on the family and the child. Families struggle with multiple issues, some of which are the frustrations of trying to maintain difficult dietary restrictions, the financial impact of medical care, and the cost of special formulas. The impact of the work performed by the parents (and the stress it engenders) to maintain a restricted diet cannot be underestimated. Dietary restrictions affect all aspects of a busy lifestyle. Family mealtime is disrupted, and eating in any other venue, such as a restaurant at school, or at a friend's or relative's home is a challenge. It is somewhat easier to control the diet and environment for preschool children at home on a restricted diet than for older children who are not consistently under the observation of responsible adults. The further loss of control over adolescents, their diet, and their medication is very common in clinical practice, and should be anticipated.

Because EoE is a chronic condition, it is important to assure that patients and their families understand the need for both immediate and sustained therapy, and the potential impact on quality of life of various treatments. Families need to be educated as to the effort that is required to maintain any therapeutic regimen.

Conclusion: A Multidisciplinary Approach

EoE can impact children and their families at many levels – at once physically, socially, emotionally, developmentally, financially. Having a team approach to support the needs of patients and their families is particularly valuable in providing comprehensive care. Core services from gastroenterology, allergy/immunology, and pathology are essential. In addition, substantial support from a dietician, social worker, and speech and language pathologist facilitates global evaluation and treatment. Ready access to other subspecialists who have experience and expertise in EoE and its comorbidities (i.e., otorhinolaryngologist, psychologist or developmental specialist, pulmonologist, and surgeon), assures consistent evaluation and clinical care of associated problems.

References

1. Pentiuk S, Putnam PE, Collins MH, Rothenberg ME. Dissociation between symptoms and histological severity in pediatric eosinophilic esophagitis. J Pediatr Gastroenterol Nutr. 2009;48(2):152–60.
2. Furuta GT, Liacouras CA, Collins MH, Gupta SK, Justinich C, Putnam PE, et al. First International Gastrointestinal Eosinophil Research Symposium (FIGERS) Subcommittees. Eosinophilic esophagitis in children and adults: a systematic review and consensus recommendations for diagnosis and treatment. Gastroenterology. 2007;133(4):1342–63.
3. Aceves SS, Newbury RO, Chen D, Mueller J, Dohil R, Hoffman H, et al. Resolution of remodeling in eosinophilic esophagitis correlates with epithelial response to topical corticosteroids. Allergy. 2010;65(1):109–16.
4. Straumann A, Spichtin HP, Grize L, Bucher KA, Beglinger C, Simon HU. Natural history of primary eosinophilic esophagitis: a follow-up of 30 adult patients for up to 11.5 years. Gastroenterology. 2003;125(6):1660–9.
5. Schoepfer AM, Gschossmann J, Scheurer U, Seibold F, Straumann A. Esophageal strictures in adult eosinophilic esophagitis: dilation is an effective and safe alternative after failure of topical corticosteroids. Endoscopy. 2008;40(2):161–4.
6. Spergel JM, Brown-Whitehorn TF, Beausoleil JL, Franciosi J, Shuker M, Verma R, et al. 14 years of eosinophilic esophagitis: clinical features and prognosis. J Pediatr Gastroenterol Nutr. 2009;48(1):30–6.
7. Orenstein SR, Shalaby TM, Di Lorenzo C, Putnam PE, Sigurdsson L, Mousa H, et al. The spectrum of pediatric eosinophilic esophagitis beyond infancy: a clinical series of 30 children. Am J Gastroenterol. 2000;95(6):1422–30. Erratum in: Am J Gastroenterol. 2001;96(7):2290.
8. Assa'ad AH, Putnam PE, Collins MH, Akers RM, Jameson SC, Kirby CL, et al. Pediatric patients with eosinophilic esophagitis: an 8-year follow-up. J Allergy Clin Immunol. 2007;119(3):731–8.
9. Franciosi JP, Tam V, Liacouras CA, Spergel JM. A case-control study of sociodemographic and geographic characteristics of 335 children with eosinophilic esophagitis. Clin Gastroenterol Hepatol. 2009;7(4):415–9.
10. Velázquez V, Camacho C, Mercado-Quiñones AE, Irizarry-Padilla J. Eosinophilic esophagitis and allergies in the pediatric population of Puerto Rico. Bol Asoc Med P R. 2009; 101(2):21–2.
11. Noel RJ, Putnam PE, Rothenberg ME. Eosinophilic esophagitis. N Engl J Med. 2004; 351(9):940–1.

12. Pentiuk SP, Miller CK, Kaul A. Eosinophilic esophagitis in infants and toddlers. Dysphagia. 2007;22(1):44–8.
13. Robles-Medranda C, Villard F, le Gall C, Lukashok H, Rivet C, Bouvier R, et al. Severe dysphagia in children with eosinophilic esophagitis and esophageal stricture: an indication for balloon dilation? J Pediatr Gastroenterol Nutr. 2010;50(5):516–20.
14. Rajagopalan J, Triadafilopoulos G. Ring(s)-related esophageal meat bolus impaction: biopsy first, dilate later. Dis Esophagus. 2009;22(5):E14–6.
15. Nurko S, Rosen R, Furuta GT. Esophageal dysmotility in children with eosinophilic esophagitis: a study using prolonged esophageal manometry. Am J Gastroenterol. 2009;104 (12):3050–7.
16. Oliveira C, Zamakhshary M, Marcon P, Kim PC. Eosinophilic esophagitis and intermediate esophagitis after tracheoesophageal fistula repair: a case series. J Pediatr Surg. 2008; 43(5):810–4.
17. Nelson SP, Chen EH, Syniar GM, Christoffel KK. Prevalence of symptoms of gastroesophageal reflux during infancy. A pediatric practice-based survey. Pediatric Practice Research Group. Arch Pediatr Adolesc Med. 1997;151(6):569–72.
18. Leslie C, Mews C, Charles A, Ravikumara M. Celiac disease and eosinophilic esophagitis: a true association. J Pediatr Gastroenterol Nutr. 2010;50(4):397–9.
19. Dauer EH, Ponikau JU, Smyrk TC, Murray JA, Thompson DM. Airway manifestations of pediatric eosinophilic esophagitis: a clinical and histopathologic report of an emerging association. Ann Otol Rhinol Laryngol. 2006;115(7):507–17.

Chapter 10
Clinical Presentation of Eosinophilic Esophagitis in Adults

Nirmala Gonsalves

Keywords Eosinophilic esophagitis • Dysphagia • Food impaction • Environmental allergens

Introduction

Over the past decade, eosinophilic esophagitis (EoE) has emerged as one of the most common causes of dysphagia and food impaction in adults. This chronic condition is characterized by increased esophageal eosinophils in the setting of esophageal symptoms. While EoE may occur in conjunction with eosinophilic gastroenteritis, the rising field is related to the subset with isolated esophageal eosinophilia [1]. Development of EoE in adults is likely due to a multitude of factors including esophageal acid exposure, food and environmental allergens, and genetic predisposition. While investigation into each of these areas is actively being studied and discussed in further detail elsewhere in this book, this chapter will highlight the clinical presentation of EoE in adults.

Epidemiology

Over the past 10 years, EoE has become a global epidemic in both adults and children. The estimated incidence of this disease in adults is 0.15 cases per 10,000 and a prevalence of 3 per 10,000 based on data from a Swiss cohort [2]. This trend has also been seen in adults in the US with incidence of adult cases in Olmsted county rising from

N. Gonsalves (✉)
Department of Medicine, Division of Gastroenterology, Northwestern University,
Feinberg School of Medicine, 676 N. St Clair St, Suite 1400, Chicago, IL 60611-2951, USA
e-mail: n-gonsalves@northwestern.edu

C.A. Liacouras and J.E. Markowitz (eds.), *Eosinophilic Esophagitis*,
Clinical Gastroenterology, DOI 10.1007/978-1-60761-515-6_10,

0.35/100,000 person-years in 1995 to 9.45/100,000 person-years in 2005 [3]. Looking at an adult patient population presenting with dysphagia, incidence of EoE has been found to be as high as 6.5% [4]. These numbers suggest that the incidence and prevalence of EoE is approximating that of other more common immunologic disorders such as inflammatory bowel disease [5]. Furthermore, these estimates likely underestimate the true incidence and prevalence of EoE, since these data are based on symptomatic patients presenting for endoscopy.

Clinical Features

The most common initial presentation of adults with EoE is solid food dysphagia. In many adults, symptoms have preceded their diagnosis by 6–7 years [6]. This delay of diagnosis was attributed previously to the lack of recognition of this disease by the medical community. Thankfully, over the past 10 years, increased awareness about this condition in gastroenterologists, allergists, and pathologist have lead to more timely diagnosis and treatment. As a result of this delay, however, many patients have become adept at accommodating for their esophageal dysfunction by chewing well, eating very slowly, drinking excessive liquids during meals, or avoiding their trigger foods. These patients may actually deny dysphagia symptoms upon initial questioning, therefore a careful history including these accommodation skills is essential in eliciting this information.

Other features such as food impaction, heartburn, and chest pain may also be seen [7]. In one series, as many as 50% of adult food impaction cases encountered in an emergency department setting were attributable to EoE and therefore esophageal biopsies performed at the time of a food impaction is advocated to make a timely diagnosis [8]. Caution must also be taken at the time of food impaction as there have been cases of endoscopic perforation during these instances [9]. Patients must also be counseled on seeking medical attention quickly in this setting because there have been cases of spontaneous esophageal perforation in patients trying to dislodge the food bolus by retching.

The patient population in EoE tends to be male predominant in both the adult and pediatric population. Among 323 adult patients in 13 reports, 76% were males with a mean age of 38 years (range 14–89) [7]. Although reports also suggest a Caucasian predilection, EoE has been described more recently in African Americans, Latin-Americans, and Asians [4, 10] There has been no geographic trend for the presentation of EoE in adults in the US as cases have been reported across the country both in rural and urban settings [11].

Historically, this diagnosis was often overlooked in adults with many patients undergoing repeated endoscopies and dilations with alternate diagnoses of Schatzki ring or gastroesophageal reflux disease (GERD) [6]. Another reason for the delay in diagnosis of EoE is that eosinophilic involvement of the esophageal mucosa previously implicated GERD. Some suggested that quantitative thresholds of eosinophilic infiltration made the distinction; lower counts were presumably related to GERD while higher counts being diagnostic of EoE [12]. Such a cut-off value has proven problematic, however, due to the high prevalence of GERD in adults and potential overlap between GERD and EoE.

Due to this dilemma, recent consensus guidelines have advocated that GERD should be adequately treated with acid suppression or ruled out with a pH-monitoring study in the diagnostic workup for EoE [7]. This is especially important because there are increasing number of adults manifesting with both GERD and EoE and the interplay between these two entities is unknown.

EoE should be considered the leading diagnosis in adults presenting with dysphagia and a history of atopic conditions such as asthma, allergic rhinitis, eczema, or atopic dermatitis. In two adult series, allergy testing was used to demonstrate the presence of atopy in adults [13, 14]. In another adult series, season variation in the presentation of EoE in adults was noted suggesting the association of aeroallergens and EoE [15]. While empiric elimination diets have been shown to be therapeutic in adults with EoE, allergy testing was not predictive in these patients [16]. Until more information is gathered on the predictive value of allergy testing in adults with EoE, it is reasonable to have patients undergo an allergic evaluation to help identify potential triggers.

Familial clustering has been recognized in adults and children with EoE, suggesting a genetic predisposition [17–19]. In a case series of 381 pediatric EoE patients, 5% had siblings with EoE and 7% had a parent with either an esophageal stricture or known EoE [20]. Therefore, an important component to include in history taking in adults with EoE is a thorough family history as additional cases may be identified.

The basis for this genetic predisposition to EoE continues to be investigated. Eotaxin-3, a gene encoding an eosinophil-specific chemoattractant, has recently been identified as the most highly induced gene in pediatric EoE patients [21]. Treatment with topical corticosteroids downregulated esophageal eotaxin-3 levels suggesting the change to be reversible [22]. While formal gene analysis has not yet been extensively studied in adults, immunohistochemical staining for eotaxin-3 in esophageal tissue of adult EoE patients was significantly increased compared to patients with reflux suggesting a similar trend to the pediatric data [23]. Another adult study further supporting a role of eotaxin-3 demonstrated increased levels of eotaxin-3 in esophageal tissue of EoE adults compared to controls and found that this gene expression decreased in response to treatment with dietary elimination [24].

Natural History

While defining the natural history and progression of EoE is critical in developing goals of treatment and management of this illness, limited natural history data exist to help guide current recommendations. Given the increased morbidity that can be associated with complications of EoE such as food impactions, a key goal of management is to prevent disease recurrence and complications. In the longest available natural history study, Straumann et al. followed 30 medically untreated adults patients for an average of 7.2 years [25]. During this time, 97% experienced continued dysphagia and one third had undergone esophageal dilation. While esophageal eosinophilia persisted, levels interestingly declined in most patients during the follow-up period. Barrett's metaplasia has been reported in patients with EoE but it is unclear as to whether or not this is a causal relationship [26]. Esophageal malignancy related to EoE has not been reported, but, again, there is limited long-term data available. In the author's experience with a series of 300 adult patients with EoE, patients tended to have symptom progression and increased frequency of food impaction as the years of dysphagia progressed [27].

Conclusion

Eosinophilic esophagitis remains an emerging clinical entity with increasing incidence in adults. Although food and aero allergens have been implicated in the disease, the natural history of the disorder is unknown. Severe complications including fibrosis, narrow caliber esophagus, and stricture are well known but predictors for which patients will develop these complications are unknown. Common symptoms in adults that implicate EoE are dysphagia, food impactions, heartburn, and atypical chest pain. It is important to ask patients about their allergic history including dietary allergies, dietary intolerance, asthma, or seasonal allergy in addition to any family history of these disorders or dysphagia. During endoscopy for suspected EoE in adults, multiple biopsies should be obtained at multiple levels in the esophagus, regardless of endoscopic features due to the patchy nature of the disease [6]. It is also helpful to alert the pathologist of your suspicion and request eosinophil counts on esophageal biopsies. Thankfully, with increased awareness by gastroenterologists, allergists and pathologists over the past several years, EoE is being recognized earlier in adults leading to more effective treatments and hopefully better outcomes for patients.

References

1. Rothenberg ME. Pathogenesis and clinical features of eosinophilic esophagitis. J Allergy Clin Immunol. 2001;108(6):891–4.
2. Straumann A, Simon HU. Eosinophilic esophagitis: escalating epidemiology? J Allergy Clin Immunol. 2005;115(2):418–9.
3. Prasad GA, Alexander JA, Schleck CD, et al. Epidemiology of eosinophilic esophagitis over three decades in Olmsted County, Minnesota. Clin Gastroenterol Hepatol. 2009;7(10):1055–61.
4. Veerappan GR, Perry JL, Duncan TJ, et al. Prevalence of eosinophilic esophagitis in an adult population undergoing upper endoscopy: a prospective study. Clin Gastroenterol Hepatol. 2009;7(4):420–6. 426.e1-2.

5. Kugathasan S, Judd RH, Hoffmann RG, et al. Epidemiologic and clinical characteristics of children with newly diagnosed inflammatory bowel disease in Wisconsin: a statewide population-based study. J Pediatr. 2003;143(4):525–31.
6. Gonsalves N, Policarpio-Nicolas M, Zhang Q, et al. Histopathologic variability and endoscopic correlates in adults with eosinophilic esophagitis. Gastrointest Endosc. 2006;64(3):313–9.
7. Furuta GT, Liacouras CA, Collins MH, et al. Eosinophilic esophagitis in children and adults: a systematic review and consensus recommendations for diagnosis and treatment. Gastroenterology. 2007;133(4):1342–63.
8. Desai TK, Stecevic V, Chang CH, et al. Association of eosinophilic inflammation with esophageal food impaction in adults. Gastrointest Endosc. 2005;61(7):795–801.
9. Shim LS, Grehan M. Oesophageal perforation during endoscopy for food impaction in patients with eosinophilic oesophagitis. J Gastroenterol Hepatol. 2010;25(2):428.
10. Assa'ad A, Putnam PE, Collins MH, et al. Eosinophilic esophagitis: association with allergic disorders. Gastrointest Endosc Clin N Am. 2008;18(1):119–32.
11. Kapel RC, Miller JK, Torres C, et al. Eosinophilic esophagitis in the US: a prevalent disease that affects all age groups. Gastroenterology. 2008;134(5):1316–21.
12. Morrow JB, Vargo JJ, Goldblum JR, et al. The ringed esophagus: histological features of GERD. Am J Gastroenterol. 2001;96(4):984–9.
13. Roy-Ghanta S, Larosa DF, Katzka DA. Atopic characteristics of adults with eosinophilic esophagitis. Clin Gastroenterol Hepatol. 2008;6(5):531–5.
14. Penfield JD, Lang DM, Goldblum JR, et al. The role of allergy evaluation in adults with eosinophilic esophagitis. J Clin Gastroenterol. 2010;44(1):22–7.
15. Almansa C, Krishna M, Buchner AM, et al. Seasonal distribution in newly diagnosed cases of eosinophilic esophagitis in adults. Am J Gastroenterol. 2009;104(4):828–33.
16. Gonsalves N, Yang G, Doerfler B, et al. A prospective clinical trial of six food elimination diet and reintroduction of causative agents in adults with eosinophilic esophagitis. Gastroenterology. 2008;134(4):A104.
17. Patel SM, Falchuk KR. Three brothers with dysphagia caused by eosinophilic esophagitis. Gastrointest Endosc. 2005;61(1):165–7.
18. Meyer GW. Eosinophilic esophagitis in a father and a daughter. Gastrointest Endosc. 2005;61(7):932.
19. Zink DA, Amin M, Gebara S, et al. Familial dysphagia and eosinophilia. Gastrointest Endosc. 2007;65(2):330–4.
20. Liacouras CA, Spergel JM, Ruchelli E, et al. Eosinophilic esophagitis: a 10-year experience in 381 children. Clin Gastroenterol Hepatol. 2005;3(12):1198–206.
21. Blanchard C, Wang N, Stringer KF, et al. Eotaxin-3 and a uniquely conserved gene-expression profile in eosinophilic esophagitis. J Clin Invest. 2006;116(2):536–47.
22. Lucendo AJ, Navarro M, Comas C, et al. Treatment with topical steroids downregulates IL-5, eotaxin-1/CCL11, and eotaxin-3/CCL26 gene expression in eosinophilic esophagitis. Am J Gastroenterol. 2008;103(9):2184–93.
23. Bhattacharya B, Carlsten J, Sabo E, et al. Increased expression of eotaxin-3 distinguishes between eosinophilic esophagitis and gastroesophageal reflux disease. Hum Pathol. 2007;38(12): 1744–53.
24. Gonsalves N, Hsu-Blatman K, Hirano I et al. The role of permeability, inflammation and proliferation genes in adults with eosinophilic esophagitis and their alteration in response to dietary therapy. Gastroenterology. 2010;S1072.
25. Straumann A, Spichtin HP, Grize L, et al. Natural history of primary eosinophilic esophagitis: a follow-up of 30 adult patients for up to 11.5 years. Gastroenterology. 2003;125(6):1660–9.
26. Wolfsen HC, Hemminger LL, Achem SR. Eosinophilic esophagitis and Barrett's esophagus with dysplasia. Clin Gastroenterol Hepatol. 2007;5(12):A18.
27. Toto E, Kern E, Moy N et al. Duration of dysphagia is associated with increased frequency of dysphagia and food impaction in adults with eosinophilic esophagitis. Gastroenterology. 2010;S1088.

Chapter 11
Relationship of Eosinophilic Esophagitis to Gastroesophageal Reflux*

Edaire Cheng, Harland S. Winter, and Stuart Spechler

Keywords Eosinophilic esophagitis • Gastroesophageal reflux disease • Proton pump inhibitor medication • Esophageal pH monitoring • Acid reflux

Introduction

In a recent consensus report sponsored by the American Gastroenterological Association Institute and the North American Society of Pediatric Gastroenterology, Hepatology, and Nutrition, eosinophilic esophagitis (EoE) is defined as "a primary clinicopathologic disorder of the esophagus, characterized by esophageal and/or upper gastrointestinal tract symptoms in association with esophageal mucosal biopsy specimens containing ≥15 intraepithelial eosinophils/HPF and *the absence of pathologic gastroesophageal reflux disease (GERD) as evidenced by a normal pH monitoring study of the distal esophagus or lack of response to high-dose proton pump inhibitor (PPI) medication* [1]. This definition implies that GERD and EoE are mutually exclusive disorders, and that GERD can be defined by an abnormal pH monitoring result or a lack of response to PPI therapy. Esophageal pH monitoring has substantial limitations as a test for GERD, and some patients who have verified reflux esophagitis can have normal esophageal pH monitoring results [2]. Lack of response to PPI therapy is, at best, a subjective index for GERD, and even a positive

*This work was supported by the Office of Medical Research, Department of Veterans Affairs and the National Institutes of Health (R01-CA134571)

S. Spechler (✉)
Department of Medicine, VA North Texas Healthcare System and the University of Texas Southwestern Medical Center, Dallas 75216, TX, USA
e-mail: SJSpechler@AOL.com

C.A. Liacouras and J.E. Markowitz (eds.), *Eosinophilic Esophagitis*, Clinical Gastroenterology, DOI 10.1007/978-1-60761-515-6_11,

response to PPI therapy may not be due to the control of acid reflux (see below). There is much evidence to suggest that the interaction between GERD and EoE can be complex, and that the notion of establishing a clear distinction between the two disorders is too simplistic [3]. Indeed, many investigators have chosen to include subjects with abnormal acid reflux documented by pH monitoring in their series of patients with EoE [4–6].

In 1982, Winter et al. were the first to report that the finding of eosinophils in the esophageal epithelium could be used as a diagnostic criterion for reflux esophagitis in children [7]. In that study, the presence of even a few intraepithelial eosinophils in the esophagus was found to correlate with abnormal acid clearance determined by overnight esophageal pH probe monitoring. Intraepithelial eosinophils could be found in all levels of the esophagus, and involvement of the proximal esophagus was associated with greater abnormalities in the pH probe study. These observations suggest that, for some patients with GERD, the immune response manifested by intraepithelial eosinophils may extend into the upper esophagus in a pattern similar to that reported for patients with EoE.

Proposed Mechanisms Underlying an Association Between Gastroesophageal Reflux and Esophageal Eosinophils

Four major mechanisms have been proposed to explain the association between GERD and esophageal eosinophils [3]: (1) GERD, through epithelial injury or stimulation, causes the production of cytokines and other molecules that attract small numbers of eosinophils to the esophagus, (2) GERD and EoE coexist but are unrelated, (3) EoE contributes to or causes GERD, or (4) GERD contributes to or causes EoE. These mechanisms are considered individually below.

GERD, Through Epithelial Injury or Stimulation, Causes the Production of Cytokines and Other Molecules that Attract Small Numbers of Eosinophils to the Esophagus

Reports have described a number of potential mechanisms whereby GERD might cause the esophageal epithelium to produce molecules that recruit eosinophils. In cultures of human esophageal microvascular endothelial cells, for example, acid exposure induces the expression of vascular cell adhesion molecule-1 (VCAM-1), an adhesion molecules recognized by ligands on the eosinophil cell surface [8, 9]. In a preparation of human esophageal mucosa, acid causes the release of platelet activating factor (PAF), a phospholipid that attracts and activates eosinophils [10]. The esophageal mucosa of patients with reflux esophagitis exhibits elevated levels of chemokines that might attract eosinophils, such as IL-8, MCP-1, and RANTES [11], and Souza has shown that esophageal squamous epithelial cells in culture secrete IL-8 when they are exposed to acidified bile salts [12]. It is not clear which, if any, of these molecules contributes to the mild eosinophilic infiltration of the esophageal squamous epithelium that can be found in patients with GERD.

GERD and EoE Coexist but Are Unrelated

Surveys suggest that approximately 20% of adults in Western countries have GERD [13, 14]. Therefore, if GERD does not protect against EoE or vice versa, then one would expect that approximately 20% of adult patients with EoE would have GERD by chance alone. It seems unlikely that either of these disorders protects against the other.

In children with EoE, reports describing the results of esophageal pH monitoring suggest that abnormal acid reflux is uncommon [15–17]. However, the validity of these reports is questionable because, in children, the sensitivity and specificity of esophageal pH monitoring as a test for GERD are not well established [18]. Factors that confound the interpretation of esophageal pH monitoring studies in children include differences in the methodology of probe placement among different medical centers, variability in the use and timing of general anesthesia before probe placement, and disruption of the child's normal activities due to the discomfort and physical restrictions imposed by the transnasal pH catheter [19–21].

In adults with EoE, the frequency of pathological acid reflux appears to be inordinately high [6, 22]. For example, 24-h esophageal pH monitoring revealed abnormal acid reflux in 10 (38%) of 26 adults with EoE in one study [22], and in 14 (56%) of 25 in another [6]. The precise frequency of GERD in patients with EoE remains unclear, and controversy regarding the definition of EoE confounds estimates of that frequency. The consensus definition of EoE mentioned above excludes patients with GERD and, therefore, strict adherence to that definition would result in a 0% frequency of GERD in patients with EoE.

EoE Contributes to or Causes GERD

Conceivably, eosinophil secretory products could cause GERD by increasing gastroesophageal reflux and by impairing the ability of the esophagus to clear itself of refluxed material. For example, eosinophils produce vasoactive intestinal peptide and PAF, agents that can relax the lower esophageal sphincter and thereby predispose to reflux [23, 24]. Eosinophils also secrete interleukin (IL)-6, which can weaken esophageal muscle contractions, an effect that might impair esophageal peristalsis and acid clearance [25, 26]. In addition, some eosinophil secretory products have cytotoxic effects that might render the esophageal epithelium more susceptible to injury by refluxed gastric material [27–29]. For example, eosinophils produce major basic protein, which has been shown to impair barrier function in monolayers of human colonic carcinoma cells [30]. In the bronchial mucosa of patients with asthma, eosinophilic infiltration is associated with damage to cellular tight junctions and dilation of the intercellular spaces [31]. Finally, eosinophils induce the mucosal remodeling with fibrosis characteristic of EoE, and such fibrosis also might affect LES function and peristalsis as it does in patients with scleroderma [32].

GERD Contributes to or Causes EoE

Mechanisms whereby GERD might cause low-grade infiltration of the esophagus by eosinophils are discussed above. In addition, GERD can cause epithelial damage that, conceivably, might predispose to the development of allergic esophagitis. Typical food allergens have a molecular weight between 3 and 90 kD [33] and, normally, the esophageal epithelium is highly impermeable to such large molecules [34]. For example, Tobey found that the normal rabbit esophagus was virtually impermeable to epidermal growth factor, a peptide with a molecular weight of 6 kD, and to dextrans with a molecular weight of 4 kD [34]. When that esophageal epithelium was exposed to acid and pepsin, however, it became permeable to epidermal growth factor and to dextrans as large as 20 kD. By increasing esophageal permeability, therefore, GERD could render the squamous epithelium permeable to allergens. It is also conceivable that GERD-induced recruitment of immune cells to the esophageal epithelium might contribute to the local development of allergies.

Anti-inflammatory Effects of PPIs

The PPIs, which block gastric acid secretion by inhibiting the proton pump of the gastric parietal cell, are widely regarded as the agents of choice for treating acid-peptic disorders, such as GERD. For patients who have gastrointestinal symptoms of uncertain etiology, improvement with PPI therapy traditionally has been considered prima facie evidence of an acid-peptic disease. However, it has not been widely appreciated that PPIs, in addition to their antisecretory effects, have antioxidant properties and direct effects on neutrophils, monocytes, endothelial cells, and epithelial cells that might prevent inflammation [35]. The mechanisms proposed to underlie the anti-inflammatory effects of the PPIs are summarized in Table 11.1.

Table 11.1 Proposed mechanisms underlying anti-inflammatory effects of proton pump inhibitors

Antioxidant effects
Direct scavenging of reactive oxygen species
Replenishment of protective sulfhydryl molecules in the gastric mucosa
Induction of heme oxygenase-1
Effects on inflammatory cells
Inhibition of oxidative burst in neutrophils
Impaired phagocytosis of microorganisms by neutrophils
Decreased expression of adhesion molecules by neutrophils and monocytes
Impaired neutrophil migration
Effects on endothelial cells
Decreased expression of adhesion molecules
Decreased production of pro-inflammatory cytokines
Effects on epithelial cells
Decreased production of pro-inflammatory cytokines
Effects on gut microflora
Growth inhibitory and killing effects on a number of bacteria and fungi

Adapted from Kedika, RR. [35]. Used with permission

Antioxidant Effects

Inflammation causes tissue damage through oxidative injuries mediated by agents like hypochlorous acid, an oxidant produced by phagocytes, and by transition metals like iron and copper [36, 37]. Omeprazole has been shown to prevent the oxidation of β-carotene by hypochlorous acid, and to inhibit the oxidation of deoxyribose sugar mediated by iron and copper [37, 38]. Similarly, lansoprazole inhibits the copper-induced oxidation of low-density lipoproteins (LDLs) [39], and both pantoprazole and lansoprazole can scavenge hydroxyl radicals generated during chemical reactions involving transition metals [38, 40]. In rats subjected to restraint and cold stress, which stimulates the gastric mucosa to produce hydroxyl radicals that cause ulceration, omeprazole prevents gastric ulcers even when it is given in doses too low to inhibit gastric acid secretion [40]. Esomeprazole has been shown to prevent gastric glutathione depletion in rats treated with indomethacin [41]. PPIs also might protect against oxidative damage in the gastrointestinal tract by inducing the enzyme heme oxygenase-1 in endothelial and epithelial cells [42]. Heme oxygenase-1 catalyzes heme degradation, thereby generating bilirubin, which has antioxidant effects, and carbon monoxide, which has cytoprotective properties.

Effects on Inflammatory Cells

In the stomach, PPIs block the p-type H^+, K^+ATPase of parietal cells that secretes acid into the gastric lumen. Some nongastric cells, like neutrophils, have vacuolar (v-type) H^+ATPases that pump acid into the extracellular space and into intracellular organelles like lysosomes [43, 44]. These v-type H^+ATPases appear to be susceptible to inhibition by PPIs [45] and, therefore, it is conceivable that PPIs might interfere with certain neutrophil functions. Indeed, PPIs have been shown to inhibit neutrophil chemotaxis and to interfere with the generation of reactive oxygen species (ROS) by neutrophils [46–49]. In neutrophils and endothelial cells, which also have v-type proton pumps, PPIs have been found to inhibit the expression of adhesion molecules that enable neutrophils to home into diseased tissues. In human umbilical vein endothelial cells stimulated with interleukin-1, for example, PPIs inhibit the expression of intercellular adhesion molecule-1 (ICAM-1) and VCAM-1, and decrease endothelial-dependent neutrophil adhesion [50]. Although these data show that PPIs can interfere with neutrophilic inflammation, it is not clear that this interference is effected by the inhibition of the v-type H^+ATPases of neutrophils and endothelial cells [51].

Effect on the Production of Pro-inflammatory Cytokines by Epithelial and Endothelial Cells

PPIs have been shown to inhibit the production of certain pro-inflammatory cytokines by epithelial and endothelial cells. Gastric mucosal production of IL-8, a potent neutrophil chemoattractant, appears to play an important role in mediating gastric inflammation mediated by infection with *Helicobacter pylori* [52]. In a human gastric cancer cell line and in human umbilical vein endothelial cells stimulated with *H. pylori* extract, for example, omeprazole and lansoprazole block the production of IL-8 [53].

Clinical Implications of Anti-inflammatory Effects of PPI's for Esophageal Eosinophilia

PPIs clearly are effective for the treatment of GERD, and there are data to suggest that PPIs also have a primary role in the treatment of esophageal eosinophilia [6]. In both disorders, it is not clear whether the beneficial effects of these agents are due solely to gastric acid inhibition, or whether the anti-inflammatory effects of the PPIs contribute as well. Nevertheless, the data discussed above raise a serious challenge to the common clinical practice of assuming that a symptomatic response to PPI treatment is proof of an underlying acid-peptic disorder. It is conceivable that the PPIs could have beneficial effects in any number of inflammatory diseases, including esophageal eosinophilia, in which acid and pepsin may or may not have a role.

An influential report published in 2006 described three pediatric patients who had profound esophageal eosinophilia and symptoms, all of which resolved completely with PPI treatment [54]. Although none of the three had a history typical of GERD, the authors concluded that the response to PPI therapy was proof for underlying reflux disease, and that the profound esophageal eosinophilia was a manifestation of peptic esophagitis. However, a positive response to PPI therapy does not necessarily distinguish GERD.

Potential Role for PPIs in the Pathogenesis of EoE

PPIs are considered a first-line therapy for patients suspected of having esophageal eosinophilia [55]. Ironically, however, recent studies also have suggested a plausible hypothesis whereby PPIs, by interfering with the peptic digestion of dietary proteins and by increasing gastric mucosal permeability, might contribute to the development of EoE [56–58].

Most recognized food allergens are glycoprotein components that have a molecular weight between 3 and 90 kD [33, 59]. Peptides smaller than 3 kD may not be capable of inducing an immunological response [60]. The class I major histocompatibility complex (MHC class I) of antigen-presenting cells typically presents peptides comprising 8–10 amino acid residues to cytotoxic T lymphocytes, and smaller peptide fragments may be ignored by the immune system [61, 62]. These observations suggest that food proteins that are rapidly digested into individual amino acids, dipeptides, and tripeptides would be unlikely to induce an immunological response.

The digestion of food proteins normally begins in the stomach through the action of pepsin proteinases in the gastric juice. The optimal pH for the enzymatic activity of the pepsins is between 1.8 and 3.2, and most of their proteinase activity ceases at pH levels above 4.5 [63, 64]. Acid suppressive medications like PPIs frequently raise the gastric pH above levels where pepsin is not active [64]. Under those circumstances, dietary proteins that normally would be partially digested in the stomach can reach the duodenum largely intact. Conceivably, that might expose the small intestine to food allergens that ordinarily would have been destroyed by peptic digestion and, thereby, predispose to the development of food allergy. In patients with GERD, furthermore, these undigested allergens could be refluxed back into the esophagus where they might initiate an immune response that contributes to the development of EoE.

A second mechanism whereby PPIs might contribute to the pathogenesis of EoE involves their effects on mucosal permeability. One group of investigators recently found that their patients with reflux esophagitis and Barrett's esophagus, many of whom were on PPIs, had abnormal sucrose permeability tests [65]. In a subsequent study, those investigators performed sucrose permeability tests in GERD patients before and after 8 weeks of treatment with esomeprazole [58]. Although the researchers originally thought that PPI treatment should improve mucosal barrier function, they were surprised to find that most patients exhibited a substantial increase in mucosal permeability to sucrose after PPI treatment. This unanticipated effect was confirmed in a group of healthy control subjects who also developed abnormal sucrose permeability tests during 9 days of PPI treatment. In patients taking

PPIs, therefore, large and potentially allergenic peptides that escape peptic digestion because of acid inhibition might be taken up through the PPI-induced mucosal leak to elicit an immunological response.

Untersmayr and her colleagues in Vienna have shown that the peptic digestion of certain food allergens is exquisitely sensitive to small variations in pH [66, 67]. They also have found that mice treated with PPIs develop allergen-specific IgE antibodies when they are fed certain fish and nut preparations [68, 69]. In a clinical study, Untersmayr assayed serum IgE levels in 152 adult outpatients who had no history of allergy and who were treated with a histamine H2-receptor antagonist or a PPI for 3 months [70]. Ten percent of these patients exhibited a rise in IgE antibody levels, and new, food-specific IgE antibodies developed in 15%. In a similar study of outpatients taking antisecretory medications for 3 months, 5 of 153 (3.3%) patients developed hazelnut-specific IgE antibodies; 4 of those developed specific skin reactivity and 2 manifested clinical food allergy to hazelnuts [69].

The PPI omeprazole was released for clinical use in the late 1980s and, today, PPIs are among the most commonly used medications in the world [71, 72]. PPIs are used regularly, not only in adults, but often in young children with GERD who might take these medications for years [73, 74]. After 5 days of conventional-dose PPI therapy, gastric pH rises to levels >4.0 for approximately 50% of the day [75]. With higher doses, as are prescribed often in clinical practice, gastric pH levels can remain >4.0 for more than 80% of the day [76]. At these pH levels, there can be little peptic digestion of a number of potential food allergens that normally would be partially degraded in the stomach. The rapid emergence of EoE approximately one decade after PPI usage became widespread would fit well with a PPI-associated, food allergic disorder.

PPIs have been a mainstay of therapy for patients with GERD for more than two decades, and they have established an excellent track record for safety. Despite the plausible mechanisms discussed above, by no means is it clear that PPIs have contributed to the rising frequency of EoE. Nevertheless, this interesting hypothesis clearly warrants further study.

References

1. Furuta GT, Liacouras CA, Collins MH, Gupta SK, Justinich C, Putnam PE, et al. First International Gastrointestinal Eosinophil Research Symposium (FIGERS) Subcommittees. Eosinophilic esophagitis in children and adults: a systematic review and consensus recommendations for diagnosis and treatment. Gastroenterology. 2007;133:1342–63.
2. Mattioli S, Pilotti V, Spangaro M, Grigioni WF, Zannoli R, Felice V, et al. Reliability of 24-hour home esophageal pH monitoring in diagnosis of gastroesophageal reflux. Dig Dis Sci. 1989;34:71–8.
3. Spechler SJ, Genta RM, Souza RF. Thoughts on the complex relationship between gastroesophageal reflux disease and eosinophilic esophagitis. Am J Gastroenterol. 2007;102:1301–6.
4. Rodrigo S, Abboud G, Oh D, DeMeester SR, Hagen J, Lipham J, et al. High intraepithelial eosinophil counts in esophageal squamous epithelium are not specific for eosinophilic esophagitis in adults. Am J Gastroenterol. 2008;103:435–42.

5. Shah A, Kagalwalla AF, Gonsalves N, Melin-Aldana H, Li BU, Hirano I. Histopathologic variability in children with eosinophilic esophagitis. Am J Gastroenterol. 2009;104:716–21.
6. Peterson KA, Thomas KL, Hilden K, Emerson LL, Wills JC, Fang JC. Comparison of esomeprazole to aerosolized, swallowed fluticasone for eosinophilic esophagitis. Dig Dis Sci. 2010;55:1313–9.
7. Winter HS, Madara JL, Stafford RJ, Grand RJ, Quinlan JE, Goldman H. Intraepithelial eosinophils: a new diagnostic criterion for reflux esophagitis. Gastroenterology. 1982;83:818–23.
8. Rafiee P, Theriot ME, Nelson VM, Heidemann J, Kanaa Y, Horowitz SA, et al. Human esophageal microvascular endothelial cells respond to acidic pH stress by PI3K/AKT and p38 MAPK-regulated induction of Hsp70 and Hsp27. Am J Physiol Cell Physiol. 2006;291:C931–45.
9. Barthel SR, Annis DS, Mosher DF, Johansson MW. Differential engagement of modules 1 and 4 of vascular cell adhesion molecule-1 (CD106) by integrins alpha4beta1 (CD49d/29) and alphaMbeta2 (CD11b/18) of eosinophils. J Biol Chem. 2006;281:32175–87.
10. Cheng L, Cao W, Behar J, Fiocchi C, Biancani P, Harnett KM. Acid-induced release of platelet-activating factor by human esophageal mucosa induces inflammatory mediators in circular smooth muscle. J Pharmacol Exp Ther. 2006;319:117–26.
11. Isomoto H, Wang A, Mizuta Y, Akazawa Y, Ohba K, Omagari K, et al. Elevated levels of chemokines in esophageal mucosa of patients with reflux esophagitis. Am J Gastroenterol. 2003;98:551–6.
12. Souza RF, Huo X, Mittal V, Schuler CM, Carmack SW, Zhang HY, et al. Gastroesophageal reflux may cause esophagitis through a cytokine-mediated mechanism, not by caustic (acid) injury. Gastroenterology. 2009;137:1776–84.
13. Locke III GR, Talley NJ, Fett SL, Zinsmeister AR, Melton III LJ. Prevalence and clinical spectrum of gastroesophageal reflux: a population-based study in Olmsted County, Minnesota. Gastroenterology. 1997;112:1448–56.
14. Shaheen N, Provenzale D. The epidemiology of gastroesophageal reflux disease. Am J Med Sci. 2003;326:264–73.
15. Sant'Anna AM, Rolland S, Fournet JC, Yazbeck S, Drouin E. Eosinophilic esophagitis in children: symptoms, histology and pH probe results. J Pediatr Gastroenterol Nutr. 2004;39:373–7.
16. Steiner SJ, Gupta SK, Croffie JM, Fitzgerald JF. Correlation between number of eosinophils and reflux index on same day esophageal biopsy and 24 hour esophageal pH monitoring. Am J Gastroenterol. 2004;99:801–5.
17. Steiner SJ, Kernek KM, Fitzgerald JF. Severity of basal cell hyperplasia differs in reflux versus eosinophilic esophagitis. J Pediatr Gastroenterol Nutr. 2006;42:506–9.
18. Vandenplas Y, Rudolph CD, Di Lorenzo C, Hassall E, Liptak G, Mazur L, et al. Pediatric gastroesophageal reflux clinical practice guidelines: joint recommendations of the North American Society for Pediatric Gastroenterology, Hepatology, and Nutrition (NASPGHAN) and the European Society for Pediatric Gastroenterology, Hepatology, and Nutrition (ESPGHAN). J Pediatr Gastroenterol Nutr. 2009;49:498–547.
19. Mahajan L, Wyllie R, Oliva L, Balsells F, Steffen R, Kay M. Reproducibility of 24-hour intraesophageal ph monitoring in pediatric patients. Pediatrics. 1998;101:260–3.
20. Michaud L, Troadec F, Beghin L, Rifai N, Guimber D, Turck D, et al. Influence of esophageal ph recording on physical activity in children. J Pediatr Gastroenterol Nutr. 2009;48:4026–430.
21. Fass R, Hell R, Sampliner RE, Pulliam G, Graver E, Hartz V, et al. Effect of ambulatory 24-hour oesophageal pH monitoring on reflux-provoking activities. Dig Dis Sci. 1999;44:2263–9.
22. Remedios M, Campbell C, Jones DM, Kerlin P. Eosinophilic esophagitis in adults: clinical, endoscopic, histologic findings, and response to treatment with fluticasone propionate. Gastrointest Endosc. 2006;63(1):3–12.
23. Cheng L, Harnett KM, Cao W, Liu F, Behar J, Fiocchi C, et al. Hydrogen peroxide reduces lower esophageal sphincter tone in human esophagitis. Gastroenterology. 2005;129:1675–85.
24. Farre R, Auli M, Lecea B, Martinez E, Clave P. Pharmacologic characterization of intrinsic mechanisms controlling tone and relaxation of porcine lower esophageal sphincter. J Pharmacol Exp Ther. 2006;316:1238–48.

25. Cao W, Cheng L, Behar J, Biancani P, Harnett KM. IL-1beta signaling in cat lower esophageal sphincter circular muscle. Am J Physiol Gastrointest Liver Physiol. 2006;291:G672–80.
26. Cao W, Cheng L, Behar J, Fiocchi C, Biancani P, Harnett KM. Proinflammatory cytokines alter/reduce esophageal circular muscle contraction in experimental cat esophagitis. Am J Physiol Gastrointest Liver Physiol. 2004;287:G1131–9.
27. Tai PC, Hayes DJ, Clark JB, Spry CJ. Toxic effects of human eosinophil products on isolated rat heart cells in vitro. Biochem J. 1982;204:75–80.
28. Motojima S, Frigas E, Loegering DA, Gleich GJ. Toxicity of eosinophil cationic proteins for guinea pig tracheal epithelium in vitro. Am Rev Respir Dis. 1989;139:801–5.
29. Young JD, Peterson CG, Venge P, Cohn ZA. Mechanism of membrane damage mediated by human eosinophil cationic protein. Nature. 1986;321:613–6.
30. Furuta GT, Nieuwenhuis EES, Karhausen J, Gleich G, Blumberg RS, Lee JJ, et al. Eosinophils alter colonic epithelial barrier function: role for major basic protein. Am J Physiol Gastrointest Liver Physiol. 2005;289:G890–7.
31. Ohashi Y, Motojima S, Fukuda T, Makino S. Relationship between bronchial reactivity to inhaled acetylcholine, eosinophil infiltration and a widening of the intercellular space in patients with asthma. Arerugi. 1990;39:1541–5.
32. Mishra A, Wang M, Pemmaraju VR, Collins MH, Fulkerson PC, Abonia JP, et al. Esophageal remodeling develops as a consequence of tissue specific IL-5-induced eosinophilia. Gastroenterology. 2008;134:204–14.
33. Untersmayr E, Jensen-Jarolim E. The effect of gastric digestion on food allergy. Curr Opin Allergy Clin Immunol. 2006;6:214–9.
34. Tobey NA, Hosseini SS, Argote CM, Dobrucali AM, Awayda MS, Orlando RC. Dilated intercellular spaces and shunt permeability in nonerosive acid-damaged esophageal epithelium. Am J Gastroenterol. 2004;99:13–22.
35. Kedika RR, Souza RF, Spechler SJ. Potential anti-inflammatory effects of the proton pump inhibitors: a review and discussion of the clinical implications. Dig Dis Sci. 2009;54:2312–7.
36. Weiss SJ. Oxygen, ischemia and inflammation. Acta Physiol Scand Suppl. 1986;548:9–37.
37. Lapenna D, de Gioia S, Ciofani G, Festi D, Cuccurullo F. Antioxidant properties of omeprazole. FEBS Lett. 1996;382:189–92.
38. Blandizzi C, Fornai M, Colucci R, Natale G, Lubrano V, Vassalle C, et al. Lansoprazole prevents experimental gastric injury induced by non-steroidal anti-inflammatory drugs through a reduction of mucosal oxidative damage. World J Gastroenterol. 2005;11:4052–60.
39. Simon WA, Sturm E, Hartmann HJ, Weser U. Hydroxyl radical scavenging reactivity of proton pump inhibitors. Biochem Pharmacol. 2006;71:1337–41.
40. Biswas K, Bandyopadhyay U, Chattopadhyay I, Varadaraj A, Ali E, Banerjee RK. A novel antioxidant and antiapoptotic role of omeprazole to block gastric ulcer through scavenging of hydroxyl radical. J Biol Chem. 2003;278:10993–1001.
41. Pastoris O, Verri M, Boschi F, Kastsiuchenka O, Balestra B, Pace F, et al. Effects of esomeprazole on glutathione levels and mitochondrial oxidative phosphorylation in the gastric mucosa of rats treated with indomethacin. Toxicol Appl Pharmacol. 2008;195:62–72.
42. Becker JC, Grosser N, Waltke C, Schulz S, Erdmann K, Domschke W, et al. Beyond gastric acid reduction: proton pump inhibitors induce heme oxygenase-1 in gastric and endothelial cells. Biochem Biophys Res Commun. 2006;345:1014–21.
43. Lafourcade C, Sobo K, Kieffer-Jaquinod S, Garin J, van der Goot FG. Regulation of the V-ATPase along the endocytic pathway occurs through reversible subunit association and membrane localization. PLoS One. 2008;3(7):e2758.
44. Harada M, Shakado S, Sakisaka S, Tamaki S, Ohishi M, Sasatomi K, et al. Bafilomycin A1, a specific inhibitor of V-type H+–ATPases, inhibits the acidification of endocytic structures and inhibits horseradish peroxidase uptake in isolated rat sinusoidal endothelial cells. Liver. 1997;17:244–50.
45. Luciani F, Spada M, De Milito A, Molinari A, Rivoltini L, Montinaro A, et al. Effect of proton pump inhibitor pretreatment on resistance of solid tumors to cytotoxic drugs. J Natl Cancer Inst. 2004;96:1702–13.

46. Wandall JH. Effects of omeprazole on neutrophil chemotaxis, super oxide production, degranulation, and translocation of cytochrome b-245. Gut. 1992;33:617–21.
47. Suzuki M, Nakamura M, Mori M, Miura S, Tsuchiya M, Ishil H. Lansoprazole inhibits oxygen-derived free radical production from neutrophils activated by Helicobacter pylori. J Clin Gastroenterol. 1995;20 Suppl 2:S93–6.
48. Suzuki M, Mori M, Miura S, Suematsu M, Fukumara D, Kimura H, et al. Omeprazole attenuates oxygen-derived free radical production from human neutrophils. Free Radic Biol Med. 1996;21:727–31.
49. Zedtwitz-Liebenstein K, Wenisch C, Patruta S, Parschalk B, Daxböck F, Graninger W. Omeprazole treatment diminishes intra- and extracellular neutrophil reactive oxygen production and bactericidal activity. Crit Care Med. 2002;30:1118–22.
50. Yoshida N, Yoshikawa T, Tanaka Y, Fujita N, Kassai K, Naito Y, et al. A new mechanism for anti-inflammatory actions of proton pump inhibitors–inhibitory effects on neutrophil-endothelial cell interactions. Aliment Pharmacol Ther. 2000;14 Suppl 1:74–81.
51. Martins de Oliveira R, Antunes E, Pedrazzoli Jr J, Gambero A. The inhibitory effects of H+ K+ ATPase inhibitors on human neutrophils in vitro: restoration by a K+ ionophore. Inflamm Res. 2007;56:105–11.
52. Smith WB, Gamble JR, Clark-Lewis I, Vadas MA. Interleukin-8 induces neutrophil transendothelial migration. Immunology. 1991;72:65–72.
53. Handa O, Yoshida N, Fujita N, Tanaka Y, Ueda M, Takagi T, et al. Molecular mechanisms involved in anti-inflammatory effects of proton pump inhibitors. Inflamm Res. 2006;55:476–80.
54. Ngo P, Furuta GT, Antonioli DA, Fox VL. Eosinophils in the esophagus–peptic or allergic eosinophilic esophagitis? Case series of three patients with esophageal eosinophilia. Am J Gastroenterol. 2006;101:1666–70.
55. Aceves SS, Furuta GT, Spechler SJ. Integrated approach to treatment of children and adults with eosinophilic esophagitis. Gastrointest Endosc Clin N Am. 2008;18:195–217.
56. Merwat SN, Spechler SJ. Might the use of acid suppressive medications predispose to the development of eosinophilic esophagitis? Am J Gastroenterol. 2009;104:1897–902.
57. Untersmayr E, Jensen-Jarolim E. The role of protein digestibility and antacids on food allergy outcomes. J Allergy Clin Immunol. 2008;121:1301–8.
58. Mullin JM, Valenzano MC, Whitby M, Lurie D, Schmidt JD, Jain V, et al. Esomeprazole induces upper gastrointestinal tract transmucosal permeability increase. Aliment Pharmacol Ther. 2008;28:1317–25.
59. Lack G. Food allergy. N Engl J Med. 2008;359:1252–60.
60. van Beresteijn EC, Meijer RJ, Schmidt DG. Residual antigenicity of hypoallergenic infant formulas and the occurrence of milk-specific IgE antibodies in patients with clinical allergy. J Allergy Clin Immunol. 1995;96:365–74.
61. Schmelzer CE, Schops R, Ulbrich-Hofmann R, Neubert RH, Raith K. Mass spectrometric characterization of peptides derived by peptic cleavage of bovine beta-casein. J Chromatogr A. 2004;1055:87–92.
62. York IA, Goldberg AL, Mo XY, Rock KL. Proteolysis and class I major histocompatibility complex antigen presentation. Immunol Rev. 1999;172:49–66.
63. Roberts NB. Human pepsins – their multiplicity, function and role in reflux disease. Aliment Pharmacol Ther. 2006;24 Suppl 2:2–9.
64. Prichard PJ, Yeomans ND, Mihaly GW, Jones DB, Buckle PJ, Smallwood RA, et al. Omeprazole: a study of its inhibition of gastric pH and oral pharmacokinetics after morning or evening dosage. Gastroenterology. 1985;88:64–9.
65. Mullin JM, Valenzano MC, Trembeth S, Allegretti PD, Verrecchio JJ, Schmidt JD, et al. Transepithelial leak in Barrett's esophagus. Dig Dis Sci. 2006;51:2326–36.
66. Untersmayr E, Poulsen LK, Platzer MH, Pedersen MH, Boltz-Nitulescu G, Skov PS, et al. The effects of gastric digestion on codfish allergenicity. J Allergy Clin Immunol. 2005;115:377–82.
67. Untersmayr E, Vestergaard H, Malling HJ, Jensen LB, Platzer MH, Boltz-Nitulescu G, et al. Incomplete digestion of codfish represents a risk factor for anaphylaxis in patients with allergy. J Allergy Clin Immunol. 2007;119:711–7.

68. Untersmayr E, Schöll I, Swoboda I, Beil WJ, Förster-Waldl E, Walter F, et al. Antacid medication inhibits digestion of dietary proteins and causes food allergy: a fish allergy model in BALB/c mice. J Allergy Clin Immunol. 2003;112:616–23.
69. Schöll I, Untersmayr E, Bakos N, Roth-Walter F, Gleiss A, Boltz-Nitulescu G, et al. Antiulcer drugs promote oral sensitization and hypersensitivity to hazelnut allergens in BALB/c mice and humans. Am J Clin Nutr. 2005;81:154–60.
70. Untersmayr E, Bakos N, Schöll I, Kundi M, Roth-Walter F, Szalai K, et al. Anti-ulcer drugs promote IgE formation toward dietary antigens in adult patients. FASEB J. 2005;19:656–8.
71. Boath EH, Blenkinsopp A. The rise and rise of proton pump inhibitor drugs: patients' perspectives. Soc Sci Med. 1997;45:1571–9.
72. Jones MI et al. Proton pump inhibitors: a study of GPs' prescribing. Fam Pract. 2001;18:333–8.
73. Tolia V, Boyer K. Long-term proton pump inhibitor use in children: a retrospective review of safety. Dig Dis Sci. 2008;53:385–93.
74. Hassall E, Kerr W, El-Serag HB. Characteristics of children receiving proton pump inhibitors continuously for up to 11 years duration. J Pediatr. 2007;150:262–7.
75. Miner Jr P, Katz PO, Chen Y, Sostek M. Gastric acid control with esomeprazole, lansoprazole, omeprazole, pantoprazole, and rabeprazole: a five-way crossover study. Am J Gastroenterol. 2003;98:2616–20.
76. Spechler SJ, Sharma P, Traxler B, Levine D, Falk GW. Gastric and esophageal pH in patients with Barrett's esophagus treated with three esomeprazole dosages: a randomized, double-blind, crossover trial. Am J Gastroenterol. 2006;101:1964–71.

Chapter 12
Radiographic Diagnosis of Eosinophilic Esophagitis

Marc S. Levine and David A. Katzka

Keywords Eosinophilic esophagitis • Barium esophagography • Esophageal mucosa • Biopsy • Endoscopy

Introduction

The diagnosis of eosinophilic esophagitis (EoE) continues to evolve as we gain a better understanding of this fascinating disease. EoE initially was diagnosed pathologically by a high number of intraepithelial eosinophils in the esophagus, but the diagnosis is now based on several histologic parameters in combination with key demographic, clinical, and endoscopic features. Despite numerous endoscopic studies on EoE, the role of barium esophagography in diagnosing this disease has received little attention in the gastroenterology literature. Lack of interest in esophagography is related to recognized advantages of endoscopy for directly visualizing the esophageal mucosa and obtaining biopsy specimens as well as the desire to avoid ionizing radiation in patients with dysphagia.

We believe, however, that endoscopy and barium esophagography should be regarded as complementary rather than competitive techniques for the evaluation of patients with dysphagia and possible EoE. In such cases, the barium study provides a global examination that can be used not only to detect esophagitis or strictures, but also to assess swallowing function, esophageal motility, and the presence and degree of gastroesophageal reflux disease (GERD) in patients with other conditions masquerading as EoE based on the clinical presentation [1].

D.A. Katzka (✉)
Department of Medicine, Mayo Clinic, 200 1st Street, S.W., Rochester, MN 55905, USA
e-mail: Katzka.david@mayo.edu

C.A. Liacouras and J.E. Markowitz (eds.), *Eosinophilic Esophagitis*,
Clinical Gastroenterology, DOI 10.1007/978-1-60761-515-6_12,

Barium esophagography may also reveal characteristic findings (including a ringed esophagus and a small-caliber esophagus) that markedly raise the pretest probability of EoE on endoscopy. In patients with a small-caliber esophagus, the radiographic findings may indicate the need for using a pediatric endoscope to traverse the narrowed esophageal lumen and guide planning for endoscopic dilation or other therapeutic interventions. In patients with tight strictures in the proximal esophagus that preclude passage of the endoscope, barium studies also enable assessment of the more distal esophagus that cannot be visualized at endoscopy. For all of these reasons, barium studies have an important role in the evaluation and treatment of patients with EoE. Our chapter describes the state of the art of barium esophagography in the diagnostic work-up of this disease.

Technique for Performing Barium Esophagography

Barium esophagograms should be performed as biphasic examinations that include double-contrast views with a high-density barium suspension and single-contrast views with a low-density barium suspension [1]. The double-contrast phase is performed by obtaining upright, left posterior oblique (LPO) double-contrast views of the esophagus using an effervescent agent (Baros; Lafayette Pharmaceuticals) and a 250% w/v high-density barium suspension (E-Z-HD; E-Z-EM Company). In patients with dysphagia, the cardia and fundus should also be visualized with the patient in a lateral, right side down position for a double-contrast view of the gastric cardia and fundus. The single-contrast phase is subsequently performed by obtaining prone, right anterior oblique (RAO) single-contrast views of the esophagus using a 50% w/v low-density barium suspension (Entrobar; Lafayette Pharmaceuticals). The double-contrast views optimize detection of esophagitis and other mucosal abnormalities, whereas the single-contrast views optimize esophageal distention for detection of rings or strictures and also improve detection of hiatal hernias.

Esophageal motility is evaluated by having the patient take multiple (usually 3–5 in number) separate swallows of low-density barium in the prone, RAO position. Esophageal motility is considered abnormal when two or more of five separate swallows fail to show normal progression of the primary peristaltic through the esophagus to the gastroesophageal junction [2].

At the end of the study, patients should routinely be evaluated for GERD by rotating them from the supine position into the right lateral position while assessing for spontaneous GERD and, if necessary, employing provocative techniques to elicit GERD, including a water siphon test or straight leg raising or a Valsalva maneuver to increase intraabdominal pressure. When reflux is observed at fluoroscopy, at least one radiograph of the esophagus should be obtained during the act of reflux for documentation.

In most radiology departments, barium esophagography is currently performed using digital fluoroscopic equipment that enables review and interpretation of the digital images at a picture archiving and communications system (PACS) workstation without the need for creation of hard-copy radiographs. This type of system has many advantages over conventional fluoroscopy, as it decreases radiation exposure to the patient, expedites patient throughput, facilitates image interpretation, and decreases the overall costs of image storage [3].

Findings on Barium Esophagography

It is estimated that as many as 25% of all patients with EoE have no abnormalities at endoscopy [4–6]. Even when endoscopy is abnormal, the most common findings are mucosal lesions, such as linear furrows, erythema, granularity, and white exudates. Such findings are found at endoscopy in 25–60% of patients with EoE [4, 5], but this mucosal disease is much more difficult to detect on barium esophagography, which therefore cannot be considered a sensitive test for the diagnosis of EoE. Nevertheless, two of the classic findings of EoE at endoscopy – a ringed esophagus and a small-caliber esophagus – can also be visualized at esophagography, and these findings are felt to be relatively specific signs of EoE on barium studies. Thus, a relatively confident diagnosis of EoE can be made when a ringed esophagus, small-caliber esophagus, or both are detected on esophagography. Strictures in the proximal, middle, or distal thirds of the thoracic esophagus are also a frequent finding in patients with EoE, but strictures may be caused by a variety of conditions, so they are less specific for this disease. The radiographic findings in EoE are considered separately in the following sections.

Strictures

Strictures are a common finding in EoE, having been reported at endoscopy in 15–57% of adult patients with this disease [4, 5, 7]. Barium esophagography is also an excellent technique for detecting strictures, which have been reported in up to 71% of adult patients with EoE [8]. Most patients have segmental strictures [8–13], but the location of these strictures is variable. In one series, 70% of radiographically diagnosed strictures were located in the upper or midthoracic esophagus (Fig. 12.1) [12], whereas in another series 64% were located in the distal thoracic esophagus or at the gastroesophageal junction (Fig. 12.2) [8]. The mean luminal diameter of these strictures is about 1 cm (with a range of 2–13 mm) and the mean length is about 5 cm (with a range of 0.5–13 cm) [8]. Interestingly, strictures in the upper or midthoracic esophagus tend to be longer than those in the distal thoracic esophagus (see Figs. 12.1 and 12.2) [8]. In general, esophageal strictures associated with EoE appear as long segments of symmetric narrowing with a smooth contour and tapered margins (see Fig. 12.1), though occasional strictures can be more focal, asymmetric, or irregular [8]. Rarely, patients with EoE may have concomitant strictures; in such

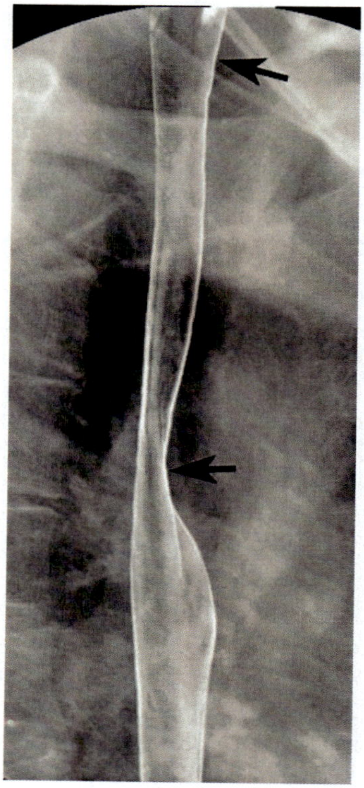

Fig. 12.1 EoE with a stricture in the upper thoracic esophagus. Spot image from a double-contrast esophagogram shows a long stricture extending from the thoracic inlet to the carina (*arrows*). Note how the stricture has a smooth contour and tapered proximal and distal margins – features characteristic of strictures in EoE

cases, the more distal stricture could be caused by simultaneous reflux disease [8]. Most patients with EoE and strictures are found to present with dysphagia.

The differential diagnosis for strictures on barium esophagography depends on the location of the stricture. Other causes of strictures in the upper or midthoracic esophagus include Barrett's esophagus, mediastinal irradiation (Fig. 12.3), caustic ingestion (Fig. 12.4), and medications, such as nonsteroidal anti-inflammatory drugs (NSAIDs), potassium chloride, and quinidine [14, 15], whereas the most common cause of strictures in the distal thoracic esophagus is scarring from reflux esophagitis (Fig. 12.5) [14]. In most cases, however, the correct diagnosis is suggested by the clinical history and presentation.

Ringed Esophagus

Esophageal rings are a frequent finding in patients with EoE; a variety of terms have been used to describe these rings in the gastroenterology literature, including "corrugation" and "trachealization" of the esophagus as well as the "ringed esophagus"

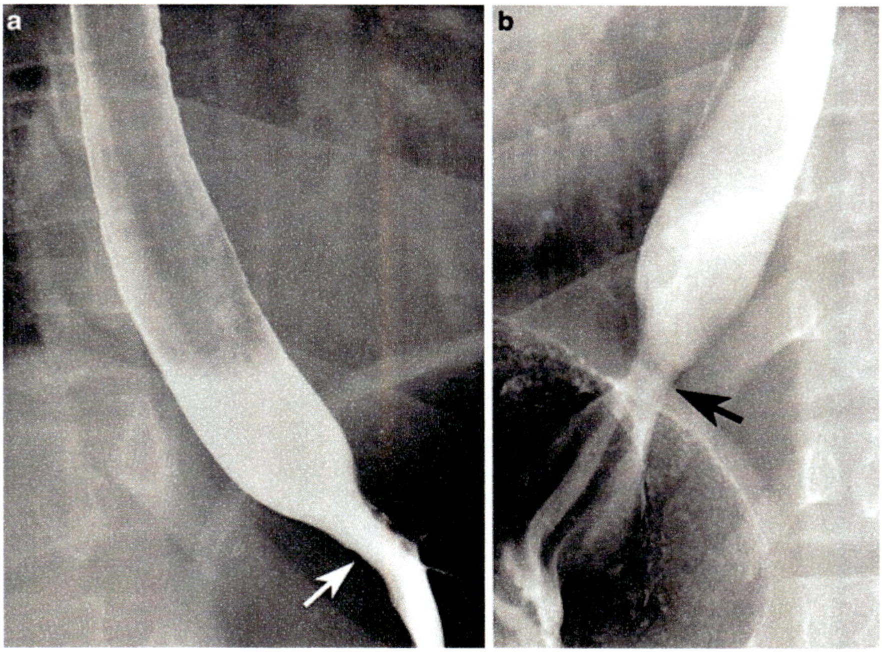

Fig. 12.2 EoE with a stricture in the distal thoracic esophagus. (**a**) Spot image from a double-contrast esophagogram shows a focal stricture (*arrow*) in the distal esophagus just above the gastroesophageal junction. (**b**) Spot image from a single-contrast esophagogram in the same patient shows a smooth, tapered stricture (*arrow*) in the distal esophagus above a hiatal hernia. Strictures in the distal esophagus in patients with EoE tend to be shorter than those in the upper or mid esophagus (see Fig. 12.1)

[5, 7, 16–18]. The extent and location of these rings are highly variable at endoscopy; they can be confined to the upper, middle, or distal thoracic esophagus or they can have a more diffuse distribution in the esophagus [5]. These rings may compromise luminal diameter to such a degree that it is difficult to advance an endoscope into the distal esophagus [5].

The ringed esophagus may be manifested on barium esophagography by distinctive ring-like indentations that are seen as multiple, closely spaced, concentric rings traversing the lumen (Figs. 12.6–12.8) [8]. In one study, the rings all occurred in the region of esophageal strictures (see Figs. 12.6 and 12.7) [8], but in another more recent study, these rings were associated with a small-caliber esophagus (see next section, Small-Caliber Esophagus) [19]. As on endoscopy, there is considerable variation in the location and extent of ring formation on barium studies in patients with EoE [8, 19]. Some patients may have rings without an associated stricture (see Fig. 12.8). Although the pathogenesis is uncertain, the ringed esophagus should be

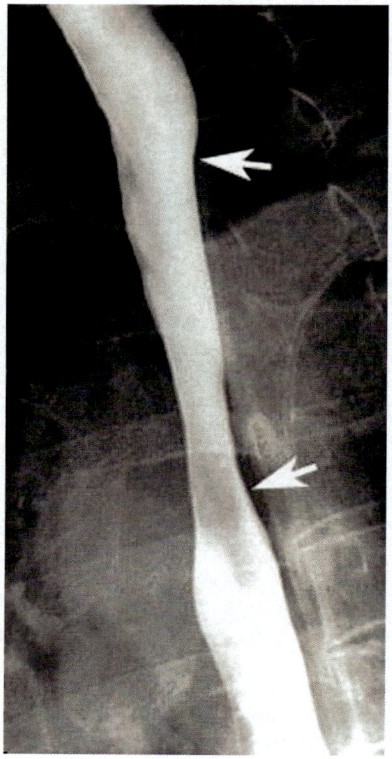

Fig. 12.3 Radiation stricture in the upper thoracic esophagus. This stricture has a smooth contour and tapered proximal and distal margins (*arrows*). Note similarity to the EoE stricture in Fig. 12.1

highly suggestive of EoE on esophagography, particularly if associated with strictures or a small-caliber esophagus.

A ringed esophagus has also been described in patients with congenital esophageal stenosis in whom barium studies or endoscopy revealed corrugated esophageal strictures containing multiple rings (Fig. 12.9) [20, 21]. In such cases, the rings have been attributed to aberrant embryologic development with tracheobronchial remnants or actual cartilaginous rings in the wall of the esophagus [20, 21]. In retrospect, however, we believe that some patients with a previous diagnosis of congenital esophageal stenosis have had unrecognized EoE as the cause of their symptoms and that patients with a ringed esophagus and esophageal strictures are far more likely to have EoE as the cause of their disease.

The differential diagnosis of the ringed esophagus also includes fixed transverse folds in patients with peptic strictures (Fig. 12.10) [22]. Unlike the rings in EoE, however, these fixed transverse folds are further apart, producing a characteristic stepladder appearance due to trapping of barium between the folds [22]. The feline esophagus could also conceivably be mistaken for the ringed esophagus of EoE

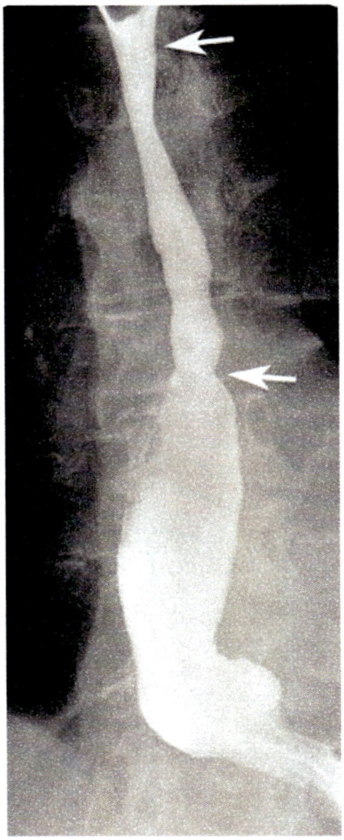

Fig. 12.4 Chronic lye stricture in the midthoracic esophagus. This patient has a long, somewhat asymmetric stricture with a smooth contour and tapered margins (*arrows*). Again note similarity to the EoE stricture in Fig. 12.1

(Fig. 12.11), but these delicate transverse striations occur as a transient phenomenon and are almost always associated with gastroesophageal reflux rather than stricture formation [23]. Finally, nonperistaltic contractions in the esophagus may occasionally produce a corrugated appearance, but this form of esophageal dysmotility is also observed as a transient finding without associated stricture formation.

Small-Caliber Esophagus

Since its original description by Vasiloupos in 2002 [24], the small-caliber esophagus has been recognized as an endoscopic sign of EoE in which there is diffuse loss of caliber of virtually the entire thoracic esophagus (Figs. 12.12 and 12.13) [25–30]. In a recent study, it was found that the small-caliber esophagus of EoE is also characterized on barium esophagography by long-segment narrowing of the thoracic esophagus; the narrowed segment has a mean length of about 15 cm with smooth,

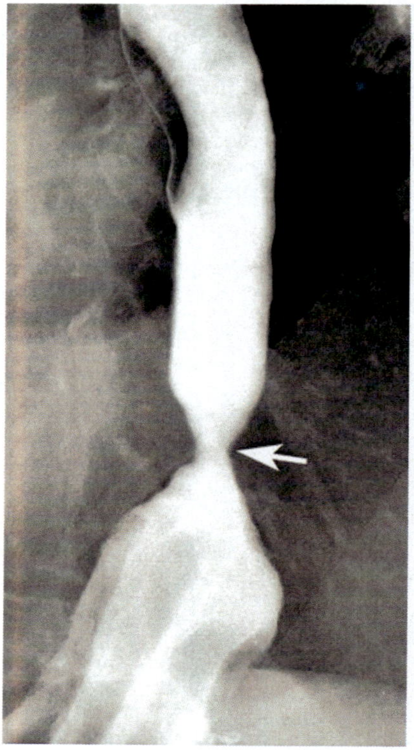

Fig. 12.5 Peptic stricture in the distal esophagus. This patient has a focal stricture (*arrow*) with smooth, tapered margins in the distal esophagus just above a hiatal hernia. Note similarity to the EoE stricture in Fig. 12.2

uniform contours and tapered margins that merge gradually with the adjacent esophagus [19]. In this study, patients with EoE all had a mean thoracic esophageal diameter of 20 mm or less, whereas control subjects all had a mean thoracic esophageal diameter greater than 20 mm, so 20 mm was a useful threshold diameter for suggesting the diagnosis of EoE [19]. In the same study, more than 90% of patients with a small-caliber esophagus on barium studies were found to have EoE on endoscopic biopsy specimens, so this finding appears to be a relatively specific radiographic sign of EoE [19]. It should be noted that the proximal extent of the small-caliber esophagus on barium studies is variable; the narrowed segment may extend proximally to the thoracic inlet, aortic arch, or even the left main bronchus, whereas it usually extends distally to the gastroesophageal junction [19].

The small-caliber esophagus should be differentiated radiographically from strictures in EoE, which are characterized by shorter, more focal segments of narrowing that have more discrete margins (see Figs. 12.1 and 12.2) [8]. Ring-like indentations

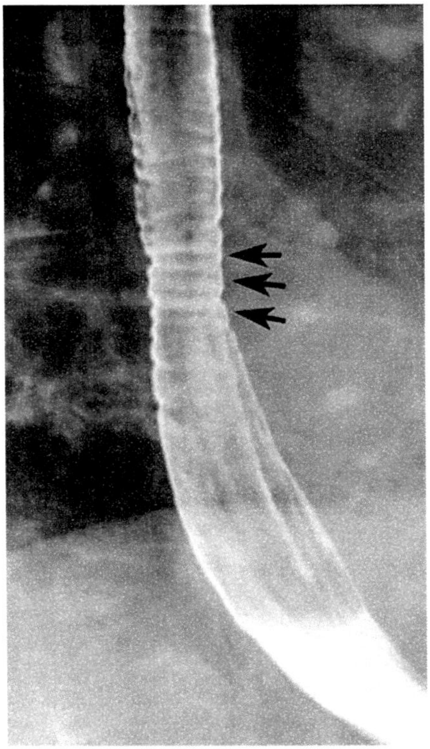

Fig. 12.6 EoE with a ringed esophagus. This patient has a smooth, tapered stricture in the lower third of the thoracic esophagus. Note multiple distinctive ring-like indentations (*arrows*) in the region of the stricture. This finding should be highly suggestive of EoE on barium studies

(i.e., the ringed esophagus) have also been observed in about 60% of patients with a small-caliber esophagus [19], so the presence of rings should further support the diagnosis of EoE when a small-caliber esophagus is diagnosed on barium studies. The degree of narrowing in some EoE patients with a small-caliber esophagus is quite subtle, however, so radiologists are more likely to diagnose a small-caliber esophagus on barium examinations if they have a low threshold for this finding when interpreting the studies.

The small-caliber esophagus of EoE has been reported on barium studies in older adolescents and adults, but to our knowledge, not in the pediatric population. We suspect this is because barium studies are more likely to be performed on adult patients with EoE and also because the small-caliber esophagus presumably represents an advanced stage of EoE that develops after years of inflammation, fibrosis, and scarring. Nevertheless, it remains unclear why some patients develop such diffuse esophageal disease while others have more localized disease manifested by rings or strictures.

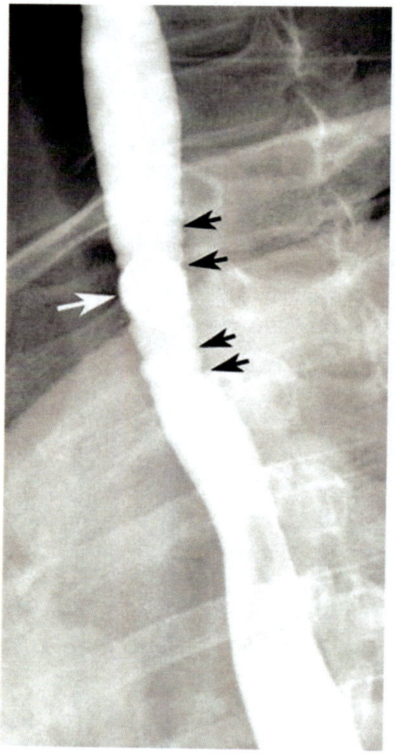

Fig. 12.7 EoE with a ringed esophagus. A prone, single-contrast esophagogram show a mild stricture in the upper thoracic esophagus with subtle ring-like indentations (*black arrows*) in the region of the stricture. A 12.5 mm in diameter barium tablet (*white arrow*) is seen to be lodged at the level of the stricture

Other Findings

A granular or nodular appearance of the mucosa has been detected on esophagography in up to 28% of patients with EoE presumably because of edema and inflammation of the mucosa (Fig. 12.14) [8]. Recently, Schatzki rings have also been reported in children with EoE. In one study, eight patients with EoE had rings that were demonstrated only on barium studies despite other typical findings of EoE at endoscopy [31]. Such observations reflect not only the subtle nature of Schatzki rings, but also the higher sensitivity of barium studies in detecting these rings compared to endoscopy [32]. Although there are no reports of Schatzki rings in adult patients with EoE, such rings may occasionally be encountered on barium studies (see Fig. 12.7).

Rarely, EoE patients with strictures or a small-caliber esophagus may also have esophageal intramural pseudodiverticula (see Fig. 12.13) [19, 33, 34]. As in other patients with pseudodiverticulosis, the pseudodiverticula presumably develop because of chronic esophagitis and stricture formation. These pseudodiverticula are typically seen in profile as tiny, flask-shaped outpouchings from the esophagus.

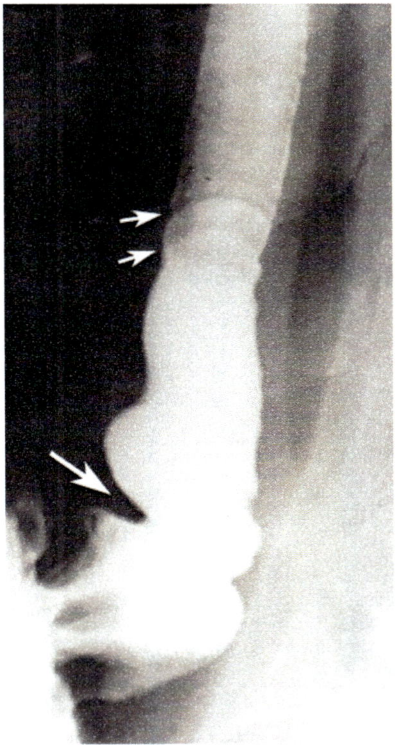

Fig. 12.8 EoE with a ringed esophagus. In this patient, a prone, single-contrast esophagogram shows the distinctive rings (*small arrows*) of EoE without a definite stricture in this region. Also note a Schatzki ring (*large arrow*) as a focal ring-like constriction at the gastroesophageal junction just above a hiatal hernia. Schatzki rings have also been described in patients with EoE

A true esophageal diverticulum has also been described in one patient with EoE, but this finding could have resulted from multiple previous esophageal dilation procedures [35]. Barium studies may also reveal hiatal hernias, gastroesophageal reflux, and esophageal dysmotility in patients with EoE, but such findings most likely have no relationship to this disease.

Other Radiologic Modalities

There is scant experience with other radiologic modalities in the diagnosis of EoE. In two case reports, CT of the chest revealed diffuse thickening of the esophageal wall in patients with the small-caliber esophagus of EoE [36, 37]. Although experience is

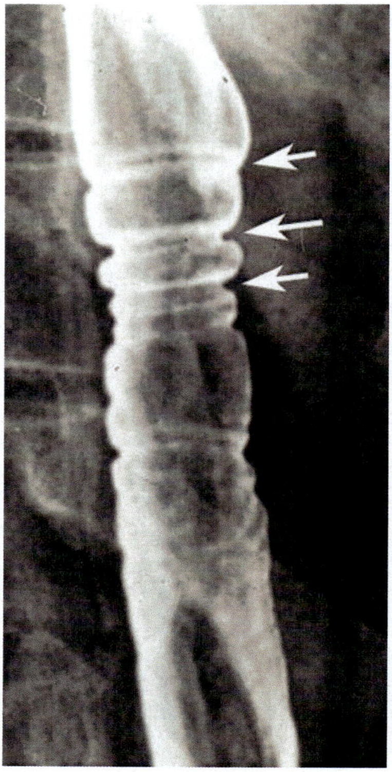

Fig. 12.9 Congenital esophageal stenosis with a ringed esophagus. This patient has distinctive ring-like constrictions (*arrows*) thought to be secondary to tracheobronchial remnants with cartilaginous rings in the wall of the esophagus. Note similarity to the ringed esophagus of EoE

limited, endoscopic ultrasound (EUS) in patients with EoE has revealed loss of the normal echo layers of the esophagus and diffuse esophageal wall thickening; these findings may be secondary to transmural fibrosis or localized thickening of the muscularis propria [38] or submucosa [39]. In other studies, EUS has revealed prominent longitudinal folds [40] and enlarged mediastinal lymph nodes that were found to be reactive with eosinophils on fine needle aspiration [41]. Nevertheless, the utility of EUS in patients with EoE remains uncertain. Also, the relatively large diameters of endoscopes used for EUS could increase the risk of perforation in patients with EoE because of the high prevalence of strictures and rings in these individuals.

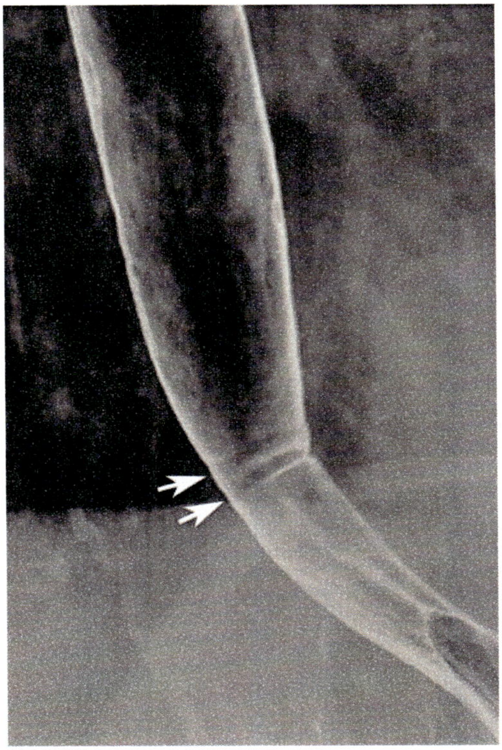

Fig. 12.10 Fixed transverse folds in the distal esophagus secondary to scarring from reflux esophagitis. This patient has a mild peptic stricture in the distal esophagus above a small hiatal hernia. Barium is also seen to be trapped between several fixed transverse folds (*arrows*) in the region of the stricture. This finding could be mistaken for the ringed esophagus of EoE

Esophagography for Suspected Esophageal Perforation

Adult patients with EoE commonly undergo dilation procedures for relief of dysphagia associated with rings and/or strictures. In the endoscopic literature, the risk of esophageal perforation during these dilation procedures appears to be greater in patients with EoE than in other patients with esophageal strictures. Patients with EoE also commonly report chest pain after dilation procedures, increasing the endoscopist's concern about a possible perforation. As a result, EoE patients often undergo esophagography with water-soluble contrast agents to rule out esophageal perforation in this clinical setting. Fortunately, when leaks occur after dilation procedures, patients with EoE are more likely to have intramural dissections or small, sealed-off leaks than other patients with esophageal perforation. Because of the often subtle nature of these leaks, the radiologist should immediately repeat the study with high-density barium if no leak is detected with a water-soluble contrast agent to increase the radiographic sensitivity for detecting subtle leaks. This approach increases the detection rate of esophageal perforation by 100% as compared to administration of water-soluble contrast agents alone [42].

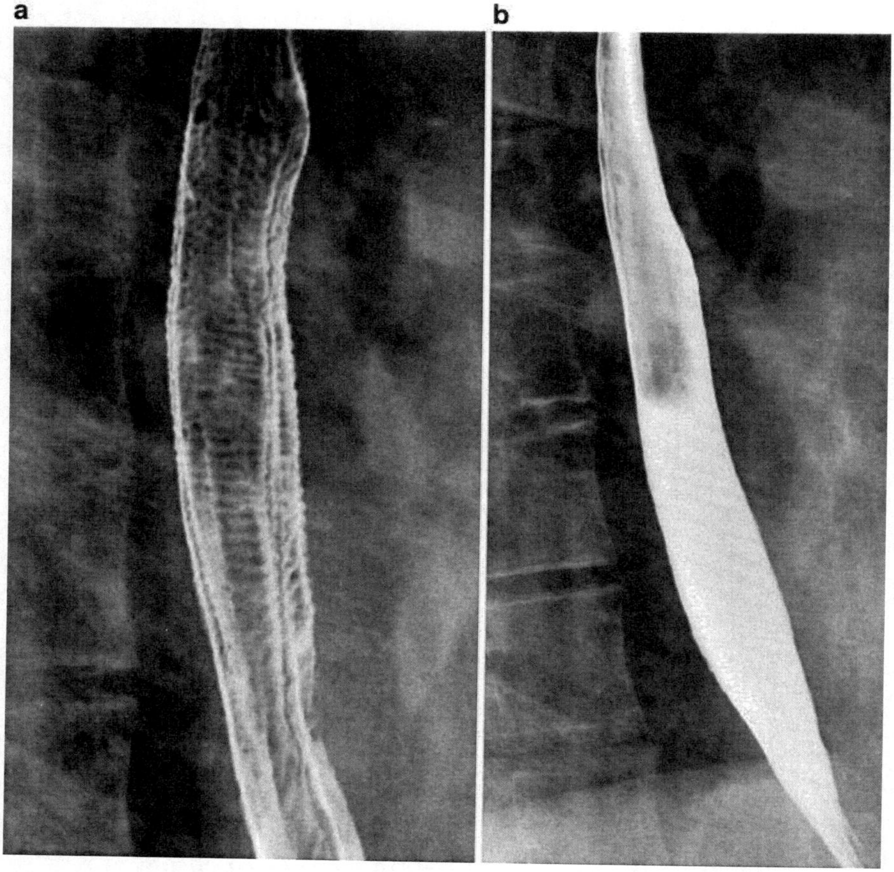

Fig. 12.11 Feline esophagus with multiple transverse striations in the esophagus. (**a**) The initial double-contrast view shows multiple, closely spaced transverse folds in the esophagus due to contraction of the longitudinally oriented muscularis mucosae. (**b**) A repeat view moments later shows no evidence of a feline esophagus. These transient transverse folds should not be mistaken for the ringed esophagus of EoE

Fig. 12.12 EoE with a small-caliber esophagus. A single-contrast esophagogram shows loss of distensibility of the entire thoracic esophagus. Note how there is diffuse luminal narrowing without a discernible stricture. This finding is characteristic of EoE

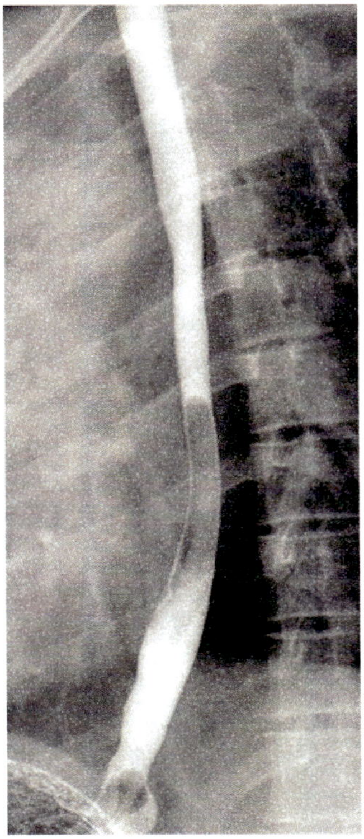

Fig. 12.13 EoE with a small-caliber esophagus. A double-contrast esophagogram shows loss of caliber of the entire thoracic esophagus indistinguishable from the small-caliber esophagus in Fig. 12.12. This patient also has tiny esophageal intramural pseudodiverticula seen as tiny outpouchings from the wall of the esophagus

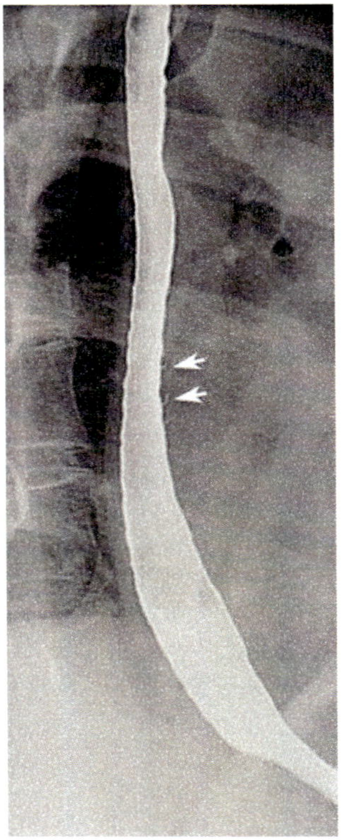

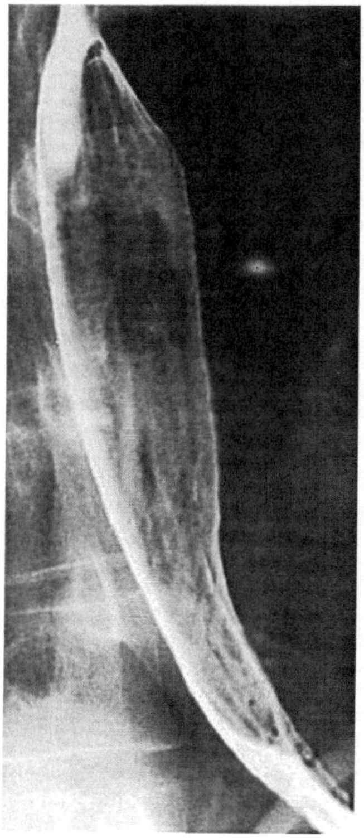

Fig. 12.14 EoE with a granular esophagus. A double-contrast esophagogram shows diffuse granularity secondary to edema and spasm of the mucosa

Conclusion

Barium esophagography can be helpful in a number of ways for evaluating patients with suspected EoE. First and foremost, it is a global examination for patients with dysphagia and can be used not only to diagnose EoE, but also a host of other abnormalities in the pharynx and esophagus. In some patients, the barium study may demonstrate relatively specific findings of EoE, such as the ringed esophagus and the small-caliber esophagus. When the barium study detects subtle strictures or diffuse esophageal narrowing not visualized at endoscopy, these findings not only may explain the patient's symptoms, but also may indicate the need for an esophageal dilation procedure. In EoE patients with severe dysphagia, the barium study may also reveal tight strictures that cannot be traversed by the endoscope and, in such cases, enable visualization of the esophagus below the stricture, facilitating treatment planning. Finally, esophagography has a critical role in assessing for possible perforation when esophageal dilation procedures are performed on these patients.

References

1. Levine MS, Rubesin SE, Laufer I. Barium esophagography: a study for all seasons. Clin Gastroenterol Hepatol. 2008;6:11–25.
2. Ott DJ, Chen YM, Hewson EG, et al. Esophageal motility: assessment with synchronous video tape fluoroscopy and manometry. Radiology. 1989;173:419–22.
3. Levine MS, Laufer I. The gastrointestinal tract: dos and don'ts of digital imaging. Radiology. 1998;207:311–6.
4. Müller S, Puhl S, Vieth M, Stolte M. Analysis of symptoms and endoscopic findings in 117 patients with histologic diagnoses of eosinophilic esophagitis. Endoscopy. 2007;39:339–44.
5. Lucendo AJ, Pasqual-Turrion JM, Navarro M, et al. Endoscopic, bioptic, and manometric findings in eosinophilic esophagitis before and after steroid therapy: a case series. Endoscopy. 2007;39:765–71.
6. Prasad GA, Talley NJ, Romero Y, et al. Prevalence and predictive factors of eosinophilic esophagitis in patients presenting with dysphagia: a prospective study. Am J Gastroenterol. 2007;102:2627–32.
7. Croese J, Fairley SK, Masson JW, et al. Clinical and endoscopic features of eosinophilic esophagitis in adults. Gastrointest Endosc. 2003;58:516–22.
8. Zimmerman SL, Levine MS, Rubesin SE, et al. Idiopathic eosinophilic esophagitis in adults: the ringed esophagus. Radiology. 2005;236:159–65.
9. Picus D, Frank PH. Eosinophilic esophagitis. AJR Am J Roentgenol. 1981;136:1001–3.
10. Matzinger MA, Daneman A. Esophageal involvement in eosinophilic gastroenteritis. Pediatr Radiol. 1983;13:35–8.
11. Feczko PJ, Halpert RD, Zonca M. Radiographic abnormalities in eosinophilic esophagitis. Gastrointest Radiol. 1985;10:321–4.
12. Vitellas KM, Bennett WF, Bova JG, Johnson JC, Caldwell JH, Mayle JE. Idiopathic eosinophilic esophagitis. Radiology. 1993;186:789–93.
13. Mahajan L, Wyllie R, Petras R, Steffen R, Kay M. Idiopathic eosinophilic esophagitis with stricture formation in a patient with long-standing eosinophilic gastroenteritis. Gastrointest Endosc. 1997;46:557–60.
14. Levine MS. Gastroesophageal reflux disease. In: Gore RM, Levine MS, editors. Textbook of gastrointestinal radiology. 3rd ed. Philadelphia, PA: Elsevier; 2007. p. 337–58.
15. Levine MS. Other esophagitides. In: Gore RM, Levine MS, editors. Textbook of gastrointestinal radiology. 3rd ed. Philadelphia, PA: Elsevier; 2007. p. 375–400.
16. Al-Hussaini AA, Semaan T, El Hag IA. Esophageal trachealization: a feature of eosinophilic esophagitis. Saudi J Gastroenterol. 2009;15:193–5.
17. Bousvaros A, Antonioli DA, Winter HS. Ringed esophagus: an association with esophagitis. Am J Gastroenterol. 1992;87:1187–90.
18. Siafakas CG, Ryan CK, Brown MR, Miller TL. Multiple esophageal rings: an association with eosinophilic esophagitis – case report and review of the literature. Am J Gastroenterol. 2000;95:1572–5.
19. White SB, Levine MS, Rubesin SE, Spencer GS, Katzka DA, Laufer I. The small-caliber esophagus: a radiographic sign of idiopathic eosinophilic esophagitis. Radiology. 2010;256(1):127–34.
20. Katzka DA, Levine MS, Ginsberg GG, et al. Congenital esophageal stenosis in adults. Am J Gastroenterol. 2000;95:32–6.
21. Oh CH, Levine MS, Katzka DA, et al. Congenital esophageal stenosis in adults: clinical and radiographic findings in seven patients. AJR Am J Roentgenol. 2001;176:1179–82.
22. Levine MS, Goldstein HM. Fixed transverse folds in the esophagus: a sign of reflux esophagitis. AJR Am J Roentgenol. 1984;143:275–8.
23. Gohel VK, Edell SI, Laufer I, Rhodes WH. Transverse folds in the human esophagus. Radiology. 1978;128:303–8.
24. Vasilopoulos S, Murphy P, Auerbach A, et al. The small-caliber esophagus: an unappreciated cause of dysphagia for solids in patients with eosinophilic esophagitis. Gastrointest Endosc. 2002;55:99–106.

25. Fox VL, Nurko S, Furuta GT. Eosinophilic esophagitis: it's not just kid's stuff. Gastrointest Endosc. 2002;56:260–70.
26. Munitiz V, Martinez de Haro LF, Ortiz A, et al. Primary eosinophilic esophagitis. Dis Esophagus. 2003;16:165–8.
27. Potter JW, Saeian K, Staff D, Komorowski RA, Shaker R, Hogan WJ. Eosinophilic esophagitis in adults: an emerging problem with unique esophageal features. Gastrointest Endosc. 2004;59:355–61.
28. Arora AS, Yamazaki K. Eosinophilic esophagitis: asthma of the esophagus? Clin Gastroenterol Hepatol. 2004;2:523–30.
29. Remedios M, Campbell C, Jones DM, Kerlin P. Eosinophilic esophagitis in adults: clinical, endoscopic, histologic findings, and response to treatment with fluticasone propionate. Gastrointest Endosc. 2006;63:3–12.
30. Sgouros SN, Bergele C, Mantides A. Eosinophilic esophagitis in adults: what is the clinical significance? Endoscopy. 2006;38:515–20.
31. Nurko S, Teitelbaum JE, Husain K, et al. Association of Schatzki ring with eosinophilic esophagitis in children. J Pediatr Gastroenterol Nutr. 2004;38:436–41.
32. Ott DJ, Chen YM, Wu WC, Gelfand DW, Munitz HA. Radiographic and endoscopic sensitivity in detecting lower esophageal mucosal ring. AJR Am J Roentgenol. 1986;147:261–5.
33. Tsai CM, Butler J, Cash BD. Pseudodiverticulosis with eosinophilic esophagitis: first reported case. Gastrointest Endosc. 2007;66:1223–4.
34. Engel MA, Raithel M, Amann K, Greess H, Hahn EG, Konturek PC. Rare coincidence of eosinophilic esophagitis with esophageal stenosis and intramural pseudodiverticulosis. Dig Liver Dis. 2008;40:700–6.
35. Mecklenburg I, Weber F, Folwaczny C. Spontaneous recovery of dysphagia by rupture of an esophageal diverticulum in eosinophilic esophagitis. Dig Dis Sci. 2006;51:1241–2.
36. Horiki N, Maruyama M, Fujita Y, Yonekura T. A case of idiopathic eosinophilic esophagitis with CT findings showing marked thickening of the esophageal wall. Jpn J Gastroenterol. 1998;95:769–76.
37. Ruiz-Rebollo ML, Atienza-Sanchez R, Perez-Alonso P. A new case of eosinophilic esophagitis. Dis Esophagus. 2004;17:176–9.
38. Stevoff C, Rao S, Parsons W, Kahrilas PJ, Hirano I. EUS and histopathologic correlates in eosinophilic esophagitis. Gastrointest Endosc. 2001;54:373–7.
39. Furuta K, Adachi K, Kowari K, et al. A Japanese case of eosinophilic esophagitis. J Gastroenterol. 2006;41:706–10.
40. Fox VL, Nurko S, Teitelbaum JE, Badizadegan K, Furuta GT. High-resolution EUS in children with eosinophilic "allergic" esophagitis. Gastrointest Endosc. 2003;57:30–6.
41. Bhutani MS, Moparty B, Chaya CT, Schnadig V, Logrono R. Endoscopic ultrasound-guided fine-needle aspiration of enlarged mediastinal lymph nodes in eosinophilic esophagitis. Endoscopy. 2007;39 suppl 1:E82–3.
42. Swanson JO, Levine MS, Redfern RO, Rubesin SE. Usefulness of high-density barium for detection of leaks after esophagogastrectomy, total gastrectomy, and total laryngectomy. AJR Am J Roentgenol. 2003;181:415–20.

Chapter 13
Endoscopic Features of Eosinophilic Esophagitis

David A. Leiman and Gary W. Falk

Keywords Eosinophilic esophagitis • Dysphagia • Food impaction • Biopsy • Endoscopy

Introduction

Eosinophilic esophagitis (EoE) is a chronic inflammatory disorder of children and adults. The disease is defined by clinicopathologic criteria, including symptoms of dysphagia and food impaction, esophageal biopsies with ≥15 eosinophils per high powered field and lack of response to antisecretory therapy [1]. Patients with eosinophilic esophagitis have a wide variety of endoscopic findings (Table 13.1) and the disease does not have a uniform endoscopic appearance. In fact, one study suggested that only 38% of individuals thought to have eosinophilic esophagitis at the time of endoscopy had histologic confirmation of the disease and a subset of patients may also have an entirely normal appearing esophagus! [2] Furthermore, endoscopic findings may vary by age [3]. Endoscopy plays a key role in the diagnosis of EoE patients and the varied endoscopic features of this disease are the focus of this chapter.

G.W. Falk (✉)
Department of Medicine, Hospital of the University of Pennsylvania, Perelman School of Medicine, Philadelphia, PA, USA

Department of Medicine, Division of Gastroenterology, Hospital of the University of Pennsylvania, 3 Ravdin, 3400 Spruce Street, Philadelphia, PA 19104, USA
e-mail: gary.falk@uphs.upenn.edu

C.A. Liacouras and J.E. Markowitz (eds.), *Eosinophilic Esophagitis*,
Clinical Gastroenterology, DOI 10.1007/978-1-60761-515-6_13,

Table 13.1 Endoscopic features associated with eosinophilic esophagitis

Normal endoscopy
Linear furrowing
Concentric rings
White exudates
Diminished vascularity
Proximal strictures
Small caliber esophagus
Crepe-paper esophagus
Schatzki's ring
Pseudodiverticula
Increased wall thickness (on EUS)

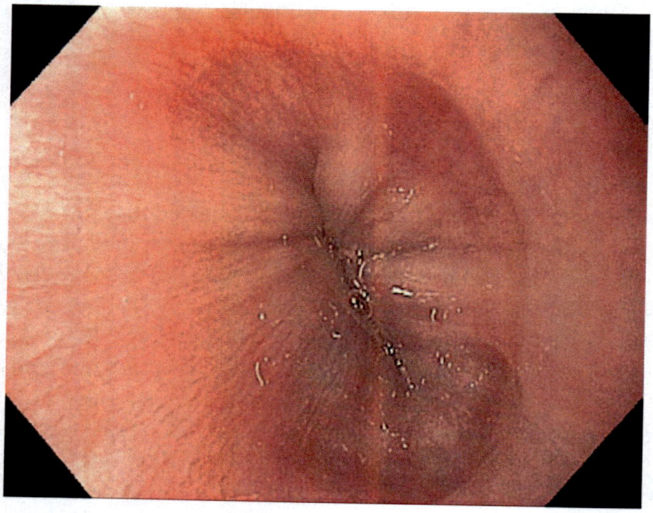

Fig. 13.1 Normal endoscopic appearance of the esophagus

Endoscopy of the Normal Esophagus

The normal squamous epithelium of the esophagus appears "pearly" white on endoscopic examination (Fig. 13.1) and terminates at a "Z-line" which serves as a demarcation from the salmon-colored columnar epithelium of the stomach. The esophagus is characterized by a fine network of subepithelial blood vessels that are more easily seen with partial air insufflation and accentuated with filters such as narrow-band imaging. The blood vessels are linearly oriented and may be more apparent in the distal esophagus.

Endoscopic Features of EoE

Linear Furrowing

Linear furrows are one of the most characteristic findings of EoE. These appear as a linear pattern of furrows that typically involve the full length of the esophagus. They can be seen with conventional white light endoscopy and are further accentuated with narrow-band imaging (Fig. 13.2). The use of chromoendoscopy with contrast-enhancing dye can make furrows appear more distinct as well [4]. Observations with endoscopic ultrasonography suggest that furrows may be related to thickening of the mucosal and submucosal layers [5]. Furrows may be seen either alone or in conjunction with other endoscopic features of EoE. It is estimated that linear furrows occur in 11–100% of EoE patients [3, 4, 6–11].

Furrows have also been described in both gastroesophageal reflux disease (GERD) patients and normal adults, but furrows in these settings tend to be more faint and limited to the distal esophagus [4]. Overall, the presence of furrows is highly suggestive of EoE in both children and adults and is an endoscopic finding that may help to distinguish EoE patients from GERD patients [3].

Concentric Rings

Perhaps the most striking endoscopic finding of EoE is that of multiple concentric rings and termed the ringed, corrugated, or "feline" esophagus (Fig. 13.3). Rings

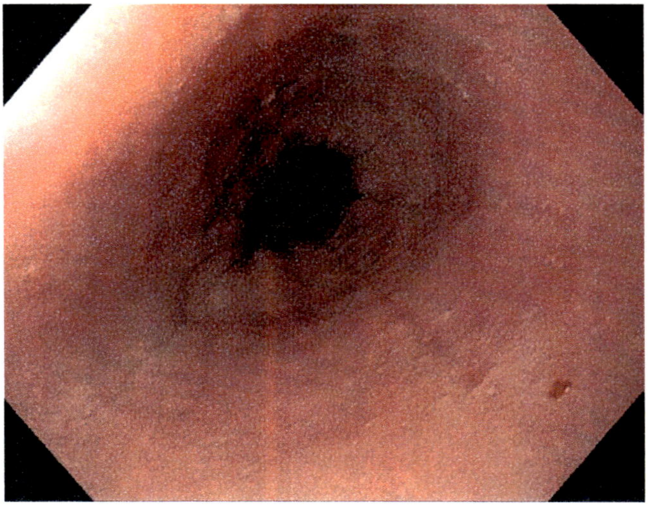

Fig. 13.2 Endoscopic appearance of linear furrows

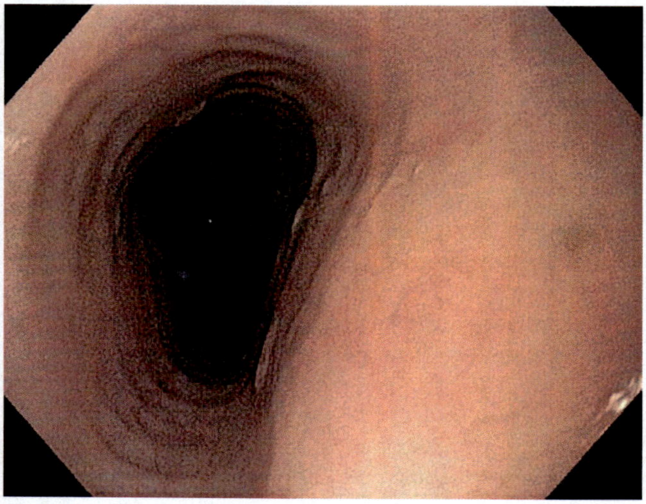

Fig. 13.3 Endoscopic appearance of concentric rings

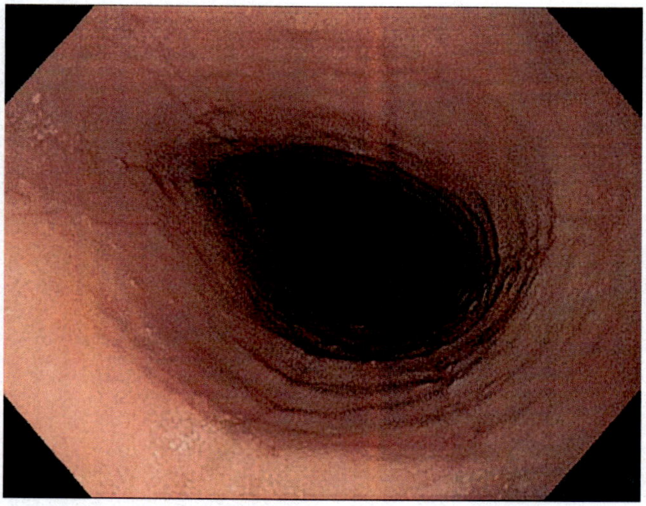

Fig. 13.4 Endoscopic appearance of concentric rings with linear furrows

can appear as the only finding or may be seen in conjunction with other endoscopic findings of EoE (Figs. 13.4 and 13.5). Concentric rings may be observed focally in esophageal segments or may involve the entire length of the esophagus. As such, they are distinctly different from a Schatzki's ring, which is typically found only at the squamocolumnar junction. Work by Dellon et al. suggests that the finding of rings is one of the features that can differentiate EoE patients from GERD patients [3]. The etiology of these esophageal rings is not completely understood and it is

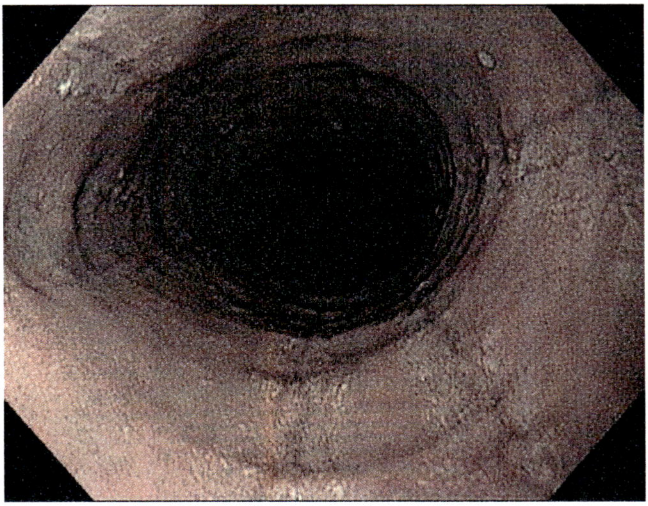

Fig. 13.5 Endoscopic appearance of concentric rings with linear furrows accentuated with narrow-band imaging

thought that rings may represent intermittent contraction of the deep muscle layer or possibly eosinophilic infiltration [12]. Interestingly these rings may resolve with appropriate therapy [9]. Estimates of the prevalence of the ringed esophagus range from 19 to 88% of EoE patients [3, 7–10, 13–15].

White Exudate

White exudates come in a variety of different shapes and sizes. Other terms used for white exudates include white specks, pinpoint nodules, patches, and scales. These vary in size from 1 to 3 mm and are typically scattered along the length of the esophagus giving the esophagus a speckled appearance and may be easily dislodged (Figs. 13.6 and 13.7). White exudates may be mistaken for *Candida* esophagitis, but in the setting of eosinophilic esophagitis, this finding corresponds to collections of eosinophils or even microabscesses in the mucosa [15]. The finding is more common in children than adults [3]. The prevalence of white exudates varies from 15 to 26% [3, 7–11, 16].

Diminished Mucosal Vascularity

The normal esophagus has a well-defined network of subepithelial blood vessels visible at the time of endoscopy as described above but mucosal inflammation may be associated with a loss of the normal vascular pattern. This appearance may be due to expansion of the basal layer of the mucosa accompanied by edema [12].

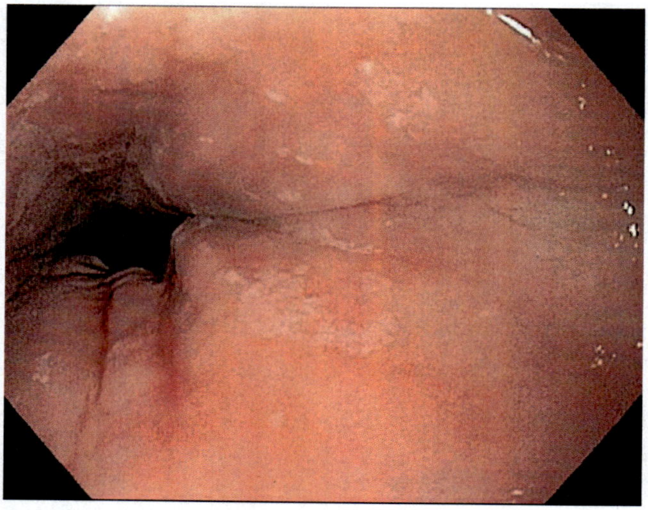

Fig. 13.6 Endoscopic appearance of white exudate

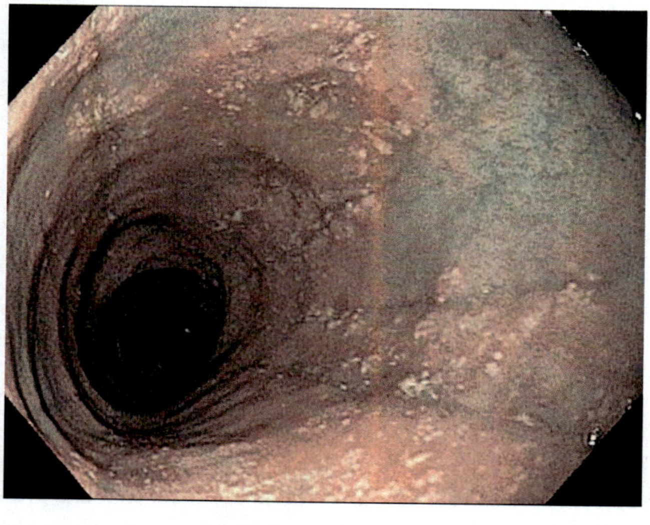

Fig. 13.7 Endoscopic appearance of white exudates combined with linear furrows and concentric rings accentuated by narrow band imaging

In a study of 30 adult EoE patients by Straumann et al., loss of the normal vascular pattern was found in 93% making it the most frequent endoscopic finding [15]. Others have described decreased vascularity in 5–26% of EoE patients [3, 7, 10]. While this finding may be subjective, current high definition white light endoscopes allow for more accurate detection of this finding, which may provide a clue for the presence of EoE.

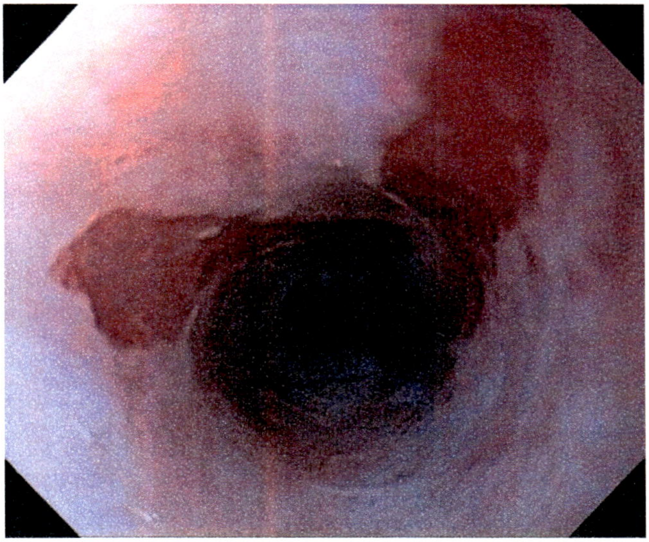

Fig. 13.8 Endoscopic appearance of the crepe-paper esophagus accompanied by a mucosal rent. (Image courtesy of Evan S. Dellon, MD, MPH)

Strictures

Focal strictures, in the absence of narrow caliber esophagus or concentric rings, may be encountered in 3–66% of EoE patients [3, 7–10, 13, 15]. These strictures are typically encountered in the proximal esophagus, may be subtle and are characterized by smooth circumferential narrowing of the esophagus. Strictures are more commonly seen in adults than in children [3, 4].

Small Caliber Esophagus

Small caliber esophagus is a unique finding in EoE and is defined as a narrow fixed internal diameter of the esophagus [13]. This feature may not be appreciated on endoscope insertion, but is characterized by extensive linear abrasions or mucosal rents best seen upon withdrawal of the endoscope or after dilation [17]. The prevalence of small caliber esophagus is estimated to be between 10 and 28% [3, 9, 10, 13].

Crepe-Paper Esophagus

The term "crepe-paper" esophagus was first suggested by Straumann et al. in a 2003 case series of five men. The mucosa of the esophagus is characterized as fragile, delicate, inelastic, and tears with little pressure (Fig. 13.8) [18].

Schatzki's Ring

Schatzki's ring, a thin diaphragm-like circumferential fold of mucosa protruding into lumen and located at gastroesophageal junction is present in 0.2–15% of the general population. It is typically associated with reflux disease but has also been described in patients with EoE [19]. Despite these reports, it remains unclear if Schatzki's rings are in fact part of the spectrum of EoE. Desai et al. described 31 adults with dysphagia and food impaction and found that 29% of those who met histologic criteria for EoE had a Schatzki's ring [11]. Gonsalves et al. reported that 14% of adult patients with EoE had incidental findings of a Schatzki's ring, but none of the patients with Schatzki's rings had significant mucosal eosinophilia [10]. However, others have failed to find a relationship between Schatzki's rings and EoE [20]. Thus the data to date suggest that there is no clear relationship between Schatzki's rings and EoE.

Pseudodiverticulosis

A more recently described finding in EoE is the presence of intramural pseudodiverticulosis. Pseudodiverticulosis is a rare finding in the esophagus characterized by multiple flask-shaped outpouchings in the esophageal wall that represent dilated excretory ducts of esophageal mucus glands [21]. These are usually seen in the setting motor abnormalities as well as in *Candida* infection, corrosive ingestion, strictures, Plummer–Vinson, and carcinoma [22]. Pseudodiverticulae have been described in two case reports to date (Fig. 13.9) [21, 22].

Normal Endoscopy in EoE

Interestingly, a completely normal endoscopy may be encountered in 10–25% of patients with EoE· [2, 3, 7, 14] In a study of 376 patients with unexplained dysphagia at the Mayo Clinic, 10 of 102 patients (9.8%) with a normal appearing esophagus had EoE on biopsies. Overall, this finding may be more common in the pediatric than the adult population [3].

Endosonographic Findings

Endosonography has been studied in a limited number of EoE patients to date. A case report of an elderly male by Stevoff et al. described circumferential but asymmetric thickening or the muscularis propria [23]. Fox et al. found significant differences in total wall thickness (2.8 mm vs. 2.1 mm), combined mucosa and

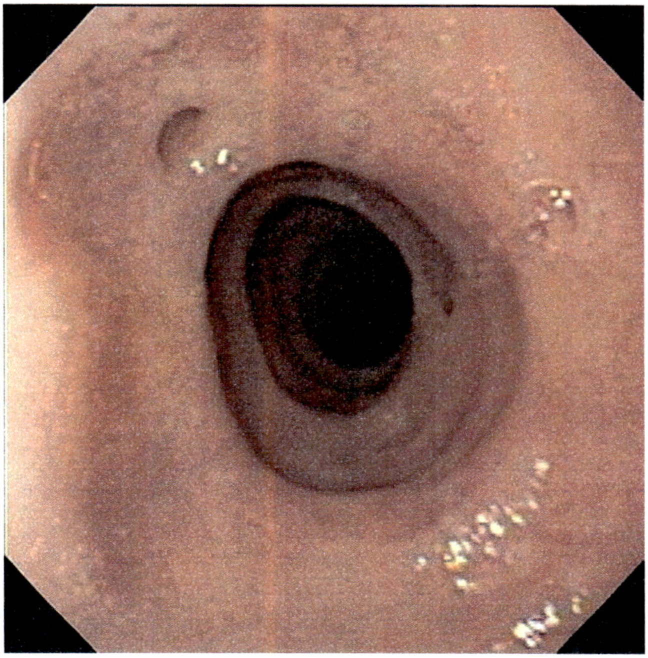

Fig. 13.9 Endoscopic appearance of the pseudodiverticulosis with concentric rings. (Image courtesy of Evan S. Dellon, MD, MPH)

submucosa thickness (1.6 mm vs. 1.1 mm), and muscularis propria thickness (1.2 mm vs. 1.0 mm) between children with EoE and control children [24]. Wall thickening has also been described in an adult case report [25].

Conclusions and Future Directions

Despite increased awareness, understanding, and evaluation of EoE, strict endoscopic criteria and terminology for defining the disease remain elusive. It seems clear that despite the growing number of endoscopic features identified and described above, these alone are not sufficient to make the diagnosis. Some features of EoE are more common in children (normal, white plaques, erythema) whereas other features are more common in adults (concentric rings, proximal strictures, crepe paper mucosa, narrow caliber esophagus) [3]. The wide variety of features described above may be found alone or in combination in EoE patients. Furthermore, one study has shown only 33% of patients with endoscopic findings thought to be compatible with EoE will receive a diagnosis of EoE and as described above, a subset of patients with EoE will have a normal endoscopy [2]. The diagnostic utility of endoscopic features of

EoE increases with the number of features present; when one feature was present EoE was diagnosed only 38% of the time vs. 40–66% of the time when more than one feature (rings) was present [2]. The inter- and intraobserver agreement for the various features described above have not been evaluated to date and are clearly in need of further study. It is hoped that standardized terminology and definitions of endoscopic findings of the esophagus in EoE become part of the new consensus guidelines under development at present.

References

1. Furuta GT, Liacouras CA, Collins MH, et al. Eosinophilic esophagitis in children and adults: a systematic review and consensus recommendations for diagnosis and treatment. Gastroenterology. 2007;133:1342–63.
2. Prasad GA, Talley NJ, Romero Y, et al. Prevalence and predictive factors of eosinophilic esophagitis in patients presenting with dysphagia: a prospective study. Am J Gastroenterol. 2007;102:2627–32.
3. Dellon ES, Gibbs WB, Fritchie KJ, et al. Clinical, endoscopic, and histologic findings distinguish eosinophilic esophagitis from gastroesophageal reflux disease. Clin Gastroenterol Hepatol. 2009;7:1305–13.
4. Croese J, Fairley SK, Masson JW, et al. Clinical and endoscopic features of eosinophilic esophagitis in adults. Gastrointest Endosc. 2003;58:516–22.
5. Fox VL, Nurko S, Furuta GT. Eosinophilic esophagitis: it's not just kid's stuff. Gastrointest Endosc. 2002;56:260–70.
6. Gupta SK, Fitzgerald JF, Chong SK, et al. Vertical lines in distal esophageal mucosa (VLEM): a true endoscopic manifestation of esophagitis in children? Gastrointest Endosc. 1997; 45:485–9.
7. Müller S, Pühl S, Vieth M, et al. Analysis of symptoms and endoscopic findings in 117 patients with histological diagnoses of eosinophilic esophagitis. Endoscopy. 2007;39:339–44.
8. Cohen MS, Kaufman AB, Palazzo JP, et al. An audit of endoscopic complications in adult eosinophilic esophagitis. Clin Gastroenterol Hepatol. 2007;5:1149–53.
9. Remedios M, Campbell C, Jones DM, et al. Eosinophilic esophagitis in adults: clinical, endoscopic, histologic findings, and response to treatment with fluticasone propionate. Gastrointest Endosc. 2006;63:3–12.
10. Gonsalves N, Policarpio-Nicolas M, Zhang Q, et al. Histopathologic variability and endoscopic correlates in adults with eosinophilic esophagitis. Gastrointest Endosc. 2006; 64:313–9.
11. Desai TK, Stecevic V, Chang CH, et al. Association of eosinophilic inflammation with esophageal food impaction in adults. Gastrointest Endosc. 2005;61:795–801.
12. Fox VL. Eosinophilic esophagitis: endoscopic findings. Gastrointest Endosc Clin N Am. 2008;18:45–57.
13. Potter JW, Saeian K, Staff D, et al. Eosinophilic esophagitis in adults: an emerging problem with unique esophageal features. Gastrointest Endosc. 2004;59:355–61.
14. Kaplan M, Mutlu EA, Jakate S, et al. Endoscopy in eosinophilic esophagitis: "feline" esophagus and perforation risk. Clin Gastroenterol Hepatol. 2003;1:433–7.
15. Straumann A, Spichtin HP, Bucher KA, et al. Eosinophilic esophagitis: red on microscopy, white on endoscopy. Digestion. 2004;70:109–16.
16. Lim JR, Gupta SK, Croffie JM, et al. White specks in the esophageal mucosa: an endoscopic manifestation of non-reflux eosinophilic esophagitis in children. Gastrointest Endosc. 2004;59:835–8.

17. Vasilopoulos S, Murphy P, Auerbach A, et al. The small-caliber esophagus: an unappreciated cause of dysphagia for solids in patients with eosinophilic esophagitis. Gastrointest Endosc. 2002;55:99–106.
18. Straumann A, Rossi L, Simon HU, et al. Fragility of the esophageal mucosa: a pathognomonic endoscopic sign of primary eosinophilic esophagitis? Gastrointest Endosc. 2003;57:407–12.
19. Nurko S, Teitelbaum JE, Husain K, et al. Association of Schatzki ring with eosinophilic esophagitis in children. J Pediatr Gastroenterol Nutr. 2004;38:436–41.
20. Sgouros SN, Bergele C, Mantides A. Schatzki's rings are not associated with eosinophilic esophagitis. Gastrointest Endosc. 2006;63:535–6.
21. Engel MA, Raithel M, Amann K, et al. Rare coincidence of eosinophilic esophagitis with esophageal stenosis and intramural pseudodiverticulosis. Dig Liver Dis. 2008;40:700–6.
22. Tsai CM, Butler J, Cash BD. Pseudodiverticulosis with eosinophilic esophagitis: first reported case. Gastrointest Endosc. 2007;66:1223–34.
23. Stevoff C, Rao S, Parsons W, et al. EUS and histopathologic correlates in eosinophilic esophagitis. Gastrointest Endosc. 2001;54:373–7.
24. Fox VL, Nurko S, Teitelbaum JE, et al. High-resolution EUS in children with eosinophilic "allergic" esophagitis. Gastrointest Endosc. 2003;57:30–6.
25. Bhutani MS, Moparty B, Chaya CT, et al. Endoscopic ultrasound-guided fine-needle aspiration of enlarged mediastinal lymph nodes in eosinophilic esophagitis. Endoscopy. 2007;39 Suppl 1:E82–3.

Chapter 14
Histologic Features of Eosinophilic Esophagitis

Margaret H. Collins

Keywords Eosinophilic esophagitis • Gastroesophageal reflux disease • Pediatric • Pathology

Introduction

Eosinophilic esophagitis (EE) is an increasingly recognized chronic inflammatory disorder of the esophagus affecting both adults and children [1–3]. EE shows a strong predilection for males, and may occur in families [4]. Esophageal biopsies from EE patients exhibit characteristic histology [5, 6] (Figs. 14.1–14.3). Gene microarray analysis of esophageal biopsies identifies a transcriptome unique to EE characterized by marked overexpression of the eotaxin-3 gene, which encodes a chemokine that attracts eosinophils into esophageal epithelium [7]. Results of an ongoing genome-wide association study strongly implicate the thymic stromal lymphopoietin (TSLP) gene as also important in the pathogenesis of EE [8]. Clinical and experimental studies demonstrate that multiple cytokines participate in numerous aspects of this disease [9–16].

M.H. Collins (✉)
Department of Pathology, University of Cincinnati, Cincinnati Children's
Hospital Medical Center, B4.180 ML 1010, 3333 Burnett Avenue, Cincinnati, OH 45229, USA
e-mail: Margaret.collins@chmcc.org

C.A. Liacouras and J.E. Markowitz (eds.), *Eosinophilic Esophagitis*,
Clinical Gastroenterology, DOI 10.1007/978-1-60761-515-6_14,

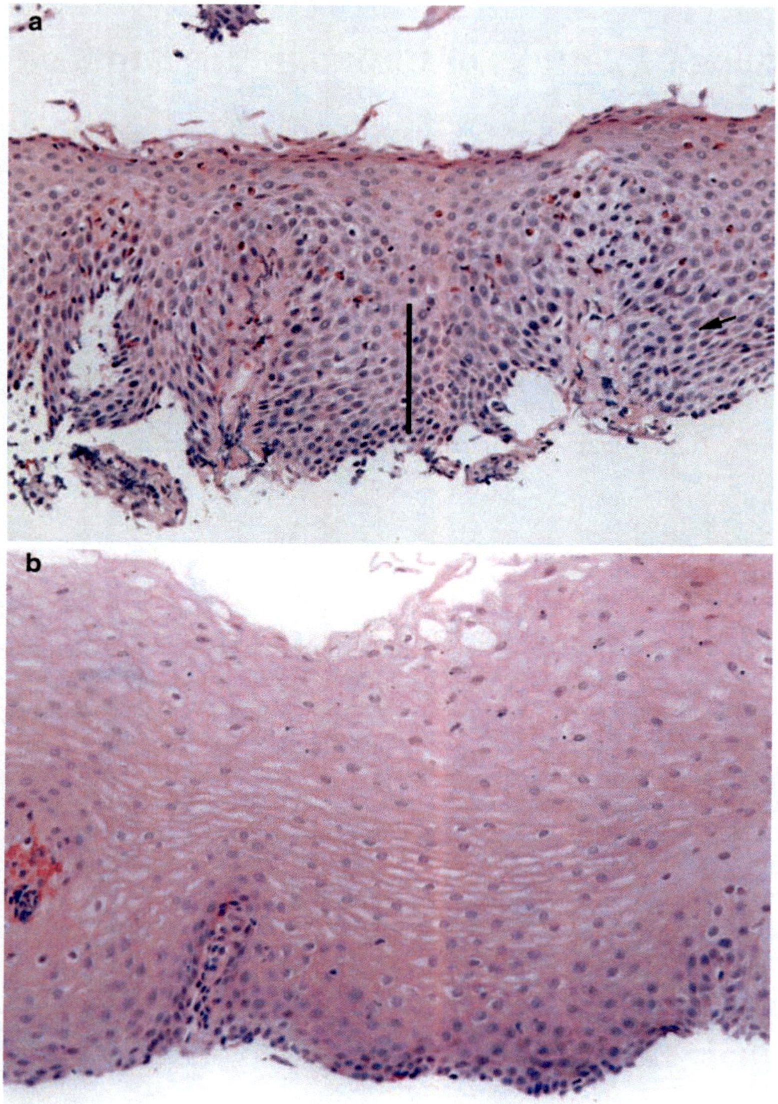

Fig. 14.1 (**a**) This esophageal biopsy illustrates many of the histologic features of eosinophilic esophagitis (EE). There are numerous intraepithelial eosinophils including at the surface (*top*), the basal layer of the epithelium is expanded (*bar*), papillae appear elongated, and intercellular spaces appear dilated (*arrow*) [hematoxylin and eosin (H&E), ×200]. (**b**) This esophageal biopsy from the same patient whose biopsy is shown in (**a**) appears normal. This is a biopsy following therapy for EE. Intraepithelial eosinophils were not found in any high power field in the biopsy, and the epithelial architecture and integrity are restored to normal (H&E, ×200)

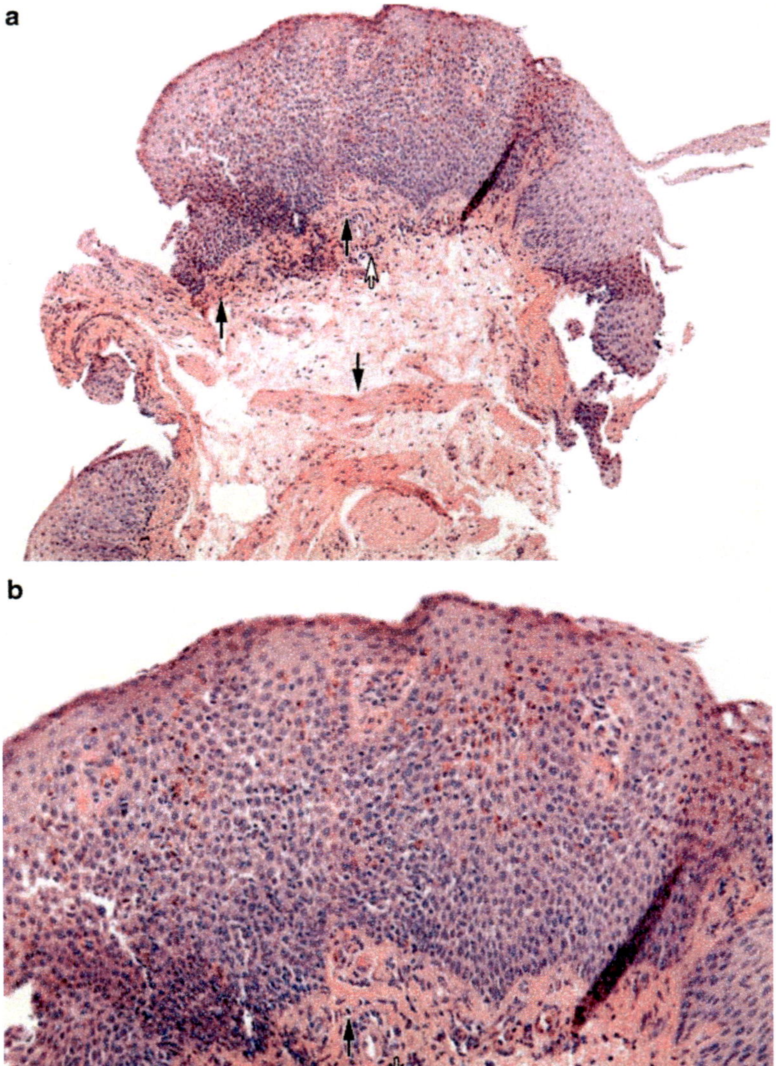

Fig. 14.2 (**a**) This biopsy includes the lamina propria (*black arrow* at left) and muscularis mucosa (*black arrow* pointing down in center) that are not seen in most esophageal biopsies. The lamina propria forms a distinct layer below the esophageal squamous epithelium, and in this case shows fibrosis. It also shows mainly chronic inflammation that includes plasma cells (*white arrow*), as well as scattered eosinophils (*outlined arrow*). The deeper lamina propria closer to the muscularis mucosa appears normal [hematoxylin and eosin (H&E), ×40]. (**b**) This is a closer view of the biopsy in (**a**). The dense fibrosis of the lamina propria is more apparent, and plasma cells (*white arrow*) and eosinophils (*outlined arrow*) are seen more clearly. An extension of the lamina propria forming a papilla is seen at the right. Also apparent is the marked basal layer expansion, dilated intercellular spaces, and numerous intraepithelial eosinophils (H&E, ×200)

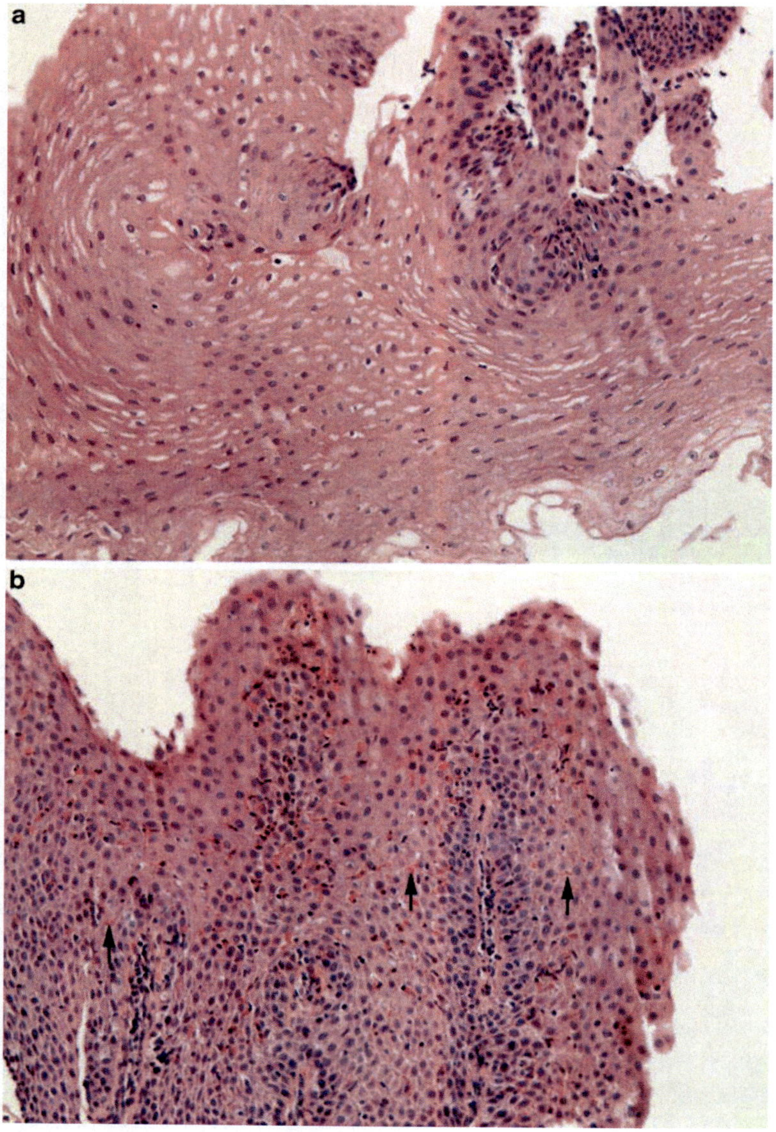

Fig. 14.3 (**a**) This piece that appears normal is from the same biopsy, the same site in the esophagus, as the piece shown in (**b**). This illustration emphasizes the patchy nature of the infiltrate in eosinophilic esophagitis (EE), and the need to submit multiple samples if EE is suspected to increase the diagnostic yield [hematoxylin and eosin (H&E), ×200]. (**b**) Although somewhat tangentially oriented, this biopsy shows many of the histologic features of EE, included trails of extracellular eosinophil granules (*arrows*). If this piece was not included in the sample, the diagnosis would be missed. This patient has inflammatory bowel disease (H&E, ×200)

Definition

EE is defined as esophageal eosinophilic inflammation that is refractory to anti-reflux therapy, or occurs in the presence of normal pH monitoring [17]. It is a clinicopathologic diagnosis. EE cannot be diagnosed by clinical signs and symptoms only. EE cannot be diagnosed by biopsy only. EE is diagnosed in patients with the appropriate clinical setting by esophageal biopsy that shows eosinophilic inflammation.

Attention continues to be focused on "THE" number that defines EE. The diagnosis of EE is not based on the number only; the clinical setting is as important to the diagnosis as the biopsy histology. The consensus statement recommends a threshold value of *at least* a peak count of 15 intraepithelial eosinophils in a ×400 high power field (hpf) in an esophageal biopsy as part of the diagnosis of EE. Clinicians and investigators may set a higher threshold value for the peak eosinophil count, if they believe that is appropriate [18, 19]. It is *not* recommended that a threshold value *lower* than 15/hpf is set for the peak esophageal eosinophil count to diagnose EE.

Indeterminate Esophagitis

Guidelines for diagnosis and treatment may not be applicable to all patients. For example, some patients who appear clinically to have EE have esophageal biopsies that contain eosinophils, but fewer than 15/hpf [20, 21]. These biopsies should be considered indeterminate for EE (Fig. 14.4). Clinicians and pathologists need to consult each other about these cases, since each provides part of the diagnosis, but neither supplies the entire diagnosis. In such cases, pathologists should be aware of the patchy nature of the infiltrates in EE and examine additional histologic sections, especially if the epithelium and lamina propria appear abnormal (Fig. 14.3). In patients whose biopsies are initially indeterminate, repeat biopsies at an appropriate time may be more informative. The goal is to treat each patient appropriately, to provide the therapy that an individual patient requires – to exercise the art of medicine. In the scenario in which the clinical setting is strongly indicative of EE, but the biopsy is equivocal, a clinician may opt to treat patients with those findings for EE, especially if other therapeutic options have failed. In this setting, patient response to therapy for EE should be communicated by the clinician to the pathologist. Reporting the outcome of cases such as these to the larger medical community will help to further define the disease.

Differential Diagnosis

EE may be classified as a primary or secondary disease [22]. The primary form is often associated with allergy. The secondary form is associated with other distinct diseases. Esophageal histology does not distinguish primary from secondary forms. It is important for pathologists and clinicians to realize that routine esophageal histology does not identify a specific etiology for EE, does not distinguish atopic from nonatopic patients, familial from sporadic cases, males from females, etc.

a

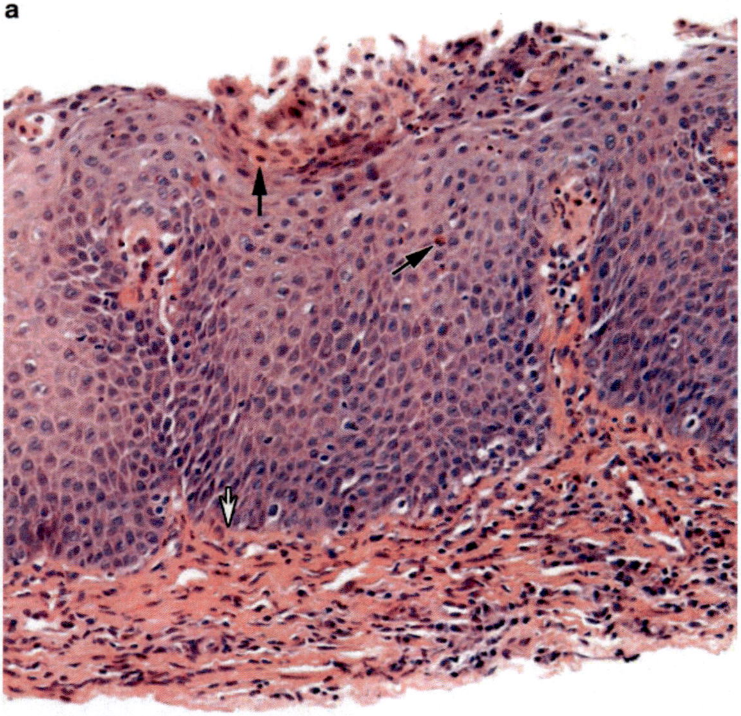

b

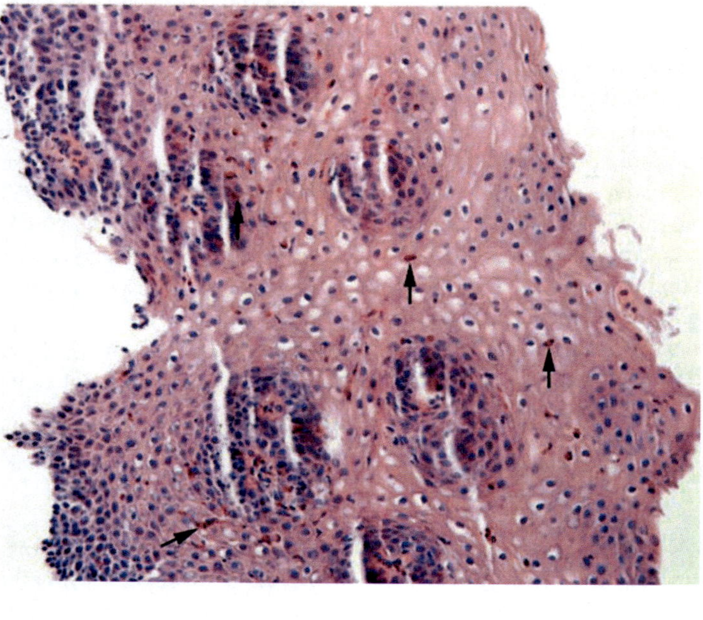

Gastroesophageal Reflux Disease

Among the causes of secondary EE, gastroesophageal reflux disease (GERD) is the most important, because it is the most common. GERD may mimic primary EE clinically and histologically. Distinguishing EE from GERD is important, because the therapy for the diseases differ. Fundoplication may be indicated for some patients who have GERD, but it is not indicated for patients who have EE. Therefore, good clinical practice is to biopsy the esophagus prior to performing fundoplication and to consider the diagnosis of EE if numerous intraepithelial eosinophils are found [23]. Indeed, 0.9–8.8% of patients who have refractory GERD (i.e., who do not respond to medical anti-reflux therapy) have EE [24, 25].

Patients who are believed clinically to have GERD are often treated empirically with medication, and if there is satisfactory resolution of signs and symptoms of GERD, endoscopy with biopsy is not performed. For example, a recent study of children who had signs and symptoms of esophageal dysfunction, with normal or abnormal pH monitoring, and a peak eosinophil count ≥15/hpf reported a substantial response rate to proton pump inhibitor (PPI) therapy, defined as <5 eosinophils/hpf on repeat esophageal biopsy; however, only 13% of the total population of patients who met the initial inclusion criteria had repeat biopsy [26]. Although in the past, intraepithelial eosinophils were considered specific indicators of abnormal esophageal reflux, it is likely that there are few if any intraepithelial eosinophils in esophageal biopsies from GERD patients who have not been treated for reflux disease. An older study in children that linked reflux to intraepithelial eosinophils in biopsies actually documented few eosinophils in patients with abnormal reflux [27]. In that study, virtually all patients who had intraepithelial eosinophils, and few eosinophils were reported or illustrated, had abnormal acid reflux, but fewer than half of the patients who had abnormal acid reflux had intraepithelial eosinophils in their esophageal biopsies.

Among patients who have GERD, biopsies demonstrating ≥15 eosinophils/hpf occur [28]. Patients who have the histologic and endoscopic features that are highly characteristic of EE including large numbers of intraepithelial eosinophils with abscesses and furrowed esophageal mucosa may respond completely, clinically and histologically, to anti-reflux medications [29, 30]. These patients should be considered to have GERD, as they do not require additional therapy. The prevalence of biopsies that have ≥15 eosinophils/hpf among untreated GERD patients is unknown since most do not have biopsies obtained prior to therapy.

Statistically significant differences exist for various aspects of the esophageal histology of patients who have GERD only compared to those who have EE only, but

Fig. 14.4 (**a**) This biopsy was taken from an adolescent male who presented with a food impaction. He had a history of allergic rhinitis and other allergies. The epithelium is thick, and there is superficial epithelial necrosis (*arrow*). The lamina propria is fibrotic (*white arrow*) and inflamed with lymphocytes, plasma cells, and eosinophils. Few intraepithelial eosinophils are seen (*outlined arrow*). This biopsy should be considered indeterminate [hematoxylin and eosin (H&E), ×200]. (**b**) The patient was treated medically for reflux disease, but continued to be symptomatic, and repeat biopsies showed fewer epithelial alterations, but numerous intraepithelial eosinophils (*arrows*) (peak count >40/hpf), consistent with eosinophilic esophagitis (H&E, ×200) there is not a histologic characteristic that occurs in one disease but not the other [31]. It is true that the histologic changes in esophageal biospies are generally more marked in EE compared to GERD, but there are exceptions [29, 30, 32].

EE is a disease that is antigen-driven, shows numerous intraepithelial eosinophils in esophageal biopsies, and is not ameliorated by therapy for reflux, whereas GERD is a disease that in most patients is responsive to acid suppression as monotherapy and shows few if any intraepithelial eosinophils in esophageal biopsies. In practice, not all patients can be clearly identified as having either one or the other disease: some patients have compelling evidence of both diseases, and many EE patients report some, but incomplete, clinical improvement with PPI therapy [33, 34]. In support of this clinical observation is in vitro data that cells from primary esophageal epithelial cell cultures significantly increase eotaxin-3 secretion at acidic pH [15]. The eotaxin-3 gene is the most upregulated gene in the EE transcriptome, is expressed in esophageal epithelial cells, and encodes a chemokine that is a powerful attractant for eosinophils [7]. Conversely, there are observations indicating that the use of acid-suppressive therapy for GERD also might contribute to the development of EE [35]. Clearly, the interaction between pathologic reflux and esophageal antigen sensitization must be explored further. Ideally, future studies should include placebo control groups, because the placebo effect may be greater than anticipated [36].

Beyond GERD

Other diseases that have been associated with esophageal biopsies showing the characteristic histology of EE include celiac disease and idiopathic inflammatory bowel disease [37] (Fig. 14.3). In patients who are suspected to have primary EE, biopsy from extra-esophageal sites should be obtained, including the lower GI tract if clinically indicated, to uncover eosinophilic disease at other sites, and to discover other pathology at those sites, such as celiac disease or idiopathic inflammatory bowel disease.

General Features

In EE, the histologic changes are typically patchy; and therefore, examining multiple biopsy pieces increases the diagnostic sensitivity of endoscopy [34, 38].

Eosinophils

The current recommendation is that eosinophils in the most intensely inflamed area in an esophageal biopsy are enumerated to generate a peak count of eosinophils/hpf. This is practical for daily surgical pathology practice. Peak values have been shown to correlate well with the results of more extensive eosinophil quantitation [39]. More extensive counting may be appropriate for research studies, and document the patchy nature of the disease in most cases.

It is recommended that eosinophils are counted at ×400 total magnification. The area on glass slides subtended by objectives varies among microscopes, and such variability affects the total eosinophil count. Optimally, sequential biopsies from a given patient are evaluated by the same pathologist using the same microscope, or any difference in the area of the various microscopes used to quantitate eosinophils is taken into account when reporting peak eosinophil counts. Reporting eosinophils as number/unit area is not currently a standard practice, but reporting counts that way would help to standardize counts among pathologists.

Eosinophils may be found dispersed in the epithelium in cases of EE, and may also form micro-abscesses and layers at the luminal surface [40] (Fig. 14.5). These features are found most often in biopsies that are the most intensely inflamed [41].

Degranulation

Extracellular granules are often seen in EE biopsies, mostly those that are intensely inflamed (Fig. 14.3b). At least some degranulation may be secondary to mechanical factors [42, 43]. Nevertheless, extracellular eosinophil granules are bound by membranes that express receptors and release protein in response to ligand binding [44, 45]. These data support the concept that extracellular granules may be important in the pathogenesis of eosinophil-related disorders including EE. Antibodies to eosinophil granule contents, such as major basic protein, eosinophil peroxidase, and eosinophil-derived neurotoxin, demonstrate more extracellular granules than are found on hematoxylin and eosin (H&E) stain [20, 30, 46, 47]. These antibodies may help ultimately to classify cases that are not easily classified, but immunohistochemistry is not currently required for diagnosis. Electron microscopy of EE biopsies has shown that the eosinophil granules are activated [48].

Epithelial Reactivity

Expansion of the basal layer is commonly found in EE (Fig. 14.5). The basal layer remains mitotically active and replenishes the remainder of the esophageal squamous epithelium normally. In EE, the degree of hyperplasia correlates with the number of eosinophils [7, 49]. The proliferation marker MIB1-antibody demonstrates that epithelial cell proliferation is increased in both EE and GERD [50]. Epithelial proliferation diminishes following therapy for EE [12, 36, 49].

There is persuasive experimental evidence that cytokines important in the pathogenesis of EE affect esophageal epithelium. For example, CD2-IL5 transgenic mice show greater basal layer hyperplasia after allergen challenge than nontransgenic

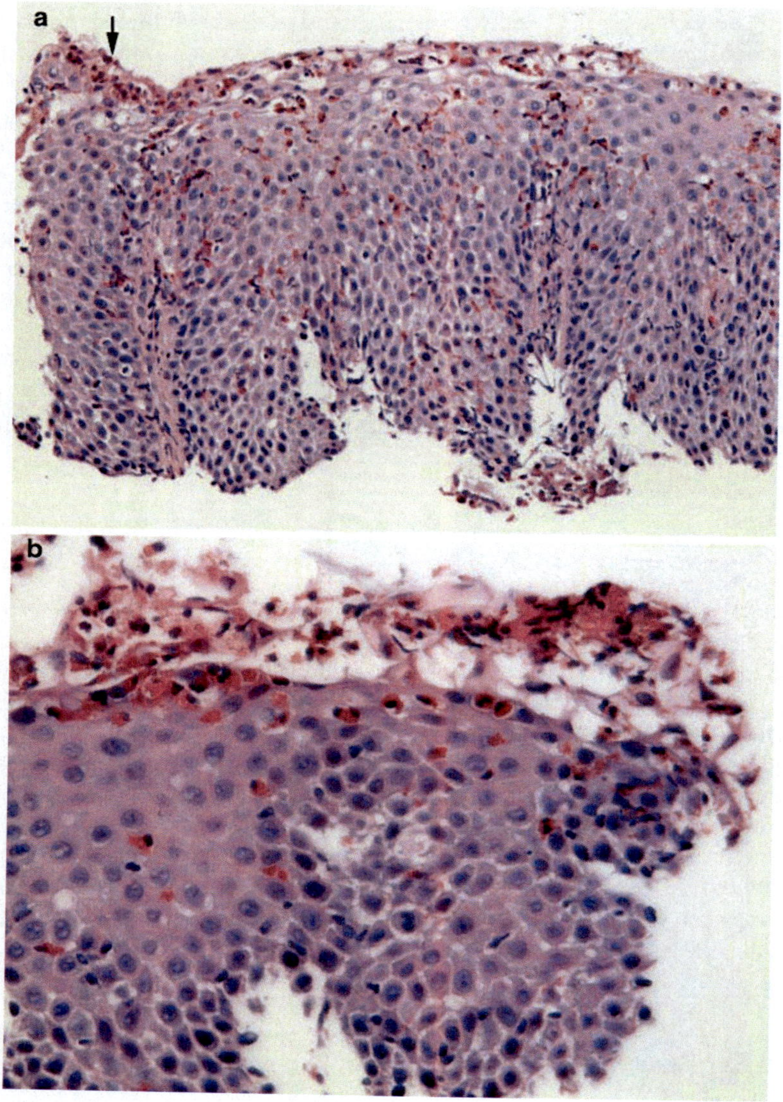

Fig. 14.5 (**a**) This biopsy of the distal esophagus from a 28-year-old symptomatic woman shows many of the features of eosinophilic esophagitis, including marked basal layer hyperplasia, dilated intercellular spaces, and numerous intraepithelial eosinophils that are concentrated at the surface. A focus of surface layering is seen at the upper left (*arrow*) [hematoxylin and eosin (H&E), ×200]. (**b**) A piece from the proximal esophagus obtained at the same endoscopic procedure shows the microscopic correlate of white streaks or patches seen on the esophageal mucosa at endoscopy: eosinophils admixed with shed necrotic epithelial cells at the surface (H&E, ×400)

mice [14]. Epithelial hyperplasia in human EE biopsies is reduced in patients who have been treated with an antibody to IL-5 [12].

Another cytokine that is overexpressed in human EE directly affects esophageal epithelium. Interleukin-13 (IL-13) increases eotaxin-3 production in vitro by cultured human esophageal epithelial cells; in vivo, the eotaxin-3 gene is upregulated in EE, mRNA levels are increased in human EE biopsies, and in situ hybridization demonstrates eotaxin-3 expression in human esophageal epithelium in EE [7, 15]. Eotaxin-3 is essential in the pathogenesis of EE, because it attracts eosinophils into esophageal epithelium. The upregulation of eotaxin-3 appears to be directed at least in part by IL-13.

In human EE, filaggrin gene expression is reduced and filaggrin mRNA levels are significantly diminished in EE esophageal biopsies, but return to normal following therapy [7, 15]. Filaggrin protein performs an important function in barrier protection in epidermis and is downregulated in atopic dermatitis, a condition that occurs in some EE patients. Furthermore, a loss of function mutation in the filaggrin gene is more prevalent among EE patients than patients without EE. IL-13 acts directly on cultured human esophageal epithelial cells to decrease the expression of the filaggrin gene [15]. These data suggest a significant IL-13-mediated alteration in epithelial barrier integrity in EE that may contribute to the chronic nature of the disease.

Other Cell Types

The esophagus is the first part of the GI tract that encounters food. Normal esophageal mucosa contains a variety of cell types that are important for immune competence.

In sections of esophageal mucosal biopsies stained with H&E, eosinophils are the predominant inflammatory cells in EE. However, special stains or antibodies may be required to detect other cell types that are also increased in esophageal epithelium in EE.

Dendritic Cells

Most EE patients have evidence of allergen sensitization, including to food, and may respond well to antigen elimination diet [51]. Dendritic cells are antigen-presenting cells that are found in skin and mucosa, and are not seen with the H&E stain. Langerhans cells are epithelial dendritic cells that stain with CD1a antibody (Fig. 14.6). Langerhans cells are found in normal esophageal epithelium, and (number expressed per unit *volume*) 5,490 ± 5,470/mm^3 have been reported in normal esophageal biopsies from adults [52]. In esophageal biopsies of adults who have GERD, 6,370 ± 6,990/mm^3 CD1a-positive cells have been reported, a nonsignificant increase from normal. Similarly, in esophageal biopsies of adults who have EE, the

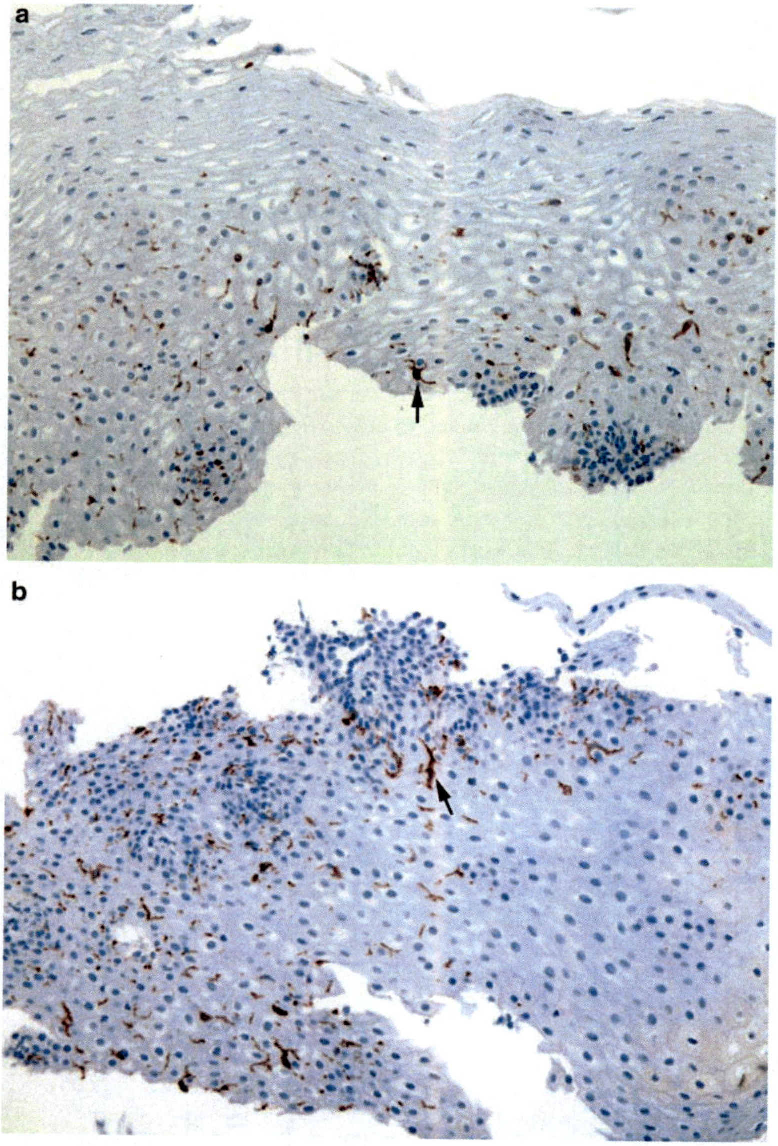

Fig. 14.6 (**a**) CD1a antibody decorates Langerhans cells, dendritic cells, in normal esophageal epithelium. The dendritic cell processes are nicely illustrated in some cells (*arrow*) (CD1a, ×200). (**b**) In eosinophilic esophagitis, dendritic cells are also seen (*arrow*) and appear more numerous in this field compared to the field from a normal biopsy in (**a**) (CD1a, ×200)

number of CD1a-positive cells has been reported as $8{,}490 \pm 17{,}550/\text{mm}^3$, also a nonsignificant increase compared to normal; after therapy with topical steroids $7{,}830 \pm 12{,}610/\text{mm}^3$ are found [52]. In contrast, the number of CD1a-positive cells in esophageal biopsies from children who have EE has decreased significantly following topical steroid therapy, from (number expressed per unit *area*) $8.6 \pm 1.6/\text{mm}^2$ to $6.4 \pm 0.8/\text{mm}^2$ in the distal esophagus, and $9.4 \pm 1.5/\text{mm}^2$ to $5.6 \pm 0.5/\text{mm}^2$ in the proximal esophagus [53]. The role of dendritic cells in the genesis and maintenance of EE should be further explored.

Mast Cells

Mast cells are virtually ubiquitous, but are generally not easily recognized in tissue sections without the use of special stains or antibodies (Fig. 14.7). Mast cells participate in allergic reactions, and in response to certain stimuli secrete preformed or newly synthesized mediators [54]. Mast cell granules contain literally hundreds of substances including the cytokines IL-5 and IL-13 that are important in the pathogenesis of EE. Other mediators contained in mast cell granules are histamine, tryptase, chymase, and carboxypeptidase. Tryptase release is considered a marker of mast cell activation. Mediators released by mast cells could potentially become biomarkers of EE and disease activity [55].

Mast cells express c-kit, a tyrosine kinase receptor encoded by the proto-oncogene ckit, and a ckit gene mutation characterizes systemic mastocytosis. Systemic mastocytosis commonly affects the gastrointestinal tract (GI) and may involve any site including, rarely, the esophagus, with esophageal strictures occurring in some patients [56, 57]. In cases of systemic mastocytosis that have the characteristic ckit mutation and involve the GI tract, the mast cell infiltrates may be accompanied by numerous eosinophils [58].

The number of mast cells detected by tryptase antibody in the epithelium of normal esophageal biopsies of children has been variable: reports have ranged from no tryptase-positive cells in the epithelium but occasional cells in the lamina propria, to 0.18 ± 0.31 mast cells/hpf, and 4.6 ± 0.3 mast cells/hpf with a peak count of 3/hpf [7, 59, 60]. Anti-c-kit (CD117) detects similar numbers of intraepithelial mast cells in esophageal epithelium [60]. The number of tryptase-positive mast cells in normal esophageal biopsies of adults has been reported as (number per unit *area*) $4 \pm 0.9/\text{mm}^2$ and (number per unit *volume*) $2{,}730/\text{mm}^3$ [52, 61].

In both children and adults who have EE, mast cells are increased in esophageal epithelium [7, 30, 36, 47, 52, 59, 61–64]. The number of tryptase-positive cells is greater in EE compared to GERD biopsies [30]. The number of tryptase-positive mast cells does not differ in biopsies of atopic patients compared to nonatopic patients, even among patients who have EE [64].

Intraepithelial mast cell density correlates with eosinophil density [7, 30, 47], basal layer hyperplasia [7], and B-cell density [64]. Mast cell number decreases with topical steroid therapy [36, 52, 63], and following anti-interleukin-5 (IL-5)

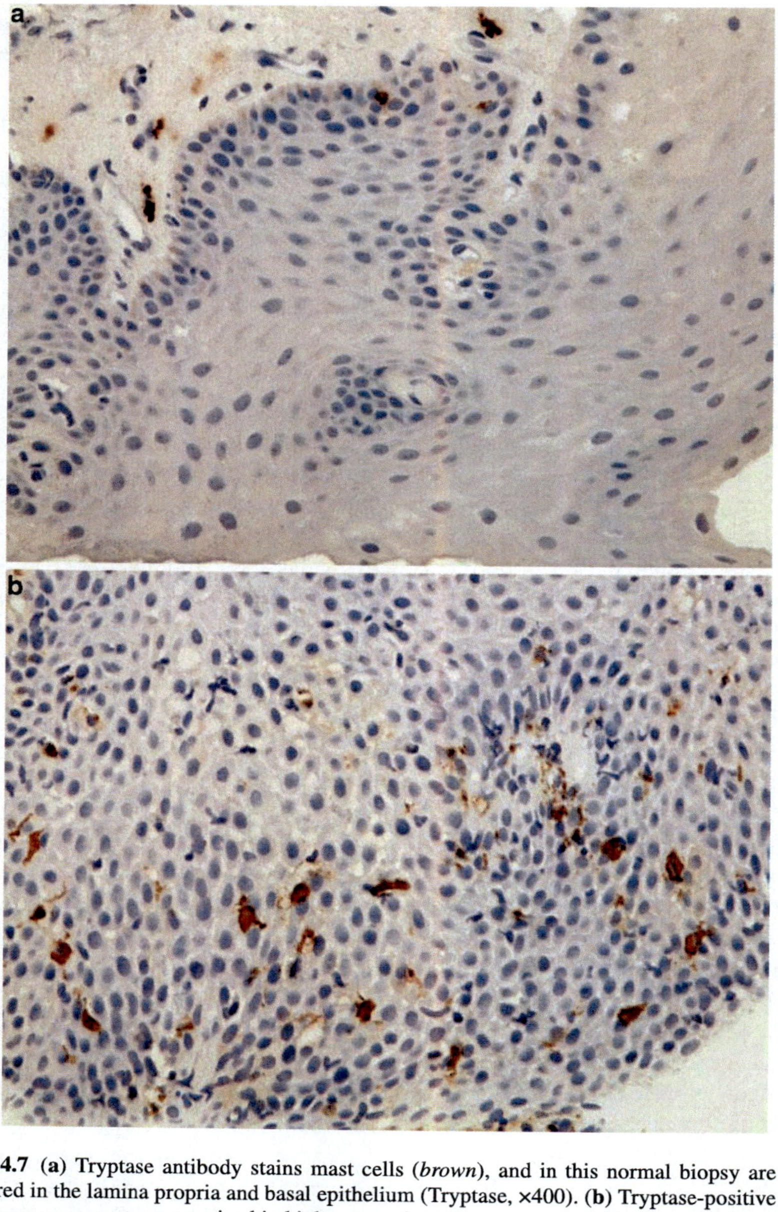

Fig. 14.7 (**a**) Tryptase antibody stains mast cells (*brown*), and in this normal biopsy are seen scattered in the lamina propria and basal epithelium (Tryptase, ×400). (**b**) Tryptase-positive mast cells appear more numerous in this high power field from an eosinophilic esophagitis biopsy (Tryptase, ×400)

(Mepolizumab) therapy in some patients [12, 65]. However, the number of mast cells in post-therapy EE biopsies may remain increased compared to normal biopsies, indicating persistent inflammation and potentially hyperactive immune responses [52].

Several observations and lines of evidence implicate immunoglobulin E (IgE) in the pathogenesis of EE, including the presence of IgE antigen-specific antibodies in the serum of many EE patients, and the overexpression of the high affinity IgE receptor gene in EE [7, 66]. IgE antibody does not decorate cells in normal esophageal biopsies, but numerous IgE-positive cells are found in EE, and none or few of these cells are found in biopsies from GERD patients [52, 59, 61, 64]. IgE-bearing mast cells are more prevalent in EE biopsies from atopic compared to nonatopic EE patients [64]. IgE-positive cells are not found in esophageal biopsies from EE patients following therapy [52].

In the EE transcriptome, five mast cell genes are highly induced including carboxypeptidase, tryptase, and FCepsilonR1, the high affinity IgE receptor. Expression of tryptase and carboxypeptidase genes correlates with mast cell numbers in suprabasilar esophageal epithelium, and both mast cell numbers and mRNA levels of carboxypeptidase decrease with therapy [67].

These data demonstrate an important role for mast cells in the pathogenesis and clinical course of EE, suggest the potential for mast cell products to be biomarkers of the disease, and potentially provide the basis for novel therapies to treat EE.

Lymphocytes

Lymphoid tissue is normally found in esophageal mucosa (Fig. 14.8). Intraepithelial lymphocytes are also normally found in esophageal squamous epithelium. In H&E stains, they appear to have irregular nuclei and are referred to as squiggle cells. In H&E-stained sections of normal esophageal biopsies, they are described as common [40] and have been quantified as 3.5 ± 1.2/hpf with a range of 2–6/hpf [7].

Intraepithelial lymphocytes are increased in EE biopsies. Lymphocytes are critical components of inflammatory and immune responses, and there is significant clinical and experimental data that support a crucial role for lymphocytes in the pathogenesis of EE. Esophageal eosinophil counts correlate with the percentage of peripheral blood T cells that express IL-5 in EE patients [68]. The EE transcriptome includes overexpression of genes (e.g., MICA, MICB, and interleukin 15 {IL-15}) that are known to stimulate intraepithelial T-cell activation [1, 7]. Activated T cells secrete IL-5 and IL-13 [1]. Lymphocyte-deficient and T-cell-deficient mice do not develop experimental EE [69]. Effector T cells are increased and regulatory T cells are decreased among total esophageal cells in allergen-challenged compared to saline-challenged mice [70].

T cells are commonly found in small numbers in esophageal epithelium and activated T cells secrete both IL-5 and IL-13 (Fig. 14.9). In normal adult esophageal biopsies, CD3-positive T cells have numbered $180 \pm 22.2/\text{mm}^2$, and in normal pediatric esophageal biopsies they have numbered 5.5 ± 2.3/hpf [53, 61]. CD3-positive

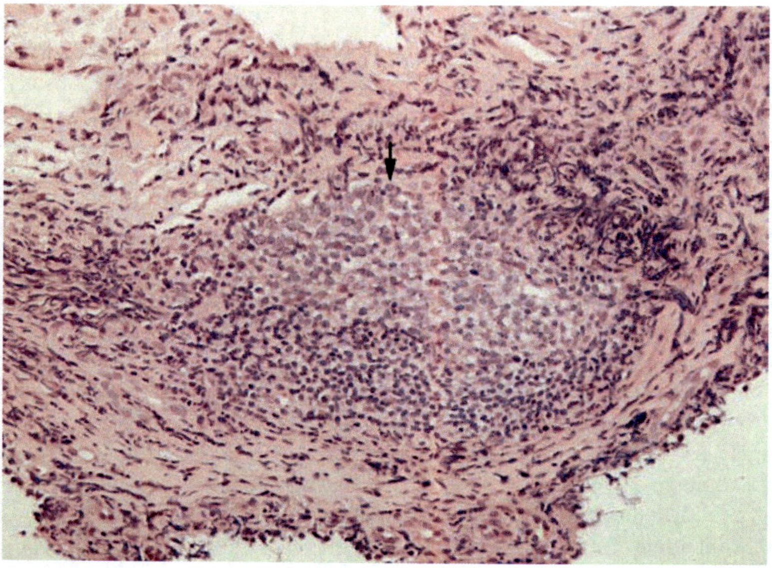

Fig. 14.8 Lymphoid tissue is a normal component of the esophageal mucosa. The *arrow* points downward to the germinal center of a lymphoid follicle in the lamina propria. The edges of the follicle are somewhat crushed, an artifact resulting from tissue handling (hematoxylin and eosin, ×200)

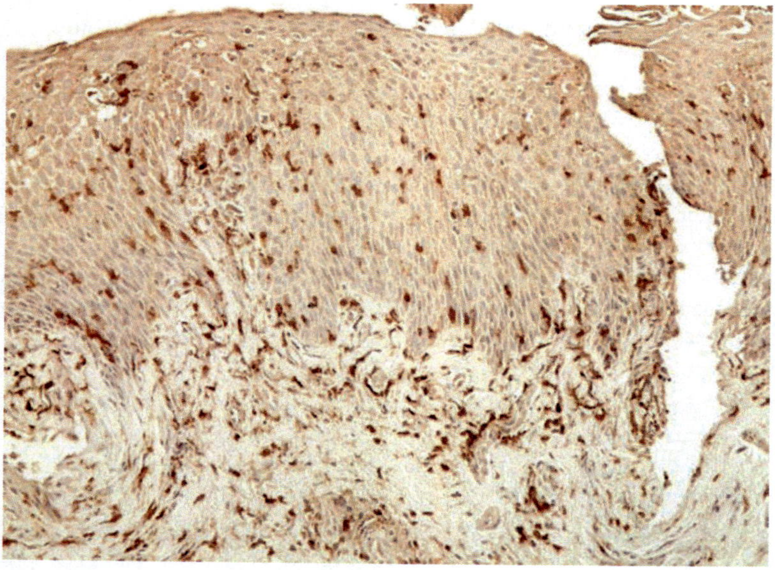

Fig. 14.9 Numerous CD3-positive T lymphocytes (*brown*) are seen in the thickened epithelium and fibrotic lamina propria in this eosinophilic esophagitis biopsy (CD3, ×200)

T cells are increased in EE biopsies compared to normal biopsies and GERD biopsies [53, 61, 63, 71]. CD3-positive cells have numbered $555 \pm 54.6/\text{mm}^2$ in EE biopsies from adults, 28.2 ± 4.5/hpf in EE biopsies from children, and 60.1 ± 11.09/hpf (range 18–105/hpf) in EE biopsies from both adults and children [53, 61, 71]. CD3-positive cells are reduced in EE biopsies after topical steroid therapy compared to pretherapy biopsies [53, 63].

Suppressor T cells (CD8-positive) are more prevalent than helper T cells (CD4-positive) in normal esophageal epithelium [52, 63] (Fig. 14.10). The number of CD8-positive cells reported in normal esophageal biopsies in children is 5.9 ± 2.8/hpf [53]. In EE, CD8-positive cells are increased [36, 49, 52, 53, 63]. The number of C8-positive T cells is also reduced following topical steroid therapy, but not placebo [36, 49, 52, 53, 63].

B cells are less prevalent than T cells in the normal esophagus (Fig. 14.11). CD20-positive B cells are not found in normal esophageal biopsies in adults [52, 61]. In children, CD20-positive B cells are rarely detected in normal esophageal biopsies, from either atopic or nonatopic patients. CD20-positive B cells are increased in EE biopsies, to a similar degree in atopic and nonatopic patients [64]. In children, CD20-positive B cells are increased in epithelium and vascular papillae, but not in lamina propria, in EE patients compared to controls [64]. In EE biopsies from children, CD20-positive B cells correlate with mast cell numbers but not eosinophil counts [64]. In adults, CD20-positive B cells are increased to a similar degree in both EE biopsies ($7.4 \pm 1.7/\text{mm}^2$) [52, 61] and GERD biopsies [52].

IgE-positive cells are found in EE, but not control esophageal biopsies [52, 61, 64]. IgE-positive cells in EE biopsies may be mast cells [61], and IgE-positive mast cells are increased in atopic compared to nonatopic EE patients [64]. However, some CD117-negative cells in EE biopsies are IgE-positive [64], and some IgE-positive cells have the morphology of plasma cells [62]. Therefore, a subset of IgE-positive cells in EE biopsies may be plasma cells, strongly implicating B cells in the immune reactions in EE. Local immunoglobulin class switching to IgE and IgE production has been recently demonstrated in esophageal tissue in EE [64]. Increased expression of B-cell-related genes is found in EE, including immunoglobulin lambda joining 3, immunoglobulin heavy chain delta, immunoglobulin J polypeptide, and B-cell RAG-associated protein [7, 64]. Therefore, B cells probably play an important role in EE, but may not contribute significantly to the initiation of EE since B-cell-deficient mice are not protected from, but are susceptible to, experimentally-induced EE [69].

Lamina Propria

In contrast to the rest of the GI tract, the lamina propria in the esophagus forms a distinct subepithelial layer and projects into the epithelial layer creating papillae (Fig. 14.2). Lamina propria is not present in all endoscopic esophageal biopsies hampering study of this layer. Although the normal cell complement of the lamina

a

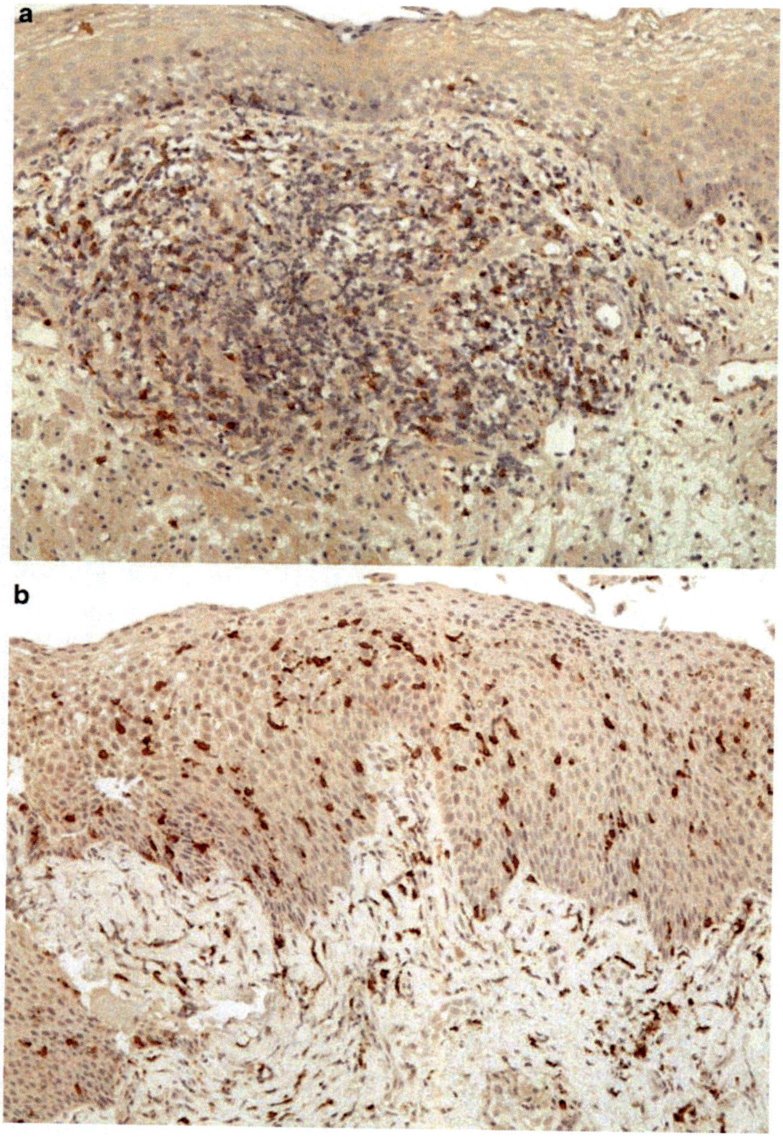

b

Fig. 14.10 (a) C8-positive suppressor cells are normally the most abundant T cells in the esophagus. Numerous cells (*brown*) are seen near a lymphoid aggregate in the lamina propria, and fewer are seen in the overlying squamous epithelium (CD8, ×200). (b) CD8-positive T cells are more numerous in the thickened epithelium and fibrotic lamina propria in field in eosinophilic esophagitis compared to normal (CD8, ×200)

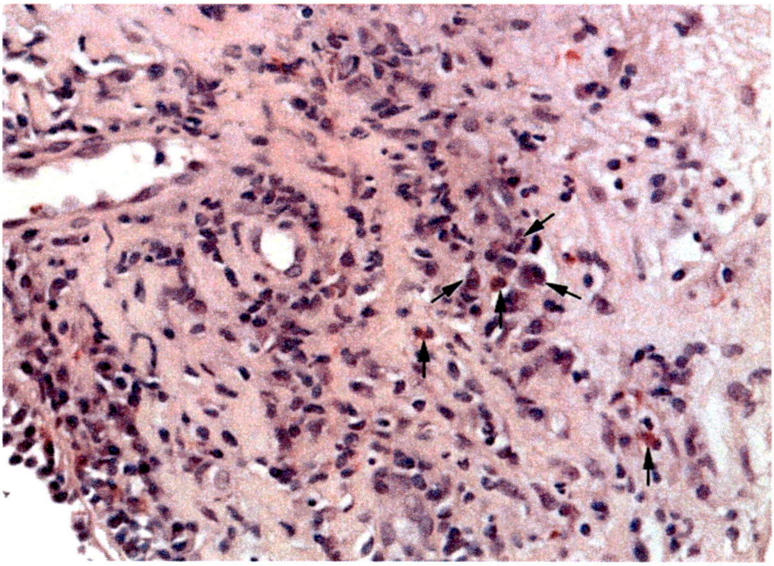

Fig. 14.11 Plasma cells (*outlined arrows*) are terminally differentiated B cells, and are seen along with eosinophils (*arrows*) in this fibrotic lamina propria in eosinophilic esophagitis (hematoxylin and eosin, ×400)

propria is not as well characterized as the esophageal epithelial layer, lymphocytes are normal components and may form lymphoid aggregates or follicles (Fig. 14.8). B cells are found in the lamina propria of normal biopsies [64]. Mast cells are also found in lamina propria of normal biopsies [47].

Eosinophils are not found in the lamina propria of normal pediatric esophageal biopsies [47]. Eosinophils are found in the lamina propria of esophageal biopsies from patients who have GERD, but are less common than among EE biopsies. In adults, lamina propria eosinophils are found in 56% of patients who have EE compared to 41% who have GERD [72]. In children, mean count ranges from 6 (range 0–23) to 17 (range 4–58) eosinophils/hpf in the lamina propria in biopsies of patients who have EE, compared to a mean count of 2 (0–9)/hpf in patients who have GERD [47, 73]. Lamina propria mast cells detected by tryptase antibody have been reported as 6 (0–64)/hpf in EE biopsies and 9.5 (7–23)/hpf in GERD biopsies in children [47].

Lamina propria fibrosis occurs in EE and may be found less commonly in other disorders. In adults, lamina propria fibrosis is found in 39% of EE biopsies and 7% of GERD biopsies [72]. It may increase in prevalence over time in esophageal biopsies of adults who have EE [74], but may resolve in children [75]. Lamina propria fibrosis correlates with dysphagia and food impactions, but not with duration of symptoms, in children [47]. Increased staining for TGFβ-1 and its downstream signaling molecule phospho-SMAD2/3 in lamina propria cells in EE biopsies showing fibrosis, including patients with strictures, strongly implicates this signaling pathway in the genesis of lamina propria fibrosis in EE [73]. Patients who respond to swallowed budesonide therapy, with reduced fibrosis and reduced staining for TGFβ-1 and phospho-SMAD2/3, are more likely to have a CC genotype at the –509 position in the TGFβ (beta)-1 promoter region [75]. This finding suggests that genotype may be important in the genesis of lamina propria fibrosis.

IL-5 is also important in the genesis of lamina propria fibrosis in EE. IL-5 levels are increased in the esophagus of EE patients, IL-5 deficient mice develop less lamina propria fibrosis than wild-type mice, and CD2-IL-5 transgenic mice showed increased fibrosis compared to nontransgenic mice [14].

A genome-wide microarray analysis of esophageal biopsies has shown increased expression of the periostin gene [7]. Periostin is a secreted protein expressed by fibroblasts that interacts with components of the extracellular matrix. Periostin is markedly overexpressed in lamina propria of EE biopsies compared to normal biopsies, and IL-13 and TGFβ increase periostin expression in primary esophageal fibrobast cultures. Periostin increases eosinophil adhesion to fibronectin in vitro, and periostin-deficient allergen-challenged mice have reduced eosinophils in lung and esophagus [76]. These data suggest that periostin plays an important role in eosinophil recruitment from the vasculature into the lamina propria.

Future Directions

Clinical and experimental studies have elucidated many aspects of the pathogenesis of EE. Studies have focused on primary or allergic EE, and efforts should be made to identify any other pathways that may be involved in the genesis of EE associated with other diseases. Experimental data have provided the basis for clinical trials [77]. The goals of therapy must be clarified. One goal should be to reduce esophageal inflammation, but the degree of reduction is not yet identified. Mechanisms of lamina propria fibrosis have been identified, and evidence is emerging that it may be reversible, but the relationship of lamina propria fibrosis to esophageal dysfunction and stricture in particular should be explored. Little is known about the natural history of EE in children. Gastroenterologists who treat adults should be aware that biopsies showing all the characteristic features of EE were obtained from children decades ago and interpreted as GERD [78]; it is possible that adults who are now diagnosed with EE had the disease in childhood, and the natural history will become clearer by reporting these patients. The goal of all these efforts is to cure EE.

References

1. Rothenberg ME. Biology and treatment of eosinophilic esophagitis. Gastroenterology. 2009;137:1238–49.
2. Vanderheyden AD, Petras RE, DeYoung BR, et al. Emerging eosinophilic (allergic) esophagitis. Increased incidence or increased recognition. Arch Pathol Lab Med. 2007;131:777–9.
3. Whitney-Miller CL, Katzka D, Furth EE. Eosinophilic esophagitis. A retrospective review of esophageal biopsy specimens from 1992 to 2004 at an adult academic medical center. Am J Clin Pathol. 2009;131:788–92.

4. Collins MH, Blanchard C, Abonia JP, et al. Clinical, pathologic, and molecular characterization of familial eosinophilic esophagitis compared with sporadic cases. Clin Gastroenterol Hepatol. 2008;6:621–9.
5. Collins MH. Histopathologic features of eosinophilic esophagitis. Gastrointest Endosc Clin N Am. 2008;18:59–71.
6. Collins MH. Histopathology associated with eosinophilic gastrointestinal diseases. Immunol Allergy Clin North Am. 2009;29:109–17.
7. Blanchard C, Wang N, Stringer KF, et al. Eotaxin-3 and a uniquely conserved gene-expression profile in eosinophilic esophagitis. J Clin Invest. 2006;116:536–47.
8. Rothenberg ME, Spergel JM, Sherrill JD, et al. Common variants at 5q22 associate with pediatric eosinophilic esophagitis. Nat Genet. 2010;42:289–91.
9. Mishra A, Hogan SP, Brandt EB, et al. IL-5 promotes eosinophil trafficking to the esophagus. J Immunol. 2002;168:2464–9.
10. Mishra A, Rothenberg ME. Intratracheal IL-13 induces eosinophilic esophagitis by an IL-5, eotaxin-1, and STAT6-dependent mechanism. Gastroenterology. 2003;125:1419–27.
11. Blanchard C, Mishra A, Saito-Akei H, et al. Inhibition of human interleukin-13-induced respiratory and oesophageal inflammation by anti-human-interleukin-13 antibody (CAT-354). Clin Exp Allergy. 2005;35:1096–103.
12. Stein ML, Collins MH, Villaneuva JM, et al. Anti-IL-5 therapy for eosinophilic esophagitis. J Allergy Clin Immunol. 2006;118:1312–9.
13. Blanchard C, Mingler MK, Vicario M, et al. IL-13 involvement in eosinophilic esophagitis: transcriptome analysis and reversibility with glucocorticoids. J Allergy Clin Immunol. 2007;120:1292–300.
14. Mishra A, Wang M, Pemmaraju VR, et al. Esophageal remodeling develops as a consequence of tissue specific IL-5-induced eosinophilia. Gastroenterology. 2008;134:204–14.
15. Blanchard C, Stucke EM, Burwinkel K, et al. Coordinate interaction between IL-13 and epithelial cell differentiation cluster genes in eosinophilic esophagitis. J Immunol. 2010;184:4033–41.
16. Zhu X, Wang M, Mavi P, et al. Interleukin-15 expression is increased in human eosinophilic esophagitis and mediates pathogenesis in mice. Gastroenterology. 2010;139:182–93.
17. Furuta GT, Liacouris CA, Collins MH, et al. Eosinophilic esophagitis in children and adults: a systematic review and consensus recommendations for diagnosis and treatment. Gastroenterology. 2007;133:1342–63.
18. Aceves SS, Newbury RO, Dohil R, et al. Distinguishing eosinophilic esophagitis in pediatric patients: clinical, endoscopic, and histologic features of an emerging disorder. J Clin Gastroenterol. 2007;41:252–6.
19. Spergel JM, Brown-Whitehorn TF, Beausolieil JL, et al. 14 Years of eosinophlic esophagitis: clinical features and prognosis. J Pediatr Gastroenterol Nutr. 2009;48:30–6.
20. Protheroe C, Woodruff SA, de Petris G, et al. A novel histologic scoring system to evaluate mucosal biopsies from patients with eosinophilic esophagitis. Clin Gastroenterol Hepatol. 2009;7:749–55.
21. Oliveira C, Zamakhashary M, Marcon P, et al. Eosinophilic esophagitis and intermediate esophagitis after tracheoesophageal fistula repair: a case series. J Pediatr Surg. 2008;43:810–4.
22. Rothenberg ME. Eosinophilic gastrointestinal disorders (EGID). J Allergy Clin Immunol. 2004;113:11–28.
23. Dellon ES, Farrell TM, Bozymski EM, et al. Diagnosis of eosinophilic esophagitis after fundoplication for "refractory reflux": implications for preoperative evaluation. Dis Esophagus. 2009; Epub ahead of print PMID: 19863640. 2010;23:191–5.
24. Poh CH, Gasiorowska A, Navarro-Rodriguez T, et al. Upper GI tract findings in patients with heartburn in whom proton pump inhibitor treatment failed versus those not receiving antireflux treatment. Gastrointest Endosc. 2010;71:23–34.
25. Foroutan M, Norouzi A, Molaei M, et al. Eosinophilic esophagitis in patients with refractory gastroesophageal reflux disease. Dig Dis Sci. 2010;55:28–31.
26. Dranove JE, Horn DS, Davis MA, et al. Predictors of response to proton pump inhibitor therapy among children with significant esophageal eosinophilia. J Pediatr. 2009;154:96–100.

27. Winter HS, Madara JL, Stafford RJ, et al. Intraepithelial eosinophils: a new diagnostic criterion for reflux esophagitis. Gastroenterology. 1982;83:818–23.
28. Rodrigo S, Abboud G, Oh D, et al. High intraepithelial eosinophil counts in esophageal squamous epithelium are not specific for eosinophilic esophagitis in adults. Am J Gastroenterol. 2008;103:435–42.
29. Ngo P, Furuta GT, Antonioli DA, et al. Eosinophils in the esophagus – peptic or allergic eosinophilic esophagitis? Case series of three patients with esophageal eosinophilia. Am J Gastroenterol. 2006;101:1666–70.
30. Mueller S, Neureiter D, Aigner T, et al. Comparison of histological parameters for the diagnosis of eosinophilic oesophagitis versus gastro-esophageal reflux disease on oesophageal biopsy material. Histopathology. 2008;53:676–84.
31. Dellon ES, Gibbs WB, Fritchie KJ, et al. Clinical, endoscopic, and histologic findings distinguish eosinophilic esophagitis from gastroesophageal reflux disease. Clin Gastroenterol Hepatol. 2009;7:1305–13.
32. Vandenplas Y, Rudolph CD, DiLorenzo C, et al. Pediatric gastroesophageal reflux clinical practice guidelines: joint recommendations of the North American Society for Pediatric Gastroenterology, Hepatology, and Nutrition (NASPGHAN) and the European Society for Pediatric Gastroenterology, Hepatology, and Nutrition (ESPGHAN). J Pediatr Gastroenterol Nutr. 2009;49:498–507.
33. Peterson KA, Thomas KL, Hilden K, et al. Comparison of esomeprazole to aerosolized, swallowed fluticasone for eosinophilic esophagitis. Dig Dis Sci. 2009; Epub ahead of print PMID: 19533356. 2010;55:1313–9.
34. Shah A, Kagalwalla AF, Gonsalves N, et al. Histopathologic variability in children with eosinophilic esophagitis. Am J Gastroenterol. 2009;104:716–21.
35. Merwat SN, Spechler SJ. Might the use of acid-suppressive medications predispose to the development of eosinophilic esophagitis? Am J Gastroenterol. 2009;104:1897–902.
36. Konikoff MR, Noel RJ, Blanchard C, et al. A randomized, double-blind, placebo-controlled trial of fluticasone propionate for pediatric eosinophilic esophagitis. Gastroenterology. 2006;131:1381–91.
37. Atkins D, Furuta GT. Mucosal immunology, eosinophilic esophagitis, and other intestinal inflammatory diseases. J Allergy Clin Immunol. 2010;125(S2):S255–61.
38. Gonsalves N, Policarpio-Nicolas M, Zhang Q, et al. Histopathologic variability and endoscopic correlates in adults with eosinophilic esopahgitis. Gastrointest Endosc. 2006;64:313–9.
39. Lai AL, Girgis S, Liang Y, et al. Diagnostic criteria for eosinophilic esophagitis: a 5-year retrospective review in a pediatric population. J Pediatr Gastroenterol Nutr. 2009;49:63–70.
40. Walsh SV, Antonioli DA, Goldman H, et al. Allergic esophagitis in children. A clinicopathologic study. Am J Surg Pathol. 1999;23:390–6.
41. Cheung KM, Oliver MR, Cameron DJS, et al. Esophageal eosinophilia in children with dysphagia. J Pediatr Gastroenterol Nutr. 2003;37:498–503.
42. Kato M, Kephart GM, Talley NJ, et al. Eosinophil infiltration and degranulation in normal human tissue. Anat Rec. 1998;252:418–25.
43. DeBrosse CW, Case JW, Putnam PE, et al. Quantity and distribution of eosinophils in the gastrointestinal tract of children. Pediatr Develop Pathol. 2006;9:210–8.
44. Neves JS, Perez SAC, Spencer LA, et al. Eosinophil granules function extracellularly as receptor-mediated secretory organelles. PNAS. 2008;105:18378–483.
45. Neves JS, Radke AL, Weller PF. Cysteinyl leukotrienes acting via granule membrane-expressed receptors elicit secretion from within cell-free human eosinophil granules. J Allergy Clin Immunol. 2010;125:477–82.
46. Kephart GM, Alexander JA, Arora AS, et al. Marked deposition of eosinophil-derived neurotoxin in adult patients with eosinophilic esophagitis. Am J Gastroenterol. 2010;105:298–307.
47. Chehade M, Sampson HA, Morotti RA, Magid MS. Esophageal subepithelial fibrosis in children with eosinophilic esophagitis. J Pediatr Gastroenterol Nutr. 2007;45:319–28.
48. Justinich CJ, Ricci Jr A, Kalafus DA, et al. Activated eosinophils in esophagitis in children: a transmission electron microscopy study. J Pediatr Gastroenterol Nutr. 1997;25:194–8.

49. Noel RJ, Putnam PE, Collins MH, et al. Clinical and immunopathologic effects of swallowed fluticasone for eosinophilic esophagitis. Clin Gastroenterol Hepatol. 2004;2:568–75.
50. Lewis CJ, Lamb CA, Kanakala V, et al. Is the etiology of eosinophilic esophagitis in adults a response to allergy or reflux injury? Study of cellular proliferation markers. Dis Esophagus. 2009;22:249–55.
51. Kelly KJ, Lazenby AJ, Rowe PC, et al. Eosinophilic esophagitis attributed to gastroesophageal reflux: improvement with an amino acid-based formula. Gastroenterology. 1995;109:1503–12.
52. Lucendo AJ, Navarro M, Comas C, et al. Immunophenotypic characterization and quantification of the epithelial inflammatory infiltrate in eosinophilic esophagitis through stereology. Am J Surg Pathol. 2007;31:598–606.
53. Teitelbaum JE, Fox VL, Twarog FJ, et al. Eosinophilic esophagitis in children: immunopathological analysis and response to fluticasone propionate. Gastroenterology. 2002;122: 1216–25.
54. Wershil BK. Exploring the role of mast cells in eosinophilic esophagitis. Immunol Allergy Clin N Am. 2009;29:189–95.
55. Gupta SK. Noninvasive markers of eosinophilic esophagitis. Gastrointest Endosc Clin N Am. 2008;18:157–67.
56. Lee JK, Whittaker SJ, Enns RA, Zetler P. Gastrointestinal manifestations of systemic mastocytosis. World J Gastroenterol. 2008;14:7005–8.
57. Sokol H, Georgin-Lavialle S, Grandpeix-Guyodo C, et al. Gastrointestinal involvement and manifestations in systemic mastocytosis. Inflamm Bowel Dis. 2010; Epub ahead of print PMID: 20162539. 2010;16:1247–53.
58. Kirsch R, Geboes K, Shepherd NA, et al. Systemic mastocytosis involving the gastrointestinal tract: clinicopathologic and molecular study of five cases. Mod Pathol. 2008;158:1–9.
59. Kirsch R, Bokhary R, Marcon MA, Cutz E. Activated mucosal mast cells differentiate allergic (eosinophilic) esophagitis from gastroesophageal reflux disease. J Pediatr Gastroenterol Nutr. 2007;44:20–6.
60. Tison BE, DeBrosse CW, Rainey HF, et al. Number and distribution of mast cells in the pediatric gastrointestinal tract. J Allergy Clin Immunol. 2010;125:AB182.
61. Straumann A, Bauer M, Fischer B, et al. Idiopathic eosinophilic esophagitis is associated with a Th2-type allergic inflammatory response. J Allergy Clin Immunol. 2001;108:954–61.
62. Gupta SK, Fitzgerald JF, Kondratyuk T, HogenEsch H. Cytokine expression in normal and inflamed esophageal mucosa: a study into the pathogenesis of allergic eosinophilic esophagitis. J Pediatr Gastroenterol Nutr. 2006;42:22–6.
63. Lucendo AJ, DeRezende L, Comas C, et al. Treatment with topical steroids downregulates IL-5, eotaxin-1/CCL11, and eotaxin-3/CCL26 gene expression in eosinophilic esophagitis. Am J Gastroenterol. 2008;103:2184–93.
64. Vicario M, Blanchard C, Stringer KF, et al. Local B cells and IgE production in the oesophageal mucosa in eosinophilic oesophagitis. Gut. 2010;59:12–20.
65. Straumann A, Conus S, Grzonka P, et al. Anti-interleukin-5 antibody treatment (mepolizumab) in active eosinophilic esophagitis: a randomized, placebo-controlled, double-blind trial. Gut. 2010;59:21–30.
66. Dehlink E, Feibiger E. The role of the high-affinity IgE receptor, FCεR1, in eosinophilic gastrointestinal disorders. Immunol Allergy Clin N Am. 2009;29:159–70.
67. Abonia JP, Blanchard C, Buckmeier-Butz BK, et al. Involvement of mast cells in eosinophilic esophagitis. J Allergy Clin Immunol. 2010;126(1):112–9.
68. Bullock JZ, Villaneuva JM, Blanchard C, et al. Interplay of adaptive th2 immunity with eotaxin-3/c-C chemokine receptor 3 in eosinophilic esophagitis. J Pediatr Gastroenterol Nutr. 2007;45:22–31.
69. Mishra A, Schlotman J, Wang M, Rothenberg ME. Critical role for adaptive T cell immunity in experimental eosinophilic esophagitis in mice. J Leukoc Biol. 2007;81:916–24.
70. Zhu X, Wang M, Crump CH, Mishra A. An imbalance of esophageal effector and regulatory T cell subsets in experimental eosinophilic esophagitis in mice. Am J Physiol Gastrointest Liver Physiol. 2009;297:G550–8.

71. Bhattacharya B, Carlsten J, Sabo E, et al. Increased expression of eotaxin-3 distinguishes between eosinophilic esophagitis and gastroesophageal reflux disease. Hum Pathol. 2007;38:1744–53.
72. Parfitt JR, Gregor JC, Suskin NG, et al. Eosinophilic esophagitis in adults: distinguishing features from gastroesophageal reflux disease: a study of 41 patients. Mod Pathol. 2006;19: 90–6.
73. Aceves SS, Newbury RO, Dohil R, et al. Esophageal remodeling in pediatric eosinophilic esophagitis. J Allergy Clin Immunol. 2007;229:206–12.
74. Straumann A, Spichtin HP, Grize L, et al. Natural history of primary eosinophilic esophagitis: a follow-up of 30 adults for up to 11.5 years. Gastroenterology. 2003;125:1660–9.
75. Aceves SS, Newbury RO, Chen D, et al. Resolution of remodeling in eosinophilic esophagitis correlates with epithelial response to topical corticosteroids. Allergy. 2010;65:109–16.
76. Blanchard C, Mingler MK, McBride M, et al. Periostin facilitates eosinophil tissue infiltration in allergic lung and esophageal responses. Mucosal Immunol. 2008;1:289–96.
77. Assa'ad A, Aceves S, Gupta S, et al. The pharmacodynamic effects of mepolizumab, a humanized monoclonal antibody against IL-5, in pediatric patients with eosinophilic esophagitis: a randomized, double-blind controlled clinical trial. J Allergy Clin Immunol. 2010;125: AB129.
78. DeBrosse CW, Collins MH, Buckmeier B, et al. The "epidemic" of eosinophilic esophagitis (EE) is due to increased recognition of a chronic disorder. J Allergy Clin Immunol. 2010;125:AB233.

Chapter 15
Complications Associated with Eosinophilic Esophagitis

Stephen E. Attwood and Glenn T. Furuta

Keywords Eosinophilic esophagitis • Esophageal narrowings • Esophageal perforations • Food impaction • Maladaptive eating behaviours

Introduction

Eosinophilic esophagitis is a chronic inflammatory disease associated with dense esophageal eosinophilia, hyperplastic epithelia and subepithelial fibrosis [1]. As clinical recognition of eosinophilic esophagitis (EoE) increases, so too do observations identifying complications of the disease and its treatments. For the purposes of this chapter, complications will be defined as unfavourable evolutions of chronic inflammation or untoward consequences of ongoing treatment. In this regard, partial or complete esophageal obstruction due to esophageal narrowings or food impaction and eating difficulties are two important complications of EoE. With respect to chronic treatment, the overall goal is to resolve symptoms and prevent EoE-related complications. But treatment endpoints have not been established and thus, the exact duration, frequency, expense and type treatments have not been formally established. Because of this lack of guidelines, clinicians are potentially faced with complications related to endoscopic procedures, medical treatments and nutritional restrictions. In this chapter, we will provide our interpretation of the literature and summary of our clinical experiences of these complications in children and adult patients with EoE.

G.T. Furuta (✉)
Gastrointestinal Eosinophilic Diseases Program, The Children's Hospital Colorado, National Jewish Health, University of Colorado Denver School of Medicine, 13123 East 16th Ave. B290, Aurora, CO 80016, USA
e-mail: glenn.furuta@childrenscolorado.org

C.A. Liacouras and J.E. Markowitz (eds.), *Eosinophilic Esophagitis*, Clinical Gastroenterology, DOI 10.1007/978-1-60761-515-6_15,

Complications Associated with EoE in Children and Adults

Esophageal Narrowings

In some patients with EoE, chronic eosinophilic inflammation can lead to partial esophageal obstruction that is manifest by symptoms of feeding difficulties, dysphagia and food impaction and endoscopic evidence of isolated esophageal strictures, narrow bore esophagus, small caliber esophagus, crepe paper esophagus, longitudinal narrowings, longitudinal rents/lacerations or mucosal tears. Clinical experience suggests that not all patients develop these problems but who and when they will develop them and identification of contributing factors toward their development are all uncertain. In addition, it is not yet clear whether any form of treatment can prevent them. Increasing clinical experience documents clinical aspects of these fibrotic changes of the esophageal mucosa.

Pediatrics

A limited body of work documents esophageal strictures and narrowings associated with EoE. Radiographic studies were the first to describe esophageal strictures in EoE and identify their propensity to develop in the proximal esophagus [2, 3]. Since then, a number of case series have identified esophageal strictures occurring in the proximal, middle and distal esophagus of children with EoE [4–10]. Age at presentation ranges from 0.6 to 11 years and longstanding histories of esophageal dysfunction with vomiting, feeding difficulties or dysphagia or past medical histories of fundoplication are not unusual suggesting that these lesions were unrecognized or that their clinical impact was underestimated. The duration of time required to form these strictures is not known but some insights were provided in a case report describing a 27-year-old man with progressive solid food dysphagia. He received an original diagnosis of eosinophilic gastroenteritis 15 years earlier at which time he presumably did not have a stricture suggesting that this lesion takes years to develop [11]. Few studies have addressed the size or frequency of esophageal strictures in EoE. In a series of four pediatric patients, the mean diameter of the stricture was 5.5 mm and in adults 14.7 mm [12].

Whether medical or nutritional treatments pre- or post-dilation are beneficial is not certain but supported by some and has been the approach in most patients in our practice [9, 13, 14]. Chronic dilation does not treat underlying inflammation associated with EoE [15–18].

Approach to Child with Suspected Esophageal Narrowing and EoE

Personal experiences and discussions with other colleagues support a thorough assessment of children in whom one suspects esophageal narrowings associated with EoE. First, a thorough history is often quite revealing. While the initial attempt to identify symptoms consistent with partial esophageal obstruction may seem non-contributory, patients often have accommodated to their longstanding problem and thus report no ongoing concerns; i.e. coping behaviours have developed to self manage their narrowings [19, 20]. In some circumstances, these behaviours have led to reduction in caloric intake, malnutrition and slowed growth. Uncovering these behaviours requires asking a few more questions related to chewing and swallowing. The question of "do you experience any problems swallowing?" may be met with a "no" response, but answers to the following series of other questions often are met with the affirmative; "Does it seem to take a long time to chew your food compared to others?" "Do you need a glass/multiple glasses of liquid to wash your food down during mealtimes?" "Do you/your parents cut your food into small pieces?" "Are you often the last person to finish your meal?" "Are you unable to finish your lunch at school?" "Do you avoid eating some foods especially meats/bagels/highly textured foods?" "Do you have problems swallowing pills?" "Do you limit going out with friends because it takes you so long to eat?" Positive responses to any of these questions will lead to a subsequent imaging study to further define the esophageal mucosa. In addition, consultation with a feeding specialist may be important to help the patient overcome these problems.

Second, a brief communication with the radiologist is often helpful to provide the rationale for the study and what lesions are suspected. Since proximal strictures are uncommon, they may be missed as the radiologist may be checking for distal strictures associated with gastroesophageal reflux disease (GERD). Narrow bore esophagus, small caliber esophagus or longitudinal narrowings may not be apparent if esophageal compliance is not assessed during a swallow.

Third, a thorough and careful endoscopic assessment of the esophageal mucosa is critical at the time of initial assessment and in follow-up [21]. While radiographic narrowings are highly suggestive of obstructive lesions, they may also represent transient esophageal contractions in children. The presence of this phenomenon is supported by two case series. In a study of 17 children with EoE, five demonstrated evidence of esophageal strictures radiographically but these were confirmed in only one endoscopically [6]. We previously reported similar findings in a retrospective study of 17 children with EoE who demonstrated radiographic evidence of Schatzki Ring but upon review of the endoscopic record, the esophageal mucosa appeared normal without any evidence of a ring [22]. Together, the studies show that radiographic evidence of esophageal narrowings may not match the endoscopic findings and thus limit the necessity for dilation.

Careful attention to the entire length and circumference of esophageal mucosa is also very important. Rapid passage of the endoscope past the upper esophageal sphincter may lead to missing a proximal narrowing. Isolated narrowings are not always readily apparent and subtle resistance to the gentle passage of an age and size appropriate endoscope may be indicative of a small caliber esophagus or diffuse esophageal edema.

Whitish exudates may be mistaken for cetacaine spray or Candida instead of eosinophilic pus. With the rapid removal of an endoscope, one may miss a longitudinal tear or mucosal rent/laceration that occurred with the initial passage of the endoscope. This tear represents the fragile nature of the esophageal mucosa in EoE or crepe paper esophagus that likely occurs following years of chronic inflammation. It may explain severe post procedure pain that has been described in some patients. Once viewed, it will not be forgotten and may represent the only pathognomonic feature of the EoE [23].

Fourth, discussions with surgical, pathology and allergy colleagues are critical to ongoing care of patients [19, 20, 24–30]. Case series from otolaryngologists and pediatric surgeons have identified children with EoE who have been referred to them primarily for feeding problems or fundoplication. Surgical specialties other than gastroenterology may perform emergency esophageal foreign body disimpactions, may be the first to identify EoE and thus need to recognize clinical and endoscopic features. Pathologists may not be aware of clinicopathological features of EoE and allergists play critical roles in caring for patients longitudinally.

Finally, dilation of EoE associated narrowings should proceed slowly and less aggressively than with GERD strictures. The precise methodology required to dilate the stenotic esophagus observed in EoE is a matter of intense discussion. Factors to consider include pre-treatment with medical or nutritional management, bougie vs. balloon dilation, and frequency of sessions. Sequential gentle dilations as opposed to rapid expansion of the narrowed lumen are preferred [15–18, 31].

To summarize, esophageal narrowing may be present at the first presentation of EoE or develop over time following an established diagnosis. Evaluation of children with any symptom suggestive of partial esophageal obstruction should begin with thorough history and a barium esophagram to allow appropriate mapping of the esophageal lumen and preparation for dilation if necessary. Close observation of the luminal surface for evidence of transient contractions prior to assigning a diagnosis of an esophageal stricture is important in patients with EoE or suspected EoE. In the patient with a known diagnosis of EoE, medical or nutritional treatment prior to endoscopic analysis may be beneficial if clinically feasible. Treatment of esophagitis before endoscopic dilation appeared to be safe in children and is the suggested approach by others in adults [9, 13, 14]. Future research studies will determine best therapeutic approaches to this manifestation of EoE in children.

Adults

Strictures in adult presentation of EoE are rare but seem to represent a severe variant of this condition. Two patterns of esophageal strictures, isolated stricture and long narrow caliber, have been seen in adults. The presence of an isolated but tight stricture seems relatively rare but has occurred in <10% of patients in published series [32–34]. These patients have often already adapted their diet and ingest only liquids or very soft foods, and eat very slowly. Such adaptation without overt symptoms suggests that their strictures developed over time although there is no observational proof of this concept.

The second variation in adults is the narrow or small caliber esophagus. This variant seems to be associated with the most severe forms of swallowing difficulty and associated malnutrition. One such patient of ours presented to her local hospital at the age of 18 years where she was initially regarded as having a psychological eating disorder. The barium esophagram was also initially misinterpreted because the overall esophageal appearance did not suggest a specific stricture and the lack of the normal distension was not something the local radiologist was sensitive to. (See section on pediatric evaluation above.) This patient was commenced on total parenteral nutrition and referred to the local surgical department for manometry to see if the dysphagia was a form of achalasia. No previous endoscopy had been performed and prior to the manometry test the endoscopy performed in our institution showed a narrow caliber esophagus that would not allow the passage of a 9-mm endoscope. Biopsies confirmed EoE and after a short course of systemic steroids swallowing was restored. Now 10 years later, that patient still remains mildly symptomatic while on medical therapy. She has recovered all her strength and successfully delivered two children. This vignette highlights the potential severity of stricture, narrow bore esophagus, or small calibre oesophagus and emphasizes that a patient may appear outwardly normal in every other way because of coping behaviours.

Another case represents other classical features of a tight stricture with a longer segment of narrow bore/small caliber esophagus. This 17-year-old male presented with a 10-year history of a swallowing disorder. His parents had been extremely supportive since they first noticed his difficulty at the age of 7 years. After 5 years of tests and unhelpful treatments (mostly acid suppression), he was referred to a surgeon who despite having the discipline of performing manometry and pH studies, decided that in the absence of acid on the pH study his stricture must be peptic and performed a Nissen fundoplication. His barium study at the age of 12 is shown in Fig. 15.1, and reveals a tight stricture in the junction of the upper and middle third of esophagus, a slightly dilated proximal esophagus, and a narrow caliber/small caliber esophagus below for 8 cm in which are classic rings. This patient was subject to a Nissen fundoplication at the age of 12 years without any improvement in his symptoms and carried on with liquid nutrition until his 17th year.

Despite never having eaten a solid meal of any kind (he lived on high calorie drinks and liquid food supplements) he had grown fit and strong and he presented to our institution when he had reached an adult age having exhausted all of the investigative possibilities in his local pediatric facilities. When he came to our institution, the diagnosis was obvious from the history and radiology, and confirmed by endoscopy and biopsy. He was treated by dilatation of his stricture from 3 to 12 mm initially, systemic steroids, followed by montelukast medication with complete symptom resolution, restoration of normal solid ingestion after having none for 10 years. Thirty months later, he experienced one recurrence of bolus obstruction that required dilatation and the addition of topical steroids for maintenance therapy.

The reason for the stricturing in these above patients has not been clearly understood. At endoscopy, the strictures appear to be covered with hyperplastic mucosae, but not endoscopically inflamed, and not overtly fibrotic. In the series of patients followed longitudinally over >5 years [32–34], there does not seem to be

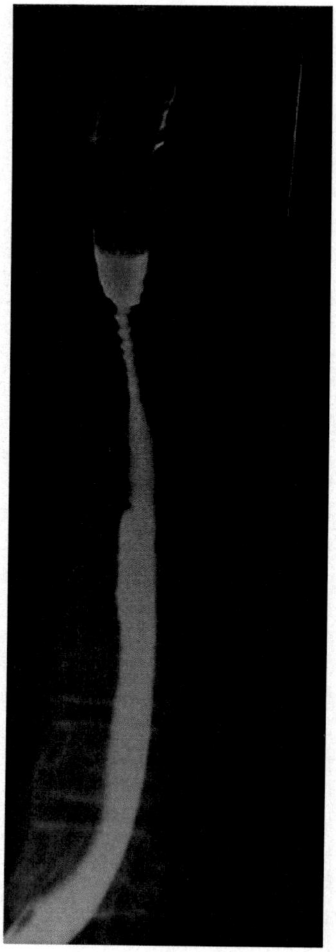

Fig. 15.1 Barium esophogram showing tight stricture at the junction of upper and middle thirds of the esophagus, with a ringed narrow calibre esophagus below, over a distance of 5 cm below, and a dilated esophagus above the stricture

progression from symptomatic dysphagia to stricture and the type of treatment used may not have any influence over the development or protection from stricturing. The use of topical steroids may reduce mucosal or even submucosal fibrosis but is unlikely to have any influence on muscular fibrosis [35]. Systemic steroids may reduce muscular fibrosis but they have generally been used to treat these patients in the early phase of their treatments, and only short courses are given to minimize side effects of long-term use. It is not clear if the use of montelukast, commonly used for this condition in the UK, has any influence on the development of strictures. Potential mechanisms of action that may be relevant to EoE relate to the fact that montelukast is a leukotriene D-4 antagonist that can stabilize eosinophil degranulation and the release of locally neuro-active mediators that may stimulate muscular dysfunction. Whether these mechanisms have any influence on the potential sporadic development of strictures is unknown.

In one American series of adults reported by Potter et al. in 2004, a much higher proportion of patients (86%) presented with rings, strictures or small caliber esophagus [36]. The reason for this much higher incidence is not clear but circumstances of referral pattern, the liberal use of barium swallows and referral after radiological identification of stricture may skew the prevalence of stricture. Although barium swallow is extremely useful it should be used to compliment, and not instead of, endoscopy and biopsy in the evaluation of dysphagia. The sensitivity and specificity of these tests in the evaluation of esophageal narrowing in EoE are not certain so that both tests offer value in the evaluation of obstructive lesions. The variation of stricture pattern seen in EoE includes mucosal fibrotic rings, which are occasionally pronounced and contribute to dysphagia at multiple levels [37]. Thus, communication with the radiologists is important so that the specific questions can be answered with the esophagram.

Food Impaction

Children and adults with EoE can experience food impaction [38–46]. Oftentimes this problem may represent the first presentation of EoE. It is not unusual to hear patients recall problems with food getting stuck after swallowing and that a variety of different maneuvers including jumping up and down, raising the arms above the head, forced gagging and attempting to swallow liquids had been used to dislodge the bolus. Often these are successful and thus the patient does not seek further attention, but eventually, the bolus remains stuck leading to a visit to the emergency room. We initially reported that 54% of adults presenting to an emergency room acutely with food impaction had findings consistent with EoE [38]. Similar findings have been reported in children and adults in other series [38–46]. Food impaction can also occur after the diagnosis of EoE has been obtained and likely relates to poorly controlled inflammation, development of an esophageal narrowing or exposure to a new food or aero-allergen. The mechanisms for food impactions are not certain but include isolated or diffuse esophageal narrowing or transient contraction of the esophageal muscularis. In support of the later mechanism is the observation that after bolus removal, an obstructing lesion may not be present.

Removal of food bolus in EoE patients also deserves comment. For a non-EoE related esophageal food impaction, a surgical approach through a rigid endoscope was preferred, with the cited advantage that retrieval of such a bolus was safer for the airway rather than with a flexible scope. However, in patients with EoE, using a Roth net or other retrieval device or placing an overtube over a flexible endoscope are alternative ways to protect the airway in such cases and the risk of perforation at a therapeutic endoscopy for bolus obstruction is likely reduced [16–18, 47]. Whether this should be performed by a gastroenterologist familiar with flexible endoscopy, or whether otolaryngologist, depends on local expertise, equipment and awareness of the relatively high frequency of EoE as a cause of bolus obstruction and its attendant risk of perforation [19, 30, 38, 48]. When a pediatric gastroenterologists performs esophageal foreign body removal, it is typically performed under general anesthesia with intubation and flexible endoscopy to protect the smaller airway anatomy.

Perforation

Spontaneous perforation. Spontaneous perforation of the esophagus in EoE is rare with the severity ranging from a full Boerhaave's rupture [44, 49–51], to partial tears [49], to circumferential dissections [52–54]. Some EoE patients may have relative fragile esophageal walls due to eosinophilic inflammation and thus may be at special risk of perforation secondary to pill ingestions. Drug-induced perforation has been suggested in relation to paracetamol use in a patient with EoE [55].

A wide range of management styles has been reported for these spontaneous perforations. A full Boerhaave type rupture requires immediate thoracotomy and repair or replacement of the esophagus. A report from Liguori et al. describes a 32-year-old man with a 3-year history of mild dysphagia followed by sudden food impaction who developed spontaneous dissection of the esophageal mucosa and an associated pneumomediastinum [53]. This patient with previously undiagnosed EoE was managed by surgical resection in the acute setting. This report allowed an interesting pathological study of the transmural effect of EoE. In contrast, patients with known EoE have been managed differently. For instance, one report described a patient with an 8-year history of EoE who developed a perforation with evidence of an air leak who was managed conservatively, without any procedural intervention. The patient was supported with parenteral nutrition and antibiotics [54]. Finally, a further variation on EoE management was the use of stent for a circumferential dissection without evidence of transmural perforation [52].

Maladaptive Eating Behaviours

During the course of chronic inflammation associated with EoE, a number of observations suggest that the patient undergoes adaptive behaviours that are directed at limiting symptoms such as pain, dysphagia and vomiting. (See section on pediatric evaluation above). In young children, these adaptive behaviours oftentimes limit food ingestion and can lead to malnutrition [20, 56–61]. In older children and adults, these adaptive behaviours, or coping strategies, may lead to altered eating habits that significantly alter lifestyles.

Pediatric. Clinical experience and a limited amount of research support the observations that children with EoE exhibit at least two forms of maladaptive feeding behaviour [20]. First, children who experience pain or discomfort with feeding and or swallowing may learn to limit the ingestion of calories and micronutrients adequate to sustain growth and development. Most often, when the inflammation is resolved, original patterns of eating will return and children will regain their growth. In some circumstances, the ingestion of adequate nutrition remains limited necessitating the use of nasogastric or gastrostomy tube supplementation. In our experience, it is rare for these interventions to be necessary but they have been utilized in some circumstances. The second type of maladaptive behaviour concerns the development of feeding difficulties. Feeding difficulties can be categorized as delayed advancement of normal eating skills or development of learned dysfunctional eating behaviours, both of which can develop as a result of an esophageal insult [20, 59]. The first problem, delayed advancement of normal eating skills, is portrayed in a 2-year-old child with EoE who does not advance through the normal developmental milestones of being able to eat more textured foods. The patient continues to eat soft foods and does not progress to ingest more highly textured foods. An example of the second problem, development of learned dysfunctional eating behaviours, is portrayed in the 6-year-old child who refuses to eat previously accepted typically high texture foods likely as a result of accommodating to an inflamed esophagus. In our recent study, learned maladaptive feeding behaviours were identified in 94% children with eosinophilic gastrointestinal diseases (EGIDs) and feeding difficulties [20]. Examples of this behaviour include food refusal, low volume or variety of intake, spitting food out, grazing, lack of mealtime structure and requiring prompting to eat. Importantly, both of these patterns may persist even when mucosal inflammation resolves [20]. Together, these kind of eating patterns can be extremely disruptive to family meals, create frustration in parent–child dynamics and, in a limited number of cases, lead to malnutrition.

Adults. The difficulties experienced by adults when eating manifest themselves in their inability to eat out in restaurants and their anxiety about the risk of the choking episodes of bolus obstruction. These fears may have marked effects by isolating patients socially, an issue clearly described by the account of Straumann et al. in his natural history of EoE [34]. In this description, he also notes the need for patients to alter their working life, even to the point of needing to change careers so that they can adapt to their eating difficulties [51].

Psychological Impacts

Unmeasured costs associated with EoE include psychological impacts related to coping with a chronic disease, undergoing repeated therapeutic evaluations and accommodating to necessary treatments. Coping with a chronic disease can bring significant disruption to any family and this is potentially compounded in EoE by repeated skin test evaluations, endoscopic procedures and anesthesia. In addition, malnutrition and social isolation related to food restriction or side effects from corticosteroid carry untold costs. See Chap. 29 [62].

Complications Associated with Treatment

Medical Treatment

Corticosteroid side effects. A number of studies document the efficacy and safety of topical corticosteroids in the treatment of allergic diseases including asthma, atopic dermatitis, allergic rhinitis and, most recently, EoE. Side effects that have been reported in association with topical steroid treatment for EoE include esophageal Candida and Herpes infection and one case of cataracts [63–66]. Other potential, but unreported, side effects of topical steroids in patients with EoE include diabetes, longitudinal growth delay, systemic infection or epithelial atrophy [67]. The systemic effects of topical steroids in EoE are minimized because of the limited systemic absorption that occurs because of first pass hepatic metabolism.

Surgical Treatment

Inappropriate surgery when EoE diagnosis is delayed. The inappropriate performance of a Nissen fundoplication for assumed GERD when the patient is actually suffering from EoE has been a recurring theme. The precise prevalence of this procedure in patients with EoE is hard to estimate but a number of case series report this occurrence in at least ten patients [24, 68–70]. Clinical experiences and these series note that in patients with EoE, anti-reflux operations provide no sustainable symptom relief.

In some practices, the presence of suitable symptoms, the observation of endoscopic inflammation or the presence of hiatus hernia is sufficient justification for fundoplication for GERD. In the authors' experiences, the use of symptoms alone to distinguish EoE from GERD is difficult at best, and endoscopic features associated with EoE are non-specific. In this light, prior to performing fundoplication, the authors will routinely use pH/impedance monitoring to insure that pathological reflux is present. In our practice, the routine use of pH probe not only identifies patients who should undergo fundoplication for recalcitrant GERD, but also permits the identification of those patients who may have EoE as an etiology for their symptoms. If GERD-like symptoms persist, despite proton pump treatment, and a normal ph monitoring of the distal esophagus is recorded when the patient is off proton pump treatment, the diagnosis of EoE is highly likely [1]. Whether non-acid reflux is a contributing cause of EoE is uncertain but at least two studies have shown that non-acid reflux is not increased in at least two studies of children with EoE [71, 72].

Perforation

Perforation as a complication of dilation. Straumann et al. have highlighted the risk of dilation of strictures in EoE; in their series, perforation occurred more often with the use of rigid endoscopy compared to flexible endoscopy [34].

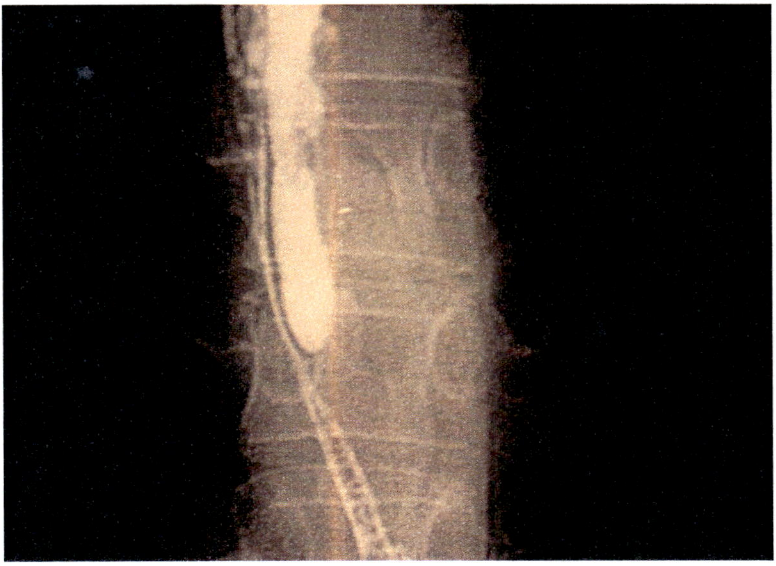

Fig. 15.2 Barium esophagram of a patient following rigid esophagoscopy for removal of a food bolus obstruction, showing a submucosal dissection and partial perforation

Among other things, this report highlights the problem of practice organization; referral patterns may send patients with EoE-related esophageal strictures to subspecialty surgeons who are not always aware of the EoE diagnosis and attendant potential predisposition to perforate. In the USA, this most commonly occurs in the emergency room setting where a patient presents acutely with an esophageal obstruction; practice organizations may either rotate the responsibility of endoscopic management between gastroenterologist and surgeon or solely refer to the surgeon. In the UK referral to an ear, nose and throat surgeon (Rhynolaryngologist) rarely if ever results in a diagnosis of EoE. In these circumstances, when the surgeon is not aware of EoE, the underlying fragile mucosa may be at increased risk of perforation with the use of a rigid endoscope.

In a subsequent report, Straumann et al. further emphasized the importance of performing a flexible endoscopy, instead of a rigid endoscopy, in EoE patients [44]. In this series, they identified the occurrence of esophageal perforation in two of ten patients undergoing rigid endoscopies compared with 0 of 124 who underwent flexible endoscopies (Fig. 15.2). Several recent studies examined practical aspects of esophageal dilation with flexible endoscopes in over 300 EoE patients [16–18, 47]. These studies report that dilation is safe when performed cautiously and despite post-procedure pain, it is well received by most patients [16]. Reported that in a study of 70 dilations performed in 36 adults with EoE, complications of mucosal tears and pain were predicted by younger patient age (23 vs. 42 years) and increased number of dilations (4 vs. 1.7) [17]. Compared 61 EoE patients treated with dilation alone to 144 patients treated with dilation and topical steroids and identified no significant differences in luminal dilation or duration of response (23 vs. 20 months dilation alone vs. dilation and treatment) [17]. No perforations were reported. A useful overview of the risk of perforation in discussed by Jacobs et al. in a recent review [31].

Perforation related to the simple passage of the endoscope. This problem lies somewhere between spontaneous perforation and that due to dilatation. The complication is relatively rare [47, 73–75]. Cohen et al. identified mucosal lacerations (7), perforations (3) in 36 adults with EoE undergoing endoscopy. The mean age of the patients was 33.9 years and dilations had been performed in six of the patients who developed complications. Again the decision on management depends on the degree of perforation, the time of discovery and the extent of the leak with the reported cases being successfully managed by esophagectomy or conservative approaches.

Muscular Involvement in EoE

Leiomyomatosis of the Esophageal Wall

A case of esophageal leiomyomatosis with eosinophilia was reported from our group by Morris et al. that showed very similar pathology to the case of Liguori et al. described above [53, 76]. In our case it was not known if the development of this complication was a direct result of mucosal esophageal eosinophilia but the dysphagia which occurred in this 61-year-old male was severe and the pathology of the section of esophageal wall removed at surgery was remarkably similar to that seen in the case of resected esophagus after perforation described by Liguori et al. The circumstance of full thickness eosinophilic infiltration in eosinophilic esophagitis was first raised by Nicholson et al. in 1997 and although their paper described the potential for a "common allergic inflammatory profile" very few other cases have been reported [77]. In the case of Morris et al., the patient had no detectable mucosal disease and at the time there was no reason to link his condition with EoE [76]. His intractable dysphagia was thought to be benign tumour on CT scan, but at surgery by thoracotomy the diffuse nature of his esophageal wall swelling was not typical of malignancy and after resecting a 2-cm wide strip of full thickness muscle from along approximately 15 cm of oesophageal myotomy, and with suitable reassurance from frozen section pathology, the esophagus was preserved and the patient swallowed comfortably for many years after.

Esophageal Muscular Inflammation

It would be of great functional interest to know if the eosinophilic involvement of muscle layers was a common phenomenon in EoE of the mucosa. The case report of Fassan published only in an abstract describing a myofibroblastic tumor as an adverse outcome of EoE may be a similar condition [78]. The work of Korsapati et al. suggests that the outer layers of esophageal longitudinal muscle show greater degrees of dysfunction but we do not know if this is secondary to mediators released from mucosal or submucosal eosinophils or it is due to eosinophil infiltration of the muscle walls [79]. At least four other studies utilizing endoscopic ultrasound and motility tracings support extension of the eosinophilia to the muscular layers in children and adults [12, 80–83]. Further research in this area would be of great interest and methods of biopsy of the deeper layers perhaps through EUS might be very revealing, as long as they can be performed safely.

Summary

The list of complications of eosinophilic esophagitis grows as clinical experience with diagnosis and treatment increases. Awareness of complications is very important given the potential seriousness of their consequences. Precautions to avoid precipitating them during therapy are paramount to the caring physicians. From a patient's perspective, Whether the first presenting with EoE is chronic dysphagia or acute bolus obstruction, the likelihood of serious complications appears to be small;this being said, the most important aspect of care of the patient with a possible complication of EoE or its treatment is attention toward prevention.

Acknowledgements Glenn T. Furuta acknowledges the insightful guidance and expertise of Victor Fox, Dan Atkins, Nancy Creskoff Maune and Angela Haas in the development and writing of this chapter.

References

1. Liacouras CA, Furuta GT, Hirano I, Atkins D, Attwood SE, Bonis PA, Burks AW, Chehade M, Collins MH, Dellon ES, Dohil R, Falk GW, Gonsalves N, Gupta SK, Katzka DA, Lucendo AJ, Markowitz JE, Noel RJ, Odze RD, Putnam PE, Richter JE, Romero Y, Ruchelli E, Sampson HA, Schoepfer A, Shaheen NJ, Sicherer SH, Spechler S, Spergel JM, Straumann A, Wershil BK, Rothenberg ME, Aceves SS Updated consensus recommendations for children and adults J Allergy Clin Immunol. 2011 Jul;128(1):3-20.e6. Epub 2011 Apr 7. PMID: 21477849.
2. Feczko P, Halpert R, Zonca M. Radiographic abnormalities in eosinophilic esophagitis. Gastrointest Radiol. 1985;10:321–4.
3. Picus D, Frank PH. Eosinophilic esophagitis. AJR Am J Roentgenol. 1981;136:1001–3.
4. Aceves SS, Newbury RO, Dohil R, Bastian JF, Broide DH. Esophageal remodeling in pediatric eosinophilic esophagitis. J Allergy Clin Immunol. 2007;119:206–12.
5. Aceves SS, Newbury RO, Dohil R, Schwimmer J, Bastian JF. Distinguishing eosinophilic esophagitis in pediatric patients: clinical, endoscopic, and histologic features of an emerging disorder. J Clin Gastroenterol. 2007;41:252–6.
6. Binkovitz LA, Lorenz EA, Di Lorenzo C, Kahwash S. Pediatric eosinophilic esophagitis: radiologic findings with pathologic correlation. Pediatr Radiol. 2010;40:714–9.

7. De Angelis P, Markowitz JE, Torroni F, Caldaro T, Pane A, Morino G, et al. Paediatric eosinophilic oesophagitis: towards early diagnosis and best treatment. Dig Liver Dis. 2006;38: 245–51.
8. Liacouras CA, Markowitz JE. Predictors of early recurrence of benign esophageal strictures: what about eosinophilic esophagitis? Am J Gastroenterol. 2004;99:182–3;author reply 184.
9. Robles-Medranda C, Villard F, le Gall C, Lukashok H, Rivet C, Bouvier R, et al. Severe dysphagia in children with eosinophilic esophagitis and esophageal stricture: an indication for balloon dilation? J Pediatr Gastroenterol Nutr. 2010;50:516–20.
10. Siafakas CG, Ryan CK, Brown MR, Miller TL. Multiple esophageal rings: an association with eosinophilic esophagitis: case report and review of the literature. Am J Gastroenterol. 2000;95:1572–5.
11. Mahajan L, Wyllie R, Petras R, Steffen R, Kay M. Idiopathic eosinophilic esophagitis with stricture formation in a patient with long-standing eosinophilic gastroenteritis. Gastrointest Endosc. 1997;46:557–60.
12. White SB, Levine MS, Rubesin SE, Spencer GS, Katzka DA, Laufer I. The small-caliber esophagus: radiographic sign of idiopathic eosinophilic esophagitis. Radiology. 2010;256:127–34.
13. Lucendo AJ, De Rezende L. Endoscopic dilation in eosinophilic esophagitis: a treatment strategy associated with a high risk of perforation. Endoscopy. 2007;39:376;author reply 377.
14. Lucendo AJ, Pascual-Turrion JM, Navarro M, Comas C, Castillo P, Letran A, et al. Endoscopic, bioptic, and manometric findings in eosinophilic esophagitis before and after steroid therapy: a case series. Endoscopy. 2007;39:765–71.
15. Bohm M, Richter JE, Kelsen S, Thomas R. Esophageal dilation: simple and effective treatment for adults with eosinophilic esophagitis and esophageal rings and narrowing. Dis Esophagus. 2010;23:377–85.
16. Dellon ES, Gibbs WB, Rubinas TC, Fritchie KJ, Madanick RD, Woosley JT, et al. Esophageal dilation in eosinophilic esophagitis: safety and predictors of clinical response and complications. Gastrointest Endosc. 2010;71:706–12.
17. Schoepfer AM, Gonsalves N, Bussmann C, Conus S, Simon HU, Straumann A, et al. Esophageal dilation in eosinophilic esophagitis: effectiveness, safety, and impact on the underlying inflammation. Am J Gastroenterol. 2010;105:1062–70.
18. Schoepfer AM, Gschossmann J, Scheurer U, Seibold F, Straumann A. Esophageal strictures in adult eosinophilic esophagitis: dilation is an effective and safe alternative after failure of topical corticosteroids. Endoscopy. 2008;40:161–4.
19. Heller JC, Freeman S, Furuta GT. Curious elements of esophageal foreign body impaction and eosinophilic esophagitis. Gastroenterol Hepatol. 2009;5:836–8.
20. Mukkada VA, Haas A, Maune NC, Capocelli KE, Henry M, Gilman N, et al. Feeding dysfunction in children with eosinophilic gastrointestinal diseases. Pediatrics. 2010;126(3):e672–7.
21. Fox VL. Eosinophilic esophagitis: endoscopic findings. Gastrointest Endosc Clin N Am. 2008;18:45–57;viii.
22. Nurko S, Teitelbaum JE, Husain K, Buonomo C, Fox VL, Antonioli D, et al. Association of Schatzki ring with eosinophilic esophagitis in children. J Pediatr Gastroenterol Nutr. 2004;38: 436–41.
23. Straumann A, Rossi L, Simon HU, Heer P, Spichtin HP, Beglinger C. Fragility of the esophageal mucosa: a pathognomonic endoscopic sign of primary eosinophilic esophagitis? Gastrointest Endosc. 2003;57:407–12.
24. Kelly KJ, Lazenby AJ, Rowe PC, Yardley JH, Perman JA, Sampson HA. Eosinophilic esophagitis attributed to gastroesophageal reflux: improvement with an amino acid-based formula. Gastroenterology. 1995;109:1503–12.
25. Thompson DM, Arora AS, Romero Y, Dauer EH. Eosinophilic esophagitis: its role in aerodigestive tract disorders. Otolaryngol Clin North Am. 2006;39:205–21.
26. Atkins D, Furuta GT. Mucosal immunology, eosinophilic esophagitis, and other intestinal inflammatory diseases. J Allergy Clin Immunol. 2010;125:S255–61.
27. Nimmons G, Van Daele DJ, Hoffman HT, Rao SS, Clark CR. Multifactorial dysphagia: diffuse idiopathic skeletal hyperostosis and eosinophilic esophagitis. Laryngoscope. 2010;120:23–5.

28. Patel N, Busler JF, Geisinger K, Hill I. Are pathologists accurately diagnosing eosinophilic esophagitis in children? A 9-year single academic institutional experience with interobserver observations. Int J Surg Pathol. 2011 Jun;19(3):290-6. Epub 2010 May 18. PMID: 20484141
29. Ramakrishnan JB. The role of food allergy in otolaryngology disorders. Curr Opin Otolaryngol Head Neck Surg. 2010;18:195–9.
30. Smith LP, Chewaproug L, Spergel JM, Zur KB. Otolaryngologists may not be doing enough to diagnose pediatric eosinophilic esophagitis. Int J Pediatr Otorhinolaryngol. 2009;73:1554–7.
31. Jacobs Jr JW, Spechler SJ. A systematic review of the risk of perforation during esophageal dilation for patients with eosinophilic esophagitis. Dig Dis Sci. 2010;55:1512–5.
32. Attwood SE, Lewis CJ, Bronder CS, Morris CD, Armstrong GR, Whittam J. Eosinophilic oesophagitis: a novel treatment using Montelukast. Gut. 2003;52:181–5.
33. Kanakala V, Lamb CA, Haigh C, Stirling RW, Attwood SE. The diagnosis of primary eosinophilic oesophagitis in adults: missed or misinterpreted? Eur J Gastroenterol Hepatol. 2010;22:848–55.
34. Straumann A, Spichtin HP, Grize L, Bucher KA, Beglinger C, Simon HU. Natural history of primary eosinophilic esophagitis: a follow-up of 30 adult patients for up to 11.5 years. Gastroenterology. 2003;125:1660–9.
35. Abu-Sultaneh SM, Durst P, Maynard V, Elitsur Y. Fluticasone and food allergen elimination reverse sub-epithelial fibrosis in children with eosinophilic esophagitis. Dig Dis Sci. 2010;56(1):97–102.
36. Potter JW, Saeian K, Staff D, Massey BT, Komorowski RA, Shaker R, et al. Eosinophilic esophagitis in adults: an emerging problem with unique esophageal features. Gastrointest Endosc. 2004;59:355–61.
37. Gonsalves N, Policarpio-Nicolas M, Zhang Q, Rao MS, Hirano I. Histopathologic variability and endoscopic correlates in adults with eosinophilic esophagitis. Gastrointest Endosc. 2006;64:313–9.
38. Desai TK, Stecevic V, Chang CH, Goldstein NS, Badizadegan K, Furuta GT. Association of eosinophilic inflammation with esophageal food impaction in adults. Gastrointest Endosc. 2005;61:795–801.
39. Luis AL, Rinon C, Encinas JL, Prieto G, Molina M, Sarria J, et al. Non-stenotic food impaction due to eosinophilic esophagitis: a potential surgical emergency. Eur J Pediatr Surg. 2006;16:399–402.
40. Byrne KR, Panagiotakis PH, Hilden K, Thomas KL, Peterson KA, Fang JC. Retrospective analysis of esophageal food impaction: differences in etiology by age and gender. Dig Dis Sci. 2007;52(3):717–21.
41. Kerlin P, Jones D, Remedios M, Campbell C. Prevalence of eosinophilic esophagitis in adults with food bolus obstruction of the esophagus. J Clin Gastroenterol. 2007;41:356–61.
42. Smith CR, Miranda A, Rudolph CD, Sood MR. Removal of impacted food in children with eosinophilic esophagitis using Saeed banding device. J Pediatr Gastroenterol Nutr. 2007;44:521–3.
43. Nonevski IT, Downs-Kelly E, Falk GW. Eosinophilic esophagitis: an increasingly recognized cause of dysphagia, food impaction, and refractory heartburn. Cleve Clin J Med. 2008;75(623–6):629–33.
44. Straumann A, Bussmann C, Zuber M, Vannini S, Simon HU, Schoepfer A. Eosinophilic esophagitis: analysis of food impaction and perforation in 251 adolescent and adult patients. Clin Gastroenterol Hepatol. 2008;6:598–600.
45. Rajagopalan J, Triadafilopoulos G. Ring(s)-related esophageal meat bolus impaction: biopsy first, dilate later. Dis Esophagus. 2009;22:E14–6.
46. Hurtado CW, Furuta GT, Kramer RE. J Pediatr Gastroenterol Nutr. 2011 Jan;52(1):43–6. PMID: 20975581
47. Cohen MS, Kaufman AB, Palazzo JP, Nevin D, Dimarino Jr AJ, Cohen S. An audit of endoscopic complications in adult eosinophilic esophagitis. Clin Gastroenterol Hepatol. 2007;5(10): 1149–53.
48. Harris R, Mitton S, Chong S, Daya H. Paediatric eosinophilic oesophagitis presenting to the otolaryngologist. J Laryngol Otol. 2010;124(1):96–100.

49. Cohen MS, Kaufman A, Dimarino Jr AJ, Cohen S. Eosinophilic esophagitis presenting as spontaneous esophageal rupture (Boerhaave's syndrome). Clin Gastroenterol Hepatol. 2007;5:A24.
50. Gomez Senent S, Adan Merino L, Froilan Torres C, Plaza Santos R, Suarez de Parga JM. Spontaneous esophageal rupture as onset of eosinophilic esophagitis. Gastroenterol Hepatol. 2008;31:50–1.
51. Straumann A. The natural history and complications of eosinophilic esophagitis. Gastrointest Endosc Clin N Am. 2008;18:99–118;ix.
52. Kim SH, Lee SO. Circumferential intramural esophageal dissection successfully treated by endoscopic procedure and metal stent insertion. J Gastroenterol. 2005;40:1065–9.
53. Liguori G, Cortale M, Cimino F, Sozzi M. Circumferential mucosal dissection and esophageal perforation in a patient with eosinophilic esophagitis. World J Gastroenterol. 2008;14:803–4.
54. Quiroga J, Prim JM, Moldes M, Ledo R. Spontaneous circumferential esophageal dissection in a young man with eosinophilic esophagitis. Interact Cardiovasc Thorac Surg. 2009;9(6):1040–2.
55. Spahn TW, Vieth M, Mueller MK. Paracetamol-induced perforation of the esophagus in a patient with eosinophilic esophagitis. Endoscopy. 2010;42 Suppl 2:E31–2.
56. Duca AP, Dantas RO, Rodrigues AA, Sawamura R. Evaluation of swallowing in children with vomiting after feeding. Dysphagia. 2008;23(2):177–82.
57. Pentiuk SP, Miller CK, Kaul A. Eosinophilic esophagitis in infants and toddlers. Dysphagia. 2007;22:44–8.
58. Flood EM, Beusterien KM, Amonkar MM, Jurgensen CH, Dewit OE, Kahl LP, et al. Patient and caregiver perspective on pediatric eosinophilic esophagitis and newly developed symptom questionnaires*. Curr Med Res Opin. 2008;24:3369–81.
59. Haas AM, Maune NC. Clinical presentation of feeding dysfunction in children with eosinophilic gastrointestinal disease. Immunol Allergy Clin North Am. 2009;29:65–75;ix.
60. Feuling MB, Noel RJ. Medical and nutrition management of eosinophilic esophagitis in children. Nutr Clin Pract. 2010;25:166–74.
61. Jarocka-Cyrta E, Wasilewska J, Kaczmarski MG. Brief report: eosinophilic esophagitis as a cause of feeding problems in autistic boy. The first reported case. J Autism Dev Disord. 2011;41(3):372–4.
62. Klinnert MD. Psychological impact of eosinophilic esophagitis on children and families. Immunol Allergy Clin North Am. 2009;29:99–107;x.
63. Karthik SV, Casson DH. Bilateral atopic cataracts in a child with eosinophilic esophagitis: an association to look out for. J Pediatr Gastroenterol Nutr. 2004;39:557–9.
64. Lindberg GM, Van Eldik R, Saboorian MH. A case of herpes esophagitis after fluticasone propionate for eosinophilic esophagitis. Nat Clin Pract Gastroenterol Hepatol. 2008;5:527–30.
65. Squires KA, Cameron DJ, Oliver M, da Fonseca Junqueira JC. Herpes simplex and eosinophilic oesophagitis: the chicken or the egg? J Pediatr Gastroenterol Nutr. 2009;49:246–50.
66. Teitelbaum J, Fox V, Twarog F, Nurko S, Antonioli D, Gleich G, et al. Eosinophilic esophagitis in children: immunopathological analysis and response to fluticasone propionate. Gastroenterology. 2002;122:1216–25.
67. Lipworth BJ. Systemic adverse effects of inhaled corticosteroid therapy: a systematic review and meta-analysis. Arch Intern Med. 1999;159:941–55.
68. Dellon ES, Gibbs WB, Fritchie KJ, Rubinas TC, Wilson LA, Woosley JT, et al. Clinical, endoscopic, and histologic findings distinguish eosinophilic esophagitis from gastroesophageal reflux disease. Clin Gastroenterol Hepatol. 2009;7(12):1305–13.
69. Lamb C, Kanakala V, Stirling R, Attwood S. Clinical lesson: eosinophilic oesophagitis, a new diagnosis to swallow. Frontline Gastroenterol. 2010;1:5–29.
70. Liacouras CA. Failed Nissen fundoplication in two patients who had persistent vomiting and eosinophilic esophagitis. J Pediatr Surg. 1997;32:1504–6.
71. Rosen R, Furuta G, Fritz J, Donovan K, Nurko S. Role of acid and nonacid reflux in children with eosinophilic esophagitis compared with patients with gastroesophageal reflux and control patients. J Pediatr Gastroenterol Nutr. 2008;46:520–3.

72. Dalby K, Nielsen RG, Kruse-Andersen S, Fenger C, Durup J, Husby S. Gastroesophageal reflux disease and eosinophilic esophagitis in infants and children. A study of esophageal pH, multiple intraluminal impedance and endoscopic ultrasound. Scand J Gastroenterol. 2010;45:1029–35.
73. Kaplan M, Mutlu EA, Jakate S, Bruninga K, Losurdo J, Keshavarzian A. Endoscopy in eosinophilic esophagitis: "feline" esophagus and perforation risk. Clin Gastroenterol Hepatol. 2003;1:433–7.
74. Riou PJ, Nicholson AG, Pastorino U. Esophageal rupture in a patient with idiopathic eosinophilic esophagitis. Ann Thorac Surg. 1996;62:1854–6.
75. Shim LS, Grehan M. Education and imaging gastrointestinal: oesophageal perforation during endoscopy for food impaction in eosinophilic oesophagitis. J Gastroenterol Hepatol. 2010;25:428.
76. Morris CD, Wilkinson J, Fox D, Armstrong GR, Attwood SE. Diffuse esophageal leiomyomatosis with localized dense eosinophilic infiltration. Dis Esophagus. 2002;15:85–7.
77. Nicholson AG, Li D, Pastorino U, Goldstraw P, Jeffery PK. Full thickness eosinophilia in oesophageal leiomyomatosis and idiopathic eosinophilic oesophagitis. A common allergic inflammatory profile? J Pathol. 1997;183:233–6.
78. Fassan M, Castoro C, Saenz AJ, Cagol M, Ninfo V, Rugge M. Inflammatory myofibroblastic tumor as adverse outcome of eosinophilic esophagitis. Endoscopy. 2009;41 Suppl 2:E95–6.
79. Korsapati H, Babaei A, Bhargava V, Dohil R, Quin A, Mittal RK. Dysfunction of the longitudinal muscles of the oesophagus in eosinophilic oesophagitis. Gut. 2009;58:1056–62.
80. Dalby K, Nielsen RG, Kruse-Andersen S, Fenger C, Bindslev-Jensen C, Ljungberg S, et al. Eosinophilic oesophagitis in infants and children in the region of Southern Denmark: a prospective study of prevalence and clinical presentation. J Pediatr Gastroenterol Nutr. 2010;51(3):280–2.
81. Nurko S, Rosen R, Furuta GT. Esophageal dysmotility in children with eosinophilic esophagitis: a study using prolonged esophageal manometry. Am J Gastroenterol. 2009;104(12): 3050–7.
82. Fox VL, Nurko S, Teitelbaum JE, Badizadegan K, Furuta GT. High-resolution EUS in children with eosinophilic "allergic" esophagitis. Gastrointest Endosc. 2003;57:30–6.
83. Lucendo AJ, Castillo P, Martin-Chavarri S, Carrion G, Pajares R, Pascual JM, et al. Manometric findings in adult eosinophilic oesophagitis: a study of 12 cases. Eur J Gastroenterol Hepatol. 2007;19:417–24.

Chapter 16
IgE- and Non-IgE-Mediated Food Allergy

Scott H. Sicherer

Keywords Eosinophilic esophagitis • Food allergies • Immunologic responses • Allergy patch tests

Introduction

Food allergy is generally defined as an immune-mediated adverse response to food [1]. In contrast, nonimmune adverse reactions to foods include intolerance, for example lactose intolerance, and pharmacologic responses, for example tachycardia from caffeine or flushing and pruritus from scombroid fish poisoning. The immunologic responses responsible for food allergies are often categorized as IgE antibody mediated, cell mediated (non-IgE), or caused by combined immune response. Food-induced eosinophilic esophagitis is typically considered to be the result of, or related to, both cellular and IgE antibody responses. This chapter focuses upon the full spectrum of food allergic disorders with less emphasis on eosinophilic esophagitis. Table 16.1 lists various types of adverse reactions to foods with examples.

There are a number of important reasons for considering a diagnosis of food allergy in those who have or may have eosinophilic esophagitis. Food is an important trigger for eosinophilic esophagitis [2]. Coexisting food allergy, or at least positive tests for food-specific IgE or positive allergy patch tests to foods [3] are frequently reported. In reports of children and adults with eosinophilic esophagitis, generally over 2/3 have positive tests for food-specific IgE [4–7]. Additionally,

S.H. Sicherer (✉)
Department of Pediatrics, Mount Sinai School of Medicine, Jaffe Food Allergy Institute,
1 Gustave L. Levy Place, 1198, New York, NY 10029, USA
e-mail: scott.sicherer@mssm.edu

C.A. Liacouras and J.E. Markowitz (eds.), *Eosinophilic Esophagitis*,
Clinical Gastroenterology, DOI 10.1007/978-1-60761-515-6_16,

Table 16.1 General overview of adverse reactions to foods with examples

Food allergy (immune responses)
IgE-mediated (e.g., anaphylaxis)
Not IgE-mediated (cell mediated, e.g., food protein-induced enterocolitis)
Mixed IgE/non-IgE (e.g., eosinophilic gastrointestinal disease, atopic dermatitis)
Intolerance (nonallergic hypersensitivity and pharmacologic responses)
Lactose intolerance (lactase deficiency)
Caffeine (jitteriness)
Toxins
Bacterial food poisoning
Scombroid (in dark-meat fish, may mimic allergy)
Neurologic and psychological/psychiatric
Auriculotemporal syndrome (facial flush with salivation)
Gustatory rhinitis (rhinitis from spicy or hot foods)
Anorexia nervosa and food aversions

6–24% of those with eosinophilic esophagitis have anaphylactic food allergies [8–11]. Thus, identification and management of IgE-mediated food allergy is an important component of care for many patients with eosinophilic esophagitis. Additionally, atopic disease such as atopic dermatitis and asthma are common co-morbidities among those with eosinophilic esophagitis and may also be related to food allergies in some patients [12]. Lastly, various food-associated gastrointestinal disorders may need to be considered in the differential diagnosis of those with possible eosinophilic esophagitis.

Pathophysiology

Food allergy is presumed to be the result of a failure to achieve, or a loss of, oral tolerance. This defect is thought to occur due to immune dysregulation associated with oral exposure to food proteins (allergens). Alternatively, a nonoral route of exposure may abrogate tolerance. For example, oral allergy syndrome/pollen-food related syndrome (a type of food allergy discussed further below) results when respiratory sensitization to protein in birch tree pollen results in oral symptoms upon ingestion of homologous proteins in specific fruits [13].

Symptoms associated with IgE antibody-mediated reactions to foods are typically sudden in onset, occurring within minutes to a few hours after exposure. These patients typically have food-specific IgE antibodies that can be demonstrated by allergy skin prick tests (SPT) or serum tests. Cell-mediated food allergies, primarily affecting the gut, cause chronic symptoms where the onset may be delayed by hours or days or may be chronic. Tests for food-specific IgE are generally negative, and in some cases researchers have demonstrated positive tests of delayed type hypersensitivity using patch testing (placement of the food on the skin under a chamber for over 24 h with evaluation of the response for several days after removal) [14].

Both eosinophilic esophagitis and food-associated atopic dermatitis are considered to be of mixed IgE/non-IgE etiology and studies have related food-responsiveness to positive tests for food-specific IgE and/or patch testing [15, 16].

Immune responses are primarily directed to proteins in foods. Relatively few protein families account for the vast majority of allergic reactions [17]. Allergic reactions to egg, milk, peanut, tree nuts, fish, shellfish, wheat, and soy account for most significant food allergies, although any food may trigger an allergic response [18]. These food allergens share a number of common features; they are water-soluble glycoproteins, 10–70 kDa in size and are relatively stable to heat, acid, and proteases. However, recent studies suggest that the carbohydrate moiety of certain glycoproteins may play a significant role in the allergenicity of specific foods. Platts-Mills and colleagues identified 24 adults who reported urticaria, angioedema, or anaphylaxis 3–6 h after ingesting beef, lamb, or pork [19]. These patients were found to have positive skin tests and serum IgE antibodies to galactose-alpha-1, 3-galactose, the carbohydrate moiety of these mammalian glycoproteins. This is the first demonstration of IgE antibodies directed at a carbohydrate epitope leading to clinical symptoms and may represent sensitization to tick bite antigens from species in the regions where these patients were observed.

Epidemiology

The epidemiology of eosinophilic esophagitis is considered in Chaps. 2 and 3. Here we focus upon general estimates of food allergy prevalence. Unfortunately, definitive studies are few and estimates vary by study design and other factors. Considering allergy to milk, egg, peanut, and seafood in a meta-analysis of 51 studies, self reported allergy ranged from 3 to 35% while estimates from 6 studies using more definitive tests such as medically supervised feedings estimated rates of 1–10.8% [20]. In a meta-analysis including 36 population-based studies focusing on allergy to fruits and vegetables (excluding peanut) [21], only 6 included supervised feeding tests and estimates of allergy varied widely from 0.1 to 4.3% for fruits and tree nuts to 0.1 to 1.4% for vegetables and under 1% for wheat, soy, and sesame.

Food allergy prevalence rates vary by age, cultural diet, and many other factors. A 2008 CDC report indicated an 18% rise in childhood food allergy from 1997 to 2007 with an estimated 3.9% of children currently affected [22]. Studies in the US and the UK have indicated at least a doubling in the rate of peanut allergy in young children within the past decade [23, 24]. Extrapolation from a US study indicates approximately 125,000 emergency room visits [25] and 53,700 episodes of anaphylaxis [26] from foods each year. Fatalities are primarily reported from allergic reactions to peanuts and tree nuts, appear to be associated with delayed treatment with epinephrine and occur more often in teenagers and young adults with asthma and a previously diagnosed food allergy [27]. Allergy to additives and preservatives, though often suspected, are uncommon (<1%) [28]. Genetic risk factors for food allergy include a family or personal history of atopic disorders (asthma, atopic dermatitis, allergic rhinitis, food allergy).

Studies to address the reasons for the apparent increased prevalence of food allergies have focused primarily on peanut. Hypotheses include: the "hygiene hypothesis" where lack of exposure to microbes results in immune dysregulation, changes in the components of the diet including antioxidants, fats, and nutrients such as vitamin D that may alter immune function, the use of antacids resulting in exposure to more intact protein, various forms of food processing, e.g., for peanut roasting and emulsification to produce peanut butter compared to fried or boiled peanut, and timing of ingestion such as exposure that is too early in life or extensively delaying [29, 30]. The latter hypothesis poses that oral exposure is tolerance inducing and lack of oral exposure may result in the opportunity to experience sensitizing exposures by nonoral routes. Evidence supporting this hypothesis is provided by a study showing peanut allergy rates in a school age cohort of Israeli Jewish children to be 0.17%, compared to a cohort of Jewish children in the UK where the rate was about tenfold higher (1.85%; $p<0.001$) in the context of data showing consumption of peanut at ages 8–14 months was 7.1 g in Israel compared to 0 g in the UK ($p<0.0001$) [31]. A case–control study additionally found that peanut allergy was associated with household peanut consumption rather than maternal or infant peanut consumption [32]. However, randomized controlled trials are needed to confirm the hypothesis that earlier ingestion of peanut is protective.

Clinical Disorders

IgE-Mediated Disorders

IgE-mediated food-allergic reactions typically result in symptoms soon after ingestion of the food. The organ system(s) affected and the specific symptom patterns, sometimes related to the route of contact or sensitization, further define the specific disorders that result from these mechanisms. The disorders generally result from the release of mediators, such as histamine and platelet-activating factor, from effector cells, e.g., mast cells and basophils, after food-specific IgE antibodies are cross-linked through interaction with the trigger proteins on the surfaces of the effector cells. The symptoms and disorders include:

Urticaria and/or angioedema. Urticaria, pruritis, and flushing are common skin manifestations of food allergy, either alone or in combination with other symptoms [1]. The rash may occur anywhere, though areas on the face are most commonly affected. A localized form of urticaria, *contact urticaria*, describes the observation that direct skin contact with the food results in hives. For a specific patient, a food that triggers contact urticaria may be tolerated when ingested without direct skin contact. *Chronic urticaria* is typically described as a period with 6 weeks or more of frequent urticaria; this disorder is not commonly associated with food allergy.

Gastrointestinal anaphylaxis. This term is used to describe isolated, acute gastrointestinal responses such as nausea, pain, vomiting and/or diarrhea induced by IgE-mediated mechanisms. Gastrointestinal anaphylaxis is uncommon, but gastrointestinal symptoms commonly accompany other organ system manifestations of acute, IgE antibody-mediated reactions to foods.

Pollen-food allergy syndrome (oral allergy syndrome). This disorder is a form of contact allergy where the primary symptoms occur in the oropharynx and lips [33]. Initial sensitization to pollen proteins may result in symptoms when homologous proteins in particular specific raw fruits/vegetables are ingested. For example, the birch pollen protein, Bet v 1, shares homology with apple, Mal d 1. Additional relationships with birch pollen proteins include other Rosaceae family fruits such as peach and plum and vegetables such as carrot. Another relationship is between ragweed pollen protein and proteins in melons such as cantaloupe and honeydew. It is estimated that 50% of pollen-allergic persons may be affected. Symptoms are typically mild and self-limited with oral pruritus and mild angioedema, but progression to a systemic reaction may occur. Causal proteins are presumably heat-labile since cooking the food typically abolishes reactions. The symptom pattern must be distinguished from mild oral reactions to stable proteins and oral reactions that may be a first symptom of a more progressive allergic response. The selfsame foods causing this oral syndrome may induce systemic reactions in persons reactive to stable proteins in them (e.g., lipid transfer proteins). Persons with eosinophilic esophagitis often have pollen allergies and the role of both respiratory exposure to the pollens and of oral-topical exposure to pollen-related proteins in raw fruits or vegetables has not been fully elucidated.

Asthma and Allergic Rhinitis. Chronic asthma and chronic allergic rhinitis are not typically solely attributable to food allergy. However, nasal respiratory symptoms of rhinorrhea, congestion, and pruritus or asthma symptoms such as cough and wheezing may accompany systemic allergic reactions from ingested food allergens. Inhalation of airborne allergenic food proteins may also induce respiratory reactions either in an occupational setting, e.g., baker's asthma from wheat, or when stable proteins become aerosolized during cooking or processing [34].

Anaphylaxis. Outside of medical settings, food is the most common trigger of anaphylaxis, a serious systemic allergic reaction that is rapid in onset and may cause death [35]. Symptoms can vary and may affect any of a combination of organ systems among the skin, respiratory tract, gastrointestinal tract, and cardiovascular system. Symptoms may also include an aura of "impending doom," and uterine contractions. While a variety of mild symptoms such as urticaria and abdominal pain may occur, life-threatening symptoms include laryngeal edema, severe asthma, and cardiovascular compromise. Fatalities are rare, but have been associated with delayed treatment, co-morbid conditions such as asthma, and reactions to foods such as peanut, tree nuts, fish, shellfish, and milk [27]. Anaphylaxis is a clinical diagnosis. Reactions may follow a biphasic course with initial symptoms waning with recurrence of severe symptoms 1–2 h later, or longer. A sub-type of food-induced anaphylaxis is *food-associated, exercise-induced anaphylaxis* [36]. This disorder is characterized by anaphylaxis occurring only when exercise follows ingestion of a specific food (or foods) that is otherwise tolerated. The syndrome of exercise-related food anaphylaxis has been attributed to a variety of specific foods, most commonly wheat and celery, but some individuals experience anaphylaxis with exercise after any meal.

Non-IgE-Mediated (Cell Mediated) Disorders

Similar to the IgE-associated disorders, these disorders may also affect various target organs [37]. However, symptoms that are associated with exposure tend to occur chronically during a period of inclusion of the food in the diet or subacutely, hours or more after an ingestion. Most of the disorders in this category affect the gastrointestinal tract.

Contact dermatitis. Eczematous eruptions from direct skin contact, often in occupational settings, represent a type IV hypersensitivity response. Fixed raised, erythematous eruptions, similar to fixed drug eruptions, have rarely been attributed to foods.

Dermatitis herpetiformis. This is a papulovesicular skin rash associated with celiac disease caused by an immune response to gluten.

Heiner's syndrome or milk-induced pulmonary hemosiderosis. This rare condition is associated with precipitating (IgG) antibodies to cow's milk. Symptoms include anemia, pulmonary infiltrates, recurrent pneumonia, and growth failure which resolve with milk elimination.

Dietary protein proctocolitis/allergic eosinophilic proctocolitis. Infants with this disorder appear generally healthy but experience mucousy, bloody stools. The disorder is attributed to an immune response directed, most commonly, against cow's milk protein. The mean age at diagnosis is approximately 60 days, with a range of 1 day to 6 months [38, 39]. Unlike bleeding associated with perirectal fissures where streaks of blood appear on formed stool, the pattern of bleeding more often results in stool that has a mixture of frothy mucous and blood. About 60% of cases occur in breastfed infants where the immune response results from maternal ingestion of the food allergen, usually cow's milk, which is passed in immunologically recognizable form into the breast milk. In formula-fed infants, the reaction is associated with cow's milk or, less commonly, soy [40–42]. Endoscopic examination is usually not needed for diagnostic purposes but, when performed, shows patchy erythema, friability, and a loss of vascularity generally limited to the rectum but sometimes extending throughout the colon [43]. Histologically, high numbers of eosinophils (5–20 per high-power field) or eosinophilic abscesses are seen in the lamina propria, crypt epithelium, and muscularis mucosa [38, 44]. The eosinophils are frequently associated with lymphoid nodules (lymphonodular hyperplasia) [38, 45].

The frequency of food allergy causing rectal bleeding in infants has not been extensively studied. Xanthakos et al. [46] performed colonoscopy and biopsy on 22 infants presenting with rectal bleeding and proved eosinophilic colitis in 14 (64%). The remainder had normal biopsies (23%) or nonspecific colitis (14%). This group recommended dietary elimination for those with eosinophilic colitis and the majority had resolution within 1–3 weeks. However, the relationship of cow's milk protein to symptoms was not proven by re-challenge in that study. Arvola et al. [47] examined 40 infants presenting with rectal bleeding. Infants were randomized to either avoid cow's milk protein or maintain their current diet. The groups were similar with regard to duration and severity of bleeding. During follow-up, cow's milk allergy was diagnosed in 18% of the infants and for these cow's milk allergic infants, there was a reduced length of bleeding if they had been randomized to an elimination diet at study outset. Atopic dermatitis and confirmed inflammation of the colonic mucosa were associated with persistence of cow's milk allergy upto the age of 1 year. These studies indicate that food allergy may not be a common cause of rectal bleeding in infants unless there are additional signs of allergy. However, a survey of 56 pediatric gastroenterologists showed that 84% prescribe empiric dietary trials [46]. In cow's milk- or soy formula-fed infants, substitution with a protein hydrolysate formula can be undertaken. Management in breastfed infants requires maternal restriction of cow's milk or possibly soy, egg, or other foods [40]. Because there is generally no risk of a severe reaction, the foods can be gradually reintroduced into the diet either as a trial to prove a causal relationship or months afterwards to monitor for resolution of the allergy.

Food protein-induced enterocolitis syndrome (FPIES). This dramatic but uncommon disorder includes a symptom complex of profuse vomiting and diarrhea usually diagnosed in the first months of life and most commonly attributable to an immune response to cow's milk or soy [48]. Both the small and large intestines are involved in the inflammatory process. When the causal protein remains in the diet, chronic symptoms can include bloody diarrhea, poor growth, anemia, hypoalbuminemia, and fecal leukocytes, and the illness may progress to dehydration and hypotension [49, 50]. Removal of the causal protein leads to resolution of symptoms but re-exposure results in a characteristic delayed, approximately 2 h, onset of vomiting, lethargy, elevation of the peripheral blood polymorphonuclear leukocyte count and possibly reduced temperature, thrombocytosis, hypotension, dehydration, acidemia, and methemoglobinemia [51, 52]. The dramatic nature of the presentation often results in evaluations for sepsis or surgical diagnoses [53], and a delay in final diagnosis until more than one episode occurs [52]. Based upon studies in the US and Israel [54–56], approximately half of infants with cow's milk reactions also react to soy and among children reacting to milk/soy, about 25% react to additional proteins such as rice or oat. Sensitivity to milk was lost in 60% and to soy in 25% of the patients after 2 years from the time of presentation. In addition, some patients maintain their allergy beyond the age of 6 years [57]. A retrospective study of 35 children from Australia evaluated over a span of 16 years showed rice (14 children), soy (12), and milk (7) to be the most common triggers and sensitivity was lost by the age of 3 years to rice and soy in about 80% [52]. In a cohort of 23 Korean infants with milk/soy FPIES, resolution rates were 64% for milk and 92% for soy by 10 months of age and all were tolerant by 20 months [58].

Various studies have implicated TNF-alpha as a mediator of interest in this disorder [59–62]. Chung et al. [62] demonstrated that the type 1, but not type 2, receptor for TGF-beta1 were decreased in duodenal biopsy specimens in patients with FPIES compared to controls. Analysis of humoral features in milk-induced enterocolitis shows milk protein-specific IgA but very low levels of specific IgG1 and IgG4, and this has been theorized to be pathogenic because IgG4 might otherwise block complement-fixing antibodies [63]. Specific IgE is sometimes noted as well, and may be a marker of persistence [51].

The diagnosis of FPIES rests on clinical and challenge criteria. Most patients would not undergo a formal challenge during infancy because the diagnosis becomes self-evident after elimination of the causal protein, and frequently patients experience inadvertent re-exposure, proving their sensitivity before a diagnostic test feeding. It must be appreciated that chronic ingestion, or re-exposure to the causal food, can result in a clinical picture that is severe and may mimic sepsis. In a review of 17 infants hospitalized with this disorder, Murray and Christie [64] reported 6 infants who presented with acidemia (mean pH 7.03) and methemoglobinemia. Follow-up medically supervised feeding may be performed at intervals to determine tolerance; dramatic reactions, including shock, can occur, so specialist care is needed. Re-evaluation for the development of antigen-specific IgE antibody before challenge may be helpful because a few children may convert to IgE-mediated reactions over time and experience more persistent symptoms and acute allergic reactions [51]. Patch testing was performed in one small study and showed 100% sensitivity and 71% specificity; [14] additional studies are needed to confirm these promising results. About half of positive challenges require treatment (usually intravenous fluids) [51]. In view of the presumed pathophysiology, corticosteroids have been administered for severe reactions. The role of epinephrine for treatment is not known, but it should be available for severe cardiovascular reactions.

Dietary protein enteropathy. This disorder is characterized by protracted diarrhea, vomiting, malabsorption, and failure to thrive. Additional features may include abdominal distention, early satiety, edema, hypoproteinemia, and protein-losing enteropathy [65]. Symptoms usually begin in the first several months of life, depending on the time of exposure to the causal proteins. The disorder was described primarily from the 1960s to 1990s and was commonly attributed to cow's milk protein, but has not been described in the literature for many years [66–69]. A decrease in prevalence was documented in Finland [70] and Spain [71] and attributed to a rise in breastfeeding and/or the use of adapted infant formula. Presentations of eosinophilic gastroenteritis with protein losing enteropathy share many features with previous descriptions of this disorder [72, 73].

Celiac disease. Because celiac disease, or gluten-sensitive enteropathy, is the result of an immune response to glutens from wheat, barley, rye, and related proteins, it is sometimes considered among allergic gastrointestinal disorders. The disorder affects approximately 1% of the population and is characterized by inflammatory injury to the small intestinal mucosa [74–76]. The classic presentation occurs in infants after weaning, at the time when cereals are introduced into the diet. Symptoms partly reflect malabsorption, with patients exhibiting failure to thrive, anemia, and muscle wasting. Additional symptoms include diarrhea, abdominal pain, vomiting, bone pain, and aphthous stomatitis. Chronic ingestion of gluten-containing grains in celiac patients is associated with increased risk of enteropathy-associated T cell lymphoma. Celiac disease is associated with autoimmune disorders and IgA deficiency. Endoscopy of the small bowel in active celiac disease typically reveals total villous atrophy and extensive cellular infiltrate. More than 90% of patients are HLA DQ2 with the remainder being HLA-DQ8 [74, 77]. Gliadin is one of the few substrates for tissue transglutaminase, which deamidates specific glutamines within gliadin, creating epitopes that bind efficiently to DQ2 gut-derived T cells [78]. The activation of DQ2 or DQ8-restricted T cells initiates the inflammatory response [76]. Elimination of gliadin from the diet results in a downregulation of the T cell-induced inflammatory process and normalizing of the mucosal histology. Tests for IgA anti-endomysial antibody (using tissue transglutaminase) are sensitive (85–98%) and specific (94–100%) with excellent positive (91–100%) and negative (80–98%) predictive values [76, 79].

"Mixed" IgE/Non-IgE-Mediated Disorders

Atopic dermatitis. Studies using double-blind, placebo-controlled oral food challenges show that approximately one in three young children with moderate to severe atopic dermatitis has food allergy [80]. There is some controversy about the role of chronic ingestion in increasing skin inflammation, as opposed to having food allergy as a co-morbid condition among those with atopic dermatitis [81–83]. However, studies have noted flaring of atopic dermatitis sometimes associated with positive tests for delayed type hypersensitivity rather than tests for food-specific IgE [16]. Most studies reveal that food-specific IgE antibody is detectable to the foods that cause symptoms. Because of the chronic nature of the disorder, and its waxing and waning course, it is difficult to associate symptoms with particular foods by history alone. Studies in children identify that over 90% of reactions are attributed to milk, egg, wheat, and soy. It is less common to verify a role for meats, fruits, or vegetables [80].

Allergic eosinophilic esophagitis/gastroenteritis. These disorders, covered extensively in this book and therefore not delineated further here, are also associated with foods with some evidence of both IgE- and cell-mediated mechanisms [2].

Additional disorders not clearly linked to food allergy. A number of publications have addressed the possibility of food allergy or nonallergic responses to foods as a trigger for reflux [84], constipation [85], or infantile colic [86]. Additional studies are needed to define these potential relationships. Food allergy is not considered a cause of behavioral symptoms [87].

Diagnosis

The diagnostic modalities to identify food allergies in persons with eosinophilic esophagitis are reviewed in Chap. 19. Here we focus on principles of general diagnosis of food allergy (Fig. 16.1). The clinical evaluation of an adverse reaction to food depends upon a careful history and physical examination to determine the type of adverse response and what food(s) may be responsible [87]. Based upon the history, adverse reactions to foods might be altogether ruled out (for example, a diagnosis of viral-induced urticaria) or nonallergic adverse reactions might be given greater consideration (for example, lactose intolerance resulting in diarrhea). Important factors to consider include the types of symptoms, the chronicity, reproducibility, and alternative reasons for symptoms. If symptoms indicate a nonimmune response is likely, additional evaluation would follow the specific suspicion. For example, lactose intolerance may be confirmed through breath hydrogen testing. If a food allergy is likely, the pattern of illness and list of possible triggers may disclose whether an IgE or non-IgE associated disorder is likely and will establish what type of testing may be appropriate. For chronic disorders such as atopic dermatitis and eosinophilic gastroenteritis, the identification of suspect foods is difficult because food is ingested throughout the day and symptoms are often chronic with a waxing and waning course. The periodic nature of the symptoms may result in misleading coincidental associations with foods. Symptom diaries are helpful but rarely diagnostic. In addition, individuals with these disorders often test positive to multiple foods that may not be causing illness. Care in selecting and interpreting the tests is paramount.

For determination of food-specific IgE antibodies, prick skin tests (PSTs) performed using a probe to introduce food protein to the superficial skin layer, or serum tests, are generally sensitive (~75–95%) and specific (~30–60%) [37]. PSTs, generally performed by allergists, are used on rash-free skin while the patient is avoiding antihistamines; intradermal skin tests should not be used. Though commercial extracts are available for performing prick skin tests for many foods, fresh extracts, particularly when testing fruits and vegetables whose proteins are prone to degradation, may be more sensitive. If IgE antibody specific for the food protein is present, a wheal and flare will occur that is compared to positive (histamine) and negative (saline-glycerine) controls. PSTs are considered positive if there is a mean wheal diameter of 3 mm or greater, after subtraction of the saline control. Another means to detect food-specific IgE antibody is a serum test. Although the term "RAST" (radioallergosorbent test) is often used, the term is antiquated and inaccurate because modern assays typically do not use radiolabels. Various assay systems are commercially available and their results may not be interchangeable [88]. Results may be expressed in a variety of measurements (units, counts, classes) that are also not interchangeable and while increasing scores or concentrations of food-specific antibody generally correlate with increasing risk of allergy, there are no absolute values that are entirely diagnostic of an allergy.

For proper diagnosis, it is therefore crucial to consider that a positive PST or serum IgE test merely indicates that food-specific IgE is present; it does not itself confirm an allergy. In a limited number of studies of a few foods in infants and/or

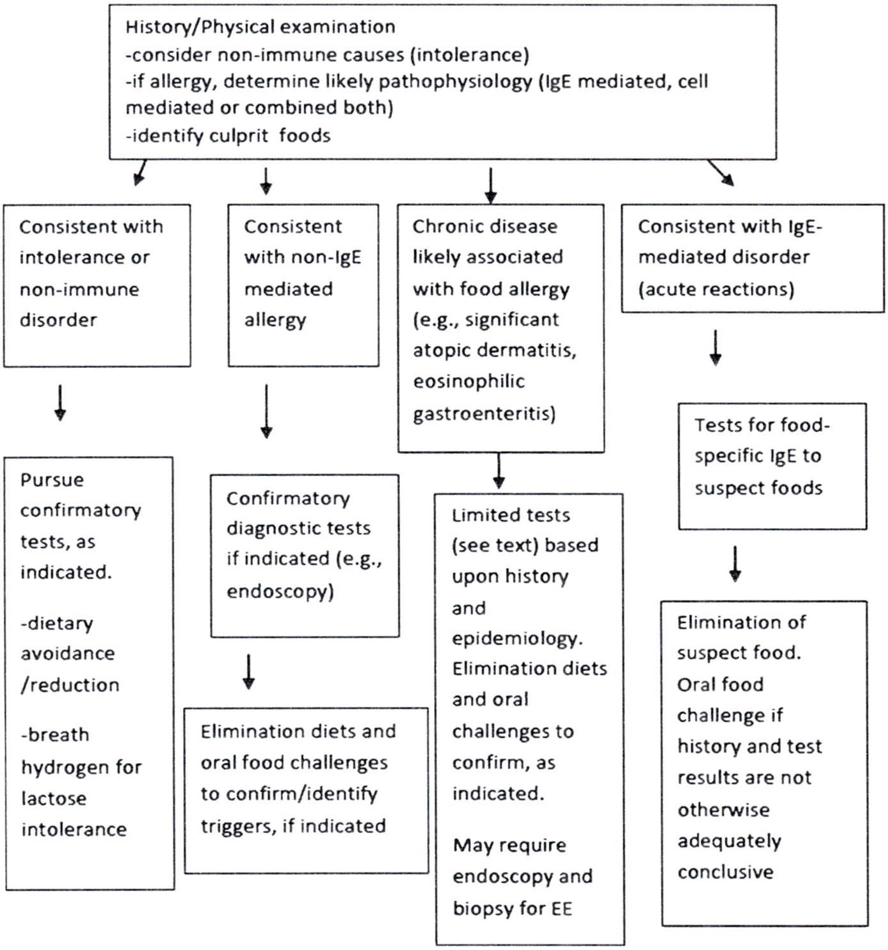

Fig. 16.1 General approach to diagnosis

children, diagnostic values associated with very high (≥95%) predictive values for reactions have been determined, though not universally confirmed. A study using PSTs in young children revealed that when wheals were particularly large (≥8 mm for milk and peanut, and ≥7 mm for egg) clinical reactions were virtually certain [89]. Studies determining the concentration of specific IgE antibody measured using a particular method (CAP-RAST FEIA® or UniCap® or ImmunoCAP® reported in kU_A/L) showed a food-specific IgE concentration of ≥7 kU_A/L to egg, ≥15 to milk, and ≥14 to peanut were 95% predictive for a reaction among 5-year-old children [90]. For children under age 2 years, the values where most reacted were lower (e.g., ≥2 kU_A/L for egg or milk). These results have not been universally confirmed [18, 87]. It must be emphasized that diagnostic concentrations are undetermined for other foods, allergic disorders, or age groups [91]. Food-specific IgE may be detected despite tolerance of a food, or may remain detectable, but typically declines, as a food allergy resolves. Obtaining "panels" of food allergy tests without consideration for the history is not a good practice because numerous irrelevant positive results may occur. The history is crucial because tests are expected to be negative when the pathophysiology of the response is consistent with non-IgE-mediated reactions; thus, a negative test may nonetheless be consistent with an allergy. A negative test is more reliable in excluding an IgE-mediated allergic reaction. However, acute anaphylactic reactions may also occasionally occur despite a negative test, so caution is needed when evaluating a patient with a convincing history despite a negative test [92].

Neither the size of the PST nor level of IgE in serum usefully predicts the type or severity of reaction. Additional diagnostic tests are being researched. Another potential pitfall is that foods with homologous proteins can result in tests that are positive among foods while an individual is not truly clinically allergic to all of the "cross-reactive" foods. For example, 95% of those with peanut allergy, a legume, can tolerate other beans and yet 50% will have positive tests to multiple beans. The rates of clinical cross-reactivity vary among foods, being high among fish and shellfish and low for grains and legumes [93].

The Atopy Patch Test (APT) which is performed by placing the food allergen on the skin under occlusion for 48 h and assessing for a delayed rash at 24–72 h shows some promise for non-IgE-mediated disorders or those with mixed etiologies including eosinophilic esophagitis. More studies are needed to determine utility [87].

For evaluation of the role of food allergy in chronic disease, the amelioration of symptoms during dietary elimination of suspected foods provides presumptive evidence of causality. Elimination diets can be undertaken by removing a defined food suspected to be causing symptoms, removing all but a defined group of foods that are rarely allergenic (oligoantigenic diet), or by giving an elemental diet of only a hypoallergenic extensively hydrolyzed formula or a nonallergenic amino acid-based formula. The elemental diet provides the most definitive trial. The type of elimination diet selected will depend upon the clinical scenario, a priori reasoning concerning offending foods, and the results of tests for IgE antibody. The length of trial depends upon the type of symptoms that have been observed, but 1–6 weeks is usually the range required. A dietitian may be needed to ensure nutritional sufficiency of trial diets. For breast-fed infants, maternal dietary elimination is required. When a food to which IgE has been demonstrated is removed from the diet during a chronic disorder, it is possible for re-introduction to induce severe reactions so caution is needed and risks/benefits (nutritional, social, immunologic) should be considered [94, 95].

When history and simple tests have not confirmed an allergy, or when tolerance is suspected after a period of avoidance, an oral food challenge (OFC) may be needed to confirm clinical allergy [95]. An oral food challenge is performed by feeding gradually increasing amounts of the suspected food under physician observation over hours or days. OFCs are performed either openly or blinded by hiding the food in another food or opaque capsules. The double-blind, placebo-controlled oral

Table 16.2 Commonly used diagnostic tests and their features

Test	Features
Medical history and examination	Defines prior probability of food allergy compared to other causes for symptoms Elucidates likely pathophysiology to provide insight on testing (IgE mediated or not) Determines, along with understanding of epidemiology, the chance of specific food(s) being implicated
Elimination diet	In the context of chronic symptoms, may implicate a food or group of foods as contributing to reactivity/disease Unlikely to be an isolated means to diagnose a specific culprit food
Prick skin tests	Provides evidence of sensitization, not necessarily intrinsically diagnostic (see text) Correlation of increasing size with increasing risk of clinical allergy
Serum food-specific IgE	Provides evidence of sensitization, not necessarily intrinsically diagnostic (see text) Correlation of increasing concentration with increasing risk of clinical allergy
Oral food challenge	Medically supervised feeding is the best test for tolerance Risk of reaction and time consuming Double-blind, placebo-controlled format is considered the "gold standard" for diagnosis

Additional types of tests are reviewed in the text. Additional details about test advantages and pitfalls are delineated in the text

food challenge is the method least prone to bias and is considered the "gold standard" to diagnose food allergy. In this format, a test food is hidden in another food and the patient and observer do not know when they are receiving active or placebo doses; feedings of the true or placebo challenge foods are separated by hours or days.

The OFC can be used to evaluate any type of suspected adverse response to foods because it is not dependent upon any particular pathophysiology. The procedure is most often needed when several foods are under consideration, tests for specific IgE are positive and elimination resulted in resolution of symptoms or when tests cannot be depended upon to confirm a diagnosis, such as non-IgE-mediated disorders. The challenge setting also provides a safe means to introduce foods that were highly suspected to cause severe reactions despite negative skin tests or IgE tests. Particularly in IgE-mediated reactions and enterocolitis syndrome, care must be taken because the OFC can result in severe reactions. The supervising clinician, usually an allergist, must have medications and supplies for resuscitation immediately available to manage reactions. Challenges may be optional or contra-indicated in certain circumstances and risks of the challenge must be weighed against the social and nutritional deficits of continued avoidance. Recent, severe anaphylaxis to an isolated ingestion, with a positive test for specific IgE antibody to the causal food is one example of a relative contraindication because this scenario represents confirmation of a convincing history. Negative challenges should always be followed by a supervised open feeding of a relevant portion of the tested food in its commonly prepared state. A summary of diagnostic tests, their utility, and limitations and listed in Table 16.2.

There are a host of tests that have been touted for the diagnosis of food allergy, but have never been found useful in blinded studies. These include measurement of IgG_4 antibody, provocation-neutralization (drops placed under the tongue or injected to diagnose and treat various symptoms), and applied kinesiology (muscle strength testing) [87].

Management

Experimental therapies designed to induce tolerance or reduce reaction severity, such as oral immunotherapy, injection immunotherapy using modified proteins, monoclonal antibodies to block immune responses and other strategies are under investigation [96]. However, the current mainstay of treatment is avoidance of the food and preparation for treatment in the event of an accidental ingestion leading to an allergic reaction, including anaphylaxis.

Dietary management of food allergy is fraught with nutritional and other pitfalls. Chapter 24 reviews dietary treatment for eosinophilic esophagitis; several principles of general dietary management of food allergy are reviewed here. Avoidance of the allergen requires care in shopping, meal preparation, and obtaining meals outside of the home. Regarding labeling of commercial food products, many countries have enacted labeling laws where specified allergens must be disclosed if they are an intended ingredient. In the US, this includes milk, egg, wheat, soy, peanut, tree nuts fish, and Crustacean shellfish. Advisory labeling in the US is not regulated, and manufacturers may voluntarily indicate if there is a possibility of inclusion of unintended allergens with statements such as "may contain peanuts" [97]. Care must be exercised for restaurant meals because cross contact with allergens during preparation, and hidden ingredients, may trigger reactions. Individuals living with food allergies should be instructed about informing others about their allergy and reviewing the above-mentioned concerns [98]. For children, dietary management in schools requires planning and communication to establish means of allergen avoidance (avoid food sharing and school projects using foods) and recognition/treatment of reactions.

In the event of an allergic reaction, antihistamines may be required to reduce itching/rash. However, for patients experiencing more severe symptoms of anaphylaxis, prompt administration of epinephrine is the indicated treatment [35, 99]. Guidelines for determining those who should have access to this medication in the form of autoinjectors are under scrutiny, but candidates include food-allergic patients with previous severe reactions, allergy to foods commonly causing severe reactions and food-allergic patients with underlying asthma. It is essential to periodically review the indications and technique of administration of self-injectable epinephrine because mistakes are common. Patients must be instructed that following the administration of the medications, prompt transportation to an emergency facility (i.e., ambulance) should be sought with prolonged observation (>4 h) since recurrence of severe symptoms is possible. Patients should obtain medical emergency bracelets identifying their allergy, and be reminded to update expired and expended epinephrine injectors. For children, an important component of the school and camp management of food allergy is to have a written emergency action plan in place, medications readily available and school personnel trained in recognizing and treating reactions. For children with food protein-induced enterocolitis syndrome, intravenous hydration and systemic steroids have been recommended for therapy [48].

Natural History

Most (~85%) children lose their sensitivity to most allergenic foods (egg, milk, wheat, soy) within the first 3–5 years of life [100]. Recent studies from a referral center present slower resolution rates for milk and egg allergy than past studies such that a majority of children were noted to continue to have the allergy at school age, but most experienced resolution by adolescence [101, 102]. In contrast, adults with food allergy may have long-lived sensitivity. Sensitivity to peanut, tree nuts, and seafood, is rarely lost. The notion that peanut and tree nut allergy is permanent derives, in part, from the observation that it is an allergy that affects adults; however, it has become apparent that about 20% of peanut allergic children under age 2 years, and about 9% of those with tree nut allergy may achieve tolerance by school age [103, 104]. Proctocolitis syndrome typically resolves in the first year of life. Food protein-induced enterocolitis usually resolves within the first 3 years [48] and eosinophilic esophagitis tends to persist [10].

Conclusions

Food allergies are common, appear to be increasing in prevalence, and account for a variety of acute and chronic disease manifestations. Although foods are a common trigger of eosinophilic esophagitis, persons with EoE may also experience other manifestations of food allergy. Understanding the underlying mechanisms and knowing the common triggers aids in selection and interpretation of diagnostic tests. Treatment includes dietary avoidance and treatment of reactions triggered by accidental ingestion. Re-evaluation is necessary because most food allergies that develop in childhood may resolve later. Future therapies may supplant avoidance and reactionary treatments of allergic reactions that are the current mainstay of treatment.

References

1. Sicherer SH, Sampson HA. Food allergy. J Allergy Clin Immunol. 2010;125(2 Suppl 2): S116–25.
2. Liacouras CA, Spergel JM, Ruchelli E, Verma R, Mascarenhas M, Semeao E, et al. Eosinophilic esophagitis: a 10-year experience in 381 children. Clin Gastroenterol Hepatol. 2005;3(12): 1198–206.

3. Spergel JM, Andrews T, Brown-Whitehorn TF, Beausoleil JL, Liacouras CA. Treatment of eosinophilic esophagitis with specific food elimination diet directed by a combination of skin prick and patch tests. Ann Allergy Asthma Immunol. 2005;95(4):336–43.
4. Orenstein SR, Shalaby TM, Di Lorenzo C, Putnam PE, Sigurdsson L, Kocoshis SA. The spectrum of pediatric eosinophilic esophagitis beyond infancy: a clinical series of 30 children [In Process Citation]. Am J Gastroenterol. 2000;95(6):1422–30.
5. Ruchelli E, Wenner W, Voytek T, Brown K, Liacouras C. Severity of esophageal eosinophilia predicts response to conventional gastroesophageal reflux therapy. Pediatr Dev Pathol. 1999; 2(1):15–8.
6. Noel RJ, Putnam PE, Rothenberg ME. Eosinophilic esophagitis. N Engl J Med. 2004;351(9): 940–1.
7. Roy-Ghanta S, Larosa DF, Katzka DA. Atopic characteristics of adult patients with eosinophilic esophagitis. Clin Gastroenterol Hepatol. 2008;6(5):531–5.
8. Sugnanam KK, Collins JT, Smith PK, Connor F, Lewindon P, Cleghorn G, et al. Dichotomy of food and inhalant allergen sensitization in eosinophilic esophagitis. Allergy. 2007;62(11): 1257–60.
9. Assa'ad AH, Putnam PE, Collins MH, Akers RM, Jameson SC, Kirby CL, et al. Pediatric patients with eosinophilic esophagitis: an 8-year follow-up. J Allergy Clin Immunol. 2007;119(3): 731–8.
10. Spergel JM, Brown-Whitehorn TF, Beausoleil JL, Franciosi J, Shuker M, Verma R, et al. 14 years of eosinophilic esophagitis: clinical features and prognosis. J Pediatr Gastroenterol Nutr. 2009;48(1):30–6.
11. Guajardo JR, Plotnick LM, Fende JM, Collins MH, Putnam PE, Rothenberg ME. Eosinophil-associated gastrointestinal disorders: a world-wide-web based registry. J Pediatr. 2002;141(4): 576–81.
12. Jyonouchi S, Brown-Whitehorn TA, Spergel JM. Association of eosinophilic gastrointestinal disorders with other atopic disorders. Immunol Allergy Clin North Am. 2009;29(1):85–97. x.
13. Fernandez-Rivas M, Bolhaar S, Gonzalez-Mancebo E, Asero R, van Leeuwen A, Bohle B, et al. Apple allergy across Europe: how allergen sensitization profiles determine the clinical expression of allergies to plant foods. J Allergy Clin Immunol. 2006;118(2):481–8.
14. Fogg MI, Brown-Whitehorn TA, Pawlowski NA, Spergel JM. Atopy patch test for the diagnosis of food protein-induced enterocolitis syndrome. Pediatr Allergy Immunol. 2006;17(5):351–5.
15. Spergel JM, Brown-Whitehorn T, Beausoleil JL, Shuker M, Liacouras CA. Predictive values for skin prick test and atopy patch test for eosinophilic esophagitis. J Allergy Clin Immunol. 2007;119(2):509–11.
16. Mehl A, Rolinck-Werninghaus C, Staden U, Verstege A, Wahn U, Beyer K, et al. The atopy patch test in the diagnostic workup of suspected food-related symptoms in children. J Allergy Clin Immunol. 2006;118(4):923–9.
17. Radauer C, Breiteneder H. Evolutionary biology of plant food allergens. J Allergy Clin Immunol. 2007;120(3):518–25.
18. Sicherer SH, Sampson HA. 9. Food allergy. J Allergy Clin Immunol. 2006;117:S470–5.
19. Commins SP, Satinover SM, Hosen J, Mozena J, Borish L, Lewis BD, et al. Delayed anaphylaxis, angioedema, or urticaria after consumption of red meat in patients with IgE antibodies specific for galactose-alpha-1,3-galactose. J Allergy Clin Immunol. 2009;123(2):426–33.
20. Rona RJ, Keil T, Summers C, Gislason D, Zuidmeer L, Sodergren E, et al. The prevalence of food allergy: a meta-analysis. J Allergy Clin Immunol. 2007;120(3):638–46.
21. Zuidmeer L, Goldhahn K, Rona RJ, Gislason D, Madsen C, Summers C, et al. The prevalence of plant food allergies: a systematic review. J Allergy Clin Immunol. 2008;121(5):1210–8.
22. Branum AM, Lukacs SL. Food allergy among U.S. children: trends in prevalence and hospitalizations. NCHS Data Brief. 2008;(10):1–8.
23. Grundy J, Matthews S, Bateman B, Dean T, Arshad SH. Rising prevalence of allergy to peanut in children: data from 2 sequential cohorts. J Allergy Clin Immunol. 2002;110(5):784–9.
24. Sicherer SH, Muñoz-Furlong A, Sampson HA. Prevalence of peanut and tree nut allergy in the United States determined by means of a random digit dial telephone survey: a 5-year follow-up study. J Allergy Clin Immunol. 2003;112(6):1203–7.

25. Ross MP, Ferguson M, Street D, Klontz K, Schroeder T, Luccioli S. Analysis of food-allergic and anaphylactic events in the National Electronic Injury Surveillance System. J Allergy Clin Immunol. 2008;121(1):166–71.
26. Decker WW, Campbell RL, Manivannan V, Luke A, St. Sauver JL, Weaver A, et al. The etiology and incidence of anaphylaxis in Rochester, Minnesota: a report from the Rochester Epidemiology Project. J Allergy Clin Immunol. 2008;122(6):1161–5.
27. Bock SA, Munoz-Furlong A, Sampson HA. Further fatalities caused by anaphylactic reactions to food, 2001–2006. J Allergy Clin Immunol. 2007;119(4):1016–8.
28. Simon RA. Adverse reactions to food additives. Curr Allergy Asthma Rep. 2003;3(1):62–6.
29. Sicherer SH, Sampson HA. Peanut allergy: emerging concepts and approaches for an apparent epidemic. J Allergy Clin Immunol. 2007;120(3):491–503.
30. Lack G. Epidemiologic risks for food allergy. J Allergy Clin Immunol. 2008;121(6):1331–6.
31. Du Toit G, Katz Y, Sasieni P, Mesher D, Maleki SJ, Fisher HR, et al. Early consumption of peanuts in infancy is associated with a low prevalence of peanut allergy. J Allergy Clin Immunol. 2008;122(5):984–91.
32. Fox AT, Sasieni P, Du Toit G, Syed H, Lack G. Household peanut consumption as a risk factor for the development of peanut allergy. J Allergy Clin Immunol. 2009;123(2):417–23.
33. Ortolani C, Ispano M, Pastorello E, Bigi A, Ansaloni R. The oral allergy syndrome. Ann Allergy. 1988;61(6 Pt 2):47–52.
34. Roberts G, Golder N, Lack G. Bronchial challenges with aerosolized food in asthmatic, food-allergic children. Allergy. 2002;57(8):713–7.
35. Sampson HA, Munoz-Furlong A, Campbell RL, Adkinson Jr NF, Bock SA, Branum A, et al. Second symposium on the definition and management of anaphylaxis: summary report – second National Institute of Allergy and Infectious Disease/Food Allergy and Anaphylaxis Network symposium. J Allergy Clin Immunol. 2006;117(2):391–7.
36. Romano A, Di Fonso M, Giuffreda F, Papa G, Artesani MC, Viola M, et al. Food-dependent exercise-induced anaphylaxis: clinical and laboratory findings in 54 subjects. Int Arch Allergy Immunol. 2001;125(3):264–72.
37. Sicherer SH, Teuber S. Current approach to the diagnosis and management of adverse reactions to foods. J Allergy Clin Immunol. 2004;114(5):1146–50.
38. Odze RD, Bines J, Leichtner AM, Goldman H, Antonioli DA. Allergic proctocolitis in infants: a prospective clinicopathologic biopsy study. Hum Pathol. 1993;24(6):668–74.
39. Wilson NW, Self TW, Hamburger RN. Severe cow's milk induced colitis in an exclusively breast-fed neonate. Case report and clinical review of cow's milk allergy. Clin Pediatr (Phila). 1990;29(2):77–80.
40. Lake AM, Whitington PF, Hamilton SR. Dietary protein-induced colitis in breast-fed infants. J Pediatr. 1982;101:906–10.
41. Anveden HL, Finkel Y, Sandstedt B, Karpe B. Proctocolitis in exclusively breast-fed infants. Eur J Pediatr. 1996;155(6):464–7.
42. Pittschieler K. Cow's milk protein-induced colitis in the breast-fed infant. J Pediatr Gastroenterol Nutr. 1990;10(4):548–9.
43. Jenkins HR, Pincott JR, Soothill JF, Milla PJ, Harries JT. Food allergy: the major cause of infantile colitis. Arch Dis Child. 1984;59(4):326–9.
44. Winter HS, Antonioli DA, Fukagawa N, Marcial M, Goldman H. Allergy-related proctocolitis in infants: diagnostic usefulness of rectal biopsy. Mod Pathol. 1990;3(1):5–10.
45. Ravelli A, Villanacci V, Chiappa S, Bolognini S, Manenti S, Fuoti M. Dietary protein-induced proctocolitis in childhood. Am J Gastroenterol. 2008;103(10):2605–12.
46. Xanthakos SA, Schwimmer JB, Melin-Aldana H, Rothenberg ME, Witte DP, Cohen MB. Prevalence and outcome of allergic colitis in healthy infants with rectal bleeding: a prospective cohort study. J Pediatr Gastroenterol Nutr. 2005;41(1):16–22.
47. Arvola T, Ruuska T, Keranen J, Hyoty H, Salminen S, Isolauri E. Rectal bleeding in infancy: clinical, allergological, and microbiological examination. Pediatrics. 2006;117(4):e760–8.
48. Sicherer SH. Food protein-induced enterocolitis syndrome: case presentations and management lessons. J Allergy Clin Immunol. 2005;115(1):149–56.

49. Hwang JB, Lee SH, Kang YN, Kim SP, Suh SI, Kam S. Indexes of suspicion of typical cow's milk protein-induced enterocolitis. J Korean Med Sci. 2007;22(6):993–7.
50. Sicherer SH. Food protein-induced enterocolitis syndrome: clinical perspectives. J Pediatr Gastroenterol Nutr. 2000;30(Suppl):S45–9.
51. Sicherer SH, Eigenmann PA, Sampson HA. Clinical features of food protein-induced enterocolitis syndrome. J Pediatr. 1998;133(2):214–9.
52. Mehr S, Kakakios A, Frith K, Kemp AS. Food protein-induced enterocolitis syndrome: 16-year experience. Pediatrics. 2009;123(3):e459–64.
53. Jayasooriya S, Fox AT, Murch SH. Do not laparotomize food-protein-induced enterocolitis syndrome. Pediatr Emerg Care. 2007;23(3):173–5.
54. Levy Y, Danon YL. Food protein-induced enterocolitis syndrome – not only due to cow's milk and soy. Pediatr Allergy Immunol. 2003;14(4):325–9.
55. Nowak-Wegrzyn A, Sampson HA, Wood RA, Sicherer SH. Food protein-induced enterocolitis syndrome caused by solid food proteins. Pediatrics. 2003;111(4 Pt 1):829–35.
56. Burks AW, Casteel HB, Fiedorek SC, Williams LW, Pumphrey CL. Prospective oral food challenge study of two soybean protein isolates in patients with possible milk or soy protein enterocolitis. Pediatr Allergy Immunol. 1994;5:40–5.
57. Busse P, Sampson HA, Sicherer SH. Non-resolution of infantile food protein-induced enterocolitis syndrome (FPIES). J Allergy Clin Immunol. 2000;105:S129.
58. Hwang JB, Sohn SM, Kim AS. Prospective follow up-oral food challenge in food protein-induced enterocolitis syndrome. Arch Dis Child. 2008;94(6):425–8.
59. Heyman M, Darmon N, Dupont C, Dugas B, Hirribaren A, Blaton MA, et al. Mononuclear cells from infants allergic to cow's milk secrete tumor necrosis factor alpha, altering intestinal function. Gastroenterology. 1994;106(6):1514–23.
60. Kapel N, Matarazzo P, Haouchine D, Abiola N, Guerin S, Magne D, et al. Fecal tumor necrosis factor alpha, eosinophil cationic protein and IgE levels in infants with cow's milk allergy and gastrointestinal manifestations. Clin Chem Lab Med. 1999;37(1):29–32.
61. Majamaa H, Aittoniemi J, Miettinen A. Increased concentration of fecal alpha1-antitrypsin is associated with cow's milk allergy in infants with atopic eczema. Clin Exp Allergy. 2001;31(4):590–2.
62. Chung HL, Hwang JB, Park JJ, Kim SG. Expression of transforming growth factor beta1, transforming growth factor type I and II receptors, and TNF-alpha in the mucosa of the small intestine in infants with food protein-induced enterocolitis syndrome. J Allergy Clin Immunol. 2002;109(1 Pt 1):150–4.
63. Shek LP, Bardina L, Castro R, Sampson HA, Beyer K. Humoral and cellular responses to cow milk proteins in patients with milk-induced IgE-mediated and non-IgE-mediated disorders. Allergy. 2005;60(7):912–9.
64. Murray K, Christie D. Dietary protein intolerance in infants with transient methemoglobinemia and diarrhea. J Pediatr. 1993;122(1):90–2.
65. Sampson HA, Anderson JA. Summary and recommendations: classification of gastrointestinal manifestations due to immunologic reactions to foods in infants and young children. J Pediatr Gastroenterol Nutr. 2000;30(Suppl):S87–94.
66. Kuitunen P, Visakorpi J, Savilahti E, Pelkonen P. Malabsorption syndrome with cow's milk intolerance: clinical findings and course in 54 cases. Arch Dis Child. 1975;50:351–6.
67. Iyngkaran N, Yadav M, Boey C, Lam K. Severity and extent of upper small bowel mucosal damage in cow's milk protein-sensitive enteropathy. J Pediatr Gastroenterol Nutr. 1988;8:667–74.
68. Yssing M, Jensen H, Jarnum S. Dietary treatment of protein-losing enteropathy. Acta Paediatr Scand. 1967;56(2):173–81.
69. Walker-Smith JA. Food sensitive enteropathies. Clin Gastroenterol. 1986;15:55–69.
70. Verkasalo M, Kuitunen P, Savilahti E, Tiilikainen A. Changing pattern of cow's milk intolerance. An analysis of the occurrence and clinical course in the 60s and mid-70s. Acta Paediatr Scand. 1981;70(3):289–95.
71. Vitoria JC, Sojo A, Rodriguez-Soriano J. Changing pattern of cow's milk protein intolerance. Acta Paediatr Scand. 1990;79(5):566–7.

72. Chehade M, Magid MS, Mofidi S, Nowak-Wegrzyn A, Sampson HA, Sicherer SH. Allergic eosinophilic gastroenteritis with protein-losing enteropathy: intestinal pathology, clinical course, and long-term follow-up. J Pediatr Gastroenterol Nutr. 2006;42(5):516–21.
73. Kondo M, Fukao T, Omoya K, Kawamoto N, Aoki M, Teramoto T, et al. Protein-losing enteropathy associated with egg allergy in a 5-month-old boy. J Investig Allergol Clin Immunol. 2008;18(1):63–6.
74. Sollid LM, Lie BA. Celiac disease genetics: current concepts and practical applications. Clin Gastroenterol Hepatol. 2005;3(9):843–51.
75. Farrell RJ, Kelly CP. Celiac sprue. N Engl J Med. 2002;346(3):180–8.
76. Green PH, Cellier C. Celiac disease. N Engl J Med. 2007;357(17):1731–43.
77. Johnson TC, Diamond B, Memeo L, Negulescu H, Hovhanissyan Z, Verkarre V, et al. Relationship of HLA-DQ8 and severity of celiac disease: comparison of New York and Parisian cohorts. Clin Gastroenterol Hepatol. 2004;2(10):888–94.
78. Anderson RP, Degano P, Godkin AJ, Jewell DP, Hill AV. In vivo antigen challenge in celiac disease identifies a single transglutaminase-modified peptide as the dominant A-gliadin T-cell epitope. Nat Med. 2000;6(3):337–42.
79. Rostom A, Dube C, Cranney A, Saloojee N, Sy R, Garritty C, et al. The diagnostic accuracy of serologic tests for celiac disease: a systematic review. Gastroenterology. 2005;128(4 Suppl 1): S38–46.
80. Sicherer SH, Sampson HA. Food hypersensitivity and atopic dermatitis: pathophysiology, epidemiology, diagnosis, and management. J Allergy Clin Immunol. 1999;104(3 Pt 2):S114–22.
81. Hanifin JM. Critical evaluation of food and mite allergy in the management of atopic dermatitis. J Dermatol. 1997;24:495–503.
82. Werfel T, Ballmer-Weber B, Eigenmann PA, Niggemann B, Rance F, Turjanmaa K, et al. Eczematous reactions to food in atopic eczema: position paper of the EAACI and GA2LEN. Allergy. 2007;62(7):723–8.
83. Hill DJ, Hosking CS, de Benedictis FM, Oranje AP, Diepgen TL, Bauchau V. Confirmation of the association between high levels of immunoglobulin E food sensitization and eczema in infancy: an international study. Clin Exp Allergy. 2008;38(1):161–8.
84. Forget PP, Arenda JW. Cow's milk protein allergy and gastroesophageal reflux. Eur J Pediatr. 1985;144:298–300.
85. Iacono G, Cavataio F, Montalto G, Florena A, Tumminello M, Soresi M, et al. Intolerance of cow's milk and chronic constipation in children [see comments]. N Engl J Med. 1998;339(16):1100–4.
86. Hill DJ, Hosking CS. Infantile colic and food hypersensitivity. J Pediatr Gastroenterol Nutr. 2000;30(Suppl):S67–76.
87. American College of Allergy, Asthma, & Immunology. Food allergy: a practice parameter. Ann Allergy Asthma Immunol. 2006;96(3 Suppl 2):S1–68.
88. Wang J, Godbold JH, Sampson HA. Correlation of serum allergy (IgE) tests performed by different assay systems. J Allergy Clin Immunol. 2008;121(5):1219–24.
89. Sporik R, Hill DJ, Hosking CS. Specificity of allergen skin testing in predicting positive open food challenges to milk, egg and peanut in children. Clin Exp Allergy. 2000;30(11):1541–6.
90. Sampson HA. Utility of food-specific IgE concentrations in predicting symptomatic food allergy. J Allergy Clin Immunol. 2001;107(5):891–6.
91. Komata T, Soderstrom L, Borres MP, Tachimoto H, Ebisawa M. The predictive relationship of food-specific serum IgE concentrations to challenge outcomes for egg and milk varies by patient age. J Allergy Clin Immunol. 2007;119(5):1272–4.
92. Hauswirth DW, Burks AW. Banana anaphylaxis with a negative commercial skin test. J Allergy Clin Immunol. 2005;115(3):632–3.
93. Sicherer SH. Clinical implications of cross-reactive food allergens. J Allergy Clin Immunol. 2001;108(6):881–90.
94. David TJ, Waddington E, Stanton RHJ. Nutritional hazards of elimination diets in children with atopic dermatitis. Arch Dis Child. 1984;59:323–5.
95. Nowak-Wegrzyn A, Assa'ad AH, Bahna SL, Bock SA, Sicherer SH, Teuber SS. Work Group report: oral food challenge testing. J Allergy Clin Immunol. 2009;123(6 Suppl):S365–83.

96. Nowak-Wegrzyn A, Sampson HA. Food allergy therapy. Immunol Allergy Clin North Am. 2004;24(4):705–25.
97. Hefle SL, Furlong TJ, Niemann L, Lemon-Mule H, Sicherer S, Taylor SL. Consumer attitudes and risks associated with packaged foods having advisory labeling regarding the presence of peanuts. J Allergy Clin Immunol. 2007;120(1):171–6.
98. Furlong TJ, DeSimone J, Sicherer SH. Peanut and tree nut allergic reactions in restaurants and other food establishments. J Allergy Clin Immunol. 2001;108((5 Part 1)):867–70.
99. Sicherer SH, Simons FE. Self-injectable epinephrine for first-aid management of anaphylaxis. Pediatrics. 2007;119(3):638–46.
100. Wood RA. The natural history of food allergy. Pediatrics. 2003;111(6 Pt 3):1631–7.
101. Savage JH, Matsui EC, Skripak JM, Wood RA. The natural history of egg allergy. J Allergy Clin Immunol. 2007;120(6):1413–7.
102. Skripak JM, Matsui EC, Mudd K, Wood RA. The natural history of IgE-mediated cow's milk allergy. J Allergy Clin Immunol. 2007;120(5):1172–7.
103. Fleischer DM, Conover-Walker MK, Christie L, Burks AW, Wood RA. The natural progression of peanut allergy: resolution and the possibility of recurrence. J Allergy Clin Immunol. 2003;112(1):183–9.
104. Fleischer DM, Conover-Walker MK, Matsui EC, Wood RA. The natural history of tree nut allergy. J Allergy Clin Immunol. 2005;116(5):1087–93.

Chapter 17
Allergic and Atopic Features of Children with Eosinophilic Esophagitis

Janet L. Beausoleil and Terri Brown-Whitehorn

Keywords Eosinophilic esophagitis • Allergies • Atopic diseases • Atopy • Topical corticosteroids

Introduction

The increased incidence of eosinophilic esophagitis has mirrored the rise in allergies over the past decade. Eosinophilic esophagitis shares many features of other atopic diseases. The inflammatory cells and cytokines secreted are similar to what is seen in the classic atopic disorders such as asthma, allergic rhinitis, and atopic dermatitis. Both environmental and food-specific IgE is present in the majority of patients with eosinophilic esophagitis. As with other atopic disorders, improvement occurs with elimination of the offending allergen or with the use of topical corticosteroids. Patients with eosinophilic esophagitis have a higher prevalence of these other atopic disorders, as well as a family history of atopy. Taken together, this implies a strong correlation between allergy, atopy, and eosinophilic esophagitis.

Atopy and Allergy

Atopy is a genetic predisposition toward the development of immediate hypersensitivity reactions against common environmental antigens. Allergy is a more broad term, and refers to an abnormal immune response to foreign proteins, and can refer to

J.L. Beausoleil (✉)
Department of Pediatrics, Division of Allergy and Immunology,
The Children's Hospital of Philadelphia, 34th Street and Civic Center Blvd,
Philadelphia, PA 19104, 610-768-9323, USA
e-mail: Janet1124@comcast.net

C.A. Liacouras and J.E. Markowitz (eds.), *Eosinophilic Esophagitis*,
Clinical Gastroenterology, DOI 10.1007/978-1-60761-515-6_17,

both immediate (IgE mediated) and delayed (non-IgE mediated) hypersensitivity reactions. Pollens, mold spores, pet dander, and dust mites may trigger allergic rhinoconjunctivitis, atopic dermatitis, or asthma. Drugs and stinging insects can trigger anaphylaxis. Food proteins, such as milk, egg, soy, peanut, and wheat can lead to a variety of reactions, including IgE-mediated reactions such as hives or anaphylaxis, cell mediated immune reactions such as colitis, or mixed IgE-mediated and non-IgE-mediated reactions that are seen in atopic dermatitis or eosinophilic esophagitis.

The presence of atopy in an individual can be defined in various ways: elevated total IgE, physician diagnosis of an atopic disease such as allergic rhinitis or atopic dermatitis, or the presence of specific IgE to a food or aeroallergen (through skin prick or serological testing). In general, atopic diseases are associated with an expansion of the Th2 cell population and subsequent secretion of cytokines such as IL-4, IL-5, and IL-13 that favor IgE synthesis and eosinophilia.

Prevalence of Atopic Diseases in Eosinophilic Esophagitis Patients

Data from the 2008 CDC National Health Interview Survey (NHIS) Summary Health Statistic for U.S. Children report a 10% prevalence of asthma in United States children. In this same report, the prevalence of hay fever was 10%, respiratory allergies were 11%, and other allergies were 14% [1]. In addition, approximately 17% of children in the United States are affected by atopic dermatitis [2]. The majority of patients with eosinophilic esophagitis are atopic. A 14-year follow up from Philadelphia of over 600 pediatric eosinophilic esophagitis patients showed that two thirds of the children were atopic, significantly higher than what would be expected in the general population. Two hundred and thirty-one of these patients had asthma (37%), 243 had allergic rhinitis (39%), and 78 had atopic dermatitis (13%) [3]. Reports from Cincinnati also demonstrate a high prevalence of environmental (79%) and food allergies (75%) in children with eosinophilic esophagitis [4] (Table 17.1). In 89 of their patients with eosinophilic esophagitis, 39% had asthma, 30% had allergic rhinitis, 19% had eczema, 9% had food-induced anaphylaxis, and 8% had allergic conjunctivitis [5]. Among 234 children from Indianapolis, 76 patients (32.5%) had a personal history of atopy, 63 (27%) of them were diagnosed with asthma/reactive airway disease, but only 15 (6%) had eczema and 4 (2%) had rhinitis [6]. In a report of 20 pediatric patients in Oregon, 35% had food allergy on either skin prick or IgE radioallergosorbent tests. Atopic diseases were common, with a 20% incidence of asthma, 15% incidence of allergic rhinitis, and 5% incidence of atopic dermatitis. The incidence of actual food-induced anaphylaxis was not reported [7]. This variation in the rate of atopy among children with eosinophilic esophagitis in the United States could represent regional differences, selection bias, or diagnostic differences. Of note, gastroenterologists

Table 17.1 Environmental and food sensitization in patients with EE

SPTs	Age (years)			Sex (%)		
Allergens	<5	>5–10	>10	Male	Female	Total patients (%)
Food						
Patient tested (*N*)	30	17	14	47	14	61
Positive	25	11	10	35 (75%)	11 (78%)	46 (75%)
Environmental						
Patient tested (*N*)	20	12	11	33	10	43
Positive	13	10	11	25 (75%)	9 (90%)	34 (79%)
Food and environmental						
Patient tested (*N*)	17	11	11	30	9	39
Both positive	11	7	8	19	7	26 (67%)
Food negative, environment positive	2	2	3	5	2	7 (18%)
Food positive, environment negative	2	2	0	4	0	4 (10%)
Both negative	2	0	0	2	0	2 (5%)

reported on those with lower prevalence of allergy, while the others were reported by allergist–immunologists.

In Australia, a similar increase in atopy among children with eosinophilic esophagitis has been reported. In 45 cases in Eastern Australia, 56% had atopic eczema, 93% had allergic rhinitis, and 67% had asthma. This is significantly increased compared to the general population in Australia, with 32% having atopic eczema, 11% having allergic rhinitis, and 11% having asthma [8]. In a world-wide-web-based registry of 109 survey respondents, including 99 from the United States, 4 from Canada, 2 from England, 1 from China, and 1 from Israel, a 64% incidence of allergic rhinoconjunctivitis, 38% incidence of asthma, 26% incidence of eczema, and 23% incidence of food-induced anaphylaxis was reported in patients with eosinophilic esophagitis. The majority of the respondents were parents of affected children (71%) [9] (Table 17.2).

Presence of Atopic Family History in Eosinophilic Esophagitis Patients

A significant number of patients with eosinophilic esophagitis have a family history of atopy. One study reported a prevalence of allergic rhinitis in 77% and asthma in 51% in immediate family members [9]. In another study, 164 out of 381 (43%) of pediatric eosinophilic esophagitis patients had a first degree relative with asthma, allergic rhinitis, or atopic dermatitis [10]. The calculated sibling risk is 80 times higher than the general population [11].

Table 17.2 Prevalence (%) of atopic disease in children with eosinophilic esophagitis

Location/year	Portland, Oregon 2009	Philadelphia. Pennsylvania 2008	Cincinnati, Ohio 2007	Queensland, Australia 2007	Indianapolis, Indiana 2007	World Wide Web 2002
# Patients with EoE	20	620	89	45	234	39
Age (years)	0.2–19.5	9.1 ± 3.1	6.2 ± 4.8	0.3–16	0.2–19.5	8 ± 12
Asthma	20%	37%	39%	66%	27%	38%
Allergic rhinitis	15%	39%	30%	93%	2%	64%
Atopic dermatitis	5%	13%	19%	55%	6%	26%
Food allergy/ anaphylaxis	35% positive allergy testing	5.7% anaphylaxis	9% anaphylaxis	24% anaphylaxis	Unknown	23% anaphylaxis

Food Allergy and Eosinophilic Esophagitis

Food allergy affects approximately 6% of young children in the United States. The most common foods are cow's milk, egg, peanut, wheat, soy, tree nuts, fish, and shellfish. Although a family history of atopic disorders is a risk factor, environmental factors modulate the expression of food allergy [12]. The expression of food allergy can be classified according to immune mechanism (IgE mediated, non-IgE mediated, or mixed) or according to the affected organ system (skin, respiratory tract, gastrointestinal tract, systemic). IgE-mediated gastrointestinal allergic disorders include oral allergy syndrome and gastrointestinal anaphylaxis. Cell-mediated gastrointestinal disorders include food protein-induced enterocolitis, food protein-induced proctocolitis, and food protein-induced enteropathy [12]. Alternatively, eosinophilic esophagitis appears to be due to a mixed IgE and non-IgE-mediated immune mechanism. After appropriate testing in these disorders, the diagnosis is confirmed by improvement after elimination of the offending foods and, when appropriate, recurrence with re-challenge to the implicated foods.

The strongest evidence for food allergy as a cause of eosinophilic esophagitis comes from the clinical response of patients who are placed on restricted or elemental diets. In 1995, ten children were described with persistent gastroesophageal reflux and esophageal eosinophilia refractory to pharmacologic treatment. Six of these patients had also received Nissen fundoplications. A dramatic decrease in esophageal eosinophilia and clinical symptoms was observed in all patients when placed on a 6-week trial of an elemental formula. Eight patients demonstrated complete resolution [13]. Further work by others has confirmed elemental diets to be successful, with a reported success rate as high as 97% [10]. In addition, 75% of children have been reported to improve on specific elimination diets of foods identified by skin prick testing and patch testing [14]. Improvement has also been reported after implementation of an empiric six-food elimination diet. Patients with eosinophilic esophagitis removed milk, soy, egg, wheat, nuts, and seafood from their diet for 6 weeks. Significant decrease in esophageal eosinophils (less than 10 per HPF) occurred in 74% of the patients compared to 88% of the patients who improved on an elemental diet [15] (Table 17.3).

In eosinophilic esophagitis, foods most commonly implicated are similar to other forms of food allergy, with milk, egg, wheat, soy, and peanut accounting for more than half of the causative foods in patients with eosinophilic esophagitis [3] (Fig. 17.1).

The majority of patients with eosinophilic esophagitis have evidence of IgE-mediated sensitization to food based on in vitro specific IgE or skin prick testing. Positive skin testing to these foods is common, with one report of 39% positive skin test to egg and peanut, 34% to soy, and 29% to cow's milk [5]. However, the reported incidence of actual food-induced anaphylaxis has been variable. Two large pediatric eosinophilic esophagitis populations in the United States have reported the incidence of anaphylaxis as 8.1 [10] and 9% [5]. In an Australian cohort of 45

Table 17.3 Effect of dietary avoidance in children with eosinophilic esophagitis

Study	Diet	% Symptoms improved	% Decrease in eosinophils
Kelly et al. [13]	Elemental	100	100
Spergel et al. [14]	Elimination based on skin prick and patch testing	75	75
Liacouras et al. [10]	Elemental	97	97
Kagalwalla et al. [15]	Empiric six-food elimination	97	74
Kagalwalla et al. [15]	Elemental	100	88

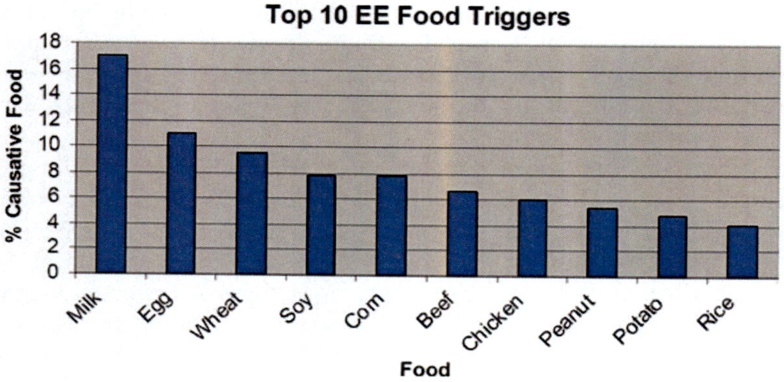

Fig. 17.1 The 10 most common food triggers of eosinophilic esophagitis confirmed by endoscopy after food allergy testing

consecutive eosinophilic esophagitis patients referred to a pediatric allergist, an even higher rate has been reported, with 24% of pediatric eosinophilic esophagitis having physician-diagnosed anaphylaxis. This number is one hundred times that reported in the general population in Australia [8].

Aeroallergens and Eosinophilic Esophagitis

There is evidence to suggest that aeroallergens may play a causative role in the development of eosinophilic esophagitis. As will be discussed later, intranasal exposure to *Aspergillus fumigatus* can induce esophageal eosinophilia in mice. A seasonal variation in the cases of newly diagnosed eosinophilic esophagitis in children has been described, with fewer cases being diagnosed in the winter, a season of low outdoor allergen exposure compared to spring, summer, and fall [6]. In a database of 620 children with eosinophilic esophagitis, 30 pollen-allergic patients had a seasonal variation in their disease, confirmed by biopsy, and an additional 16 had a potential seasonal influence, correlating with a spring or fall pollen season. Food allergies were still the primary cause of disease in all but one of these patients. However, exacerbation of disease was documented during the spring or fall pollen season. Full disease control was achieved on proper dietary avoidance during non-pollen seasons [3]. From the same institution, one female was reported with a temporal association with eosinophilic esophagitis and pollen exposure. This patient had mild to no esophagitis in the winter, and moderate to severe esophagitis during pollen seasons (Figs. 17.2 and 17.3) [16]. In Australia, a positive relationship between increasing patient age and degree of aeroallergen sensitization, and a negative relationship between increasing patient age and food allergen sensitization was found [8]. This suggests that aeroallergen sensitization may play a more important role in adolescents with eosinophilic esophagitis compared to younger children. However, since this was based on skin prick and patch testing only, the clinical relevance of these findings is not clear.

Increase in Eosinophilic Esophagitis and Other Atopic Diseases in the General Population

The reported prevalence of allergic diseases (asthma, allergic rhinitis, atopic dermatitis, and food allergy) as well as eosinophilic esophagitis has increased over the last few decades. The reported prevalence of asthma rose from 3% in 1990 to 7.7% in 2007 [17]. The prevalence of pediatric atopic dermatitis rose from 7.3% in 1998 to 10% in 2006 [18] and the prevalence of allergic rhinitis in the United States now approaches 16% [19]. An estimated 25–30% of the population in industrialized countries has atopic dermatitis, food allergy, or allergic rhinitis [20]. Although the prevalence of eosinophilic esophagitis does not approach that of other atopic diseases, the numbers are clearly on the rise [21]. The disease has been reported in every continent except Africa. In Western Australia, an 18-fold increase in cases between 1995 and 2004 has been reported [22]. At The Children's Hospital of Philadelphia, there was a 35-fold increase in newly diagnosed eosinophilic esophagitis cases in a 10-year period, from 2 cases in 1994 to 72 cases in 2003 [10]. This number further increased in 2006 to 124 new cases [3] (Fig. 17.4). There are likely to be other cases undiagnosed, with an estimated 5–10% of pediatric patients with poorly controlled gastroesophageal reflux thought to have eosinophilic esophagitis [23–25].

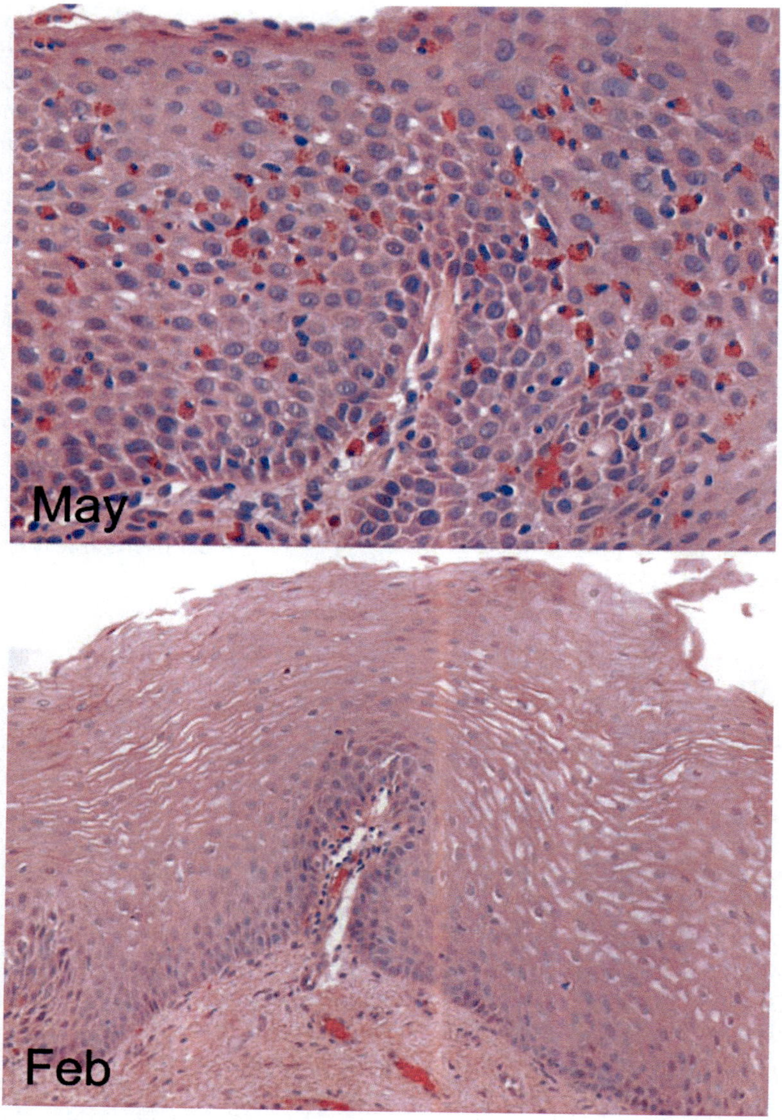

Fig. 17.2 Eosinophils in biopsy. Esophageal biopsy specimens obtained in the spring and winter. Numerous eosinophils and hyperplasia of the basal layer were seen in the biopsy obtained in May. The inflammation had entirely subsided by February, and the squamous epithelium had a normal appearance

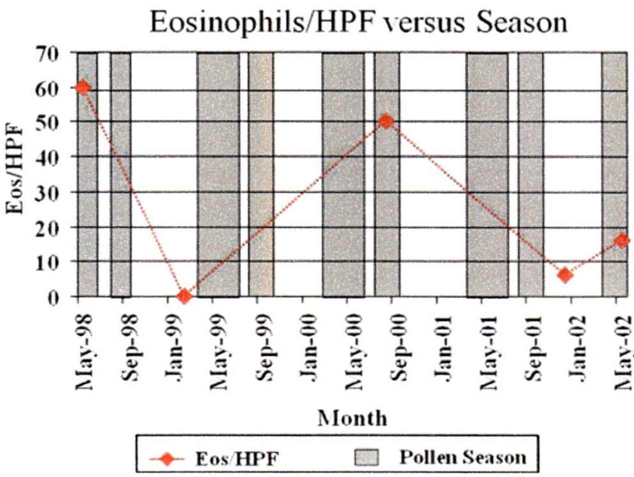

Fig. 17.3 Eosinophils/high-power field plotted against month of biopsy. Pollen seasons are indicated in *gray*: mid-March to June and mid-August to October

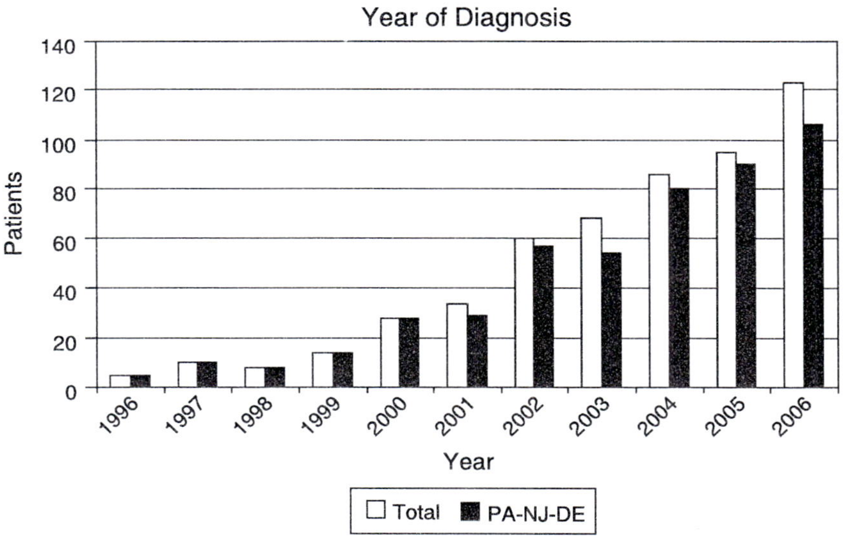

Fig. 17.4 The incidence of new cases of eosinophilic esophagitis diagnosed on an annual basis. *PA–NJ–DE* Pennsylvania, New Jersey, and Delaware

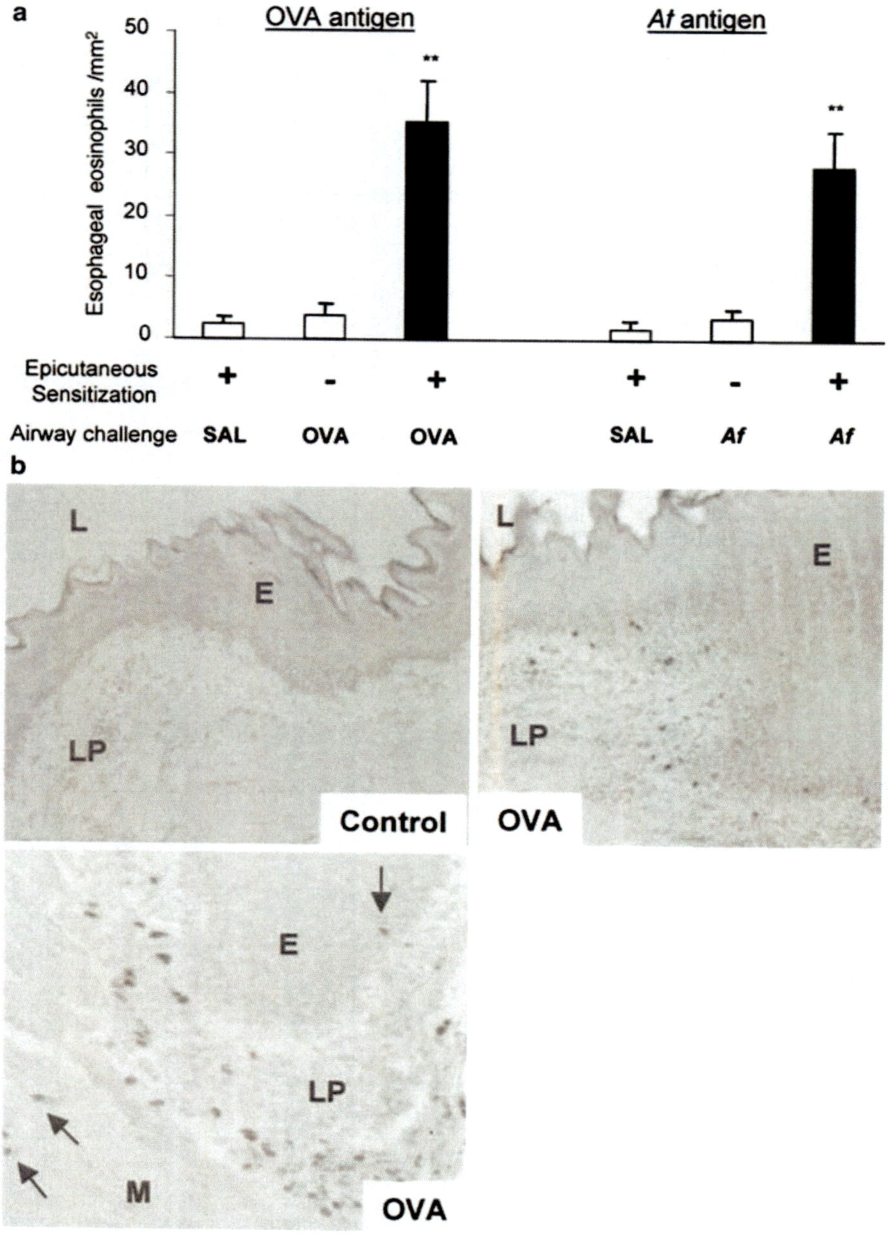

Fig. 17.5 Esophageal eosinophilia in epicutaneously sensitized mice. (**a**) The eosinophil level in the esophagus of mice sensitized with OVA or *A. fumigates* (+) or control vehicle (–). Mice were exposed to epicutaneous antigen for 1 week; following a rest period of 2 weeks, this procedure was repeated over the course of 7 weeks (OVA) and 4 weeks (*A. fumigatus*). Two days following the last day of epicutaneous antigen exposure, mice were exposed to intranasal allergen or control

Link Between Allergen Sensitization and Eosinophilia in the Skin, Lung, and Esophagus in Murine Models

Sensitization in mice can lead to allergic inflammation in the skin, airway, and esophagus depending on the route of exposure. A mouse model was able to link asthma and eosinophilic esophagitis. In this model, repeated intranasal exposure to *A. fumigatus* produced eosinophilia in both the airway and the esophagus, but not the stomach or small intestine. Oral exposure of the same allergen did not lead to eosinophilia in the airway or the esophagus [26]. In another study, mice were sensitized to *A. fumigatus* or ovalbumin epicutaneously, which led to atopic dermatitis-like skin changes without esophageal changes. Following a single intranasal challenge to the same allergen, these mice developed significant eosinophilic esophagitis [27] (Fig. 17.5).

Similar Pathophysiology in Eosinophilic Esophagitis and Other Atopic Diseases

Th2-driven inflammation is present in the end-organs of atopic conditions. The inflammatory cells found in patients with asthma, allergic rhinitis, atopic dermatitis, and IgE-mediated food allergies are similar to those found in patients with eosinophilic esophagitis. Activation of mast cells by cross linking of allergen-specific IgE leads to an increase in Th2 cells, eosinophils, and neutrophils. Eosinophils are found in nasal secretions of those with allergic rhinitis [28]. Th2 cells and eosinophils are found in asthma and early lesions of atopic dermatitis [29, 30]. The esophagus of patients with eosinophilic esophagitis have 300 times the density of eosinophils compared to controls and significantly higher levels of T cells and mast cells compared to patients with gastroesophageal reflux [31].

Th2 cytokines, such as IL-4, IL-5, and IL-13, are present in atopic diseases including eosinophilic esophagitis [32] (Fig. 17.6). Th2 chemokines and their receptors are also important in atopic diseases including eosinophilic esophagitis. The gene encoding for eotaxin 3, a chemokine important for trafficking of eosinophils, was highly induced in patients with eosinophilic esophagitis. A single nucleotide polymorphism was associated with increased susceptibility to eosinophilic esophagitis [33]. Another molecule that may be associated with the development of atopic diseases is filaggrin. Mutations in filaggrin lead to increased atopic dermatitis and

Fig. 17.5 (continued) saline (SAL). Data are expressed as mean ± SEM with 8 mice/group. $^{**}P<0.01$ compared with control or saline group. (**b**) Eosinophils were identified by immunostaining with anti-major basic protein. Representative eosinophils are indicated by *arrows*. Significant eosinophilia was observed in the OVA group but not in the control group. Eosinophils were observed mainly in the lamina propria (LP), but occasional eosinophils were observed in epithelial (E) or muscle layers (M). L, lumen. (Original magnification: upper figures, 100×; lower figure, 400×)

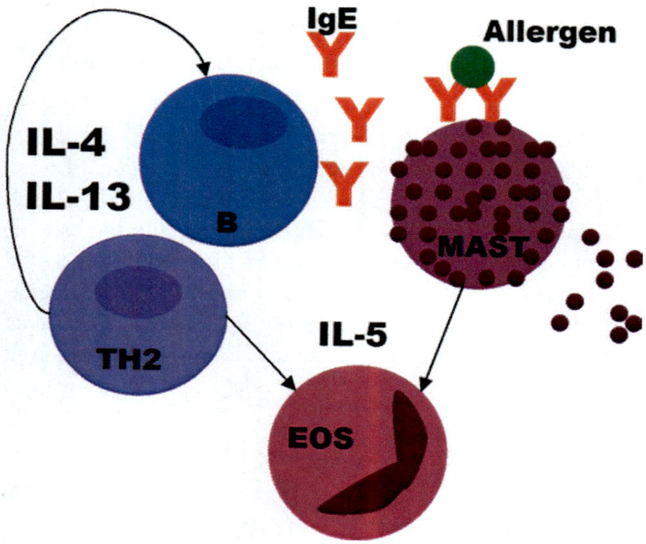

Fig. 17.6 Th2-driven inflammation is present in the end-organs of atopic conditions. Th2 cytokines, such as IL-4, IL-5, and IL-13, are present in atopic diseases including eosinophilic esophagitis. Activation of mast cells by cross linking of allergen-specific IgE releases mediators and cytokines leading to allergic inflammation including an increase in eosinophils

possibly asthma and allergic rhinitis [34]. In addition, functional impairment in filaggrin expression may be associated with eosinophilic esophagitis [35].

In atopic diseases, chronic inflammation may lead to more fixed structural changes referred to as remodeling. In some asthmatics, thickening of the bronchial mucosa may lead to a permanent decline in lung function [36]. In atopic dermatitis, lichenification of the skin may occur [30]. Similarly, in eosinophilic esophagitis, a narrowing or stricture may occur in the esophagus [3, 10]. Patients with untreated eosinophilic esophagitis have basement membrane thickening and increased vascular activation similar to changes seen in asthmatic airway remodeling [37].

Summary

Most children with eosinophilic esophagitis have evidence of concomitant asthma, allergic rhinitis, atopic dermatitis, and/or IgE-mediated food allergy. All atopic conditions, including eosinophilic esophagitis, are thought to be chronic and on the rise. Both the underlying pathophysiology and current approaches to management are similar. Future research in all atopic diseases is important as the more we learn, the more we will be able to help our patients.

References

1. Bloom B, Cohen RA, Freeman G, National Center for Health Statistics. Summary health statistics for U.S. children: National Health Interview Survey, 2008. Vital Health Stat. 2009;10(244):1–81.
2. Akdis CA, Akdis M, Bieber T, et al. Diagnosis and treatment of atopic dermatitis in children and adults: European Academy of Allergology and Clinical Immunology/American Academy of Allergy, Asthma and Immunology/PRACTALL Consensus Report. Allergy. 2006;61(8):969–87.
3. Spergel J, Brown-Whitehorn TF, Beausoleil JL, et al. 14 years of eosinophilic esophagitis: clinical features and prognosis. J Pediatr Gastroenterol Nutr. 2009;48:30–6.
4. Noel RJ, Putnam PE, Ropthenberg ME. Eosinophilic esophagitis. N Engl J Med. 2004;351:940–1.
5. Assa'ad AH, Putnam PE, Collins MH, et al. Pediatric patients with eosinophilic esophagitis: an 8-year follow-up. J Allergy Clin Immunol. 2007;119:731–8.
6. Wang FY, Gupta SK, Fitzgerald JF. Is there a seasonal variation in the incidence or intensity of allergic eosinophilic esophagitis in newly diagnosed children? J Clin Gastroenterol. 2007;41(5):451–3.
7. Eroglu Y, Lu H, Terry A, et al. Pediatric eosinophilic esophagitis: single-center experience in northwestern USA. Pediatr Int. 2009;51(5):612–6.
8. Sugnanam KK, Collins JT, Smith PK, et al. Dichotomy of food and inhalant allergen sensitization in eosinophilic esophagitis. Allergy. 2007;62:1257–60.
9. Guajardo J, Plotnick L, Fende J, et al. Eosinophil-associated gastrointestinal disorders: a world-wide-web based registry. J Pediatr. 2002;141:576–81.
10. Liacouras CA, Spergel JM, Ruchelli E, et al. Eosinophilic esophagitis: a 10-year experience in 381 children. Clin Gastroenterol Hepatol. 2005;3:1198–206.
11. Rothenberg ME, Spergel JM, Sherrill JD, et al. Common variants at 5q22 associate with pediatric eosinophilic esophagitis. Nat Genet. 2010;42(4):289–91.
12. Sicherer SH, Sampson HA. 9. Food allergy. J Allergy Clin Immunol. 2006;117 Suppl 2:S470–5.
13. Kelly KJ, Lazenby AJ, Rowe PC, et al. Eosinophilic esophagitis attributed to gastroesophageal reflux: improvement with an amino acid-based formula. Gastroenterology. 1995; 109:1503–12.
14. Spergel JM, Beausoleil JL, Mascarenhas M, et al. The use of skin prick tests and patch tests to identify causative foods in eosinophilic esophagitis. J Allergy Clin Immunol. 2002;109(2):363–8.
15. Kagalwalla AF, Sentongo TA, Ritz S, et al. Effect of six-food elimination diet on clinical and histologic outcomes in eosinophilic esophagitis. Clin Gastroenterol Hepatol. 2006;14:1097–102.
16. Fogg MI, Ruchelli E, Spergel JM. Pollen and eosinophilic esophagitis [letter]. J Allergy Clin Immunol. 2003;12(4):796–7.
17. Brim SN, Rudd RA, Funk RH, et al. Asthma prevalence among US children in underrepresented minority populations: American Indian/Alaska Native, Chinese, Filiipino, and Asian Indian. Pediatrics. 2008;122(1):e217–22.
18. Laughter D, Istvan JA, Tofte SJ, et al. The prevalence of atopic dermatitis in Oregon schoolchildren. J Am Acad Dermatol. 2000;43(4):649–55.
19. Plaut M, Valentine MD. Clinical practice. Allergic rhinitis. N Engl J Med. 2005; 353(18):1934–44.
20. Kiyohara C, Tanaka K, Miyake Y. Genetic susceptibility to atopic dermatitis. Allergol Int. 2008;57(1):39–56.
21. Orenstein SR, Shalaby TM, Di Lorenzo C, et al. The spectrum of pediatric eosinophilic esophagitis beyond infancy: a clinical series of 30 children. Am J Gastroenterol. 2000;95(6):1422–30.
22. Cherian S, Smith NM, Forbes DA. Rapidly increasing prevalence of eosinophilic oesophagitis in Western Australia. Arch Dis Child. 2006;91(12):1000–4.

23. Blanchard C, Wang N, Rothenberg ME. Eosinophilic esophagitis: pathogenesis, genetics, and therapy. J Allergy Clin Immunol. 2006;118(5):1054–9.
24. Markowitz JE, Spergel JM, Ruchelli E, et al. Elemental diet is an effective treatment for eosinophilic esophagitis in children and adolescents. Am J Gastroenterol. 2003;98(4):777–82.
25. Fox VL, Nurko S, Furuta GT. Eosinophilic esophagitis: it's not just kid's stuff. Gastrointest Endosc. 2002;56(2):260–70.
26. Mishra A, Hogan SP, Brandt EB, et al. An etiologic role for aeroallergens and eosinophils in experimental esophagitis. J Clin Invest. 2001;107(1):83–90.
27. Akei HS, Mishra A, Blanchard C, et al. Epicutaneous antigen exposure primes for experimental eosinophilic esophagitis in mice. Gastroenterology. 2005;129(3):985–94.
28. Durham SR. The inflammatory nature of allergic disease. Clin Exp Allergy. 1998;28 Suppl 6:20–4.
29. Robinson D, Hamid Q, Ying S, et al. Predominant Th2-like bronchoalveolar T-lymphocytes population in atopic asthma. N Engl J Med. 1992;326:298–304.
30. Bieber T. Atopic dermatitis. N Engl J Med. 2008;358(14):1483–94.
31. Lucendo AJ, Navarro M, Comas C, et al. Immunophenotypic characterization and quantification of the epithelial inflammatory infiltrate in eosinophilic esophagitis through serology: an analysis of the cellular mechanisms of the disease and the immunologic capacity of the esophagus. Am J Surg Pathol. 2007;31(4):598–606.
32. Straumann A, Bauer M, Fischer B, et al. Idiopathic eosinophilic esophagitis is associated with a T(H)2-type allergic inflammatory response. J Allergy Clin Immunol. 2001;108(6):954–61.
33. Blanchard C, Wang N, Stringer KF, et al. Eotaxin-3 and a uniquely conserved gene-expression profile in eosinophilic esophagitis. J Clin Invest. 2006;116(2):536–47.
34. Weidinger S, O'Sullivan M, Illig T, et al. Filaggrin mutations, atopic eczema, hay fever, and asthma in children. J Allergy Clin Immunol. 2008;121(5):1203–9. e1.
35. Rothenberg ME. Biology and treatment of eosinophilic esophagitis. Gastroenterology. 2009;137(4):1238–49.
36. Hoshino M, Nakamura Y, Sim J, et al. Bronchial subepithelial fibrosis and expression of matrix metalloproteinase-9 in asthmatic airway inflammation. J Allergy Clin Immunol. 1998;102(5):783–8.
37. Aceves SS, Newbury RO, Dohil R, et al. Esophageal remodeling in pediatric eosinophilic esophagitis. J Allergy Clin Immunol. 2007;119(1):206–12.

Chapter 18
Atopic and Allergic Features of Adults with Eosinophilic Esophagitis

Javed Sheikh and Katherine N. Cahill

Keywords Allergen exposure • Atopy • Pathophysiology of EoE • Skin prick testing • Specific IgE testing

Introduction

Allergen exposure has been well documented to have a role in the pathogenesis of pediatric eosinophilic esophagitis (EoE). A 1995 case series of pediatric patients demonstrated a dramatic clinical response to an elemental diet and subsequent clinical relapse upon reintroduction of foods. In the adult population, it has been hypothesized that allergen exposure plays a role in the pathophysiology of adult EoE, supported by high rates of personal and family history of atopy. Although published reports of successful resolution of clinical symptoms or eosinophilic infiltrates on biopsy as the result of food or aeroallergens identified through any of the below measures discussed are limited in adults, there is increasing evidence for a role for food and aeroallergens in the pathophysiology of adult EoE and a potential for future diagnostic and therapeutic implications.

J. Sheikh (✉)
Center for Eosinophilic Disorders, Beth Israel Deaconess Medical Center,
Harvard Medical School, One Brookline Place, Suite 623, Brookline, MA 02132, USA
e-mail: jsheikh@bidmc.harvard.edu

C.A. Liacouras and J.E. Markowitz (eds.), *Eosinophilic Esophagitis*,
Clinical Gastroenterology, DOI 10.1007/978-1-60761-515-6_18,

Background

Over the past 15 years, allergen exposure has been well documented to have a role in the pathogenesis of pediatric eosinophilic esophagitis (EoE). When children with long-standing reflux failed to respond to anti-reflux therapies, attention shifted toward a possible role for allergens as the cause of the dense eosinophilic infiltrates found on endoscopic biopsies of the esophagus. In 1995 a case series of pediatric patients demonstrated a dramatic clinical response to an elemental diet and subsequent clinical relapse upon reintroduction of foods [1]. Since that time, food sensitization has been shown to be present in 96% of pediatric EoE patients [2]. As we shift our attention to the adult population, it has been hypothesized that allergen exposure plays a role in the pathophysiology of adult EoE. High rates of personal and family history of atopy, repeatedly demonstrated in case series of adult patients, provide supporting clues. With few epidemiological studies, reports of elimination diet outcomes, and no large-scale systematic allergy testing of the adult EoE population published to date, a role for food allergy in the adult population is not clear. Children and adults are known to have different clinical presentations of EoE, and the natural history of food allergy is one that decreases with age, suggesting there may be more than food allergy at play in the adults. Clinical histories of significant allergic rhinitis, case reports of seasonal variation in symptom severity, mouse models of EoE triggered by aeroallergen exposure and incomplete response to elimination diets in the adult population have prompted further evaluation into the role aeroallergen (as compared to food allergen) exposure has in adult EoE.

In the pediatric literature clinical observation supports that eosinophilic esophagitis represents a spectrum of clinical presentations [3]. This spectrum is anchored on one end by atopic individuals and non-atopic on the other. At the one extreme, the profoundly atopic pediatric patient presents in early childhood with a constellation of atopic features including asthma, atopic dermatitis, and food and environmental allergy associated with eosinophilic esophagitis that responds to an elemental diet. Reintroduction of any food causes a flare in symptoms. Their co-occurring atopic conditions are often quite severe and do not respond to dietary modification alone. On the other extreme, are the non-atopic patients who lack evidence of food allergy on formal testing, do not respond to an elemental diet, and often respond to topical corticosteroid treatment. Discontinuation of swallowed corticosteroids often results in a relapse. In between, the largest number of patients present with a few food allergies associated with mild atopic asthma, eczema, and/or environmental allergen sensitivity, and are usually successfully treated with an elimination diet. The presence of a similar spectrum in adults has not yet been established but is suggested by a number of adult EoE case series which highlight that many but not all patients carry the atopic phenotype to varying levels of severity and have documented sensitization to food and aeroallergens when tested [4–7].

This chapter focuses on the allergic phenotypic of the adult with EoE; the overlap with the pediatric population, and individual case reports, case series, and clinical trials that focus directly on the adult with EoE and the unique allergic qualities this population demonstrates. In this emerging body of literature, you will find sound evidence for a role of food and aeroallergens in the pathogenesis of adult EoE.

Demographics

Adult patients with EoE could be arbitrarily classified into two categories, the first consisting of pediatric patients with EoE who have brought their childhood disease characteristics and associated food allergy into adulthood. In the second category are adult patients with symptoms that began after age 18. Most published studies to date do not distinguish between these two groups when reporting demographic data. In a review of all adult series of patients with EoE, male predominance is universal with the average ratio of 2.4 to 1 and a peak incidence around the fourth to fifth decade of life [5, 8, 9]. When reviewing racial and ethnic distribution, one adult study of 94 patients from a Cincinnati OH teaching hospital showed an overwhelming predominance in the white population at 96% (91 of 94) [10]. In our unpublished population of 93 adult patients, the predominance in the white male population with peak incidence in their fourth decade of life holds true. We found a male to female ratio of 2.9 to 1, 95% were self-identified as white, and median age at onset of symptoms was 26. The demographics of adult EoE patients are outlined in Table 18.1.

Family History

The current literature is limited to self-reporting statistics for rates of atopy among family members of adults with EoE. Adult patients report high rates of food allergy, asthma, allergic rhinitis, and atopic dermatitis among their family members. Family history of atopy in a series of 30 adult patients was approximately 20% [6]. Our data in a larger population support a higher rate of familial atopic disease at 55% which is more consistent with rates found in the pediatric population of 40–50% [11]. Most data published are limited by lack of clinical validation of these self-reports. As the disease prevalence has increased and more attention has been paid to differentiating reflux esophagitis from EoE by pathologists and endoscopists, self-reporting of family members with EoE has increased over the past 10 years. Straumann et al. in their follow-up of 30 adult patients with EoE, found five cases involving two families with EoE [6]. One case series in 2005 reported three adult siblings with EoE [12] and a second communication identified two adults, father aged 80 and daughter aged 52, diagnosed with EoE who both reported long-standing dysphagia for 30 and 12 years, respectively [13]. Noel et al. in 2004 reported 6.8% of their pediatric population of 103 patients had a first degree relative with EoE [14]. In 381 pediatric patients, 5% had a sibling with EoE; 7% had a parent with EoE or history of an esophageal stricture [11].

Table 18.1 Allergic characteristics of adult eosinophilic esophagitis patients

Study	Year	No. of patients	Age		Male gender		Personal history of atopy					
			Mean	Range	No.	%	Any	Allergic rhinitis	Asthma	Atopic dermatitis	Food allergy	EoE
Croese et al.	2003	31	34.0	14–77	24	77	13 of 28	#	#	#	7	#
Pasha et al.	2007	42	44.0	21–74	31	74	18 of 42	#	15	#	#	#
Roy-Ghanta et al.	2008	23	35.2	18–57	14	61	18 of 23	18	6	1	#	#
Simon et al.	2005	31	37.0	18–66	25	81	21 of 31[a]	Most common	#	#	#	#
Straumann et al.	2003	30	33.4	6–65	22	73	18 of 30	17[b]	#	3	4	#
Penfield et al.	2010	26	41.4	20–74	17	65	25 of 26	24 of 26	9	3	#	#
Cahill and Sheikh[c]	2010	93	41.0	19–78	69	74	71 of 93	66	25	18	18	#

Study	Year	No. of patients	Family history of atopy					
			Any	Allergic rhinitis	Asthma	Atopic dermatitis	Food allergy	EoE
Croese et al.	2003	31	12 of 28	#	12	#	#	#
Pasha et al.	2007	42	5 of 42	#	5	#	#	#
Straumann et al.	2003	30	5 of 30	#	#	#	#	5
Cahill and Sheikh[c]	2010	93	51 of 93	#	#	#	#	#

[a]Physician diagnosed
[b]Any respiratory allergy
[c]Data unpublished to date
#=no data

Personal History of Atopy

In both the pediatric and the adult population with EoE, an overlap with atopic disease independent of cause is clear. Incidence of personal history of asthma, atopic dermatitis, or other extra-esophageal allergy ranges from 29 to 96%, with asthma and allergic rhinitis being most often associated [4, 8]. In a systematic review of adult EoE papers published between 1993 and 2005, 102 of 185 patients (55%; CI, 48–62%) had associated atopic or allergic disease [9]. In a more recent series of 26 adult patients with EoE who were referred for and completed allergy evaluation, 96% had concomitant atopic disorders with allergic rhinitis being the most common at 92% followed by asthma at 35% [4]. The challenge with interpreting this information is that EoE patients who follow through with allergy evaluation may be biased toward seeking care by the presence of other allergic symptoms. Self-reported atopy was found in 21 of 31 (68%) adult EoE patients, again with allergic rhinitis being the most commonly reported, in a case series from Switzerland in 2005 [7]. In 2007, a case series of 42 adults had self-reported rates of atopy or allergy in 43%, and asthma in 36% [9]. Clinician-documented atopic disease was found in 18 of 23 adult patients in a case series from 2008 [5]. In this study, all atopics were found to have allergic rhinitis with six diagnoses of asthma and one of atopic dermatitis. In our series of adult patients who completed allergy evaluation, 76% had a personal history of atopic disease with allergic rhinitis being the most prevalent at 71%. Table 18.1 summarizes these findings.

Food Allergens

A connection between EoE and food allergens was first described after an amino-acid diet was successful in eliminating symptoms in a case series of ten pediatric patients [1]. Two subsequent studies in the pediatric population support a role for food antigens in the pathogenesis of EoE: Markowitz et al. in 2003 evaluated the use of elemental diets and Kagalwalla et al. in 2006 employed empirical elimination of milk, soy, wheat, egg, peanut, and seafood in the diet (six food elimination diet) [2, 15]. Ninety five to ninety eight percent of pediatric EoE patients were found to respond to an elemental diet even in absence of identification of the specific offending food antigens [2, 11]. The extent to which food antigens are responsible for symptoms and pathologic findings of the adult EoE population is not clear. This is due primarily to a lack of dietary modification studies that have demonstrated clinical improvement. In a negative study, Simon et al. removed wheat, rye, and barley for 6 weeks from the diet of six adult patients who demonstrated sensitization, and documented no clinical improvement in symptoms [16]. Gonsalves et al. in 2007 used the same empiric six-food elimination diet as Kagalwalla et al. and found that only 30% of the adult population studied versus 70% of the pediatric population showed a clinical response [17]. In 2008, they published preliminary data from 23 adult patients who completed a six food elimination diet with 94% reporting decreases in symptom scores, and histological improvement in 78% [18]. These studies suggest a smaller role for food allergy in adult EoE as compared with the pediatric population, but certainly do not exclude it entirely.

Historically, the definitive diagnosis of food allergy is made through direct observed food challenge that results in an immediate hypersensitivity reaction, such as urticaria, angioedema, vomiting, or diarrhea within minutes to 2 h of ingestion [19]. Very few patients in either the pediatric or adult EoE population demonstrate such a reaction, yet clearly their EoE can often be treated through dietary avoidance of the offending food antigen(s). One good example of this comes from a case report from Spain of a 37-year-old male with a history of allergic rhinoconjunctivitis and sensitization to dust mite and grass pollen, who was diagnosed with EoE after 2 years of reflux, dysphagia, and epigastric pain symptoms [20]. Allergy evaluation including skin prick testing (SPT) to food (fish, shellfish, nuts, legumes, wheat flour, egg, milk, almond, apple peel, apple pulp and pear) and aeroallergens (dog and cat dander, dust mite, Alternaria, aspergillus, grasses, trees, weeds, olive, cypress, latex, and Anisakis) and prick-prick testing to egg white, egg yolk, milk, and apple peel and pulp were performed. In addition to positive dust mite, grass, and olive results on SPT, prick-prick testing was positive for egg white. Serum-specific IgE testing was also positive for egg white (class 2). Despite these findings, the patient had not self-identified any change in his symptoms with eggs or any egg containing foods. Treatment with an egg-free diet, Montelukast, and Ketotifen resulted in symptom resolution.

The current hypothesis of the mechanism of food sensitivity in EoE is thought to be a combination of IgE-mediated (as demonstrated by serum specific IgE or SPT and delayed non-IgE-mediated (as might be demonstrated by food atopy patch testing) hypersensitivity responses. Clinical observations of patients with negative SPT results to foods despite symptoms with reintroduction in diet served as a clue to a non-IgE mediated process. A few studies have highlighted the observation of non-IgE mediated reactions to food(s) that were not demonstrated through SPT which result in symptomatic improvement once eliminated.

There are many challenges in evaluating the role of food antigens for both the individual as well as the adult EoE population as a whole, and subsequently, elucidating the role of food antigens in the pathophysiology of adult EoE is complex. With evidence to support both an IgE and a non-IgE mediated pathway for food antigens, the clinical community often struggles to identify, even after performing an exhaustive search, which food or foods are triggering the cascade of cytokines that eventually lead to eosinophilic infiltration of the esophagus. Due to a lack of standardized methods for establishing responsible food antigens in adults, the large number of potential offending agents or combinations thereof, poor adult compliance with elimination diets, a possible role of aeroallergens that is not being addressed, and a disease process that may be less food responsive in the adult patient, we are far from understanding the role of food antigen exposure in adult EoE.

Food Skin Prick Testing

Skin prick testing (SPT) is used to identify IgE-mediated sensitization and is generally considered the more sensitive test for determining a true allergen over specific IgE testing [14, 19]. It is currently the recommended means of performing allergy evaluation in adult EoE patients [21]. A review of the published studies employing SPT to foods reveals there is not one established panel of foods used in evaluation, and SPT is often not sufficient to identify all possible food sensitizations.

In one of the earliest series evaluating the use of SPT in adult EoE patients, Simon et al. evaluated 31 adult EoE patients from Switzerland in 2005 who underwent SPT to 14 food allergens (ALK Denmark) and three native probes from wheat grain, rye grain, and soy milk, as well as evaluation of specific IgE levels to cow's milk, egg white, wheat flour, rye flour, and gluten [7]. Nineteen of 31 patients had positive SPT to food allergens; 12 of those 19 had SPT reactions to cross-reacting aeroallergens. Looking specifically at wheat and rye results, 16 of 31 were identified as sensitized to either or both through SPT and specific IgE results. Eight patients had positive SPT results to either or both foods, and 14 of the 16 had a specific-IgE response to either or both foods. Fifteen of the 16 were noted to be cross-sensitized to grass pollen on SPT. In a follow-up study, six of these patients who were identified on the basis of specific-IgE testing results to be sensitized to wheat or rye but not positive on SPT underwent an unsuccessful elimination diet [16].

A more recent study of 26 adult EoE patients referred by their gastroenterologist for allergy evaluation underwent SPT to a standard panel of foods plus any other foods to which clinical history supported a reaction [4]. Half of the patients (13/26) had a positive result to one or more foods tested: egg white (27%), cow's milk (19%), soybean (23%), peanut (38%), English walnut (19%), wheat (4%), shrimp (4%), halibut (0%), and others based on supporting clinical history (almond, Brazil nut, pistachio, filbert nut, and cantaloupe). There was no mention of the use of these data to direct an elimination diet and/or symptom or pathologic response to food elimination.

In a preliminary report on the use of a six food elimination diet (milk, egg, soy, wheat, nuts, and seafood) in 23 adult patients, 18 patients were reported to have completed the trial [18]. All patients underwent SPT to food and aeroallergens prior to the start of the empiric six food elimination diet with 55% having a positive SPT to food and 72% to aeroallergens. After 6 weeks of the elimination diet, they had a 94% decrease in symptom scores and a 78% improvement on histology. On reintroduction, the most common food triggers were milk and wheat and these food triggers were only predicted 22% of the time by SPT results.

In adult EoE patients evaluated with food SPT, one half to two thirds (depending on the population studied) showed at least one food sensitization (see Table 18.2). The reports, although limited in number, on use of these to successfully direct elimination diets show only modest success.

Table 18.2 Food allergen characteristics of adults with eosinophilic esophagitis

Study	Year	No. of patients	Age		Food sensitization	
			Mean	Range	Positive RAST	Positive SPT
Roy-Ghanta et al.	2008	23	35.2	18–57	19 of 23	#
Simon et al.	2005	31	37	18–66	#	19 of 30
Penfield et al.	2010	26	41.4	20–74	#	13 of 26

Results of specific food allergens

Study	Wheat	Rye	Egg white	Cow's milk	Peanut	Soybean	Walnut	Shrimp	Other	Fish
Roy-Ghanta et al.	9 of 23	3 of 23	7 of 23	7 of 23	6 of 23	5 of 23	2 of 23	#	#	#
Penfield et al.	1 of 24	#	7 of 26	5 of 26	10 of 26	6 of 26	5 of 26	1 of 25	9 of 26	0 of 26

= no data

Food Specific IgE Testing

There has been attention toward the use of specific IgE testing, in complement to or in place of SPT, in hopes of more fully evaluating the numerous potential food sensitizations in adult EoE and then better guiding treatment through elimination diets. One argument for the use of specific IgE testing is the ease and large number of tests that can be performed, in a population that tends to have greater variability in their diet [5]. One case series of 23 adult patients who underwent food-allergen specific testing reported results from specific IgE testing to common foods and spices [5]. Specific IgE testing was guided by a 96 food list from which patients self-identified foods they ate most often and those which cause symptom exacerbation. Nineteen of 23 had one or more positive food-specific IgE with a median of five (mean, 10.3±12.8) and a range of 0–55. The foods most commonly sensitized to were wheat and carrots (39%) and onions and tomatoes (35%). Following closely behind were cow milk, egg white, sesame seed, banana, and apple at 30%. Notable was the absence of sensitization to fish or shellfish, one of the most common food allergens in the adult population. No information on effect of elimination diet following the determination of food sensitization or control population for comparison of sensitization rates was offered in this study.

In a small series of six adult EoE patients identified by specific IgE results to have sensitization to wheat and rye, a double-blind placebo-controlled food challenge and an elimination diet were performed [16]. The food challenge revealed one patient of the six who had provocation of dysphagia with solid wheat ingestion on the blinded food challenge. Following a 6-week elimination diet, one patient reported a decrease in frequency of dysphagia attacks but in the absence of histological improvement on repeat biopsy, while the remainder saw no change in their symptoms. Notably, this one patient also was found to have 2+ positive SPT reactions to both wheat and rye but did not develop symptoms on the blinded food challenge. The authors concluded that sensitization to food allergens is not a major cause of symptoms in adult EoE and that elimination diets are less helpful in adults than in their pediatric counterparts. The authors suggested that a cross-reaction with grass pollen extracts may have led to false positive results as all of the patients enrolled also were sensitized to grass pollen on SPT or specific IgE results. Given the small sample of adult patients and short duration of the elimination diet, we feel that these findings should be interpreted with caution when thinking about the role of specific-IgE testing in the evaluation and subsequent treatment of the adult EoE patient. Anecdotal reports from others suggest that specific IgE testing is of low yield in identifying causative agents of EoE [22]. One major challenge with the use of specific IgE results is which ones and how many to test. In the study by Roy-Ghanta, positive tests ranged from 0 to 55.

Another consideration for the failure of the rye and wheat elimination diet in the 2006 study from Simon et al. is incomplete identification of food allergens through SPT and specific-IgE testing. Studies from the pediatric population have shown that not all foods are identified by SPT alone and the use of atopy patch testing (APT) is necessary to evaluate for food antigens responsible for a delayed-type hypersensitivity reaction [22, 23].

Atopy Patch Testing

More recent evidence to support a role of non-IgE mediated immune response has lead clinicians to evaluate adult EoE patients with APT to food antigens. APT is primarily used by non-U.S. clinicians in the evaluation of atopic dermatitis patients to identify possible delayed-type hypersensitivity reactions. Foods are applied to the skin under occlusion under a small disc and left in place for at least 48 h, with subsequent readings to look for delayed onset skin reactions. Support for the use of APT comes from a few clinical trials which have documented that patients with negative SPT may have a positive APT to a particular food antigen. A study of 146 pediatric patients found that most patients had positive reactions on SPT and APT, with different foods reacting on the different tests [23]. This combination method was able to identify the causative food in approximately 67% of patients who would clinically and pathologically respond to an elimination diet. The success of SPT and APT testing rises to 82% if you include those who responded clinically but had only a partial pathologic response. Of the food tests found to be positive on SPT (810), only 57 were also positive on APT. It is noted, however, that large SPT reactions of >15 mm were not repeated on APT in this study. In the adult EoE population data on the use of APT are limited to anecdotal evidence. In our evaluation of 93 patients with EoE, APT has been reserved for patients with negative SPT and specific IgE testing or incomplete symptom resolution after food specific elimination diets, and in the 14 patients evaluated, the yield has been low with only three positive results (with unclear clinical significance of these findings to date).

Environmental Allergens

Food allergen sensitization in the pediatric EoE population is established to be very high. Continued investigation in the adult population suggests that there is a role of food allergen sensitization, but lower than in the pediatric population. However, a larger role for aeroallergens in the adult EoE population compared to the pediatric population has a growing body of evidence. It has been proposed that the "atopic march" is important in pathophysiology of adult EoE, its evaluation, and treatment. In a case series of pediatric EoE patients, age 3 months to 16 years, who underwent SPT to food and aeroallergens and APT to select food allergens, a positive relationship between rates of aeroallergen sensitization based on SPT results and age, and a negative relationship between food sensitization based on SPT and APT results and age were identified [24]. Data supporting this continued trend with age in the adult EoE population, although established for other atopic diseases, have not yet been published.

More recently a potential role for environmental allergens in the pathogenesis of adult eosinophilic esophagitis has been raised. Patient reports of symptoms that fluctuate with the seasons and predominate in spring and fall, and the increase in food impaction and diagnosis in the spring months support the concept of an environmental allergen exposure as a possible trigger for EoE [25, 26]. Histological studies have demonstrated that patients with allergic rhinitis have higher numbers of eosinophils per high-power field in their esophagus during pollen season as compared with biopsies performed out of the pollen season [27]. Ten of 38 adult patients with allergic rhinitis during pollen season, 5 of 24 with gastroesophageal reflux disease (GERD), and zero of 25 healthy controls had eosinophils present in their esophagus. Although the incidence of patients with eosinophils present in the esophagus was not different between those with allergic rhinitis or those with GERD the number of eosinophils trended toward being higher in the allergic rhinitis population. A case report of a 21-year-old female who presented with symptomatic and biopsy proven exacerbations of EoE during the pollen season and resolution of symptoms during the winter is particularly interesting [25]. She had a history of asthma and allergic rhinitis when she developed reflux symptoms that were not responsive to aggressive medical therapy. Initial biopsy in May was consistent with EoE and repeat biopsy in February, a time of symptom improvement, showed only rare eosinophils. Repeated biopsies in August, December, and July of subsequent years revealed the same pattern. SPT and APT to foods were negative. SPT to aeroallergens were positive for multiple trees, grasses, ragweed, aspergillus, cat, dog, and dust mite. Another interesting case report is that of a 91-year-old man who presented with dysphagia to liquids and solids and was found to have greater than 100 eosinophils per HPF on biopsy. SPT and APT were performed and revealed sensitization to multiple trees, grass, molds, dust mites, and cat dander with a negative food panel [28]. In a series of 41 adult patients diagnosed with EoE, the majority of patients were diagnosed in the spring and summer seasons, with May and June having the highest number of EoE diagnoses made via endoscopy [26].

Additionally, there are mouse models that support the role of aeroallergens in the development of EoE. Mishra et al. showed mice exposed to intranasal respiratory allergen (*Aspergillus fumigates*) develop esophageal eosinophils, free eosinophil granules, and epithelial cell hyperplasia [29]. Intragastric or oral allergen exposure was insufficient to promote these changes in the esophagus. The role of aeroallergen sensitivity in EoE might also be supported by studies in adults where the onset of symptomatic environmental allergy has been shown to precede the onset of EoE symptoms [7].

Environmental Skin Prick Testing

SPT is standard of care for the evaluation of aeroallergens in the adult and pediatric population, but the place it has in evaluation of the adult patient with EoE has limited supporting evidence. Straumann et al. reported rates of aeroallergen sensitization of over 58% (17 patients) in their series of 30 adult patients [6]. Penfield et al. performed aeroallergen SPT evaluation on a subset of 15 patients in a case series of

26 adults with EoE referred on for allergy evaluation on an ad hoc basis by their gastroenterologist [4]. The subpopulation was selected based on coexisting allergic rhinitis and/or asthma who had not previously undergone aeroallergen testing at an outside institution. Fourteen of 15 (93%) patients tested had one or more positive SPT. SPT results included cat (67%), dog (53%), cockroach (31%), dust mite (69%; *Dermatophagoides farinae* and *Dermatophagoides pteronyssinus)*, mold spores (64%), tree mix (73%), grass (87%), weed mix (93%; including ragweed). See Table 18.3 for a summary of aeroallergen sensitization in adult EoE patients.

The reports we have at our center of adult patients with EoE who have undergone SPT to aeroallergens have been limited to those with concomitant allergic rhinitis or asthma. This has been based on the assumption that SPT to aeroallergens in the absence of upper or lower airway symptoms is of low yield in revealing clinically meaningful sensitizations in rhinitis and asthma. With more data to support that aeroallergens may play a direct role in producing eosinophilic inflammation in the esophagus, more comprehensive testing of EoE patients without airway symptoms will need to be carried out in a large clinical trial. Until this is performed, we will continue to have an incomplete understanding of any role aeroallergens have in the pathogenesis of adult EoE.

Environmental Specific IgE Testing

Although SPT is considered standard of care in the evaluation of aeroallergens (unless otherwise contraindicated), one study evaluated the use of specific IgE testing for aeroallergens in a subset of patients. Roy-Ghanta et al. looked at 21 adults with EoE and a history of allergic rhinitis who underwent specific IgE evaluation for aeroallergens. The panels included the common tree, grass, and weed pollens of the northeastern United States, cat and dog dander, and dust mite. Those with negative IgE results underwent skin prick testing with the same environmental panel and confirmed the negative results. Eighteen of the 21 patients had at least one positive result with 17 of these patients having a positive result in three or more of the tested categories. Their results suggested that adult EoE patients with environmental allergens are polysensitized [5].

Despite the above data from both SPT and specific IgE testing, there have not been any clinical trials to date demonstrating that aeroallergen avoidance results in disease modification in adult or pediatric patients with EoE [30]. In addition, the use of immunotherapy or medical treatment for aeroallergens has not yet been well studied.

Role of Allergen Avoidance and Implications for Treatment

In the adult population with EoE, reports of successful resolution of clinical symptoms or eosinophilic infiltrates on biopsy as the result of avoidance of food or aeroallergens identified through any of the above measures discussed are limited [18]

Table 18.3 Aeroallergen characteristics of adults with eosinophilic esophagitis

Study	Year	No. of patients tested	Age		Aeroallergen sensitization			Specific aeroallergens						
			Mean	Range	All	RAST positive	SPT positive	Birch	Timothy and ryegrass	Ragweed	Dust mite	Pet dander	Cockroach	Molds
Roy-Ghanta et al.	2008	21	35.2	18–57	18	18	#	17	16	16	15	15	#	#
Simon et al.	2005	30	37	18–66	23	#	#	#	15 of 16	#	#	#	#	#
Penfield et al.	2010	15	41.4	20–74	14	#	14	11	13	14[a]	9 of 13	10 cat 8 dog	4 of 13	9 of 14

[a]All weeds

= no data

or unsuccessful [16] in the published literature. One case from 2006 reported symptom improvement and decrease in peripheral blood eosinophilia with the elimination of egg, and treatment with Montelukast after prick-prick testing and SPT identified egg white and dust mite, grass, and olive sensitization from the diet of a 37-year old male patient [20]. To our knowledge there are no large studies reporting the efficacy of an elimination diet guided by SPT results alone. However, it is the clinical experience of the authors that identification through SPT of food allergens for individual patients and subsequent initiation of elimination diets is successful for some patients and a worthy attempt prior to subjecting a patient to life-long swallowed corticosteroids. The data on the success of aeroallergen identification, avoidance, and treatment is very limited and is inconclusive to date. Many studies have documented that the typical adult patient with EoE is sensitized to aeroallergens (see Table 18.3), which typically predates the onset of their EoE symptoms [7]. The idea of cross sensitization between aeroallergens and food allergens as a causative model for EoE has also been raised [4, 5, 16]. It remains a challenge to tease out the interplay between aeroallergen and food allergen sensitization, and designing large trials of adults who have undergone comprehensive food and aeroallergen testing followed by a combination of intervention measures will be necessary in order to establish the best treatment plan for our adult patients.

In 2007, a consensus statement published in *Gastroenterology* recommended a complete evaluation by a well-informed allergist including SPT for food and aeroallergens for all adult EoE patients [21].With studies and case reports documenting the clear benefit of food allergen avoidance in some adult patients with EoE and an emerging body of literature that clearly documents the presence of aeroallergen sensitization, we have a modest amount of evidence to base a recommendation for routine food and aeroallergen testing in the adult patient with EoE.

Summary

EoE is an inflammatory disorder characterized by eosinophilic infiltration into the lamina propria of the esophagus. EoE presents in both children and adults with different clinical features. It was first diagnosed and is well characterized in the pediatric population. In the adult population, current knowledge on the role of food and aeroallergens is limited to case reports, retrospective case series, and a few prospective trials. The adult population demonstrates high rates of familial and personal atopy, which is not limited to food. Observational data have suggested a seasonal variation in symptoms and diagnosis [25, 26]. A growing number of case-series demonstrate that aeroallergens and food allergens co-occur in the adult with EoE [4, 5, 7]. Although published reports of successful resolution of clinical symptoms or eosinophilic infiltrates on biopsy as the result of food or aeroallergens identified through any of the above measures discussed are limited in adults, there is growing evidence for a role for food and aeroallergens in the pathophysiology of adult EoE and a potential for future diagnostic and therapeutic implications.

References

1. Kelly KJ, Lazenby AJ, Rowe PC, Yardley JH, Perman JA, Sampson HA. Eosinophilic esophagitis attributed to gastroesophageal reflux: improvement with an amino acid-based formula. Gastroenterology. 1995;109(5):1503–12.
2. Markowitz JE, Spergel JM, Ruchelli E, Liacouras CA. Elemental diet is an effective treatment for eosinophilic esophagitis in children and adolescents. Am J Gastroenterol. 2003;98(4): 777–82.
3. Putnam PE. Eosinophilic esophagitis in children: clinical manifestations. Gastrointest Endosc Clin N Am. 2008;18(1):11–23. vii.
4. Penfield JD, Lang DM, Goldblum JR, Lopez R, Falk GW. The role of allergy evaluation in adults with eosinophilic esophagitis. J Clin Gastroenterol. 2010;44(1):22–7.
5. Roy-Ghanta S, Larosa DF, Katzka DA. Atopic characteristics of adult patients with eosinophilic esophagitis. Clin Gastroenterol Hepatol. 2008;6(5):531–5.
6. Straumann A, Spichtin HP, Grize L, Bucher KA, Beglinger C, Simon HU. Natural history of primary eosinophilic esophagitis: a follow-up of 30 adult patients for up to 11.5 years. Gastroenterology. 2003;125(6):1660–9.
7. Simon D, Marti H, Heer P, Simon HU, Braathen LR, Straumann A. Eosinophilic esophagitis is frequently associated with IgE-mediated allergic airway diseases. J Allergy Clin Immunol. 2005;115(5):1090–2.
8. Katzka DA. Demographic data and symptoms of eosinophilic esophagitis in adults. Gastrointest Endosc Clin N Am. 2008;18(1):25–32. viii.
9. Pasha SF, DiBaise JK, Kim HJ, et al. Patient characteristics, clinical, endoscopic, and histologic findings in adult eosinophilic esophagitis: a case series and systematic review of the medical literature. Dis Esophagus. 2007;20(4):311–9.
10. Assa'ad AH, Putnam PE, Collins MH, et al. Pediatric patients with eosinophilic esophagitis: an 8-year follow-up. J Allergy Clin Immunol. 2007;119(3):731–8.
11. Liacouras CA, Spergel JM, Ruchelli E, et al. Eosinophilic esophagitis: a 10-year experience in 381 children. Clin Gastroenterol Hepatol. 2005;3(12):1198–206.
12. Patel SM, Falchuk KR. Three brothers with dysphagia caused by eosinophilic esophagitis. Gastrointest Endosc. 2005;61(1):165–7.
13. Meyer GW. Eosinophilic esophagitis in a father and a daughter. Gastrointest Endosc. 2005;61(7):932.
14. Noel RJ, Putnam PE, Rothenberg ME. Eosinophilic esophagitis. N Engl J Med. 2004;351(9): 940–1.
15. Kagalwalla AF, Sentongo TA, Ritz S, et al. Effect of six-food elimination diet on clinical and histologic outcomes in eosinophilic esophagitis. Clin Gastroenterol Hepatol. 2006;4(9):1097–102.
16. Simon D, Straumann A, Wenk A, Spichtin H, Simon HU, Braathen LR. Eosinophilic esophagitis in adults – no clinical relevance of wheat and rye sensitizations. Allergy. 2006;61(12):1480–3.
17. Gonsalves N. Food allergies and eosinophilic gastrointestinal illness. Gastroenterol Clin North Am. 2007;36(1):75–91. vi.
18. Gonsalves N, Yang G, Doerfler B, Ritz S, Ditto AM, Hirano I. 727 A Prospective Clinical Trial of Six Food Elimination Diet and Reintroduction of Causative Agents in Adults with Eosinophilic Esophagitis (EE). Gastroenterology. 2008;134(4 Suppl 1):A-104–5.
19. Bernstein IL, Li JT, Bernstein DI, et al. Allergy diagnostic testing: an updated practice parameter. Ann Allergy Asthma Immunol. 2008;100(3 Suppl 3):S1–148.
20. Anton Remirez J, Escudero R, Caceres O, Fernandez-Benitez M. Eosinophilic esophagitis. Allergol Immunopathol (Madr). 2006;34(2):79–81.
21. Furuta GT, Liacouras CA, Collins MH, et al. Eosinophilic esophagitis in children and adults: a systematic review and consensus recommendations for diagnosis and treatment. Gastroenterology. 2007;133(4):1342–63.
22. Spergel JM. Eosinophilic esophagitis in adults and children: evidence for a food allergy component in many patients. Curr Opin Allergy Clin Immunol. 2007;7(3):274–8.

23. Spergel JM, Andrews T, Brown-Whitehorn TF, Beausoleil JL, Liacouras CA. Treatment of eosinophilic esophagitis with specific food elimination diet directed by a combination of skin prick and patch tests. Ann Allergy Asthma Immunol. 2005;95(4):336–43.
24. Sugnanam KK, Collins JT, Smith PK, et al. Dichotomy of food and inhalant allergen sensitization in eosinophilic esophagitis. Allergy. 2007;62(11):1257–60.
25. Fogg MI, Ruchelli E, Spergel JM. Pollen and eosinophilic esophagitis. J Allergy Clin Immunol. 2003;112(4):796–7.
26. Almansa C, Krishna M, Buchner AM, et al. Seasonal distribution in newly diagnosed cases of eosinophilic esophagitis in adults. Am J Gastroenterol. 2009;104(4):828–33.
27. Onbasi K, Sin AZ, Doganavsargil B, Onder GF, Bor S, Sebik F. Eosinophil infiltration of the oesophageal mucosa in patients with pollen allergy during the season. Clin Exp Allergy. 2005;35(11):1423–31.
28. Spiegel A, Wolf DC, Sperber K, Gimenez C. An unusual presentation of eosinophilic esophagitis. Gastrointest Endosc. 2009;70(2):382–3. discussion 383.
29. Mishra A, Hogan SP, Brandt EB, Rothenberg ME. An etiological role for aeroallergens and eosinophils in experimental esophagitis. J Clin Invest. 2001;107(1):83–90.
30. Assa'ad A. Eosinophilic esophagitis: association with allergic disorders. Gastrointest Endosc Clin N Am. 2008;18(1):119–32. x.

Chapter 19
Allergy Testing in Eosinophilic Esophagitis

Antonella Cianferoni and Jonathan Spergel

Keywords Food allergy • Allergy testing • Skin testing • Patch testing • Eosinophilic esophagitis

Introduction: Allergy Testing

Atopy and allergic responses have been strongly implicated in the etiology of Eosinophilic Esophagitis (EoE) based on several lines of epidemiological, molecular biology and clinical and evidences.

1. From an epidemiologic prospective, the prevalence of EoE is the highest and continues to rise in the western country mirroring the demographics of atopic disease [1–5].
2. Substantial evidence is accumulating that EoE is associated with T helper cell (Th) 2 type immune responses (the type of T helper cell polarization seen in allergic individuals). In particular, elevated levels of eosinophil-active Th2 cytokines [e.g., interleukin (IL)-4, IL-5, and IL-13] as well as mast cells are present in the esophagus of EoE patients [6–8]. In addition, experimental animal models of EoE can be induced in mice by allergen exposure, as well as by over-expression of Th2 cytokines (IL-5 and IL-13) [9–12] Collectively, these data demonstrate an intimate connection between the development of eosinophilic inflammation in the respiratory tract and esophagus not only in response to external allergic triggers but also to intrinsic Th2 cytokines.
3. Clinically up to 80% of patients with EoE have been reported to be atopic based on the coexistence of atopic dermatitis (AD), allergic rhinitis (AR), food allergy

J. Spergel (✉)
Department of Pediatrics, Division of Allergy and Immunology, The Children's Hospital of Philadelphia, 34th Street and Civic Center Blvd, Philadelphia, PA 19104, USA
e-mail: spergel@email.chop.edu

C.A. Liacouras and J.E. Markowitz (eds.), *Eosinophilic Esophagitis*, Clinical Gastroenterology, DOI 10.1007/978-1-60761-515-6_19,

(FA) and/or asthma and the presence of allergic antigen sensitization based on skin prick testing or measurement of plasma antigen-specific IgE [13]. It is interesting to note that patients with EoE sometimes report seasonal variations in their symptoms and/or seasonal changes in esophageal eosinophil levels [14]. Even more importantly, most patients become symptom free and the esophageal lesions greatly improve on allergen-free elemental diets, providing supportive evidence that food-allergens are triggering the disease [4, 15].

EoE and Atopic Diseases

Atopy involves an exaggerated immune response to common environmental allergens. Atopic diseases, such as asthma, AR, FA, or AD, have common features: inflammation (often eosinophilic), hyperresponsiveness to stimuli, remodeling of tissues, and Th2 cellular production [16–19].

We and others have reported that the prevalence of atopy among children and adults with EoE is greater than in the general population. Indeed in patients with EoE, atopy has been reported with a prevalence between 40 and 93% [4, 20–24] vs. only 20% of adults and children in the general population in western countries [25–27].

At our institution, a 14-year follow-up of more than 600 pediatric patients who had EoE showed that two thirds had evidence of other allergic disease, approximately threefold greater than the general population [4]. Data from Cincinnati also indicated a high prevalence of environmental (79%) and food allergies (75%) in children who had EoE [23]. Simon et al. have described a similar pattern of increased atopy in 31 adult patients who had EoE. Of these adult patients who had EoE, 68% experienced asthma, AD, or AR [28]. The reported incidence of actual food-induced anaphylaxis has been between 8.1 and 24% [4, 21, 23, 24], with an incidence similar to the one reported in AD [29], which has a similar mechanism suggesting a non-IgE-mediated reaction or mixed reactions for both diseases.

EoE and Food Allergens

Foods have been shown to be the cause of EoE through the use of elimination diets or elemental formulas [4, 15]. Elemental diets have demonstrated resolution of symptoms and normalization of biopsies in greater than 95% of the patients [4, 13]. Such efficacy of the elemental diet was originally reported by Kelly et al., who examined ten children who had persistent gastroesophageal reflux disease (GERD) and esophageal eosinophilia refractory to pharmacotherapy and/or Nissen fundoplication as a treatment of medically resistant GERD. Following a 6-week trial of elemental formula, a significant decrease in esophageal eosinophils and clinical symptoms was observed in all of the patients, with eight patients demonstrating complete resolution [15]. At our institution, in our last published report of 381 EoE patients treated with an elemental diet, 97% achieved symptom resolution and esophageal biopsy normalization [4, 13], which remains consistent in our current population of nearly 900 EoE patients. Because of the poor palatability of elemental formulas, elimination diets based on skin prick tests (SPTs) and atopy patch tests (APTs) [30, 31] or removal of the most common food allergens [32] have been tried with rates of improvement of 70–80%. Indeed the use of specific elimination diets of foods identified by skin prick testing and patch testing led to improvement in 75% of cases [13]. Kagalwalla et al. [32], demonstrated improvement of EoE after implementation of an empiric six-food elimination diet. After a 6-week elimination of six most common food allergens (milk, soy, egg, wheat, peanuts, tree nuts, and seafood) from the diets of 35 EoE patients, they found significant improvement in 74% of patients on the six-food elimination group, as compared with an 88% response in children treated with an elemental diet. However, removal of the most common food allergens did not reduce eosinophils to a normal range (13.6 eosinophils/HPF) [32] whereas elimination diets when effective based on SPT and APT testing reduce counts to 1.1 eosinophils/HPF [30, 31] and elemental diets [13] reduced eosinophil counts to a normal range of 0 eosinophils/HPF.

The mechanism underlying the immunologic reaction to foods in EoE is not only IgE mediated but also cell mediated, as in atopic AD. Indeed, after ingestion of the offending food, symptoms may develop within 2 h, as with anaphylaxis or certain type of AD, can be delayed several hours, as reported by Kelly et al. [15], or even days or months. Moreover, Kelly et al. [15] demonstrated that the introduction of skin test – negative foods into the diet could induce clinical disease. To help address this issue, we have used patch testing as a tool for identifying delayed, cell-mediated allergic reactions in EoE. In pediatric patients, this testing method, along with skin prick testing, has been shown to be effective in guiding management. The combination of skin prick and patch testing had a negative predictive value of 88–100% for 20 foods (except milk), whereas the positive predictive value was greater than 74% for the most common foods causing EoE [33].

The link between foods and EoE is not as clear in adult patients because limited data exist regarding the use and efficacy of elemental and elimination diets. In one study, six adults with EoE and sensitization (shown by skin tests positivity) to wheat/rye wheat failed to respond to antigen removal [34]. However, these patients were also sensitized to grass pollen, which can account for the wheat/rye sensitization due to cross reactivity. Moreover, a series of case reports published in an abstract form indicate that diet may be helpful in adults. For example, Gonsalves reported a 50% response rate in adults on a six food elimination diet and near 100% resolution on an elemental diet [35].

EoE and Aeroallergens

Some evidence suggests that aeroallergens may play a causative role in the development of EoE in humans. A seasonal variation in cases of newly diagnosed EoE has been described, with fewer cases being diagnosed in the winter when the air contains less pollen [36]. During pollen season there is an increased number of eosinophils in patients with AR compared to normal controls, although the number of eosinophils observed was lower than values typically seen in patients who have EoE [14]. In our EoE population, we have confirmed seasonal/pollen variation in 55 patients, with worsening symptoms and esophageal eosinophilia during pollen seasons. Food allergies were still the primary cause of disease in these patients. However, during pollen season in the spring or fall, an exacerbation of disease (confirmed by biopsy) was documented. Full disease control was achieved only during non-pollen seasons and on proper dietary therapy [4]. Although direct deposition of pollens onto the esophageal mucosa is one potential mechanism for inflammation, experimental evidence points toward other potential mechanisms such as eotaxin secretion upon aeroallergen stimulation resulting in eosinophil migration into the esophagus. Indeed, eotaxin is over-expressed in patients with EoE and during the pollen season they may have excessive production that facilitates the recruitment of eosinophils in the esophagus [37]. Interestingly, intranasal steroid therapy has been shown to decrease nasal secretion of eotaxin in patients who have AR [38]. Hence, aggressive treatment of AR with topical steroids is highly recommended in a patient with EoE [39].

Allergic Evaluation of EoE Patients

History

History is very important in management of EoE. The patient's history must focus on possible triggers or seasonal variation of EoE. The patient needs to be asked specifically if any food seems to trigger the EoE. Many times, patients intuitively avoid foods that may exacerbate their disease, so even if the patient cannot cite any offending foods, the caregiver also needs to ask if the patient is limiting the intake of any particular food [4]. Because of the high rate of allergic rhinitis, asthma, and/or eczema in EoE patients, a complete evaluation by a well-informed allergist for food allergy and other atopic diatheses is recommended [40].

Skin Prick Testing for Antigen Sensitization

Skin prick testing for foods and environmental allergens should be considered so that potential allergens and the atopic status of EoE patients are identified. Skin prick tests should be performed using commercially available extracts. Using a needle, the operator should prick through a drop of the extract, which will be then absorbed. Positive histamine and negative diluent controls need also be used.

Reactions need to be recorded on the basis of the largest diameter (in millimeters) of the wheal and flare at 15 min. A wheal of 3 mm greater than the negative control is considered positive. Fifteen studies involving 12 case series and 3 case reports have examined skin prick testing in EE patients. In adults, positive skin tests to food allergens have been difficult to elicit, whereas positive skin tests to environmental allergens are more frequently found than positive reactions to food antigens [28]. In pediatric patients, more comprehensive studies have been reported [4, 30]. Approximately two thirds of patients have positive skin tests to at least one food allergen. The most common foods reported to be positive by skin prick tests included common food allergens – cow's milk, eggs, soy, wheat – in addition to potato, corn, chicken, rice, and beef. Peanuts and nuts were reported positive in a small subgroup of patients.

As history is often not enough to delineate which food may be implicated in triggering EoE, large food panels are recommended that should include all the foods suspected by history, plus the common food allergens – cow milk, eggs, peanuts, soy, wheat – as well as representative members of classes of foods including grains (oat, rye, barely, corn, rice), meats (chicken, beef, turkey, pork), seafood (seafood and fish mix), fruits (apple, peach), and vegetables (carrots, potato). If there is a clinical history of EoE triggered by vegetable and/or fruit that come back negative by SPT using commercially available extracts, the prick by prick technique using fresh vegetables and/or fruit should be tried, as the commercially available extracts may contain degraded allergens [41]. All foods that are positive should be eliminated from the diet. Those that are negative from this panel should be tested as Atopy Patch Tests.

Atopy Patch Testing in EoE

Atopy patch testing (APT) has been used for the diagnosis of non-IgE, cell-mediated immune responses in which T cells are thought to play a prominent role. Indeed, their role is well established in the evaluation of contact dermatitis. In the evaluation of food allergy, APT has been most extensively studied in AD. After the first controlled trial on patch testing in eczema published in 1982 [42], several studies have found that APT is better in identifying late reactions and GI reactions in children with atopic dermatitis [43–45]. APT involves prolonged contact of the allergen to the skin with the goal of mimicking a similar immune response to AD. In fact, biopsy specimens of the patch test sites typically show an initial Th2 cell infiltration followed by a predominance of Th1 cytokines and eosinophils [46] similar to the biopsy findings that have been observed in the skin of atopic dermatitis patients in acute and chronic lesions [18]. The food to be tested is typically placed in aluminum cups (Finn Chambers on Scanpore; Allerderm Laboratories, Inc. Petaluma, CA) and then applied to uninvolved areas of the patient's back in the 12-mm chambers [30]. Similar to patch testing for contact dermatitis, a 48-h occlusion time is used, and the patches are subsequently read at 24 h after removal of the Finn chamber, examining for erythema, papules, and induration [47, 48]. Any food can be assessed with patch testing, although cow's milk, egg, wheat, and soy have been studied most extensively [33]. We have used APT diagnosis of food allergies in EoE extensively [30, 33]. We examined 361 children in our last published series on this topic with biopsy specimen-diagnosed EoE, and eliminated foods based on positive skin test and atopy patch test. We found that 77% of the patients had resolution of their esophageal biopsy abnormalities based on these results (including 14% that required elemental formulas because of the multiple positive food allergies). Greater than 98% of the population responded to an elemental diet [13] suggesting that patients who failed testing did not have the correct foods identified. The same panel of food used in SPT should be used, less those foods that came back positive at SPT.

The combined positive values of SPT and APT should guide the diagnosis of food allergy. We have calculated the positive and negative predictive values (PPV and NPV) of the single and combined testing and found that the combination of the two tests yielded the best PPV and NPV [49]. Indeed, when we examined a subgroup of patients in whom we could definitively identify the foods that were causing the disease and calculated the negative predictive values (NPVs), positive predictive values (PPVs), specificity, and sensitivity for SPT and APT. All patients in this cohort had EoE on the basis of >20 eosinophils per HPF after at least 1 month treatment with a proton pump inhibitor. The group used for statistical evaluation were patients for whom we could identify the individual foods that caused EoE on the basis of the following:

1. Removal of an individual food led to normal esophageal biopsy (0 eosinophils/HPF), and/or
2. Addition of an individual food led to increased esophageal eosinophils (greater than 20 eosinophils/HPF) on biopsy after a previously normal biopsy.

This subgroup was similar to our entire EoE cohort of 316 patients who have undergone APT and SPT. However, these patients had biopsies 1–2 months after single food introduction or removal of an individual food. The most common foods for APT in the entire cohort and the subcohort were the same: milk, wheat, corn, beef, egg, potato, chicken, soy, barley, oat, and rice. The PPVs and NPVs along with specificity and sensitivity were calculated on the basis of identification of single foods causing increased eosinophils in biopsies. The values are listed for the 12 most common foods in Tables 19.1 and 19.2. Milk and egg were the most common foods causing EoE in 46 and 39 patients, respectively. The PPV for SPT was greater than 75% for milk, egg, beef, and peanut. This is better than traditional skin testing for IgE-mediated reactions, with PPV reported around 50% [50]. The predictive value for APT ranged from 94% for beef to 54% for potato. The specificity for APT ranged from 43 to 89%, lower than the reported 91% for APT in atopic dermatitis (AD) [51]. Like all allergy testing, SPT and APT are not perfect but serve as a guide for diet evaluation.

Table 19.1 Predictive values for SPT and APT

	SPT				APT			
Food	PPV (%)	NPV (%)	Specificity (%)	Sensitivity (%)	PPV (%)	NPV (%)	Specificity (%)	Sensitivity (%)
Milk (n=46)	95.7	57.7	42.3	97.6	83.3	58.7	43.5	90.2
Egg (n=39)	84.8	75.4	65.1	90.2	78.3	82.8	62.1	91.4
Soy (n=28)	70.0	68.9	37.8	89.5	66.7	87.3	66.7	87.3
Wheat (n=26)	77.8	64.7	18.9	96.5	74.2	83.9	71.9	85.5
Corn (n=26)	57.1	71.3	13.8	95.4	65.8	93.9	89.3	78.0
Beef (n=23)	81.8	74.7	30.0	96.9	94.4	87.0	65.4	98.4
Chicken (n=15)	50.0	83.3	26.3	93.3	66.7	95.7	80.0	91.7
Rice (n=14)	50.0	85.6	13.3	97.5	59.1	96.9	86.7	87.5
Potato (n=11)	60.0	89.9	25.0	97.6	53.8	94.6	63.6	92.1
Peanut (n=10)	77.8	97.6	77.8	97.6	75.0	97.6	60.0	98.8
Oat (n=9)	33.3	90.1	10.0	97.6	47.4	98.5	90.0	87.0
Barley (n=9)	42.9	90.8	27.3	95.2	90.0	98.7	90.0	98.7

n = number of patients with positive change in biopsy after diet modification

Table 19.2 Predictive values for the combination of SPT and APT

Food	Combined SPT and APT			
	PPV (%)	NPV (%)	Specificity (%)	Sensitivity (%)
Milk	92.0	40.9	63.9	81.8
Egg	84.8	87.5	86.7	85.7
Soy	73.7	92.9	87.5	83.9
Wheat	76.5	90.0	81.3	87.1
Corn	63.4	92.5	86.7	76.6
Beef	85.2	92.5	82.1	93.9
Chicken	62.5	98.6	93.8	88.5
Apple	57.1	97.7	66.7	96.6
Rice	60.9	100.0	100.0	88.8
Potato	61.1	97.4	84.6	91.4
Peanut	71.4	100.0	100.0	95.2
Oat	50.0	100.0	100.0	89.4
Barley	73.3	100.0	100.0	95.2

Because EoE is most likely a mixed IgE and non-IgE food-mediated reaction, the combination of SPT and APT in the management of EoE has been found to be effective and indeed the combination of the two testing methods had an excellent NPV (88–100%) for all foods except milk, which was very low at 41% (Table 19.2). The PPV was greater than 74% for the most common foods (milk, egg, and soy), but dropped off as the food became a less common cause of EoE. Similarly, the sensitivity for identification of foods causing EoE ranged from 77 to 97%, depending on the food. Therefore, the combination of SPT and APT in designing a diet plan has a high success rate for food elimination or food reintroduction in EoE with the exception of milk. Milk's NPV was unacceptably low, suggesting that a negative test to milk on SPT and APT does not rule out milk triggering EoE.

Assessment of Atopy by Analysis of Blood Samples

Peripheral eosinophil count. Overall, 10–50% of adults and 20–100% of children had elevated peripheral eosinophil counts but usually only modestly elevated (less than twofold). In all studies, there was a high percentage of concurrent allergic sensitization, and it is likely that concurrent allergic diatheses in conjunction with EoE play a role in the elevated eosinophil counts found in these patients. One study demonstrated that persistent blood eosinophilia correlated with persistent dysphagia [52]. In another study, the degree of elevation of serum eosinophils correlated with the severity of EoE [53]. Following treatment with fluticasone, 88% of patients demonstrated decreased blood eosinophil counts [54]. In another study of oral corticosteroids, most patients demonstrated decreased blood eosinophils following treatment [55]. However, there are no studies that define the PPVs and the NPVs of blood eosinophilia and has majority of EoE patients, variation in their eosinophilia can be due to changes in other atopic diseases. Moreover, most of the cited studies involve only few patients and had significant amount of variability in the defining level for "peripheral eosinophilia" (range of eosinophils reported as abnormal ranged from greater than 350 eosinophils per mm^3 to greater than 800 eosinophils per mm^3). Hence, routine checking of blood eosinophils is not recommended in children with EoE.

Total IgE

Similar to peripheral blood eosinophilia, only few studies with a limited number of patients have reported the total level of IgE and the defining criteria for abnormal values varied among studies, thus making broad conclusions difficult. Overall, 71–78% of pediatric EoE patients and 60–69% of adult EoE patients had elevated total IgE levels [8, 28, 33, 52, 54, 55]. The high rate of concurrent atopic diatheses in these patients suggests that elevated IgE levels were likely not linked specifically to EoE. No published studies document whether or not total IgE can serve as a surrogate marker for disease progression or resolution, hence we are not currently routinely measuring their levels.

Food-Specific IgE

Currently there are no positive or negative predictive values for food-specific IgE level testing in EoE. Indeed only a limited number of studies have used specific serum IgE in the evaluation of food allergy in children with EoE [56–58]. No studies were able to design a successful food specific-based elimination diet based on the food specific serum IgE levels. Hence, in vitro food allergy testing is not supported in the evaluation of EoE patients at this time, and empiric food testing should utilize skin prick tests. In case of impossibility of performing skin test (specific IgE for example, severe atopic dermatitis or unable to stop antihistamines) can substitute for skin testing.

Food-Specific IgG

Food-specific IgG is part of a normal physiological response to food and is not useful in testing for any allergy. It is not recommend by any of the national/international allergy societies [59]. There is no evidence for using other methods including lymphocyte proliferation, basophil release, facial thermography, gastric juice analysis, cytotoxic assays, electrodermal test, or mediator Release Assay (LEAP diet).

Aeroallergen-Specific IgE

Although the presence of allergic rhinitis is cited in multiple studies, one adult study specifically delineates the presence of antigen-specific IgE to specific allergens (grass, a potential cross-reacting allergen to wheat and rye) in a patient with EoE and symptoms [28]. However, several studies point to the role of aeroallergen in EoE. In fact, aeroallergens have been shown to lead to esophageal eosinophilia [14] and EoE [39] in two different studies. In addition, Sugnanman found an increased sensitization to aeroallergens with older patients [24]. Finally, there appears to be seasonality in the diagnosis of EoE with increased diagnosis in the pollen season. Given the high rate of other allergic diatheses (50–80%) in EoE patients and the potential of aeroallergens to have a role in the instigation of EoE, it is important to evaluate EoE patients for aeroallergen sensitivity. Evaluation should be done via SPT or serum-specific IgE, although SPT are generally cheaper and more sensitive in the diagnosis of aeroallergen sensitivity [60, 61].

Conclusion

There is strong clinical and mechanistic evidence that allergies play a key role in the EoE. Food Allergies have been found to be consistent trigger in the majority of both pediatric and adult patients. However, the food allergies are not "classic" food allergies as they are not IgE-mediated as the symptoms are delayed and removal of IgE-positive foods do not lead to resolution of symptoms and normalization of biopsies. Therefore, EoE appears to be a mixed IgE and non-IgE mediated food reaction.

The testing for allergies in particular food allergies is not perfect. Skin testing and atopy patch testing can have both false positive and negatives. But, in general, if a food is negative on both skin and atopy patch testing, it is unlikely that food is causing disease with the exception of milk. We use SPT and APT to guide us in developing a treatment plan (Fig. 19.1). If history and/or skin test confirm environmental allergies, they should be treated aggressively with inhaled/nasal steroids, to minimize the potential facilitation of Eosinophils recruitment in the esophagus, due to a concomitant airways inflammation and consequent eotaxin production.

As per the food allergy, an extensive SPT and APT panel should be performed and a trial of food-specific elimination diet should be tried. Patients should be re-scoped after 6 weeks. When EoE is in clinical remission (i.e., no symptoms), food should be reintroduced either individually or as select groups. Food-specific elimination diets are equally effective in causing EoE remission. If food-specific diet is not effective, alternative therapies such as Elemental diet or pharmacological therapy should be explored (Fig. 19.1).

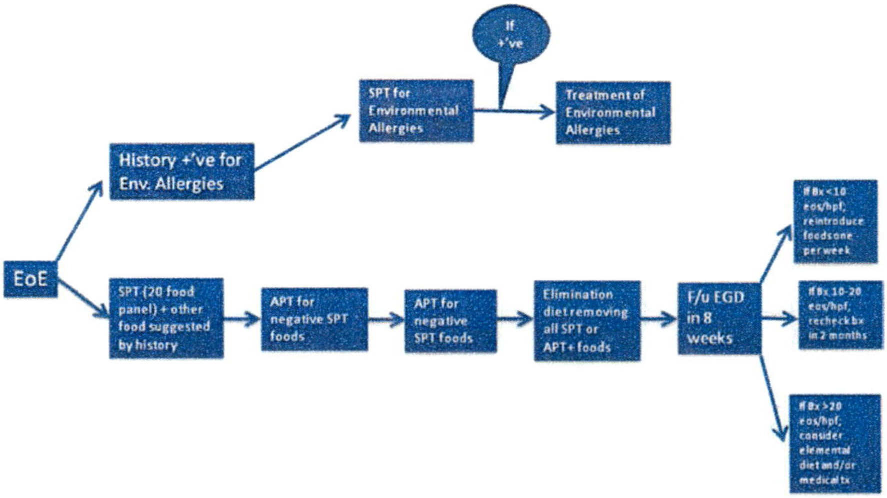

Fig. 19.1 Flow chart of EoE allergic evaluation and treatment decisions

References

1. Noel RJ, Putnam PE, Rothenberg ME. Eosinophilic esophagitis. N Engl J Med. Aug 2004;351(9):940–1.
2. Cherian S, Smith NM, Forbes DA. Rapidly increasing prevalence of eosinophilic oesophagitis in Western Australia. Arch Dis Child. Dec 2006;91(12):1000–4.
3. Franciosi JP, Tam V, Liacouras CA, Spergel JM. A case-control study of sociodemographic and geographic characteristics of 335 children with eosinophilic esophagitis. Clin Gastroenterol Hepatol. Apr 2009;7(4):415–9.
4. Spergel JM, Brown-Whitehorn TF, Beausoleil JL, et al. 14 years of eosinophilic esophagitis: clinical features and prognosis. J Pediatr Gastroenterol Nutr. Jan 2009;48(1):30–6.
5. Gupta R, Sheikh A, Strachan DP, Anderson HR. Time trends in allergic disorders in the UK. Thorax. Jan 2007;62(1):91–6.
6. Straumann A, Kristl J, Conus S, et al. Cytokine expression in healthy and inflamed mucosa: probing the role of eosinophils in the digestive tract. Inflamm Bowel Dis. Aug 2005;11(8):720–6.
7. Gupta SK, Fitzgerald JF, Kondratyuk T, HogenEsch H. Cytokine expression in normal and inflamed esophageal mucosa: a study into the pathogenesis of allergic eosinophilic esophagitis. J Pediatr Gastroenterol Nutr. Jan 2006;42(1):22–6.
8. Straumann A, Bauer M, Fischer B, Blaser K, Simon HU. Idiopathic eosinophilic esophagitis is associated with a T(H)2-type allergic inflammatory response. J Allergy Clin Immunol. Dec 2001;108(6):954–61.
9. Akei HS, Brandt EB, Mishra A, et al. Epicutaneous aeroallergen exposure induces systemic TH2 immunity that predisposes to allergic nasal responses. J Allergy Clin Immunol. Jul 2006;118(1):62–9.
10. Mishra A, Hogan SP, Brandt EB, Rothenberg ME. An etiological role for aeroallergens and eosinophils in experimental esophagitis. J Clin Invest. Jan 2001;107(1):83–90.
11. Mishra A, Hogan SP, Brandt EB, Rothenberg ME. IL-5 promotes eosinophil trafficking to the esophagus. J Immunol. Mar 2002;168(5):2464–9.

12. Mishra A, Rothenberg ME. Intratracheal IL-13 induces eosinophilic esophagitis by an IL-5, eotaxin-1, and STAT6-dependent mechanism. Gastroenterology. Nov 2003;125(5):1419–27.
13. Liacouras CA, Spergel JM, Ruchelli E, et al. Eosinophilic esophagitis: a 10-year experience in 381 children. Clin Gastroenterol Hepatol. Dec 2005;3(12):1198–206.
14. Onbasi K, Sin AZ, Doganavsargil B, Onder GF, Bor S, Sebik F. Eosinophil infiltration of the oesophageal mucosa in patients with pollen allergy during the season. Clin Exp Allergy. Nov 2005;35(11):1423–31.
15. Kelly KJ, Lazenby AJ, Rowe PC, Yardley JH, Perman JA, Sampson HA. Eosinophilic esophagitis attributed to gastroesophageal reflux: improvement with an amino acid-based formula. Gastroenterology. Nov 1995;109(5):1503–12.
16. Robinson DS, Hamid Q, Jacobson M, Ying S, Kay AB, Durham SR. Evidence for Th2-type T helper cell control of allergic disease in vivo. Springer Semin Immunopathol. 1993;15(1):17–27.
17. Spergel JM. Atopic march: link to upper airways. Curr Opin Allergy Clin Immunol. Feb 2005;5(1):17–21.
18. Bieber T. Atopic dermatitis. N Engl J Med. Apr 2008;358(14):1483–94.
19. Sampson HA. Food allergy. Part 1: Immunopathogenesis and clinical disorders. J Allergy Clin Immunol. May 1999;103(5 Pt 1):717–28.
20. Noel RJ, Putnam PE, Collins MH, et al. Clinical and immunopathologic effects of swallowed fluticasone for eosinophilic esophagitis. Clin Gastroenterol Hepatol. Jul 2004;2(7):568–75.
21. Guajardo JR, Plotnick LM, Fende JM, Collins MH, Putnam PE, Rothenberg ME. Eosinophil-associated gastrointestinal disorders: a world-wide-web based registry. J Pediatr. Oct 2002;141(4):576–81.
22. Roy-Ghanta S, Larosa DF, Katzka DA. Atopic characteristics of adult patients with eosinophilic esophagitis. Clin Gastroenterol Hepatol. May 2008;6(5):531–5.
23. Assa'ad AH, Putnam PE, Collins MH, et al. Pediatric patients with eosinophilic esophagitis: an 8-year follow-up. J Allergy Clin Immunol. Mar 2007;119(3):731–8.
24. Sugnanam KK, Collins JT, Smith PK, et al. Dichotomy of food and inhalant allergen sensitization in eosinophilic esophagitis. Allergy. Nov 2007;62(11):1257–60.
25. Ait-Khaled N, Pearce N, Anderson HR, Ellwood P, Montefort S, Shah J. Global map of the prevalence of symptoms of rhinoconjunctivitis in children: The International Study of Asthma and Allergies in Childhood (ISAAC) Phase Three. Allergy. Jan 2009;64(1):123–48.
26. Pearce N, Ait-Khaled N, Beasley R, et al. Worldwide trends in the prevalence of asthma symptoms: phase III of the International Study of Asthma and Allergies in Childhood (ISAAC). Thorax. Sep 2007;62(9):758–66.
27. Bernardini R, Novembre E, Lombardi E, et al. Prevalence of and risk factors for latex sensitization in patients with spina bifida. J Urol. Nov 1998;160(5):1775–8.
28. Simon D, Marti H, Heer P, Simon HU, Braathen LR, Straumann A. Eosinophilic esophagitis is frequently associated with IgE-mediated allergic airway diseases. J Allergy Clin Immunol. May 2005;115(5):1090–2.
29. Eigenmann PA, Sicherer SH, Borkowski TA, Cohen BA, Sampson HA. Prevalence of IgE-mediated food allergy among children with atopic dermatitis. Pediatrics. Mar 1998;101(3):E8.
30. Spergel JM, Beausoleil JL, Mascarenhas M, Liacouras CA. The use of skin prick tests and patch tests to identify causative foods in eosinophilic esophagitis. J Allergy Clin Immunol. Feb 2002;109(2):363–8.
31. Spergel JM, Brown-Whitehorn T. The use of patch testing in the diagnosis of food allergy. Curr Allergy Asthma Rep. Jan 2005;5(1):86–90.
32. Kagalwalla AF, Sentongo TA, Ritz S, et al. Effect of six-food elimination diet on clinical and histologic outcomes in eosinophilic esophagitis. Clin Gastroenterol Hepatol. Sep 2006;4(9):1097–102.
33. Spergel JM, Andrews T, Brown-Whitehorn TF, Beausoleil JL, Liacouras CA. Treatment of eosinophilic esophagitis with specific food elimination diet directed by a combination of skin prick and patch tests. Ann Allergy Asthma Immunol. Oct 2005;95(4):336–43.
34. Simon D, Straumann A, Wenk A, Spichtin H, Simon HU, Braathen LR. Eosinophilic esophagitis in adults – no clinical relevance of wheat and rye sensitizations. Allergy. Dec 2006;61(12):1480–3.

35. Gonsalves N. Food allergies and eosinophilic gastrointestinal illness. Gastroenterol Clin North Am. Mar 2007;36(1):75–91. vi.
36. Wang FY, Gupta SK, Fitzgerald JF. Is there a seasonal variation in the incidence or intensity of allergic eosinophilic esophagitis in newly diagnosed children? J Clin Gastroenterol. May-June 2007;41(5):451–3.
37. Blanchard C, Wang N, Stringer KF, et al. Eotaxin-3 and a uniquely conserved gene-expression profile in eosinophilic esophagitis. J Clin Invest. Feb 2006;116(2):536–47.
38. Greiff L, Petersen H, Mattsson E, et al. Mucosal output of eotaxin in allergic rhinitis and its attenuation by topical glucocorticosteroid treatment. Clin Exp Allergy. Aug 2001;31(8):1321–7.
39. Fogg MI, Ruchelli E, Spergel JM. Pollen and eosinophilic esophagitis. J Allergy Clin Immunol. Oct 2003;112(4):796–7.
40. Furuta GT, Liacouras CA, Collins MH, et al. Eosinophilic esophagitis in children and adults: a systematic review and consensus recommendations for diagnosis and treatment. Gastroenterology. Oct 2007;133(4):1342–63.
41. Webber CM, England RW. Oral allergy syndrome: a clinical, diagnostic, and therapeutic challenge. Ann Allergy Asthma Immunol. Feb 2010;104(2):101–8. quiz 109–110, 117.
42. Mitchell EB, Crow J, Chapman MD, Jouhal SS, Pope FM, Platts-Mills TA. Basophils in allergen-induced patch test sites in atopic dermatitis. Lancet. Jan 1982;1(8264):127–30.
43. Kalach N, Soulaines P, de Boissieu D, Dupont C. A pilot study of the usefulness and safety of a ready-to-use atopy patch test (Diallertest) versus a comparator (Finn Chamber) during cow's milk allergy in children. J Allergy Clin Immunol. Dec 2005;116(6):1321–6.
44. Isolauri E, Turjanmaa K. Combined skin prick and patch testing enhances identification of food allergy in infants with atopic dermatitis. J Allergy Clin Immunol. Jan 1996;97(1 Pt 1):9–15.
45. Kekki OM, Turjanmaa K, Isolauri E. Differences in skin-prick and patch-test reactivity are related to the heterogeneity of atopic eczema in infants. Allergy. Jul 1997;52(7):755–9.
46. Darsow U, Drzezga A, Frisch M, et al. Processing of histamine-induced itch in the human cerebral cortex: a correlation analysis with dermal reactions. J Invest Dermatol. Dec 2000;115(6):1029–33.
47. Rance F. What is the optimal occlusion time for the atopy patch test in the diagnosis of food allergies in children with atopic dermatitis? Pediatr Allergy Immunol. Feb 2004;15(1):93–6.
48. Heine RG, Verstege A, Mehl A, Staden U, Rolinck-Werninghaus C, Niggemann B. Proposal for a standardized interpretation of the atopy patch test in children with atopic dermatitis and suspected food allergy. Pediatr Allergy Immunol. May 2006;17(3):213–7.
49. Spergel JM, Brown-Whitehorn T, Beausoleil JL, Shuker M, Liacouras CA. Predictive values for skin prick test and atopy patch test for eosinophilic esophagitis. J Allergy Clin Immunol. Feb 2007;119(2):509–11.
50. Verstege A, Mehl A, Rolinck-Werninghaus C, et al. The predictive value of the skin prick test weal size for the outcome of oral food challenges. Clin Exp Allergy. Sep 2005;35(9):1220–6.
51. Darsow U, Laifaoui J, Kerschenlohr K, et al. The prevalence of positive reactions in the atopy patch test with aeroallergens and food allergens in subjects with atopic eczema: a European multicenter study. Allergy. Dec 2004;59(12):1318–25.
52. Straumann A, Spichtin HP, Grize L, Bucher KA, Beglinger C, Simon HU. Natural history of primary eosinophilic esophagitis: a follow-up of 30 adult patients for up to 11.5 years. Gastroenterology. Dec 2003;125(6):1660–9.
53. Konikoff MR, Blanchard C, Kirby C, et al. Potential of blood eosinophils, eosinophil-derived neurotoxin, and eotaxin-3 as biomarkers of eosinophilic esophagitis. Clin Gastroenterol Hepatol. Nov 2006;4(11):1328–36.
54. Esposito S, Marinello D, Paracchini R, Guidali P, Oderda G. Long-term follow-up of symptoms and peripheral eosinophil counts in seven children with eosinophilic esophagitis. J Pediatr Gastroenterol Nutr. Apr 2004;38(4):452–6.
55. Liacouras CA, Wenner WJ, Brown K, Ruchelli E. Primary eosinophilic esophagitis in children: successful treatment with oral corticosteroids. J Pediatr Gastroenterol Nutr. Apr 1998;26(4):380–5.
56. Teitelbaum JE, Fox VL, Twarog FJ, et al. Eosinophilic esophagitis in children: immunopathological analysis and response to fluticasone propionate. Gastroenterology. May 2002;122(5): 1216–25.

57. Orenstein SR, Shalaby TM, Di Lorenzo C, et al. The spectrum of pediatric eosinophilic esophagitis beyond infancy: a clinical series of 30 children. Am J Gastroenterol. Jun 2000;95(6):1422–30.
58. Croese J, Fairley SK, Masson JW, et al. Clinical and endoscopic features of eosinophilic esophagitis in adults. Gastrointest Endosc. Oct 2003;58(4):516–22.
59. Stapel SO, Asero R, Ballmer-Weber BK, et al. Testing for IgG4 against foods is not recommended as a diagnostic tool: EAACI Task Force Report. Allergy. Jul 2008;63(7):793–6.
60. Sistek D, Tschopp JM, Schindler C, et al. Clinical diagnosis of current asthma: predictive value of respiratory symptoms in the SAPALDIA study. Swiss Study on Air Pollution and Lung Diseases in Adults. Eur Respir J. Feb 2001;17(2):214–9.
61. Tschopp JM, Sistek D, Schindler C, et al. Current allergic asthma and rhinitis: diagnostic efficiency of three commonly used atopic markers (IgE, skin prick tests, and Phadiatop). Results from 8329 randomized adults from the SAPALDIA Study. Swiss Study on Air Pollution and Lung Diseases in Adults. Allergy. Jun 1998;53(6):608–13.

Chapter 20
Esophageal Dilation for Eosinophilic Esophagitis

Matthew Bohm and Joel E. Richter

Keywords Esophageal dilation • Proton pump inhibitors • Esophageal remodeling • Elemental diets

Introduction

Eosinophilic esophagitis (EoE) is a chronic inflammatory disorder of the esophagus characterized by the proton pump inhibitor-refractory accumulation of eosinophils in the esophageal epithelium (>15 intraepithelial eosinophils/HPF) in combination with a range of symptoms including dysphagia, food impaction, chest pain, abdominal pain, and vomiting [1–3]. The clinical manifestations of EoE vary with age. Children under the age of 2 years commonly present with feeding disorders; children under the age of 12 present with vomiting, abdominal pain, or vague gastroesophageal reflux disease (GERD) symptoms; and patients over the age of 12 have similar presentation to adults [1]. Nearly all adults complain of solid food dysphagia with many being "slow eaters" who meticulously chew their food. More than 50% give a history of food impaction.

The endoscopic features of EoE suggest a chronic disease progressing from the inflammatory features of furrows, microabscesses, and plaques seen predominantly in pediatric patients to esophageal remodeling characterized by the narrow caliber esophagus, strictures, and ring formation more commonly seen in adult EoE patients. The most efficacious treatment for these early inflammatory changes and their associated

J.E. Richter (✉)
Department of Medicine, Section of Gastroenterology, Temple University School of Medicine, 3401 N. Broad Street, 801 Parkinson Pavilion, Philadelphia, PA 19140, USA
e-mail: jrichter@temple.edu

C.A. Liacouras and J.E. Markowitz (eds.), *Eosinophilic Esophagitis*, Clinical Gastroenterology, DOI 10.1007/978-1-60761-515-6_20,

symptoms are anti-inflammatory medications (swallowed fluticasone, budesonide, prednisone) or restrictive and elemental diets [4–18]. On the other hand, adult EoE patients' esophageal changes typically show a lesser degree of active inflammation and more fibrotic changes due to collagen deposition in the epithelium and lamina propria. In treating adult EoE patients, esophageal dilation is often necessary to correct this fixed stenosis caused by esophageal remodeling. Dilation relieves the major symptom of solid food dysphagia and alleviates the fear of food impaction which improves quality of life. Potential side effects of too aggressive dilation are of concern, but the long-term relief seems to outweigh these complications.

This chapter will review the underlying pathophysiology producing strictures and remodeling, review in detail the available case series, discuss the role and technique of esophageal dilation in the management of adult EoE patients and its potential complications.

Pathophysiology

The structural changes of the esophagus arise from a cascade of events that begins with an influx of inflammatory cells, most importantly eosinophils into the mucosa of the esophagus, where normally they are rarely observed. These changes are discussed in more detail earlier in this book. In addition to the local inflammatory process caused by eosinophils and major basic protein (MBP), some believe GERD causes acid-peptic damage to the epithelial tight junctions increasing permeability and leading to the recruitment and exposure to inflammatory cells, including eosinophils [19–24]. Tobey and Barlow et al. first described in GERD patients the damage acid and pepsin do to the tight junctions between epithelial cells [23, 24]. The increased permeability also allows deeper penetration of gastric acid causing further injury and tissue damage leading to structural changes (fibrosis) which may affect the lower esophageal sphincter (LES) and peristalsis.

The chronic exposure to inflammatory cells from either allergic mediators or acid reflux leads to lamina propria and subepithelial fibrosis on microscopic examination and a narrowed lumen, strictures, and rings on endoscopy. Mishra et al. first reported an impressive accumulation of collagen in the epithelial mucosa, basal layer and lamina propria in the esophagus of EoE patients as well as mice with experimental EoE compared to controls [19–21]. The induction of collagen deposition was dependent on IL-5 and eotaxin as mice that were devoid of these cytokines did not display collagen deposition in their esophagus. Later, Aceves et al. examined esophageal biopsies for remodeling in seven children with EoE (average age 10.5 years, all male), seven children with GERD (average age 8.4 years, 57% male), and seven children that were normal controls (average age 11.2 years, 84% male) [25]. They found increased levels of subepithelial fibrosis and increased expression of TGF-b1 and its signaling molecule phospho-SMAD2/3 compared with patients with GERD and normal control patients. All seven patients with EoE demonstrated subepithelial fibrosis (four severe, three moderate) on hematoxylin-eosin staining

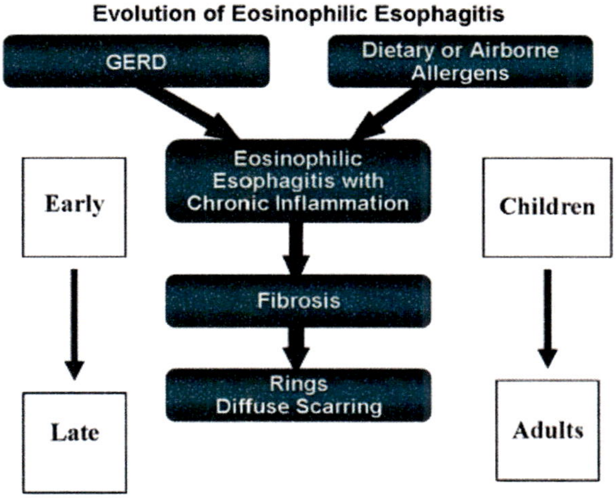

Fig. 20.1 The pathogenesis of EoEs arises from either GERD, dietary, or airborne allergens or a combination of the two. This figure illustrates the progressive evolution of EoE from a predominantly inflammatory process early on in pediatric patients leading to rings, esophageal narrowing, and stricture formation seen later in the disease in the adult population

and/or trichrome staining. Interestingly, the two youngest patients with EoE (ages five and six) had no strictures as opposed to the older EoE children whom all had strictures (range 10–14), but none had esophageal rings. However, even the two patients with EoE without strictures had increased fibrosis compared with patients with GERD and normal patients, suggesting that the remodeling process is occurring even in the absence of stricture formation.

Ultimately, the subepithelial fibrosis leads to esophageal strictures, rings, and a narrow caliber lumen which serves as a marker for disease chronicity. The ongoing inflammatory response and more importantly, the fibrotic changes produce the chronic symptoms of solid food dysphagia and food impaction characterizing the adult presentation of EoE. Thus, from childhood to adulthood, there seems to be a progressive process caused by the eosinophil infiltration that begins with inflammation and ultimately leads to fibrosis (Fig. 20.1).

Current Case Series

There are numerous pediatric EoE prospective case reports, comparison treatment studies, and even a placebo-controlled trial, but these studies rarely involve esophageal dilation. Most medical treatments are anti-inflammatory drugs targeting the reduction of mucosal eosinophilia, but sustained clinical remission is infrequent after therapy is stopped. Even the advocates of steroid therapy for EoE have found that mucosal eosinophilia and dysphagia symptoms return to baseline in at least

35% of cases over the subsequent 3–12 months after stopping anti-inflammatory drugs [10–18]. In adults, treatment studies are scarce and nearly all are case series. However, long-term clinical resolution of dysphagia symptoms has been reported with esophageal dilation and PPI therapy (Table 20.1) [26–36].

The first case series treating EoE patients with esophageal dilation appeared before the disease was well known in adults. Morrow et al. conducted a retrospective study of 19 patients (17 males; median: 35 years) diagnosed with what they called "ringed esophagus" treating them with serial esophageal dilations [26]. Of these patients, 11 (58%) reported heartburn, 17 (89%) patients had a prior food impaction, 7 (37%) had reflux on a barium swallow study and 11 (58%) had erosive esophagitis at the time of endoscopy [26]. The characteristic endoscopic appearance was a poorly distensible esophagus with multiple concentric rings located in the mid-esophagus causing significant stenosis. Esophageal biopsies showed extensive mucosal eosinophilia associated with basal cell hyperplasia and prolongation of rete pegs; the latter findings at that time considered pathognomonic of early GERD. Most patients required several sessions of esophageal dilation with Savory bougie gradually increasing dilator size to a goal diameter of 14–15 mm. No perforations occurred, but deep mucosal tears were common with several patients requiring temporary narcotic analgesia after dilation. Telephone follow-up was performed on average 19 months (±2.4 months) later with 16 (84%) patients reporting that their dysphagia improved dramatically. Using the following dysphagia scale (0 = no dysphagia, 1 = less than once a month, 2 = several times a month, 3 = several times a week, 4 = every day, not every meal and 5 = every meal), the average patient score improved from 4 to 1.2. After the initial series of dilations and the addition of PPI therapy, only one patient required repeat dilations. This patient was subsequently treated with oral prednisone and did well.

Two years after the Morrow study was published, Straumann et al. reported their prospective case series of 30 adult EoE patients (average age 40 years, 22 males) with intermittent solid food dysphagia followed for an average 7.2 years [27]. The decision to dilate was based on the frequency and severity of dysphagia symptoms with the actual dilation technique not reported. Success was evaluated with two different scales: a frequency scale where: 0 = no attacks during the last year, 1 = 1 or 2 attacks/year, 2 = 1 attack/3 months, 3 = 1 attack/month, 4 = 1 attack/week, and 5 = at least 1 attack/day; and an intensity scale where 1 = swallowing unhindered and without pain, 2 = slight retching disappearing spontaneously (spontaneous anterograde removal), 3 = short periods of obstruction necessitating intervention such as drinking, deep breathing, or retching (induced anterograde removal), 4 = longer-lasting obstruction only removable by vomiting (forced retrograde removal), and 5 = continuous complete obstruction not removable by the patient (requiring endoscopic intervention). Patients sustaining at least one attack of dysphagia per week (frequency scores 4 and 5) and those with severe attacks (intensity scores 4 and 5) were treated with esophageal dilation. Overall, 11 (37%) patients required esophageal dilation. Seven had a single dilation and four required repeat dilations. Six patients reported being free of dysphagia post-procedure and four reported a 50% reduction in their symptoms. Dysphagia improvement lasted

Table 20.1 Summary of esophageal dilation reports

Reference	Form of treatment	Type of study	No. of patients	Outcome	Complications
Morrow et al. [26]	Dilation and PPI	Case study	19 Adults	16/19 Improved clinically	Several mucosal tears; no perforations
Vasilopoulos et al. [31]	Dilation	Case study	3 Adults, 2 adolescents	5/5 Clinically improved	5/5 Mucosal tear; no perforations
Straumann et al. [27]	Dilation	Case study	11 Adults	6/11 Clinically improved at 2 year F/U	Several mucosal tears; no perforations
Croese et al. [28]	Dilation	Case study	17 Adults	16/17 Improved clinically	13/17 mucosal tears; no perforations
Potter et al. [35]	Dilation and PPI	Case study	13 Adults	7/13 Clinically improved	10/13 Mucosal tear; no perforations
Cantu et al. [29]	Dilation	Case study	2 Adults	2/2 Improved clinically	1/2 Mucosal tear; no perforations
Zimmerman et al. [30]	Dilation	Retrospective study	8 Adults	8/8 Clinically improved	Not reported
Pasha et al. [34]	Dilation	Case study	13 Adults	11/13 Adults improved clinically	6/18 Mucosal tears; no perforations
Schoepfer et al. [33]	Dilation	Case study	10 Adults	10/10 Improved clinically	7/10 Odynophagia; no perforations
Schoepfer et al. [32]	Dilation	Retrospective study	63 Adults	60/63 Clinically improved	53/63 Chest pain; no perforations
Bohm and Richter [36]	Dilation and PPI	Case study	10 Adults	8/10 Clinically improved at 2 year average F/U	1/10 Mucosal tear; no perforations

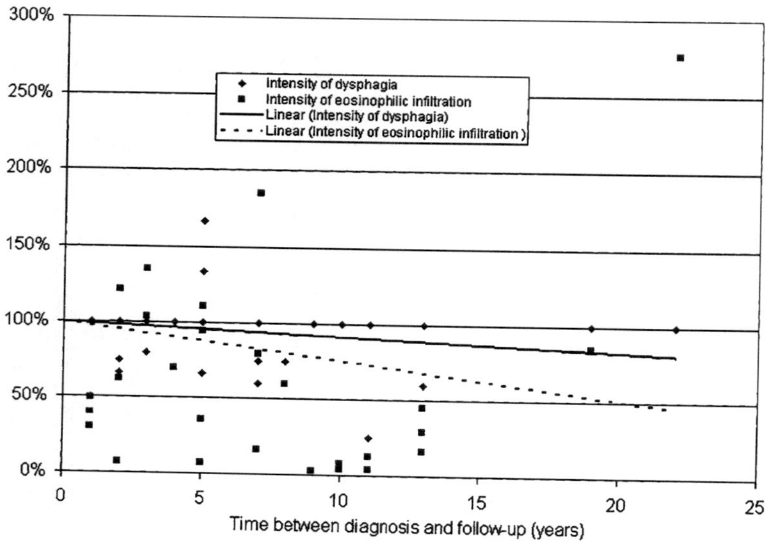

Fig. 20.2 This graph compares the intensity of dysphagia and maximum eosinophils/HPF between the time of diagnosis and follow-up of 11 EoE patients. For all patients, baseline levels of dysphagia and eosinophilic infiltration were 100% at time zero. The trends at follow-up showed a marked decrease in eosinophilic infiltration and only a slight decrease in dysphagia. Thus, the improvement in eosinophilic infiltration did not correlate with an improvement in dysphagia. From Straumann A, Spichtin HP, et al. Gastroenterology. 2003;125:1660–9, with permission

from 1 to 24 months (average 8.6 months). It was not reported if patients were using other therapies, such as PPIs. Severe mucosal tearing occurred frequently, but no perforations were noted. The average eosinophilic infiltration over the observation period decreased significantly in the proximal (78 to 40 hpf) and distal esophagus (117 to 41 hpf) (Fig. 20.2). In addition, the basal zone hyperplasia and the papillary size decreased over time. Interestingly, histological examination of the subepithelial compartments showed an impressive increase in fibrous tissue with thickening and alteration of the architecture of these layers in 6/7 patients. The patients with more dense eosinophilic infiltration (>350 eos/hpf) and more pronounced esophageal narrowing at baseline endoscopy showed a trend of more attacks and need for dilation. No dysplasia or cancer was detected during the careful follow-up of these patients.

Pasha et al. conducted a retrospective review of 42 adult EoE patients (31 men; mean age 44 years) [34]. The predominant symptom was solid food dysphagia and 23 patients had a history of food impaction. Eighteen patients underwent esophageal dilation (mean two dilations, range 1–5) ranging from 15 to 20 mm. Eleven of the 13 (85%) patients available for follow-up had improvement of their symptoms. Of these, 12 had balloon and one had bougie dilation. Five patients were dilated to a diameter of 15 mm, four dilated to 18 mm, and three dilated to 20 mm. The remaining patient was dilated with a 50 Fr Maloney bougie. One third of the patients had superficial mucosal tears, but no perforations occurred.

Croese et al. performed a retrospective review of 31 patients with EoE (all Caucasian; 24 men; mean age 34 years) [28]. Esophageal dilations were done in 17 adult patients (mean 3.4 dilations, range 1–13). This provided relief of 16 (94%) patients' chest pain, dysphagia, and dyspepsia symptoms. Mucosal tears occurred in 13 (87%) patients but no perforations occurred.

Potter et al. performed esophageal dilation in 13 adult EoE patients. Bougienage was performed by passage of polyvinyl filiform dilators under fluoroscopic monitoring in 12; a through-the-scope balloon dilator was used in one patient [35]. The dilations ranged from 30 Fr to 45 Fr with a mean of 39 Fr depending on resistance and more importantly mucosal disruption. Longitudinal mucosal tears occurred in 10/13 patients. Moderate chest pain was experienced by most patients. There were no esophageal perforations despite extensive esophageal trauma. Improvement was seen in 7/13 patients at the 3-month follow-up.

Schoepfer et al. reported a retrospective series of ten adult EoE patients with symptomatic esophageal stenosis unresponsive to topical corticosteroids [33]. Nine of the patients received swallowed fluticasone (1–2 mg/day) and one patient received swallowed budesonide (0.4 mg/day) for at least 8 weeks. Two patients were concomitantly receiving oral steroids. Eight patients had a single esophageal stricture, one patient had two strictures, and another had three strictures. The mean stricture length measured by endoscopy was 2.1 cm (range 1–6 cm). All patients were dilated using Savory bougies in millimeter increments (average number dilations: 2.7 range: 1–5 sessions). The mean diameter after dilation was 15.3 mm (range 12–19 mm). The progression of bougie diameter per session was limited to 3 mm or less to prevent complications. Bougienage led to prompt symptom relief. The average decrease in dysphagia score was 1.7–0.4 (0 = no dysphagia, 1 = able to eat solid food, 2 = semi-solids only, 3 = liquids only, 4 = complete dysphagia). Every patient had a decrease in their dysphagia score by at least one point. All patients had visible mucosal tears after upper endoscopy dilation, but no perforations occurred. Transient post-procedural odynophagia occurred in seven patients which resolved in all patients by 3 days. During the follow-up period (mean 6 months; range 2–11 months), all patients were asymptomatic with the average dysphagia score remaining at 0.4.

In the largest study to date, Schoepfer et al. utilizing a combined database from Switzerland and Northwestern Hospital in Chicago, recently reported a retrospective review of 207 adult EoE patients divided into two cohorts that underwent esophageal dilation [32]. Cohort 1 comprised 63 adult EoE patients (53 male; average age 48 years) treated only with esophageal dilation. All patients complained of solid food dysphagia, 48% had a history of prior food impaction, 17% were taking PPIs and 62% reported a history of allergies. All patients had stopped anti-inflammatory medications for a minimum of 3 months prior to esophageal dilation. Forty-four patients (70%) were diagnosed with focal esophageal strictures, three patients had a small caliber esophagus (5%), and among the remaining 16 patients' (25%) the length of esophageal narrowing was not described. Forty-six patients were dilated with Savary bougies and 17 (26%) by through-the-scope balloons. There was a median of two esophageal dilations with an improvement of esophageal diameter from an average of 11–16 mm ($p < 0.001$). This corresponded with an improvement in the dysphagia score from an average score of 1.7–0.9 ($p<0.001$). (0 = no dysphagia, 1 = able to eat solid food, 2 = semisolids only, 3 = liquids only, 4 = complete dysphagia). After dilation, 45% of patients reported complete resolution of their dysphagia and 50% complained of only minor swallowing difficulties. Dysphagia complaints slowly returned on average 23 months after dilation, but 45% were still dysphagia-free after 24 months or longer. Nearly half of the patients experienced moderate to severe pain following esophageal dilation, but there were no perforations, hospitalizations, or severe bleeding. Chest discomfort persisted for 1 day in 36% of patients, up to 3 days in 32% and 4 days or more in 32%. All patients, regardless of their level of discomfort post-procedure, were willing to undergo further esophageal dilations. Review of serial esophageal biopsies ($n=42$) allowed the investigator to assess the influence of esophageal dilation on mucosal histology. As previously reported, there was no striking change in intraepithelial eosinophil infiltration in their serial esophageal biopsies. Giemsa stains of esophageal tissues before and after dilations detected an increase in subepithelial collagen deposition in patients with longer disease duration.

Cohort 2 (114 males; mean age 42 years) included 144 adolescent and adult EoE patients treated with the combination of dilation and anti-eosinophilic medical therapy. The anti-eosinophilic treatments included topical steroids (97%), systemic steroids (6%), immunomodulators (2%), and montelukast (6%). Esophageal diameter was retrieved in 118/144 dilated patients with 78 having a pre-dilation diameter <11 mm and 70 >11 mm. Focal strictures were seen in 70 (59%) patients, extensive strictures in 14 (12%) patients, and stricture details were not recorded in 34 (29%) patients. Eighty percent of the patients were dilated with Savary bougies and 20% with through-the-scope balloons. Patients underwent an average of two dilations (range 1–8) with the average esophageal diameter increasing from 10 to 17 mm. Post-dilation the mean dysphagia score decreased from 1.9 to 1.0 ($p<0.001$). No major complications occurred. Long-term follow-up was not reported in this cohort. Therefore, both cohorts seemed to have a similar response to esophageal dilation.

We recently reported a prospective follow-up of ten adult EoE patients treated primarily with esophageal dilation [36]. All patients underwent a follow-up phone interview, office visit, repeat endoscopy with biopsies and photographs, and comprehensive allergy testing (two patients phone interviews only). Of the ten patients (eight men, two women between the ages of 27 and 58 years), eight had esophageal dilation (average: 17 mm: range 15–20 mm) at their baseline visit. Nine patients were initially treated with a PPI, usually in the morning; one patient was treated with a restrictive diet; and one patient was treated with prn swallowed fluticasone as well as a PPI. At follow-up, nine patients were still taking PPIs and one patient was on a restrictive diet attempting to eliminate soy, wheat, and nuts from his diet. All ten adult EoE patients (average 22 months; range 12–40 months) improved with our primary treatment regimen of esophageal dilation. Eight patients reported complete resolution of their dysphagia exemplified by the decrease of the group's average dysphagia scores from 2.1 to 0.3. In addition, none had a recurrent food impaction. As reported by others, the improvement in dysphagia symptoms occurred despite

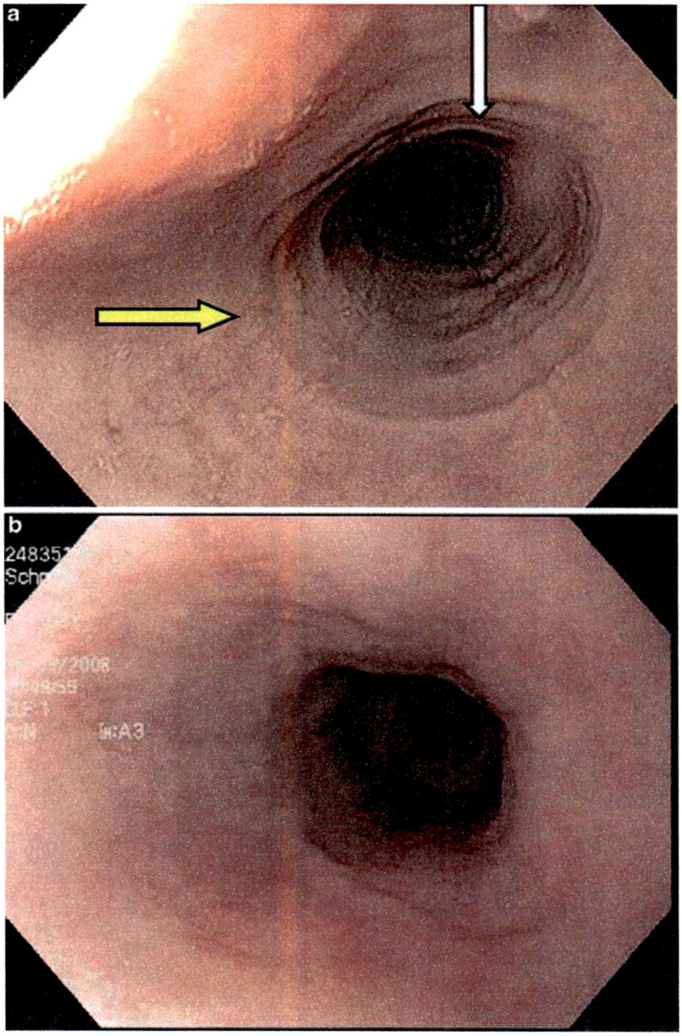

Fig. 20.3 (**a**) Endoscopic image of patient at baseline with classic rings (*white arrow*) and longitudinal furrows (*yellow arrow*). Distal eosinophil counts was 185/HPF. (**b**) At 27 months follow-up, only on PPI and after dilation to 15 mm, the endoscopic features of EoE has resolved, despite the eosinophil count still being abnormal (400/HPF proximally and 37/HPF distally)

the general absence of changes in the gross appearance of the esophagus or the eosinophilic infiltration on biopsies of the proximal and distal esophagus. However, one patient had normalization of the gross appearance of the esophagus on endoscopy (Fig. 20.3).

Overall, our review of the literature finds that a remarkable 149/160 (93%) patients treated by esophageal dilation had improvement in their dysphagia symptoms for up to 1 to 2 years with minimal complications. Three of the case series clearly showed that clinical resolution of dysphagia symptoms was independent of the degree of subepithelial eosinophil infiltration, which was unchanged after dilation. This suggests that in adult EoE patients symptom resolution rather than eosinophilic infiltration maybe a better endpoint of treatment.

Dilation Approach

There are no recommendations from our GI societies about esophageal dilation in patients with EoE. The following comments are based on our review of this literature and the senior author's experience dilating over 50 EoE patients during the last 15 years. All patients should be forewarned that pain, sometimes persisting several days, may be a problem after esophageal dilation, but true perforation with the need for hospitalization is rare. The pain responds well to reassurance and mild analgesics with infrequent need for narcotics. Since the esophageal lumen can be narrowed in multiple sites and sometimes diffusely, Savary or Maloney bougies are the dilators of choice. Dilations are performed after careful endoscopy to identify the areas of maximum narrowing and to generally size the esophageal lumen diameter. At the initial endoscopy, multiple biopsies are taken from the proximal and distal esophagus – this does not increase the chance of complications. The guiding rules are to start with a small diameter bougie, progress slowly and dilate to 15–18 mm. These esophageal diameters will allow the patient to eat a modified regular diet (15 mm – 45 Fr) or a full regular meal (18 mm – 54 Fr) [37]. As the recent literature suggests and our experience confirms, the more severely narrowed esophagus (resistance with passage of a standard 9 mm endoscope) will require 2–3 dilation sessions generally separated by several weeks. Other patients can be dilated to the desired lumen in a single session if the degree of resistance with passage of the bougie is minimal. Some authors limit the progression of bougie diameter per session to 3 mm or less [32]. Some monitor the dilations with repeating endoscopy to look for mucosal tears. This is not our approach since there is no evidence that the degree of mucosal tear correlates with chest pain or need for hospitalization. Rather, our subsequent management is guided by the post-dilation clinical scenario monitored by telephone calls, if necessary. Post-procedure Gastrograffin/barium esophagrams are reserved for the rare patient with severe pain and/or fever.

Safety and Potential Complications

The fear of esophageal perforation seems to be the area of greatest concern, limiting the use of esophageal dilation by community gastroenterologists. This is in striking contrast to the relative comfort level that gastroenterologists have in dilating peptic esophageal strictures. In patients with EoE, the esophageal wall has reduced elasticity from the extensive deposition of collagen, is fragile like "crepe paper," and prone to deep mucosal tears [38].

The most common complication of esophageal dilation and endoscopy in EoE is mucosal tears associated with a few days of chest pain or odynophagia [28, 32, 34]. Cohen et al. conducted a retrospective review over a 5-year span at a tertiary care center of endoscopic complications among 36 adult patients with EoE [39]. Complications were defined as mucosal lacerations or radiographic evidence of perforation. The mean age at presentation was 33.9 years and 28 (78%) of the patients were men. Complications occurred in 11 (31%) patients: 7 mucosal lacerations, 3 perforations with pneumomediastinum, and 1 emesis-induced rupture. Strictures were reported in 7/11 complicated cases compared with 2/25 of uncomplicated cases. Among the complicated cases with strictures, through-the-scope balloon dilators were used in four cases, bougienage dilator in one case and an endoscope as a dilator in one case. Unfortunately, the report did not mention the therapeutic interventions implemented after these complications or the final outcome. The risk of complication was higher in those with a longer duration of symptoms (13.2 years complication group vs. 6.7 years uncomplicated group) and more pronounced eosinophilic infiltration (7/9 patients with a complication showed 40 or more eosinophils/HPF compared to 12/25 patients with uncomplicated EoE).

Despite the numerous case reports of EoE patients treated with esophageal dilation, there have been only 13 reports of esophageal perforation. Four perforations were related to passage of the endoscope and six were spontaneous perforations (Boerhaave's syndrome) [41–46]. Cohen et al. reported the remaining three perforations in his retrospective review, but it is unclear what intervention or clinical scenario precipitated them [39].

Straumann et al. reported a retrospective review of 251 adolescents and adults with EoE in which three patients experienced an esophageal perforation [40]. Two of the cases were procedure related involving ENT physicians using rigid esophagoscopy to remove an impacted food bolus. The third case was elicited by retching resulting in a Boerhaave's syndrome. Eisenbach reported a case of esophageal perforation in a 17-year old girl with EoE after dilation. She was dilated to 11 mm, and post-dilation endoscopy revealed minor bleeding and mucosal lacerations. A CT scan post-procedure showed air in the para-esophageal space. Four weeks after the procedure, the air resolved and the patient remained clinically stable with no therapeutic intervention. Additionally, Kaplan et al. performed a retrospective review reporting an esophageal perforation in an adult with EoE after the passage of an endoscope. Spontaneous perforations unrelated to endoscopy or esophageal dilation have been reported in EoE patients with some patients being treated conservatively and others requiring surgery [43–46]. There have been no deaths reported in the literature from esophageal perforations suffered in EoE patients.

Conclusion

Esophageal dilation is a safe and efficacious treatment of adult EoE patients with solid food dysphagia giving more long-term relief than other available treatments. Dilation is essential to stretch the fibrosis resulting from esophageal remodeling. We believe the treatment of EoE in adults should be re-evaluated and esophageal dilation considered first-line therapy in patients with solid food dysphagia and esophageal stenosis. An algorithm for EoE patients is outlined in Fig. 20.4 with two treatment pathways depending on the appearance of the esophagus at endoscopy. Patients with active inflammation and dense eosinophilic infiltration evident endoscopically by furrows, plaques, and microabcesses are more likely to benefit from anti-inflammatory (topical or systemic) or disease-modifying immunomodulator medications. On the other hand, patients with esophageal remodeling and fibrotic changes visualized on endoscopy by strictures, rings, or a narrowed lumen achieve the greatest clinical improvement with esophageal dilation because it directly stretches and expands the esophageal lumen. Pain may be an expected side effect, but this side effect seems to be outweighed in patient satisfaction by the prolonged symptom improvement with esophageal dilation.

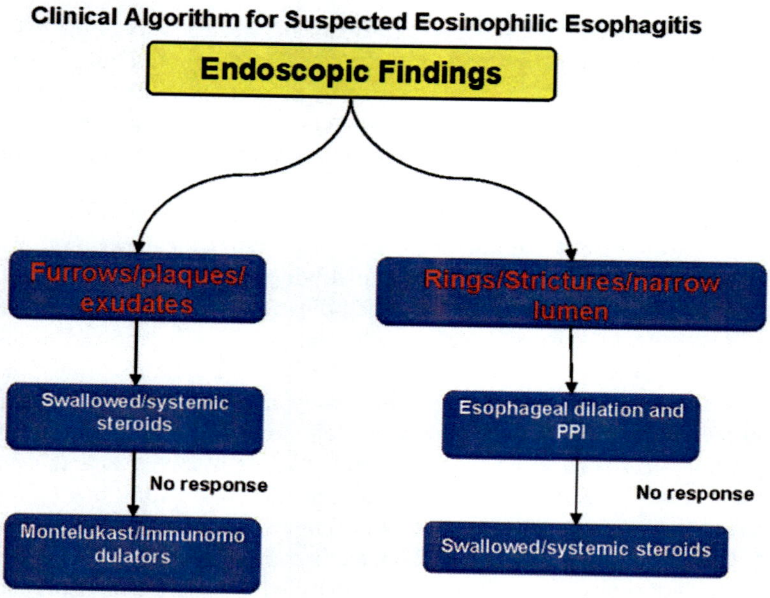

Fig. 20.4 Proposed algorithm for the treatment of patients with EoE based on initial endoscopic appearance. Those with predominantly an inflammatory process at endoscopy characterized by the presence of furrows, plaques, exudates, and microabscesses should be treated with anti-inflammatory medications or immunomodulators. On the other hand, patients with predominantly rings, strictures, or a narrowed lumen should be treated first-line with esophageal dilation and a PPI

References

1. Furuta GT, Liacouras CA, Collins MH, et al. Eosinophilic esophagitis in children and adults: a systematic review and consensus recommendations for diagnosis and treatment. Gastroenterology. 2007;133:1342–63.
2. Parfitt JR, Gregor JC, Suskin NG, et al. Eosinophilic esophagitis in adults: distinguishing features from gastroesophageal reflux disease: a study of 41 patients. Mod Pathol. 2006;19:90–6.
3. Rothenberg ME. Eosinophilic gastrointestinal disorders. J Allergy Clin Immunol. 2004;113: 11–28.
4. Spergel JM, Andrew T, Brown-Whiteorn TF, et al. Treatment of eosinophilic esophagitis with specific food elimination diet directed by a combination of skin prick and patch tests. Ann Allergy Asthma Immunol. 2005;95:336–43.
5. Kagalwalla AF, Sentongo TA, Ritz S, et al. Effects of six-food elimination diet on clinical and histological outcomes in eosinophilic esophagitis. Clin Gastroenterol Hepatol. 2006;4:1097–102.
6. Kelly K, Lazenby A, Rowe P, et al. Eosinophilic esophagitis attributed to gastroenterology reflux: improvement with amino acid based formula. Gastroenterology. 1995;109:1503–12.
7. Markowitz JE, Spergel JM, Ruchelli E, et al. Elemental diet is an effective way treatment for eosinophilic esophagitis in children and adolescents. Am J Gastroenterol. 2003;98:777–82.
8. Liacouras CA, Spergel JM, Ruchelli E, et al. Eosinophilic esophagitis: a 10-year experience in 381 children. Clin Gastroenterol Hepatol. 2005;3:1198–206.
9. Gupta S, Fitzgerald J, Davis M. Treatment of allergic eosinophilic esophagitis with oral prednisone and swallowed fluticasone: a randomized prospective study in children. Gastroenterology. 2003;124:A-19.
10. Faubion W, Perrault J, Burgart L, et al. Treatment of eosinophilic esophagitis with inhaled corticosteroids. J Pediatr Gastroenterol Nutr. 1998;27:90–3.
11. Langdon DE. Corrugated ringed esophagus. Am J Gastroenterol. 1993;88:1461.
12. Teitelbaum JE, Fox VL, Twaroj FJ, et al. Eosinophilic esophagitis in children: immunopathological analysis and response to fluticasone propionate. Gastroenterology. 2002;122:1216–25.
13. Noel RJ, Putnum PE, Collins MH, et al. Clinical and immunopathologic effects of swallowed fluticasone for eosinophilic esophagitis. Clin Gastroenterol Hepatol. 2004;2:568–75.
14. Remedios M, Campbell C, Jones DM, et al. Eosinophilic esophagitis in adults: clinical, endoscopic, histologic findings, and response to treatment with fluticasone propionate. Gastrointest Endosc. 2006;63:3–12.
15. Arora AS, Yamazaki K. Eosinophilic esophagitis: asthma of the esophagus? Clin Gastroenterol Hepatol. 2004;2:523–30.
16. Aceves SS, Bastian J, Newbury RO, Dofil R. Oral viscous budesonide: a potential new therapy for eosinophilic esophagitis in children. Am J Gastroenterol. 2007;102:2271–9.
17. Schaefer ET, Fitzgerald J, Molleston JP, et al. Comparison of oral prednisone and topical fluticasone in the treatment of eosinophilic esophagitis: a randomized trial in children. Clin Gastroenterol Hepatol. 2008;6:165–73.
18. Konikoff MR, Noel RJ, Blanchard C, et al. A randomized, double-blind, placebo-controlled trial of fluticasone propionate for pediatric eosinophilic esophagitis. Gastroenterology. 2006;131:1281–91.
19. Mishra A, Hogan SP, Brandt EB, Rothenberg ME. An etiological role for aeroallergens and eosinophils in experimental esophagitis. J Clin Invest. 2001;107:83.
20. Mishra A, Hogan SP, Brandt EB, Rothenberg ME. IL-5 promotes eosinophil trafficking to the esophagus. J Immunol. 2002;168:2464.
21. Mishra A, Rothenberg ME. Intratracheal IL-13 induces eosinophilic esophagitis by an IL-5, eotaxin-1, and STAT6-dependent mechanism. Gastroenterology. 2003;125:1419.
22. Spechler SJ, Genta R, Souza RF. Thoughts on the complex relationship between gastroesophageal reflux disease and eosinophilic esophagitis. Am J Gastroenterol. 2007;102:1301–6.
23. Tobey NA, Carson JL, Alkiek RA, et al. Dilated intercellular spaces: a morphological feature of acid reflux-damaged human esophageal epithelium. Gastroenterology. 1996;111:1200–5.

24. Barlow WJ, Orlando RC. The pathogenesis of heartburn in non-erosive disease: a unifying hypothesis. Gastroenterology. 2005;128:771–8.
25. Aceves SS, Newbury RO, Dohil R, et al. Esophageal remodeling in pediatric eosinophilic esophagitis. J Allergy Clin Immunol. 2007;119(1):206–12.
26. Morrow JB, Vargo JJ, Goldblum JR, et al. The ringed esophagus: histological features of GERD. Am J Gastroenterol. 2001;96:984–9.
27. Straumann A, Spichtin HP, Grize L, et al. Natural history of primary eosinophilic esophagitis: a follow-up of 30 adult patients for up to 11.5 years. Gastroenterology. 2003;125:1660–9.
28. Croese J, Fairley SK, Masson JW, et al. Clinical and endoscopic features of eosinophilic esophagitis in adults. Gastrointest Endosc. 2003;58:516–22.
29. Cantu P, Velio P, Prada A, et al. Ringed esophagus and idiopathic eosinophilic esophagitis in adults: an association in two cases. Dig Liver Dis. 2005;37:129–34.
30. Zimmerman SL, Levine MS, Rubesin SE, et al. Idiopathic eosinophilic esophagitis in adults: the ringed esophagus. Radiology. 2005;236:159–65.
31. Vasilopoulos S, Murphy P, Auerbach A, et al. The small-caliber esophagus: an unappreciated cause of dysphagia for solids in patients with eosinophilic esophagitis. Gastrointest Endosc. 2002;55:99–106.
32. Schoepfer AM, Gonsalves N, Bussmann C, et al. Esophageal dilation in eosinophilic esophagitis: effectiveness, safety, and impact on the underlying inflammation. Am J Gastroenterol. 2010;105(5):1062–70.
33. Schoepfer AM, Gschossmann J, Scheurer U, et al. Esophageal strictures in eosinophilic esophagitis: dilation is an effective and safe therapeutic alternative after failure of topical corticosteroids. Endoscopy. 2008;40:161–4.
34. Pasha SF, Sharma K, Crowell MD. Current concepts and treatment options in eosinophilic esophagitis. Curr Opin Investig Drugs. 2006;7:992–6.
35. Potter JW, Saeian K, Staff D, et al. Eosinophilic esophagitis in adults: an emerging problem with unique esophageal features. Gastrointest Endosc. 2004;59:355–61.
36. Bohm M, Richter JE, Kelsen SG, Thomas R. Esophageal dilation: a simple and effective treatment for adults with eosinophilic esophagitis and esophageal rings and narrowing. Dis Esophagus. 2010;23(5):377–85.
37. Goldschmid S, Boyce Jr HW, Brown JI, et al. A new objective measurement of esophageal lumen patency. Am J Gastroenterol. 1989;84(10):1255–8.
38. Straumann A, Rossi L, Simon HU, et al. Fragility of the esophageal mucosa: a pathognomonic endoscopic sign of primary eosinophilic esophagitis? Gastrointest Endosc. 2003;57:407–12.
39. Cohen MS, Kaufman AB, Palazzo JP, et al. An audit of endoscopic complications in adult eosinophilic esophagitis. Clin Gastroenterol Hepatol. 2007;5:1149–53.
40. Straumann A, Bussmann C, Zuber M, et al. Eosinophilic esophagitis: analysis of food impaction and perforation in 251 adolescent and adult patients. Clin Gastroenterol Hepatol. 2008;6:598–600.
41. Eisenbach C, Merle U, Schirmacher P. Perforation of the esophagus after dilation treatment for dysphagia in a patient with eosinophilic esophagitis. Endoscopy. 2006;38 Suppl 2:E43–4.
42. Lucendo AJ, De Rezende L. Endoscopic dilation in eosinophilic esophagitis: a treatment strategy associated with a high risk of perforation. Endoscopy. 2007;39(4):376. author reply 377.
43. Kaplan M, Mutlu EA, Jakate S, et al. Endoscopy in eosinophilic esophagitis: "feline" esophagus and perforation risk. Clin Gastroenterol Hepatol. 2003;1:433–7.
44. De la Santa E, Lazo MD, Cordero C, et al. Esofagi – tis eosinoffllica. Presentación de tres casos y reflexión sobre el papel de la endoscopia en una enfermedad probablemente infradiag – nosticada. In: Libro de comunicaciones de la XXVI Jornada Nacional de la Sociedad Espaæo – la de Endoscopia Digestiva. Madrid 1989; 48.
45. Riou PJ, Nicholson AG, Pastorino U. Esophageal rupture in a patient with idiopathic eosinophilic esophagitis. Ann Thorac Surg. 1996;62(6):1854–6.
46. Liguori G, Cortale M, Cimino F, et al. Circumferential mucosal dissection and esophageal perforation in a patient with eosinophilic esophagitis. World J Gastroenterol. 2008;14(5):803–4.

Chapter 21
Steroid Therapy of EoE in Children

Paola De Angelis and Luigi Dall'Oglio

Keywords Corticosteroids • Prednisone • Eosinophilic esophagitis

Introduction

The current practice guidelines for the diagnosis and management of EoE are based on retrospective studies and expert opinion. The primary goal of treatment is a combination of symptom reduction and resolution of histologic inflammation wherever possible; this aim is best achieved by proper identification of the underlying cause of the symptoms. However, there remain questions as to the exact cause of this disorder. While a growing body of evidence has established that this disease represents an immune-mediated response involving several pro-inflammatory mediators and chemo-attractants known to regulate eosinophilic accumulation in the esophagus, such as IL-4, IL-5, and IL-3 and eotaxin-1, -2, and -3, to date the specific etiology remains in debate [1].

Development of diagnostic guidelines based on a combination of symptoms as well as endoscopic and histopathologic criteria has improved the awareness among clinicians for the diagnosis of EoE. The clinically challenging discrimination of EoE from gastroesophageal reflux disease (GERD) has become more apparent and has evoked the need for more individualized therapy options [2]. EoE remains an emerging disorder whose pathogenesis involves food allergy and TH_2 type immune response; the relationship between EoE and GERD remains a subject of investigation.

P. De Angelis (✉)
Digestive Surgery and Endoscopy Unit, Pediatric Hospital Bambino Gesu,
Piazza S. Onofrio, 4, Rome 00165, Italy
e-mail: paola.deangelis@opbg.net

C.A. Liacouras and J.E. Markowitz (eds.), *Eosinophilic Esophagitis*,
Clinical Gastroenterology, DOI 10.1007/978-1-60761-515-6_21,

In fact, EoE and GERD may coexist; the esophagus of EoE patients may have enhanced sensitivity to acid, even in the absence of pathologic reflux [3]; EoE could therefore be considered one of the causes of refractory GERD [4].

Dietary Treatment

Many therapies are available for EoE; they address symptoms and histopathology. One of the effective treatment approaches is dietary management, which aims to eliminate exposure to food allergens. Approaches to dietary management include the use of elemental diets, elimination diets, and tailored elimination diets, each of which poses potential nutrition risks [5].

Corticosteroids

As a complete understanding of the mechanisms underlying the inflammatory process is yet to be delineated, steroids still play a significant role in enabling patients with recurrent symptoms to lead a more normal life. This pharmacological treatment represents the oldest medical therapy for EoE, still used both as acute and maintenance therapy.

Corticosteroids act against eosinophils, through induction of apoptosis, downregulation of chemotactic factors, and inhibition of proinflammatory mediators [3]. Systemic corticosteroids are a mainstay of treatment for eosinophilic gastroenteritis and as such were among the first used in pediatric EoE, leading to widespread recognition over the past decade [6].

Risk factors associated with long-term use of systemic steroids include growth abnormalities, bone abnormalities, mood disturbance, adrenal axis suppression, in addition to others. The effective dosage for relieving clinico-pathologic abnormalities are similar to those used in inflammatory bowel disease (1–2 mg/kg/die of prednisone, maximum 60 mg/die), with a similar schedule for discontinuation [3].

Symptomatic and histologic remission of EoE has been documented in more than 95% of children treated with systemic corticosteroids for 4 weeks, although symptoms and esophageal eosinophilia come back within 6 months of stopping therapy in most cases [7, 8]. The well-known side effects of protracted treatment with systemic steroids have limited their usefulness for long-term therapy, leading to trials with topical steroids such as fluticasone propionate, less frequently associated with adrenal suppression and systemic absorption. In both adults and children, symptomatic improvement has been demonstrated using swallowed fluticasone propionate, with a consequent positive histologic response. Esophageal candidiasis and dry mouth are the most reported side effects during brief therapy; recurrence of disease after treatment discontinuation is common, although the features that confer higher risk of relapse are not clear [9].

Schaefer et al. in 2008 performed an important comparison between oral and topical steroids in the treatment of pediatric EoE: in a prospective randomized trial, 80 patients were enrolled to receive oral prednisone (40 children) and swallowed fluticasone (40 children) for 4 weeks. Systemic adverse effects were present in 40% of patients treated with prednisone, while esophageal candidiasis was the most common adverse event (15%) seen in those receiving fluticasone. There was a greater degree of histologic improvement in patients treated with prednisone, but no significant difference in time to symptomatic relapse was found, highlighting the need for maintenance treatment with either treatment approach [10].

Systemic corticosteroids, in our clinical experience, are most appropriate in urgent symptom treatment and in emergent cases, such as severe dysphagia, dehydration, weight loss, esophageal strictures, and small caliber esophagus at high risk of perforation; we do not recommend them for long-term use. While topical steroids are also effective in inducing EoE remission, their use for maintenance treatment has not been well elucidated [3]. Follow-up data regarding use of swallowed steroids in children are lacking; a 3-year follow up of topical corticosteroids for EoE in adults was recently published by Helou et al. and confirmed the necessity of repeated cycles of topical treatment. EoE is a chronic relapsing condition resembling bronchial asthma; it is of interest that the esophagus and bronchial tree are derived from the same embryological foregut. That topical, aerosolized steroids are well tolerated and appear to be effective for treating both conditions with rapid onset of response and limited side effects may be more than coincidental [11].

Whether topical esophageal corticosteroids can reverse strictures or decrease the necessity or frequency of esophageal dilations remains to be evaluated, but in our experience only systemic steroid therapy has been shown so far to be successful in this role. It is not yet clear whether topical therapy has a rapid enough onset to preclude the need for dilation in severe cases. In cases where systemic steroids fail, or when critical narrowing of the esophagus is present, dilation plays an important role. In an adult series, after failure of topical corticosteroids, Shoepfer et al. demonstrated that dilations led to prompt symptom relief and did not lead to severe complications, apart from transient odynophagia. Nevertheless, esophageal perforation remains a concern when dilation is performed in patients with EoE, as the long-term efficacy and safety of topical corticosteroids and of dilation of eosinophilic esophagitis-associated strictures have not yet been thoroughly clarified [12].

Conclusion

In summary, most patients with EoE can be treated successfully with corticosteroids.

Several unresolved questions remain, however: how many cycles of steroids are appropriate and how long will they be tolerated; what is the role of topical steroids together with anti-reflux drugs (GERD therapy) in patients affected by EoE and GERD ("overlap" EoE); how do steroids fit in with seasonal flares, in mild-moderate symptoms, in severe histology with few clinical features, in maintenance therapy? Regardless, corticosteroids remain one of the most studied and detailed therapeutic options for EoE, and will likely continue to have a role despite the ongoing discovery of other treatments.

References

1. Mishra A. Mechanism of eosinophilic esophagitis. Immunol Allergy Clin North Am. 2009;29:29–40. viii.
2. Straumann A, Hruz P. What's new in the diagnosis and therapy of eosinophilic esophagitis? Curr Opin Gastroenterol. 2009;25:366–71.
3. Furuta GT, Liacouras CA, Collins MH, Gupta SK, Justinich C, Putnam PE, et al. Eosinophilic esophagitis in children and adults: a systematic review and consensus recommendations for diagnosis and treatment. Gastroenterology. 2007;133:1342–63.
4. Liu JJ, Saltzman JR. Refractory gastro-oesophageal reflux disease: diagnosis and management. Drugs. 2009;69:1935–44.
5. Santangelo CM, McCloud E. Nutritional management of children who have food allergies and eosinophilic esophagitis. Immunol Allergy Clin North Am. 2009;29:77–84. ix–x.
6. Yan BM, Shaffer EA. Primary eosinophilic disorders of the gastrointestinal tract. Gut. 2009;58:721–32.
7. Liacouras CA, Wenner WJ, Brown K, Ruchelli E. Primary eosinophilic esophagitis in children: successful treatment with oral corticosteroids. J Pediatr Gastroenterol Nutr. 1998;26:380–5.
8. Liacouras CA, Spergel JM, Ruchelli E, Verma R, Mascarenhas M, Semeao E, et al. Eosinophilic esophagitis: a 10-year experience in 381 children. Clin Gastroenterol Hepatol. 2005;3:1198–206.
9. Aceves SS, Furuta GT, Spechler SJ. Integrated approach to treatment of children and adults with eosinophilic esophagitis. Gastrointest Endosc Clin N Am. 2008;18:195–217. xi.
10. Schaefer ET, Fitzgerald JF, Molleston JP, Croffie JM, Pfefferkorn MD, Corkins MR, et al. Comparison of oral prednisone and topical fluticasone in the treatment of eosinophilic esophagitis: a randomized trial in children. Clin Gastroenterol Hepatol. 2008;6:165–73.
11. Helou EF, Simonson J, Arora AS. 3-yr-follow-up of topical corticosteroid treatment for eosinophilic esophagitis in adults. Am J Gastroenterol. 2008;103:2194–9.
12. Schoepfer AM, Gschossmann J, Scheurer U, Seibold F, Straumann A. Esophageal strictures in adult eosinophilic esophagitis: dilation is an effective and safe alternative after failure of topical corticosteroids. Endoscopy. 2008;40:161–4.

Chapter 22
Medical Treatment for Pediatric Eosinophilic Esophagitis

James P. Franciosi

Keywords Eosinophilic esophagitis • Treatment • Medication • Children • Gastroesophageal reflux disease

Introduction

Treatments for eosinophilic esophagitis (EoE) are divided into broad categories of dietary restrictions and medications. Dietary elimination and elemental diets as therapies for EoE will be discussed separately. Medication for EoE generally falls into acid suppression therapy, steroid medications, and additional therapies.

The current 2007 Consensus Guidelines for EoE define this condition as present only with the exclusion of other conditions such as gastroesophageal reflux disease (GERD) [1]. Exclusion of GERD is achieved by persistent clinicopathologic findings consistent with EoE despite negative pH probe testing or 8 weeks of proton pump inhibitor (PPI) therapy in the distal esophagus. With regard to impedance testing, a retrospective case–control study demonstrated that children with GERD had significantly higher acid reflux events compared to children with EoE, and pediatric EoE patients did not have an increase in acid or non-acid reflux compared to healthy children [2]. However, use of PPI therapy to treat esophageal eosinophilia has shown varying degrees of symptomatic and histologic success in pediatric patients [3–6]. In a retrospective cohort study, Dranove et al. described that 17 of 43 (40%) pediatric patients histologically responded (≤5 eos/hpf) and 16 of 17 (94%)

J.P. Franciosi (✉)
Division of Gastroenterology, Hepatology and Nutrition, Cincinnati Children's Hospital Medical Center, 3333 Burnet Avenue, ML 2010, Cincinnati, OH 45229, USA
e-mail: James.Franciosi@cchmc.org

C.A. Liacouras and J.E. Markowitz (eds.), *Eosinophilic Esophagitis*, Clinical Gastroenterology, DOI 10.1007/978-1-60761-515-6_22,

had improved or resolved symptoms in response to PPI therapy (mean dose 1.06 mg/kg/day, range 0.5–1.88) [7]. In another pediatric retrospective cohort study, Sayej et al. [8] showed similar results with 3 months of high dose PPI therapy (maximum dosing Lansoprazole 30 mg BID; Omeprazole or Esomeprazole 20–40 mg BID) with 14 of 36 (39%) showing a histologic response and 15/22 (78%) reported a resolution of symptoms [32]. In a small prospective adult EoE comparative effectiveness trial between esomeprazole and swallowed Fluticasone Proprionate, esomeprazole at 40 mg once per day was suggested to achieve symptomatic improvement in 3/12 (25%), partial histologic resolution (≤15 eos/hpf) in 6/12 (50%), and complete histologic resolution (≤5 eos/hpf) in 33% (4/12). However, none of these endpoints achieved statistical significance likely due to a small sample size (a type II error) [9]. It is clear that both adult and pediatric well-designed randomized, double-blind, placebo-controlled clinical trials are needed to assess the efficacy of high dose acid suppression therapy to treat the symptoms and esophageal pathology associated with esophageal eosinophilia [10].

Swallowed Steroid Therapies

Topical esophageal corticosteroid treatment is a current standard of care for pharmacologic treatment of EoE. The advantage of using topical steroids as maintenance therapy is that their side effects are significantly less than systemic steroids. Fluticasone propionate can be sprayed into the pharynx and swallowed to topically coat the esophagus and reduce inflammation. Patients do not eat, drink, or rinse their mouth for 30 min after using this medication. When using topical, swallowed corticosteroids, the initial dose varies from 110 to 880 μg, twice daily, depending on patient's age, degree of clinical symptoms, and the preference of the practitioner. Konikoff et al. [11] conducted a randomized, double-blind, placebo-controlled trial of a low dose of swallowed fluticasone (220 μg, 2 puffs BID) in 36 pediatric patients with active EoE. Of these, 50% of the fluticasone-treated patients achieved complete histologic remission compared to 9% of patients who received placebo. Resolution of clinical symptoms also occurred more frequently with fluticasone compared to placebo. A recent study demonstrated similar clinical and histologic efficacy in excess of 90% for both oral prednisone (1 mg/kg/dose BID, max 30 mg BID) and high dose swallowed Fluticasone proprionate (2 puffs QID; 110 μg/puff 1–10 years of age, 220 μg/puff 11–18 years of age) for EoE [12].

An equally effective alternative swallowed steroid formulation to Fluticasone proprionate is swallowed Budesonide [13–17]. Budesonide is administered in a slurry formulation that is made using Splenda® (five packets per 500 μg) to improve taste and consistency for topical esophageal administration. Dohil et al. [14] recently conducted a pediatric randomized, double-blind, placebo-controlled trial using Budesonide. Dosing of the Budesonide was 1 and 2 mg divided BID based on the respective height classification of < or ≥5 ft tall. In this study, all subjects were concomitantly treated with PPI therapy for 3 months, and there was an 86.7% histologic response rate in the Budesonide group compared to none of the controls. Symptom scores were also significantly improved.

From the current pediatric EoE literature, it is clear that the majority of EoE patients will respond histologically and symptomatically to steroid administration. However, intermittent dosing will likely lead to disease relapse, and the majority of patients require chronic maintenance therapy [9, 11–14]. Depending on the clinical scenario, the clinician should decide whether to start with high dose formulations and titrate down, or to begin at lower formulations and increase if not effective. Regardless of the strategy, endoscopic assessment is necessary to determine histologic response rate that is best assessed after 3 months of therapy [15].

As clinical and histologic efficacy of swallowed steroid formulations in pediatric EoE has been demonstrated, appropriate consideration should be given to the side effect profile of maintenance swallowed steroid medication therapy. Several concerns include, but are not limited to, esophageal candidiasis as well as overall growth and development. The risk of esophageal candidiasis is approximately 10–15%, but is usually easily treated with antifungal medications [1]. Typically, Fluconazole is used as a 6 mg/kg/day (max dose, 200 mg) on day 1 followed by 3 mg/kg/day (max dose, 100 mg) to complete a 21-day course. Recurrent candidiasis may be treated with prophylaxis or alternative therapies for EoE may be needed.

With regard to the impact of long-term swallowed steroids used to treat EoE, there is currently no direct literature to address this important question. Steroids are known to affect bone mineralization by a direct inhibitory action on osteoblast activity, reduction of intestinal absorption of calcium, stimulation of parathyroid hormone release, and by adverse effects on growth hormone action [19]. The minimum dose associated with steroid-induced bone loss is unknown; reduced bone density has occurred with doses as low as 5 mg of prednisone per day [19], while fracture risk has been shown to increase with daily doses of prednisone equivalent to 2.5–7.5 mg [20]. However, not all diseases managed with steroids are associated with clinically significant bone disease and growth retardation.

Given that both asthma and EoE utilize fluticasone or budesonide corticosteroid medications for maintenance therapy, some speculation can be drawn from this literature. In that regard, there is a growing body of evidence that suggests the current management of asthma with inhaled corticosteroids have little if any short-term effects on bone health, linear growth, and development [21–23]. Yet it would be premature to assume that the same would be found in patients with EoE managed with fluticasone or budesonide therapies. Major differences exist between the treatments for asthma and EoE. Where asthma treatments are designed for inhalation and absorption via the pulmonary system, EoE treatment with swallowed steroid interacts with the esophageal mucosa lining and the remainder of the GI tract. Additionally, treatment for EoE with swallowed steroids is typically at much higher daily doses than are typically used for asthma maintenance therapy (Fluticasone propionate: 440, 880, or 1,780 μg; Budesonide 0.5, 1, or 2 mg). It should also be noted that budesonide in particular undergoes extensive first-pass hepatic metabolism, which may limit systemic effects when absorbed enterally. The effects of these higher dose treatments localized to the esophageal mucosa on bone health, bone development, and growth has yet to be appropriately studied. It is also important to mention that the current alternative to swallowed steroid therapy, dietary elimination, has also not been well studied with regard to long-term nutritional, psychological and developmental effects [24].

Additional Therapies

As EoE has some features in common with allergic rhinitis, asthma, and inflammatory bowel disease, it is reasonable to question whether several therapies utilized for other inflammatory conditions may be successful in EoE patients. Cromolyn sodium is a mast cell stabilizer and anti-inflammatory agent utilized for allergic rhinitis and asthma. In a small case series of 14 EoE patients, cromolyn sodium did not demonstrate any histologic or clinical improvement in a series of 14 patients [25]. Additional case series data for the use of Leukotriene receptor antagonists with doses of 10–100 mg/day were prescribed with reports of symptomatic but not histologic improvement [25].

In refractory and severe EoE cases, some clinicians have drawn from the experience in inflammatory bowel disease and suggested immunomodulator therapy. One case series of only three adult patients with steroid dependent eosinophilic esophagitis were symptomatically and histologically treated with 6-Mercaptopurine for a period of 3–8 years with relapse upon successful discontinuation of the medication [26]. In an attempt to use other successful therapies in inflammatory bowel disease for EoE, an Anti-TNF-alpha agent (infliximab) was not able to induce histologic remission after two infusions of the 5 mg/kg dosing in a case series of three adult patients [27]. However, caution should be exercised in interpreting these very small case series, and larger randomized clinical trials are warranted.

Other biologic therapies are a source of current active investigation. Basic science and molecular investigations have determined that IL-5 and IL-13 cytokines are important in the pathogenesis of EoE [32–35]. The natural extension of this important mechanistic research is to determine whether agents that block these cytokines will be clinically effective in addressing the symptomatic and histologic outcomes in EoE. Stein studied the use of anti-IL-5 in four patients identified with EoE [28]. These patients had long-standing dysphagia and esophageal strictures. After receiving monthly intravenous infusions of anti-IL-5 for three consecutive months, clinical symptoms and repeat upper endoscopy were evaluated. Anti-IL-5 therapy was associated with marked decreases of peripheral blood and esophageal eosinophilia along with improved clinical symptoms and significant resolution of dysphagia. In a small adult double blind, randomized clinical trial, six patients tolerated mepolizumab infusions of up to 1,500 mg, with reduction in eosinophilia but not complete remission (<5 peak eosinophil number/hpf) and minimal symptomatic improvement [29]. Other biologic therapies in various stages of development include biologic therapies directed toward IL-13 and eotaxin [30–35].

Conclusion

In conclusion, medical therapies for EoE currently are limited to various steroid formulations, but with active investigations into immunomodulator and biologic therapies. Future therapies for chronic EoE will seek to effectively induce sustained histologic remission, positively impact patient reported outcomes of symptoms as well as quality of life, and optimize growth with minimal side effects and medication toxicity profiles.

References

1. Furuta GT, Liacouras CA, Collins MH, et al. Eosinophilic esophagitis in children and adults: a systematic review and consensus recommendations for diagnosis and treatment. Gastroenterology. 2007;133:1342–63.
2. Rosen R, Furuta G, Fritz J, et al. Role of acid and nonacid reflux in children with eosinophilic esophagitis compared with patients with gastroesophageal reflux and control patients. J Pediatr Gastroenterol Nutr. 2008;46:520–3.
3. Ngo P, Furuta GT, Antonioli DA, et al. Eosinophils in the esophagus – peptic or allergic eosinophilic esophagitis? Case series of three patients with esophageal eosinophilia. Am J Gastroenterol. 2006;101:1666–70.
4. Attwood SE, Lewis CJ, Bronder CS, et al. Eosinophilic oesophagitis: a novel treatment using Montelukast. Gut. 2003;52:181–5.
5. Meyer GW. Eosinophilic esophagitis in a father and a daughter. Gastrointest Endosc. 2005;61:932.
6. Morrow JB, Vargo JJ, Goldblum JR, et al. The ringed esophagus: histological features of GERD. Am J Gastroenterol. 2001;96:984–9.
7. Dranove JE, Horn DS, Davis MA, et al. Predictors of response to proton pump inhibitor therapy among children with significant esophageal eosinophilia. J Pediatr. 2009;154:96–100.
8. Sayej WN, Patel R, Baker RD, et al. Treatment with high-dose proton pump inhibitors helps distinguish eosinophilic esophagitis from noneosinophilic esophagitis. J Pediatr Gastroenterol Nutr. 2009;49(4):393–9.
9. Peterson KA, Thomas KL, Hilden K, et al. Comparison of esomeprazole to aerosolized, swallowed fluticasone for eosinophilic esophagitis. Dig Dis Sci. 2010;55:1313–9.
10. Debrosse CW, Franciosi JP, King EC, et al. Long-term outcomes in pediatric-onset esophageal eosinophilia. J Allergy Clin Immunol. 2011;128(1):132–8. Epub 2011 Jun 2.
11. Konikoff MR, Noel RJ, Blanchard C, et al. A randomized, double-blind, placebo-controlled trial of fluticasone propionate for pediatric eosinophilic esophagitis. Gastroenterology. 2006;131:1381–91.
12. Schaefer ET, Fitzgerald JF, Molleston JP, et al. Comparison of oral prednisone and topical fluticasone in the treatment of eosinophilic esophagitis: a randomized trial in children. Clin Gastroenterol Hepatol. 2008;6:165–73.
13. Straumann A, Conus S, Degen L, et al. Budesonide is effective in adolescent and adult patients with active eosinophilic esophagitis. Gastroenterology. 2010;139:1526–37.
14. Dohil R, Newbury R, Fox L, et al. Oral viscous budesonide is effective in children with eosinophilic esophagitis in a randomized, placebo-controlled trial. Gastroenterology. 2010;139:418–29.
15. DeBrosse CW, Collins MH, Buckmeier Butz BK, et al. Identification, epidemiology, and chronicity of pediatric esophageal eosinophilia, 1982–1999. J Allergy Clin Immunol. 2010; 126(1):112–9.

16. Maples KM, Henderson SC, Graham M, et al. Treatment of eosinophilic esophagitis with inhaled budesonide in a 7-year-old boy with concomitant persistent asthma: resolution of esophageal submucosal fibrosis and eosinophilic infiltration. Ann Allergy Asthma Immunol. 2007;99:572–4.
17. Aceves SS, Bastian JF, Newbury RO, et al. Oral viscous budesonide: a potential new therapy for eosinophilic esophagitis in children. Am J Gastroenterol. 2007;102:2271–9.
18. Aceves SS, Dohil R, Newbury RO, et al. Topical viscous budesonide suspension for treatment of eosinophilic esophagitis. J Allergy Clin Immunol. 2005;116:705–6. quiz 80.
19. Lukert BP, Raisz LG. Glucocorticoid-induced osteoporosis. Rheum Dis Clin North Am. 1994;20:629–50.
20. Van Staa TP, Leufkens HG, Abenhaim L, et al. Use of oral corticosteroids and risk of fractures. J Bone Miner Res. 2000;15:993–1000.
21. Boot AM, de Jongste JC, Verberne AA, et al. Bone mineral density and bone metabolism of prepubertal children with asthma after long-term treatment with inhaled corticosteroids. Pediatr Pulmonol. 1997;24:379–84.
22. Tattersfield AE, Town GI, Johnell O, et al. Bone mineral density in subjects with mild asthma randomised to treatment with inhaled corticosteroids or non-corticosteroid treatment for two years. Thorax. 2001;56:272–8.
23. Allen DB, Bronsky EA, LaForce CF, et al. Growth in asthmatic children treated with fluticasone propionate. Fluticasone Propionate Asthma Study Group. J Pediatr. 1998;132:472–7.
24. Franciosi JP, Hommel KA, Debrosse CW, et al. Quality of life in paediatric eosinophilic oesophagitis: what is important to patients? Child Care Health Dev. 2011 Jun 15. doi: 10.1111/j.1365–2214.2011.01265.
25. Liacouras CA, Spergel JM, Ruchelli E, et al. Eosinophilic esophagitis: a 10-year experience in 381 children. Clin Gastroenterol Hepatol. 2005;3:1198–206.
26. Netzer P, Gschossmann JM, Straumann A, et al. Corticosteroid-dependent eosinophilic oesophagitis: azathioprine and 6-mercaptopurine can induce and maintain long-term remission. Eur J Gastroenterol Hepatol. 2007;19:865–9.
27. Straumann A, Bussmann C, Conus S, et al. Anti-TNF-alpha (infliximab) therapy for severe adult eosinophilic esophagitis. J Allergy Clin Immunol. 2008;122:425–7.
28. Stein ML, Collins MH, Villanueva JM, et al. Anti-IL-5 (mepolizumab) therapy for eosinophilic esophagitis. J Allergy Clin Immunol. 2006;118:1312–9.
29. Straumann A, Conus S, Grzonka P, et al. Anti-interleukin-5 antibody treatment (mepolizumab) in active eosinophilic oesophagitis: a randomised, placebo-controlled, double-blind trial. Gut. 2010;59:21–30.
30. Bhattacharya B, Carlsten J, Sabo E, et al. Increased expression of eotaxin-3 distinguishes between eosinophilic esophagitis and gastroesophageal reflux disease. Hum Pathol. 2007;38:1744–53.
31. Fujiwara H, Morita A, Kobayashi H, et al. Infiltrating eosinophils and eotaxin: their association with idiopathic eosinophilic esophagitis. Ann Allergy Asthma Immunol. 2002;89:429–32.
32. Blanchard C, Wang N, Stringer KF, et al. Eotaxin-3 and a uniquely conserved gene-expression profile in eosinophilic esophagitis. J Clin Invest. 2006;116:536–47.
33. Mishra A, Rothenberg ME. Intratracheal IL-13 induces eosinophilic esophagitis by an IL-5, eotaxin-1, and STAT6-dependent mechanism. Gastroenterology. 2003;125:1419–27.
34. Blanchard C, Stucke EM, Burwinkel K, et al. Coordinate interaction between IL-13 and epithelial differentiation cluster genes in eosinophilic esophagitis. J Immunol. 2010;184:4033–41.
35. Blanchard C, Mingler MK, Vicario M, et al. IL-13 involvement in eosinophilic esophagitis: transcriptome analysis and reversibility with glucocorticoids. J Allergy Clin Immunol. 2007;120:1292–300.

Chapter 23
Corticosteroid Treatment of Eosinophilic Esophagitis in Adults

Karthik Ravi and Amindra S. Arora

Keywords Eosinophilic esophagitis • Fluticasone • Budesonide • Prednisone • Topical corticosteroids • Systemic corticosteroids

Case Presentation

A 36-year-old Caucasian gentleman is referred to his local gastroenterologist for dysphagia. The patient reports a 4-year history of intermittent solid food dysphagia. His previous evaluations, including endoscopy, have been unremarkable. Despite a lack of heartburn or reflux, the patient has been on twice daily proton pump inhibitor therapy for the past 6 months with no change in symptoms. His health has previously been excellent aside from childhood asthma.

An esophagram reveals no structural abnormalities. Endoscopic evaluation is unremarkable, with a normal appearing esophagus with no esophagitis noted. Middle and distal esophageal biopsies are obtained with reveal 40 eos/HPF in the mid and 55 eos/HPF in the distal esophagus.

The patient is started on a trial of swallowed fluticasone 220 μg/puff, 4 puffs twice daily for 6 weeks. At the completion of this medication trial, his symptoms have completely resolved and the fluticasone is discontinued. The patient returns 8 months later with recurrent problems with solid food dysphagia and another trial of swallowed fluticasone is initiated with subsequent resolution of symptoms.

A.S. Arora (✉)
Department of GIH, Mayo Clinic, 200 First Street SW, Rochester, MN 55905, USA
e-mail: Arora.amindra@mayo.edu

C.A. Liacouras and J.E. Markowitz (eds.), *Eosinophilic Esophagitis*, Clinical Gastroenterology, DOI 10.1007/978-1-60761-515-6_23,

Introduction

Eosinophilic esophagitis (EoE) was first described by Landres et al. [1] and is characterized by eosinophils in the squamous epithelium or deeper layers of the esophagus. The exact pathogenesis of EoE remains unclear, limiting the optimization of treatment strategies for the disease. Eosinophils, while present at low levels throughout the body, including the gastrointestinal tract, are absent from the esophagus in health. However, eosinophils are seen in conditions other than EoE, including gastroesophageal reflux, collagen vascular diseases, Crohn's disease, infections, and achalasia.

Eosinophils release inflammatory mediators which cause mucosal injury and lead to a chronic inflammatory state. This in turn leads to structural and functional abnormalities in the esophagus and likely the clinical manifestations of EoE. However, the exact pathogenesis of this inflammatory response remains poorly understood, with most investigators supporting an allergen-related immune response. Consequently, treatment strategies have focused on this pathway, with strategies including elimination diet, leukotriene receptor inhibitors, and monoclonal antibodies showing variable success. This chapter will focus on the role of corticosteroids in the treatment of EoE in the adult population.

The role of corticosteroids in other eosinophilic inflammatory conditions such as asthma is well described. Corticosteroids are believed to be effective in the treatment of eosinophil-derived inflammation by a variety of proposed mechanisms [2, 3]. Consequently, its use has been extended to the treatment of EoE.

Systemic Corticosteroids

Liacouras et al. were the first to demonstrate that systemic corticosteroids were an effective treatment strategy in the pediatric population. In this study, 20 children with presumed eosinophilic esophagitis were treated with oral methylprednisolone at a dose of 1.5 mg/kg/day divided into twice daily doses for a total of 4 weeks, with clinical and histological improvement demonstrated in all but one patient [4], with all patients tapered off of steroids after 6 weeks. However, long term follow up of these patients at 12 months found that of the 19 patients who responded to systemic corticosteroid therapy, only 10 remained asymptomatic.

A similar clinical experience has been seen in the adult population. While effective, the relapsing course of EoE with discontinuation of systemic corticosteroids has proven problematic. This relapsing course requires repeated courses of systemic corticosteroids, increasing the risk for adverse effects such as bone abnormalities, mood abnormalities, and adrenal suppression. These significant adverse effects have limited the use of systemic corticosteroids for acute exacerbations in select patient populations. In the 2007 Eosinophilic Esophagitis consensus recommendation statement, systemic corticosteroids were restricted to patients in whom urgent symptom relief was required. This patient population was defined as those with severe dysphagia, dehydration, significant weight loss, or esophageal strictures as well of those with small caliber esophagus deemed to be high risk for perforation with endoscopic dilation [5]. Prednisone is typically the formulation used, at a dose of 1–2 mg/kg/day with a maximum of 60 mg/day, with subsequent appropriate tapering.

Topical Corticosteroids

The significant side-effect profile and long-term complications associated with systemic corticosteroids suggested the need for a more localized administration of steroids for the treatment of EoE. This void was filled by the use of topical corticosteroids.

While the initial studies of topical corticosteroids in EoE were done in the pediatric population, efficacy in the adult population has been demonstrated (Table 23.1). Faubion and colleagues reported the first use of topical corticosteroids, describing the use of swallowed fluticasone or beclomethasone in four children with EoE, with clinical improvement seen in all cases [6]. Since that time, the use of topical corticosteroids in EoE has been extended to the adult population.

Arora et al. reported the clinical experience of 21 adult patients with EoE and solid food dysphagia for a minimum of 6 years [7]. All patients were treated with 4 puffs of fluticasone (220 µg/puff) twice daily for a total of 6 weeks. All patients had complete resolution of solid food dysphagia at 4 months after completion of topical corticosteroid therapy. Remedios et al. described similar results in 19 patients treated with 2 puffs of fluticasone (250 µg/puff) twice daily for a total of 4 weeks [8]. All 19 patients had significant improvement of symptoms at the end of the 4-week treatment period, with 11 being asymptomatic. Additionally, 18 demonstrated histological response with significantly reduced eosinophil counts.

Topical corticosteroids have traditionally been delivered in the form of fluticasone. Administration is typically given via a metered-dose inhaler (MDI) without the use of the spacer. The patient is instructed to insert the MDI into their mouth and spray with lips sealed around the device. The powder is to be swallowed, with patients abstaining from eating or drinking for a minimum of 30 min. Doses range from 880 to 1,760 µg/day, typically for a duration of 6–8 weeks.

As would be expected, adverse effects with topical corticosteroids are minimal compared to those associated with use of systemic corticosteroids. In the combined experience of 40 patients from the above noted studies, adverse effects were noted in only 4 patients. These side effects were relatively mild; with asymptomatic oral candidiasis identified during endoscopic evaluation in three and severe dry mouth in one patient. However, a meta-analysis in asthmatic patients suggested that use of inhaled fluticasone at doses greater than 75 µg/day may be associated with bone loss [9]. Furthermore, at least one case report of HSV esophagitis has been reported in a patient treated with topical corticosteroids for EoE [10].

Table 23.1 Corticosteroid treatment in adults with eosinophilic esophagitis

Study	Number of subjects	Medication	Follow up	Response to treatment
Arora et al. [5]	21	Fluticasone 4 puffs 220 μg BID × 6 weeks	12–18 months	Dysphagia resolution in all at 4 months. Dysphagia recurrence in 3/21 at 12–18 months
Remedios et al. [6]	19	Fluticose 2 puffs 250 μg BID × 4 weeks	3 months	Dysphagia resolution in all and histological improvement in 18/19 at treatment completion. Recurrent symptoms in 14 of 19 at 3 month follow-up
Straumann et al. [10]	36	Budesonide 1 mg twice daily × 15 days	None	Histologic remission in 72.2% vs. 11.1% and clinic improvement in 84% vs. 33% in budesonide and placebo groups, respectively
Neumann et al. [12]	16	Budesonide 3 mg twice daily × 1 week, then either 3 mg twice daily ($n=5$) or once daily ($n=11$) × 5 weeks	None	All 16 patients with at least 75% improvement in dysphagia, with 9 reporting complete resolution

Similar to those treated with systemic corticosteroids, patients treated with topical corticosteroids frequently have recurrent symptoms following discontinuation of therapy. Of the 21 patients reported by Arora et al., 3 had relapse of dysphagia 12–18 months after completion of therapy [5]. Similarly, Remedios et al. reported recurrent symptoms in 14 patients at 3 months following completion of topical corticosteroids [8]. Arora et al. prospectively described the natural history of EoE in 32 patients treated with the same fluticasone [11]. Twenty-nine patients reported recurrent dysphagia occurring at a mean of 8.8 months following completion of treatment. Twenty-two of 29 patients required repeated treatment courses with swallowed fluticasone with 12 of these requiring two or more repeated treatments and 4 requiring four or more repeated treatments over a mean follow up of 3.3 years. However, these patients required less frequent esophageal dilations following treatment with swallowed fluticasone.

Similarly, a study presented in abstract form by Straumann et al. demonstrated treatment efficacy of budesonide in this patient population [12]. Thirty-six patients with EoE were treated with either budesonide 1 mg twice daily via nebulizer or placebo. They reported histologic remission in 72.2% of patients treated with budesonide compared to 11.1% in the placebo group, with a reduction in tissue eosinophilia from 62 to 4 eos/HPF. Further, symptomatic improvement was noted in 84% of patients treated with budesonide vs. 33% in the placebo group.

More recently, oral viscous budesonide formulations have been developed specifically for the treatment of EoE. The primary benefit of oral formulations has been thought to be the relative ease of administration and the potential beneficial effects on patient compliance. Aceves and colleagues reported on the use of oral viscous budesonide in a pediatric population [13]. Viscous budesonide was made by mixing a liquid formulation of budesonide with sucralose. Twenty children were given 1–2 mg of oral viscous budesonide daily for a period of 3–4 months, with histologic response noted in 80% of patients and symptomatic improvement in all patients.

The use of an oral gel combining budesonide and the mucosal adherent rincinol has also been reported upon in the adult population by Neumann et al. [14]. Sixteen patients with EoE were treated with 3 mg of budesonide twice daily for 1 week with this oral gel. Eleven patients reported symptomatic improvement and the frequency was decreased to once daily, while the other five patients were continued on twice daily therapy. All patients completed a 6-week course of treatment. At the conclusion of treatment, all patients reported at least a 75% improvement in dysphagia, with 56% reporting complete resolution.

Proton Pump Inhibitors

More recently, evidence has emerged to suggest that proton pump inhibitors (PPIs) are an effective treatment option in patients with esophageal eosinophilia. Ngo et al. described three patients with clinical and endoscopic features of EoE with greater than 20 eos/HPF. After 2 months of treatment with PPI, all three patients had clinical, endoscopic, and histologic response [15]. Desai et al. reported on patients presenting with food bolus impaction and greater than 20 eos/HPF. Of 16 patients treated with 4–8 weeks of PPI therapy, 8 reported symptomatic improvement while 8 did not. Of the latter group, five of six patients subsequently treated with topical corticosteroids reported symptomatic improvement [16]. Gastroesophageal reflux is often associated with eosinophilic esophagitis. While the above studies demonstrate that PPIs may be effective in treating symptoms associated with secondary reflux, Peterson et al. reported a randomized trial of 25 patients with EoE treated with omeprazole 40 mg daily vs. fluticasone 440 μg twice daily. He showed that there was no significant difference in clinical or histological response in either treatment group [17] thus helping to confirm the distinct difference between GERD and EoE.

Conclusion

Corticosteroids, both systemic and topical formulations, are effective treatments for EoE in the adult population. The use of systemic corticosteroids is limited by significant adverse effects with continued use, and should be limited to acute emergent symptoms related to EoE. Topical corticosteroids are also an effective treatment strategy for EoE with less associated adverse effects. Symptoms of EoE tend to relapse following discontinuation of corticosteroids, and repeat treatment courses are typically necessary. Future directions in therapy may include formulations specifically developed for EoE with simplified delivery and increased patient compliance.

References

1. Landres RT, Kuster GG, Strum WB. Eosinophilic esophagitis in a patient with vigorous achalasia. Gastroenterology. 1978;74:1298–301.
2. Jeffery PK, Godfrey RW, Adelroth E, et al. Effects of treatment on airway inflammation and thickening of basement membrane reticular collagen in asthma: a quantitative light and electron microscopic study. Am Rev Respir Dis. 1992;145:890–9.
3. Djukanovic R, Wilson JW, Britten KM, et al. Effects of an inhaled corticosteroids on airway inflammation and symptoms in asthma. Am Rev Respir Dis. 1992;145:669–74.
4. Liacouras CA, Wenner WJ, Brown K, Ruchelli E. Primary eosinophilic esophagitis in children: successful treatment with oral corticosteroids. J Pediatr Gastroenterol Nutr. 1998;26:380–5.
5. Furuta FT, Liacouras CA, Collis MH, et al. Eosinophilic esophagitis in children and adults: a systematic review and consensus recommendations for diagnosis and treatment. Gastroenterology. 2007;133:1342–63.
6. Faubion Jr WA, Perrault J, Burgart LJ, et al. Treatment of eosinophilic esophagitis with inhaled corticosteroids. J Pediatr Gastroenterol Nutr. 1998;27:90–3.
7. Arora AS, Perrault J, Smyrk TC. Topical corticosteroid treatment of dysphagia due to eosinophilic esophagitis in adults. Mayo Clin Proc. 2003;78:830–5.
8. Remedios M, Campbell C, Jones DM, et al. Eosinophilic esophagitis in adults: clinical, endoscopic, histologic findings, and response to treatment with fluticasone propionate. Gastrointest Endosc. 2006;63:3–12.
9. Lipworth BJ. Systemic adverse effects of inhaled corticosteroid therapy: a systematic review and meta-analysis. Arch Intern Med. 1999;159:941–55.
10. Lindberg GM, Van Eldik R, Saboorian MH. A case of herpres esophagitis after fluticasone propionate for eosinophilic esophagitis. Nat Clin Pract Gastroenterol Hepatol. 2008;5: 527–30.
11. Helou EF, Simonson J, Arora AS. 3-Yr-follow-up of topical corticosteroid treatment for eosinophilic esophagitis in adults. Am J Gastroenterol. 2008;103:2194–9.
12. Straumann A, Degen L, Felder S, et al. Budesonide as induction treatment for active eosinophilic esophagtis in adolescents and adults: a randomized, double-blind, placebo-controlled study. Gastroenterology. 2008;134:A-104.
13. Aceves S, Bastian JF, Newbury RO, et al. Oral viscous budesonide: a potential new therapy for eosinophilic esophagitis in children. Am J Gastroenterol. 2007;102:2271–9.
14. Neumann DA, Alexander GL, Farrugia G, et al. A new therapy for eosinophilic esophagitis in adults: efficacy of budesonide – rincinol gel for 6 weeks in patients with dysphagia. Am J Gastroenterol. 2009;103(S8):S19.
15. Ngo P, Guruta GT, Antonioli DA, et al. Eosinophils in the esophagus-peptic or allergic eosinopilic esophagitis? Case series of three patients with esophageal eosinophilia. Am J Gastroenterol. 2006;101:1660–70.
16. Desai TK, Stecevic V, Chang CH, et al. Association of eosinophilic inflammation with esophageal food impaction in adults. Gastrointest Endosc. 2005;61:795–801.
17. Peterson KA, Samuelson WM, Ryujin DT, et al. The role of gastroesophageal reflux in exercise triggered asthma: a randomized controlled trial. Dig Dis Sci. 2009;54:564–72.

Chapter 24
Dietary Treatment of Eosinophilic Esophagitis

Amir F. Kagalwalla and Sally Ritz

Keywords Eosinophilic esophagitis • Food antigens • Elemental diet • Anaphylactic food allergies

Introduction

Eosinophilic esophagitis (EoE) is an immune-mediated chronic inflammatory disorder that, in most children and many adults, is triggered by food antigens. In 1995, Kelly et al. first described EoE in children and also demonstrated that clinical symptoms and eosinophilic esophageal inflammation was reversed with exclusive amino acid-based elemental diet and exclusion of all food antigens [1]. The authors also identified specific food antigens including cow's milk, soy, wheat, egg, and peanuts as potential proteins that induced the esophageal inflammation. These initial important observations from that first pediatric study form the basis of the different dietary approaches currently offered to treat EoE.

The goals of treatment in EoE, as for most other chronic disorders, include: (1) resolution of clinical symptoms, (2) maintenance of remission or prevention of disease relapse, (3) prevention of complications such as fibrosis and strictures by maintaining histological remission, (4) prevention of iatrogenic treatment-related adverse reactions such as nutritional deficiencies as in dietary treatment, and (5) maintenance of quality of life (QOL).

A genome-wide microarray expression study of esophageal tissue from EoE patients demonstrated that, within the unique EoE transcript signature, the gene for

A.F. Kagalwalla (✉)
Division of Gastroenterology, Hepatology, and Nutrition, Northwestern University Feinberg School of Medicine, Children's Memorial Hospital, John H. Stroger Hospital of Cook County, 2300 Children's Plaza, 65, Chicago, IL 60614, USA
e-mail: Akagalwa@childrensmemorial.org

C.A. Liacouras and J.E. Markowitz (eds.), *Eosinophilic Esophagitis*, Clinical Gastroenterology, DOI 10.1007/978-1-60761-515-6_24,

Table 24.1 Outcome of various dietary approaches in eosinophlic esophagitis

Author	No.	Allergy tests	Diet	Outcome	Residual eosinophil count
Kelly [1]	10	SPT 6/9	Elemental diet	Clinical improvement 10/10 (100%)	0.5
				Histologic improvement 9/10 (90%)	
Teitelbaum [9]	11	SPT/RAST	Allergy test based elimination	No improvement	
Noel [10]	10	SPT	Elimination diet	No response	
Spergel [6]	146	SPT and APT	Elimination diet	Significant improvement 112 (77%)	1.1±2.1
				Partial improvement 19 (13%)	12.0±3.2
				Treatment failure 15 (10%)	36.3±14.9
Laicouras [3]	172		Elemental diet	Significant clinical and histologic improvement 160/164 (98%)	1.1±0.6
Kagalwalla [4]	60	Allergy tests not utilized	SFED	Significant improvement SFED=26/35 (74%)	3.1±3.2
	ELED 25 SFED 35		Elemental diet	Significant improvement ELED=22/25 (88%)	1.6±2.1
Gonsalves [7]	18		SFED	Significant clinical and histologic improvement 14/18 (78%)	

eotaxin-3 was most highly induced and high levels of eotaxin-3 correlated with disease severity [2]. It is speculated that eotaxin-3 may be induced in response to innate signaling and could be triggered by ingested stimuli such as food antigens and it could be further speculated that perhaps this induction can be reversed by eliminating the external stimuli, i.e., food antigen. The dietary approach is based on the hypothesis that food antigens trigger eosinophilic inflammation, and clinical along with histological remission can be induced by identifying and excluding the causative food antigens. It is believed that eliminating causative food antigens targets the cause and thus induces long-term remission. There are no prospective controlled double-blind studies assessing and demonstrating the efficacy of the different dietary approaches. The current recommendation for treatment of EoE with diet are based on a number of retrospective and observational studies [3–7]. The available dietary approaches include: (1) elemental diet with an amino acid-based complete liquid formulation [1, 3–5], (2) directed elimination diet based on the results of allergy testing [6], and (3) standard or nondirected elimination diet where a number of common food antigens are excluded from the diet [4]. The type of treatment selected should be individualized and tailored to the needs of the patient and should depend on the presence or lack of anaphylactic food allergies, the age of the child, and the comfort and acceptance of the elimination diet by the family. Outcomes of all the different, successful as well as unsuccessful, dietary approaches are summarized in Table 24.1.

Elemental Diet

Crystalline amino acid-based (exclusive) elemental diet was first successfully used to treat ten children with gastroesophageal reflux disease (GERD)-like symptoms resistant to acid suppression [1]. Clinical and histological remission occurred with introduction of exclusive amino acid-based formula in lieu of regular diet. Subsequent controlled reintroduction of solid foods resulted in recurrence of gastrointestinal symptoms specific to individual foods. A clear link between food allergy and esophageal injury was established in these patients [1]. Since this seminal publication by Kelly et al., two series of 172 and 25 cases reported a remission rate of 96 and 88%, respectively, in children treated with elemental diet (Neocate, Neocate EO28, Neocate 1+, SHS International, Liverpool, UK; or Elecare, Ross Pediatrics, Abbott Laboratories, Abbott Park, Illinois) [3, 4]. This treatment outcome was achieved without any reported complications. The likelihood of achieving mucosal healing has been shown to be higher with this modality than other dietary interventions or with corticosteroids. The added advantages are the much lower residual eosinophil counts and thus almost complete remission with elemental diet. The disadvantage of this approach is the poor taste, patient compliance, and impaired QOL due to elimination of regular foods. This limits the ability to ingest it orally and many of these children require either nasogastric or gastrostomy tubes to deliver adequate nutrients. The tube placement is also a source of patient discomfort and parental distress. Limiting a child to an exclusive elemental diet restricts the child's participation in social activities, since many childhood activities involve food, which can lead to impaired QOL. Elemental formulas are expensive and not always covered by most traditional insurance plans thereby placing significant financial and social burden on the families. There may also be additional costs related to tubes, pumps, bags, and other supplies. Several states are covering or working toward providing coverage for the elemental formulas for EoE, but it continues to be a struggle for most families to get reimbursement for the cost of these formulations.

Once histological remission is established, as demonstrated with repeat endoscopy performed 4–6 weeks after exclusive elemental diet, food reintroduction is initiated beginning with the least allergenic foods from vegetable or fruit groups; a single food is introduced every 5–7 days, followed by a single food from within the grain, meat, and nut groups as outlined by Markowitz et al. [5]. In this algorithm the most allergic food group which includes foods such as cow's milk, soy, wheat, egg, chicken, and corn are the last foods reintroduced. Single foods from a specific food group labeled

Table 24.2 Dietary introduction approach to food reintroduction in eosinophilic esophagitis

A	B	C	D
Vegetables (non-legume): Carrots, squash (all types), sweet potato, white potato, string beans, broccoli, lettuce, beets, asparagus, cauliflower, brussel sprouts *Fruit (non-citrus, nontropical)*: Apple, pear, peaches, plum, apricot, nectarine, grape, raisins *Vegetables*: Tomatoes, celery, cucumber, onion, garlic, any other vegetables	*Citrus fruits*: Orange, grapefruit, lemon, lime *Tropical fruits*: Banana, kiwi, pineapple, mango, papaya, guava, avocado *Melons*: Honeydew, cantaloupe, watermelon *Berries*: Strawberry, blueberry, raspberry, cherry, cranberry *Grains*: Rice, millet, quinoa	*Legumes*: Lima beans, chickpeas, white/black/red beans *Grains*: Oat, barley, rye, other grains *Meat*[a]: Lamb, chicken, turkey, pork	Fish/shellfish Corn Peas Peanut Wheat Beef Soy Egg Milk

Modified with permission from Table 2 published by Spergel and Shuker. Gastrointest Endosc Clin N Am. 2008;18:179–94

[a]Progress from well cooked to rarer

from A to D as shown in Table 24.2 are reintroduced in the diet every 5–7 days [8]. Following successful reintroduction of all foods in one food group, endoscopic esophageal biopsies are performed to demonstrate continuing remission before introducing the next single food from the next food group. However, if the patient is symptomatic following ingestion of any given food, that food is excluded from the diet and the patient proceeds to the next food in that group once the symptoms have resolved.

Directed Elimination Diets Based on Results of Allergy Testing

Children treated with elimination diets based only on radioallergosorbent test (RAST) and/or skin prick test (SPT) results have failed to demonstrate clinical and histological remission [9, 10]. In a prospective study in which adults were treated with standard elimination diet, the predictive value of SPT for causal foods was only 22% in subjects [7]. RAST testing and SPT alone or together fail to correctly identify foods causing esophageal inflammation in most patients. However, when patients underwent both skin prick and atopic patch testing (APT) and were treated with an elimination diet based on the results of a combination of SPT and APT to common foods, 78% demonstrated significant clinical and histological remission [6]. Patients in this series underwent testing to common foods including meats (chicken, turkey, beef, and pork), vegetables (peas, string beans, squash, sweet potatoes, potatoes, and carrots), fruits (apples, pears and peaches), and grains (wheat, rice, rye, oats, barley, and corn). Patients were also tested to milk protein, soy, eggs, and peanuts. Milk, soy, wheat, chicken, and beef were the foods most frequently identified by both APT and SPT. Of the 146 children treated with an elimination diet based on the results of both APT and SPT, 112 (78%) responded with both clinical and histological improvement. Within this group, 39 subjects were allergic to specific foods including milk, egg, soy, and beef. Patch skin test lacks standardization for food allergies and is currently a research tool awaiting results of further studies to validate it [11].

Standard Elimination Diet

The advantage of standard or nondirected elimination diet, as also in the case of elemental diet, is that it does not require allergy testing to determine foods for elimination from the diet. In a retrospective study, six-food elimination diet (SFED) was utilized to treat a cohort of 35 children [4]. Cow's milk protein, soy, wheat, egg, peanut/tree nut, fish, and shellfish were the only foods excluded from the diet while all other solid foods were allowed. Twenty-six (74%) children experienced significant clinical and histological improvement (esophageal eosinophil count ≤10/HPF). There was complete mucosal healing with 0–1 eosinophil/HPF documented in esophageal biopsies in 7 of these 26 (27%) children. Complete histological remission induced by elimination diet is shown in Fig. 24.1. This treatment approach has since been validated by a recent prospective study in which 78% of adults treated with SFED demonstrated histological improvement [7]. The primary advantage of elimination diet over exclusive elemental diet is that it allows intake of a variety of table foods including meats, grains, fruits, vegetables, and legumes compared to a

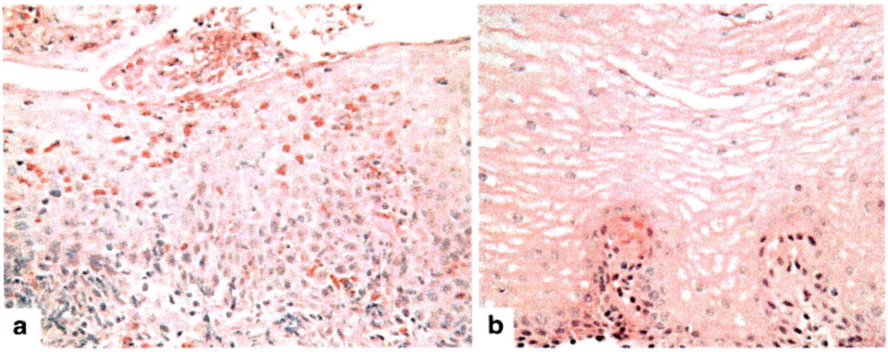

Fig. 24.1 Esophageal biopsies. (**a**) Before treatment, demonstrating high eosinophil count; (**b**) after treatment with elimination diet, demonstrating complete resolution of eosinophils and inflammation

single nutrient source taken orally or via a tube. In situations where allergy testing is not easily accessible, and where elemental diet is not a consideration, this approach is the dietary treatment of choice. In addition, this diet is not a significant drain on the families' budget.

Once clinical and histological remission with SFED is achieved, single food reintroduction in the diet is begun. Patients are evaluated after 4–6 weeks of new food reintroduction by endoscopy with esophageal biopsy. The next food is reintroduced after the histology establishes remission. In a cohort of 21 children who had achieved clinical and histological remission with SFED, cow's milk was the most common food triggering disease recurrence in patients (81%), followed by soy (19%) and wheat (14%) based on data presented by Shah et al. during an oral session at the Children's Digestive Health and Nutrition Foundation (CDHNF) Annual Meeting in San Diego, CA on November 14, 2008.

Food Substitutions and Cross-Contamination in Elimination Diets

Directed and nondirected food elimination diets require more than the physician just directing the patient to eliminate the food(s) in question. Multiple concerns are raised including the fact that eliminating major foods such as milk, soy, wheat, and egg from the diet of a growing child may have deleterious consequences. The foods removed should be adequately substituted to ensure the diet is nutritionally complete. This requires knowledge and understanding of the nutrient deficiencies caused by elimination of specific food as well as the appropriate substitution for that food as shown in Table 24.3.

Another important aspect of eliminating foods from the diet involves food cross-contamination. Cross-contamination can transform a naturally occurring antigen-free food, into an antigen-containing food. Cross-contamination can occur during processing, preparing, cooking, or serving food. Many processed foods as well as fast foods maybe cross-contaminated with one or more foods such as milk, soy, wheat, or nuts. Cross-contamination can also occur during the process of food preparation at home and can be avoided by simple measures such as using different utensils and strict hand washing between cooking different foods. Tips for avoiding cross-contamination are summarized in Table 24.4.

Individuals on elimination diets must read food labels to ensure that those products are allowed in the diet. Food labels should be reviewed each time the product is consumed because manufacturing or processing may have changed, and a food that was formerly antigen-free may now contain the excluded antigen. The US Food and Drug Administration Food Allergen Labeling and Consumer Protection Act (FALCA) of 2004 has helped consumers identify foods that are potential allergens and if cross-contamination is a concern. This act requires that all foods made with any of the eight most common food allergens (cow milk, soy, egg, wheat, peanut, tree nut, fish, and shellfish) must be clearly labeled to indicate the presence of these ingredients [12].

Table 24.3 Potential nutritional deficiencies

Food	Nutrients	Alternative food sources
Milk	Protein, calcium, vitamin D, vitamin A, B12, riboflavin, pantothenic acid, potassium	Meats, legumes, whole grains, nuts, fortified foods (with B vitamins, calcium, vitamin D)
Egg	Protein, vitamin B12, pantothenic acid, biotin, selenium	Meat, chicken, legumes whole grains
Soy	Protein, iron, zinc, magnesium, thiamin, riboflavin, pyridoxine, folate	Meats, allowed grains
Wheat	Iron, thiamin, riboflavin, niacin, folic acid	Alternative grains that are fortified
Peanut/tree nut	Vitamin E, niacin, magnesium, manganese, chromium, folic acid, B6, copper, zinc, selenium, phosphorus, potassium	Legumes, whole grains, vegetable oils
Fish/shellfish	Vitamin E, B6, niacin, phosphorus, selenium, omega 3 fatty acids	Whole grains, meats, soybean, flaxseed, nuts, oils

Table 24.4 Tips to avoid cross-contamination

- Follow proper hand-washing procedures
- Prepare antigen free foods first, then cover
- Clean surfaces and utensils before/after preparing antigen-free foods
- Separate antigen-free from antigen-containing foods
- Seal or wrap antigen-free foods
- Separate condiments (to avoid double dipping) or use squeeze bottles/sprays

Nutritional Assessment

Nutritional assessment of children with EoE, by a registered dietitian, prior to initiating the elimination diet is warranted. This assessment involves obtaining a detailed nutritional history including descriptions of food and supplements being consumed (including brand names of foods), preparation methods and eating environment, to improve compliance of prescribed nutritional therapy. Although, not very common, some children may present with malnutrition. This is typically seen in younger children whose symptoms may include vomiting and food aversion or children with multiple IgE-mediated food allergies. The initial assessment may identify preexisting nutritional deficiencies which can be addressed concurrently when prescribing an elimination diet. Children who are on elimination diets for a prolonged period will need to have their nutritional intake monitored. In addition to anthropometric measurements including weight, height, and body mass index (BMI), some children, especially those who have a large number of foods excluded, will require biochemical tests including complete blood count, prealbumin, iron, calcium, and vitamin D levels to monitor for deficiencies [13, 14].

Potential Nutritional and Other Consequences of Elimination Diets

It is important to be cautious when recommending elimination diets, since exclusion of important food elements from a growing child's diet can have disastrous consequences including impaired growth, rickets, and vitamin deficiencies [15, 16]. A recent report demonstrated several cases of Kwashiorkor caused by protein malnutrition of toddlers suspected of having a milk protein allergy that were subsequently put on a diet excluding only milk protein [17]. Frequently it is not a specific food per se that is a cause of nutritional deficiency as is the concurrent exclusion of a large number of processed foods that may contain that particular food antigen as a contaminant. Elimination diets with emphasis on excluding milk, wheat, soy, and nuts among other foods also can be challenging for children on a vegetarian diet. Participation of a registered dietitian is extremely important to ensure a calorically adequate diet for growth, to provide education on appropriate food substitutions, prevent contamination with excluded food antigens and to be an ongoing resource for families as they learn to adapt to the diet modification. Tips for successful elimination diet are shown in Table 24.5.

Other issues related to elimination diet include behavioral problems including refusal to comply with the diet since some of the younger children in daycare or elementary school settings do not want to appear or seem different from their peers. This, in our unpublished experience, has been a cause of treatment noncompliance. Depression, cheating, lying, and stealing foods from other children are other behavioral consequences of diet therapy that have been reported in children on elimination diets for celiac disease and presumed food induced severe eczema. Proper patient selection for elimination dietary therapy can minimize these consequences.

Table 24.5 Tips for successful elimination diet

Problem	Potential solution
Unfamiliar foods	Involve child in preparation, serve variety of safe foods using different preparations, safe spices for different tastes
Cooking	Food allergy and anaphylaxis network (FAAN) cookbooks, newsletters, online, cooking shows/cooking magazines-adapt ideas to special foods
Eating out/ socialization	Have plan, call ahead to restaurants, go off peak times, talk to chef/manager. Bring own food if unable to meet needs
Traveling	Bring own food staples, if possible stay in hotel with kitchenette, call hotel, restaurants ahead regarding dietary restrictions
Holidays/birthday party	Plan gatherings around non-meal times, have nonfood related activities, i.e., "non-cake" cake
Sneaking foods	Make sure child understands consequences – cheating can cause harm to body. Let EoE team know so can postpone endoscopy
Other caregivers/ relatives	Provide a written explanation of what EoE is and what the diet is. Provide list of acceptable and unacceptable foods. Consider providing snacks/ meals when outside home

Summary

Elimination of food proteins that are triggering esophageal inflammation often leads to resolution of symptoms and sustained healing of the esophagus. This treatment approach of eliminating the cause of esophageal damage is a logical cause and effect way to managing EoE. However, the different dietary treatments can be challenging and are often difficult to implement. Elemental diet with complete elimination of all intact food antigens offers the best outcome results as well as most complete healing but subsequent food reintroduction is long, tedious, and often frustrating. Directed and standard or nondirected dietary treatments are less effective than elemental diet; both options offer good outcomes but directed elimination diet has the drawback that patch testing remains to be validated and is not universally available. When contemplating dietary options, it is important to remember that one size does not fit all and that dietary approach needs to be tailored to the needs of the individual patient.

References

1. Kelly KJ, Lazenby AJ, Rowe PC, Yardley JH, Perman JA, Sampson HA. Eosinophilic esophagitis attributed to gastroesophageal reflux: improvement with amino acid-based formula. Gastroenterology. 1995;109:1503–12.
2. Blanchard C, Wang N, Stringer KF, Mishra A, Fulkerson PC, Abonia JP, et al. Eotaxin-3 and a uniquely conserved gene-expression profile in eosinophilic esophagitis. J Clin Invest. 2006;116:536–47.
3. Liacouras CA, Spergel JM, Ruchelli E, Verma R, Mascarenhas M, Semeao E, et al. Eosinophilic esophagitis: a 10-year experience in 381 children. Clin Gastroenterol Hepatol. 2005;3:1198–206.
4. Kagalwalla AF, Sentengo TS, Ritz S, Hess T, Nelson SP, Emerick KM, et al. Effect of six-food elimination diet on clinical and histological outcomes in eosinophilic esophagitis. Clin Gastroenterol Hepatol. 2006;4:1097–102.
5. Markowitz JE, Spergel JM, Ruchelli E, Liacouras A. Elemental diet is an effective treatment for eosinophilic esophagitis in children and adolescents. Am J Gastroenterol. 2003;98:777–82.
6. Spergel JM, Andrews T, Brown-Whitehorn TF, Beausoleil JL, Liacouras CA. Treatment of eosinophilic esophagitis with specific food elimination diet directed by a combination of skin prick and patch tests. Ann Allergy Asthma Immunol. 2005;95:336–43.
7. Gonsalves N, Yang G, Doerfler B, Ritz S, Ditto A, Hirano I. A prospective clinical trial of six food elimination diet and reintroduction of causative agents in adults with eosinophilic esophagitis. Gastroenterology. 2008;134:727.
8. Spergel JM, Shuker M. Nutritional management of eosinophilic esophagitis. Gastrointest Endosc Clin N Am. 2008;18:179–94.
9. Tietelbaum JE, Fox VL, Twarog FJ, Nurko S, Antonioli D, Gleich G, et al. Eosinophilic esophagitis in children: immunopathological analysis and response to fluticasone propionate. Gastroenterology. 2002;122:1216–25.
10. Noel RJ, Putnam PE, Collins MH, Assa'ad AH, Guajardo JR, Jameson SC, et al. Clinical and immunopathologic effects of swallowed fluticasone for eosinophilic esophagitis. Clin Gastroenterol Hepatol. 2005;2:568–75.

11. Assa'ad A. Detection of causative foods by skin prick and atopy patch tests in patients with eosinophilic esophagitis: things are not what they seem. Ann Allergy Asthma Immunol. 2005;95:309–11.
12. Food Allergen Labeling and Consumer Protection Act of 2004. (Title II of Public law 168–282) USC 343,303.
13. Salman S, Christie L, Burks W, Mccabe-Sellers B. Dietary intakes of children with food allergies: comparison of the food guide pyramid and the recommended dietary allowances. J Allergy Clin Immunol. 2002;109:S221.
14. Monfdi A. Nutritional management of pediatric food hypersensitivity. Pediatrics. 2003;111:1645–53.
15. Carvalho NF, Kenney RD, Carrington PH, Hall DE. Severe nutritional deficiencies in toddlers resulting from health food milk alternatives. Pediatrics. 2001;107:e46.
16. Noimark L, Cox HE. Nutritional problems related to food allergy in childhood. Pediatr Allergy Immunol. 2008;19:188–95.
17. Liu T, Howard RM, Mancini AJ, Weston WL, Paller AS, Drolet BA, et al. Kwashiorkor in the United States fad diets, perceived and true milk allergy and nutritional ignorance. Arch Dermatol. 2001;137:630–6.

Chapter 25
Nutritional Management of Eosinophilic Esophagitis in Pediatric Patients

Mimi Girten, Elizabeth Goldberg, and Michele Shuker

Keywords Eosinophilic esophagitis • Dietary therapy • Elimination diets • Skin prick testing • Atopy patch testing

Introduction

Dietary therapy is the primary method of treatment of EoE in the pediatric population. The nutritional management of children with EoE is therefore an essential component of care and underscores the important role played by the pediatric nutritionist.

Currently, three nutritional or dietary approaches exist for EoE, including guided elimination diets, empiric elimination diets, and total elemental diets. Foods can be selectively eliminated from the diet using either guided removal based on allergy testing or on empiric removal of the most common foods known to cause EoE. Guided food removal utilizes the combined results of both skin prick testing (SPT) and atopy patch testing (APT) to direct dietary therapy [1].

An alternate method is the empiric removal of the most common food allergens (milk, soy, wheat, egg, fish, shellfish, peanuts, treenuts) [2]. Other foods also noted as common causes include corn, beef, and chicken [3]. Both the guided and empiric methods of food removal have resulted in similar rates of improvement, with normalization of biopsies occurring about 75% of the time [1, 2]. The third method is the total elemental diet that is the replacement of all foods with an elemental formula.

This chapter will examine these approaches with emphasis on the nutritional risks, and advantages and disadvantages of each method. A discussion of the role of the registered dietitian in managing the pediatric patient with EoE as well as information on enteral feedings and patient/family education and resources will also be included.

M. Shuker (✉)
Division of Allergy and Immunology, The Children's Hospital of Philadelphia, 3550 Market Street, 3rd Floor, Philadelphia, PA 19104, USA
e-mail: shuker@email.chop.edu

C.A. Liacouras and J.E. Markowitz (eds.), *Eosinophilic Esophagitis*, Clinical Gastroenterology, DOI 10.1007/978-1-60761-515-6_25,

Elimination Diet

Overall Nutrition Assessment of the EoE Patient

Each of the three proposed methods for dietary treatment of EoE presents potential nutritional risks. A thorough nutrition assessment with a registered dietitian (RD) experienced in food allergy is therefore advisable for all patients after diagnosis. The challenge to the RD is not only educating the patient and family as to which foods and ingredients to avoid, but helping them to identify appropriate substitutions to replace nutrients lost when major allergens are removed.

A detailed nutritional assessment must include:

Medical history/family history
Anthropometric data and growth trends
Biochemical data
Clinical data
Dietary history including psychosocial assessments.

A complete diet history should be obtained and include food preferences, brand names of food, amounts consumed at meals, eating behaviors, number of caregivers involved in food shopping and preparation, and methods of food preparation. All of these factors can affect adherence to the prescribed diet and a careful review can help identify potential barriers to successful nutrition therapy.

Assessment of growth is important for all children. The majority of the children living in the United States have adequate intakes of most nutrients. However, children at risk for nutritional deficiencies include those on medically prescribed diets such as allergen-free, gluten-free, or tube feedings [4]. Standard measurements of height, weight, weight-to-height ratios, and head circumference as plotted on the appropriate growth charts may not provide enough information about a child's growth. It has been proposed that monitoring the growth charts for a change in the child's growth velocity is an important assessment for nutritional deficiency. This is especially necessary in infants and young children who present with failure to thrive. Christie found that children with milk allergy or children with two or more food allergies were shorter, based on height-for-age percentiles than those with only one food allergy [5].

Estimating Nutritional Requirements

Estimated nutritional requirements are determined via established methods for the pediatric population: Recommended Dietary Allowances (RDAs) and Dietary Reference Intakes (DRIs) [6, 7]. Nutritional requirements for children with EoE are generally the same as for healthy children without allergies. Additional calories, protein and/or micronutrients may be required in certain situations for children with a history of poor weight gain and/or growth, atopic dermatitis, or other accompanying diagnoses which increase nutritional requirements.

Carbohydrates should provide 45–55% of total calories, with an emphasis on whole grains, fruits, and vegetables for micronutrients and fiber. Consumption of whole grains and fresh fruits and vegetables should be emphasized not only for the nutrient value but also to provide fiber to the diet. Wheat is often removed from the diet of children with EoE, which necessitates the use of alternate grain sources. High-quality sources of protein should make up for 15–20% of the diet.

Provisions must be made to supply adequate essential amino acids by ensuring sufficient intake of complete proteins and/or complimentary proteins [8]. Fat should provide the remaining 30–35% of total calories. Adequate dietary fat helps to ensure appropriate energy intake, normal growth, and prevention of essential fatty acid deficiency. A variety of dietary fat is encouraged so that appropriate amounts of monounsaturated, polyunsaturated, and saturated fats are consumed. Normal growth in infants is dependent on adequate amounts of Essential Fatty Acids (EFA). Vegetable oils, except for coconut oil, are mostly unsaturated fats. Vegetable oils such as safflower, canola, corn, soybean, and olive oil supply monounsaturated and polyunsaturated fats and EFA to allergic individuals. Animal proteins provide saturated fats.

The RDA and DRI for vitamins, minerals, and trace elements can serve as a guideline for children with food allergies. Micronutrient intake will vary according to the severity of diet restrictions. Salman noted that the intake of children with food allergies was low in calcium, iron, vitamin D, vitamin E, and zinc. The need for supplementation should be continually assessed when diet modifications change throughout treatment [9].

Nutritional Concerns with an Elimination Diet

The risk of dietary inadequacy will increase with the number and type of foods removed from the diet, a poor nutritional status at the time of diagnosis and the presence of dysfunctional eating behaviors such as food refusal, selective eating, or texture aversion.

Elimination diets pose significant challenges to patients and families. Some foods are easier to omit from the diet than others, but the removal of even one dietary staple can make for a difficult adjustment. The diet of the average child in our population would likely not be severely altered by the removal of soy, peanut, and seafood (assuming they were on an open diet prediagnosis). Milk and wheat proteins are generally the most difficult allergens to remove as they are present in the diets of so many children and their removal often has the greatest nutritional impact (Table 25.1).

For example, those on a dairy-free diet may need to replace calcium and protein. Fiber supplements may be needed if grains are removed and intake of fruits and vegetables is suboptimal. Vitamin and mineral supplements may be necessary. A thorough evaluation of the supplement is essential when determining the type to be

Table 25.1 Nutrients in major food allergens and appropriate substitutes

Food	Nutrients	Substitutions
Milk	Protein, calcium, phosphorus, vitamin D, riboflavin, pantothenic acid vitamin B12	Meats, legumes, whole grains, nuts, fortified foods, and beverages (ex: enriched soy milk, fortified orange juice)
Wheat	Iron, niacin, riboflavin, thiamin, folate, fiber	Fortified foods, fruits, vegetables, other fortified grains (barley, oat, corn, rice, rye), alternative grains such as buckwheat, quinoa, soy, amaranth (if fortified)
Egg	Protein, choline, vitamin A, riboflavin, pantothenic acid, biotin, selenium	Meats, legumes, whole grains, dairy
Soy	Protein, thiamin,, riboflavin, pyridoxine, folate, calcium, phosphorus, magnesium, iron, zinc	Meats, other legumes, fortified beverages

given. The "complete" type of pediatric multivitamin/mineral suggests that diet contains a wide variety of both vitamins and minerals ; it does not signify that it contains 100% of the recommended dietary allowance for each nutrient. For example, gummy-type products tend to have fewer nutrients than the complete chewable type [4].

When a food or food group is eliminated from the diet, consideration to types of nutrients lost, whether other components of the diet can make up for the lost nutrients and what dietary alterations are needed to replace the lost nutrients must be made. A 3-day diet record can be kept by the family once the patient has transitioned to his or her restricted diet. Analysis of the recorded intake is useful in determining nutritional adequacy and the need for nutritional supplementation. Supplementation with an elemental formula may be necessary at the outset of treatment if numerous diet restrictions are required, or later if intake of solid foods eventually proves inadequate.

Additional calories, when needed, can be provided from a variety of sources. The most efficient way to add calories is with dietary fat (vegetable oils), which is generally not restricted for most patients. Commercial modular supplements, such as Duocal (Nutricia, Gaithersburg, MD 20884) or Polycose (Ross Products Division, Abbott Laboratories, Columbus, OH 43215) can also be used for most patients.

Milk Avoidance

Milk is a leading dietary source of protein, calcium, phosphorus, vitamin D, riboflavin, pantothenic acid and vitamin B12. Enriched soymilk can substitute for cow's milk, as it provides protein, calcium, vitamin D, and riboflavin [8]. If soy is also restricted from the diet, enriched rice milk can be used. Rice milk is not a significant source of protein, however, and the remainder of the diet should be reviewed by the RD to ensure that protein needs can be met by solid foods. Rice milk is also low in fat and other sources of dietary fats such as vegetable oils may need to be added to the diet [8]. The same concerns hold true for beverages derived from oat, potato, and some hemp-based beverages, but these products, if accepted, can be used as significant source of calories in an otherwise balanced diet. Use of enriched products can also help meet calcium requirements. Table 25.2 provides information on some currently available dairy alternatives products such as Ultracare for Kids (Metagenics, Inc., San Clemente, CA) and MimicCreme Non-Dairy Cream Substitute (MimicCreme, Albany, NY) can be used to provide calories or missing nutrients to a child's diet. Careful analysis of the diet is required on an ongoing basis (Table 25.2).

Wheat Avoidance

Wheat and enriched wheat products provide iron, niacin, riboflavin, thiamin, folate, and fiber. The removal of wheat and other grains can significantly affect the intake of dietary fiber. Patients should be encouraged to increase fruits and vegetables, if allowed in the diet. Wheat alternatives such as amaranth, arrowroot, barley, buckwheat, corn, oat, potato, rice, soybean, tapioca, and quinoa flour may be used if permitted in the diet and tolerated by the patient. There are many wheat and gluten-free products available today and families should receive information on how to obtain them and how to incorporate alternative grains into recipes.

Egg Avoidance

Eggs provide protein, choline, vitamin A, riboflavin, pantothenic acid, biotin, and selenium. Most of these can usually be provided by other foods, depending on what remains in the diet. Both egg whites and egg yolks must be avoided. Eggs are also an important ingredient in baked goods, providing leavening and structure. Instructions on how to replace eggs in baking can be found at The Food Allergy and Anaphylaxis Network (http://www.foodallergy.org). Cholesterol-free egg substitutes such as Egg Beaters (ConAgra Foods, Inc., Omaha, NE) contain egg whites and are not appropriate for use. Energ-G Foods (http://www.ener-g.com) produces an egg replacer that is safe for many restricted diets.

Soy Avoidance

Soy provides protein, thiamin, riboflavin, pyridoxine, folate, calcium, phosphorus, magnesium, iron, and zinc. Its removal may not present a nutritional risk unless it has already been used as a replacement for dairy products or other foods and was a

Table 25.2 Dairy-free beverages

	Product	Calories per 8 oz serving	Protein per serving (g)	Available with added calcium/other micronutrients?	Suitable as sole source of nutrition?	Additional flavors available?
Soy-based	Soy dream[a]	140	7	Yes	No	Yes
	Kidz dream[a]	100	4	Yes	No	Yes
	Silk soy, vanilla[b]	100	6	Yes	No	Yes
	Bright beginnings soy pediatric drink[c]	240	7	Yes	Yes	No
Rice based	Rice dream[a]	120	1	Yes	No	Yes
Hemp-based	Hemp dream[a]	100	4	Yes	No	Yes
	Living harvest hempmilk[d]	100	2	Yes	No	Yes
	Pacific foods hemp milk (contains rice)[e]	140	4	Yes		
Coconut-based	So delicious original coconut milk[f]	80	1	Yes	No	Yes
Oat-based	Pacific foods organic oat milk[e]	130	4	Yes		
Nut-based	Almond dream[a]	50	1	Yes	No	Yes
	Pacific foods hazelnut milk (contains rice)[e]	110	2	Yes	No	Yes

Availability may vary based on geographical area. Please remember that ingredients can change at any time. Carefully read ingredient lists and periodically contact manufacturers to ensure safety

[a]The Hain Celestial Group, Inc., Boulder, CO 80301

[b]Whitewave Foods, Broomfield, CO 80021

[c]PBM Products, Gordonsville, VA 22942

[d]Living Harvest Foods, Inc., Portland, OR 97208

[e]Pacific Foods of Oregon, Tualatin, OR 97062

[f]Turtle Mountain, LLC, Eugene, OR 97402

significant part of the diet prior to diagnosis. As mentioned above, fortified rice milks or other grain and/or nut-based beverages can replace the calories and some of the nutrients that soy products provide. Soy is a significant source of protein, and care must be taken to ensure that protein requirements can be met by the remainder of the diet. Soy oil and soy lecithin are typically not restricted as they contain very little protein. Studies show that most soy allergic individuals can safely consume soy oil and soy lecithin [10].

The elimination of soy, egg, peanut, and seafood from an already open diet does not usually present major nutrient losses, as these foods are not typically eaten in similar amounts and frequency as milk and/or wheat. If the diet is already restricted, however, the removal of these foods can result in significant challenges toward ensuring adequate intake. Micronutrient supplementation will likely be needed and elemental formula or modular supplementation with vegetable oils or other commercially available products may be required to provide optimal intake of calories, protein, and fat.

Nutritional Concerns with Elemental Diet

The success of elemental diets in treating EoE has been demonstrated numerous times and the use of amino acid-based formulas as the sole source of nutrition has been shown to resolve esophageal eosinophilia almost all of the time [2, 11–13].

An elemental diet requires the replacement of all solid foods with a nutritionally complete elemental formula, where the protein source entirely comprises synthetic amino acids. Elemental formulas contain free essential and non-essential amino acids, corn syrup solids, safflower, coconut, soy oils, and medium chain triglycerides (MCT) oil. They are sucrose, lactose, and milk-free. Some of the more commonly used formulas are Neocate Infant, Neocate Junior, E028 Splash (Nutricia, Gaithersburg, MD 20884) Elecare (Ross Products Division, Abbott Laboratories, Columbus, OH 43215), and Nutramigen AA (Mead Johnson, Evansville, IN 47721). Neocate Nutra (Nutricia) is an elemental semisolid food that can be used to supplement elemental formula, but is not intended for use as a sole source of nutrition. Hydrolyzed protein or semi-elemental formulas such as Nutramigen (Mead Johnson, Evansville, IN 47721) or Peptamen (Nestle Nutrition, Glendale, CA 91203) or Alimentum (Ross Products Division, Abbott Laboratories, Columbus, OH 43215) are not acceptable for use as they contain small amounts of milk proteins.

Other Nutrients/Vitamins/Protein/Fat

Micronutrient supplementation may be required on an elemental diet, depending upon the volume of formula consumed. Most additional needs can be met using over-the-counter supplements, which are free of major allergens. Kirkman (http://www.kirkmanlabs.com) and Freeda (http://www.freedavitamins.com) sell many hypoallergenic products, as do numerous other companies. Product ingredients should be reviewed on a regular basis to ensure safety.

It is important to note that most elemental formulas do not contain dietary fiber. An exception to this is Neocate Junior with Prebiotics (Nutricia North America, Gaithersburg, MD). A temporary lack of dietary fiber should not pose long-term health issues. Fiber supplements are useful for those children who develop or are prone to constipation, or for those who remain dependent on elemental formula for longer periods of time if solid foods cannot be reintroduced. Supplements should be free of known allergens. Guar-gum, psyllium, and inulin-based supplements can be used by most patients.

Palatability

One of the most frequently encountered barriers to success with an elemental diet is the acceptance of the formulas by patients. The use of amino acids as the main protein source renders the formulas significantly less palatable than their intact protein counterparts. The flavors of these formulas have improved in recent years, although this remains, as expected, largely a matter of opinion. It can indeed be overwhelming to be faced with the prospect of drinking at least a liter of these formulas per day. Flavored and unflavored formulas are available, and different strategies can be employed to enhance palatability, such as using the sugar-based flavor packets provided by the manufacturer or adding protein-free flavorings of the patient's choice (allergen-free chocolate/strawberry syrup, powdered drink mixes). Any flavorings should be discussed with the allergist before use to ensure their safety, although the use of sugar-based or artificially sweetened products that do not contain protein are likely to pose little allergenic risk. Sugar-based candies, Gatorade, and artificially flavored waters may be permitted for some patients.

If a patient is unable or unwilling to consume the required volume of elemental formula, enteral tube feedings may be necessary. This is, of course, a concept foreign to most patients and families, but with proper training, the feedings can be provided successfully in almost all cases. An experienced Registered Dietitian can help in managing tube feeding regimens.

A recent review of patients seen in the Center for Pediatric Eosinophilic Disorders revealed that 15% of the population received more than half of their nutritional requirements from elemental formula. Of these patients, 62% took the formula by mouth and 38% via enteral tube feedings.

Enteral Tube Feedings

There are many contributing reasons why children with EoE may require enteral tube feedings. Food refusal, dysphagia, and reduced volume or variety of intake, including the avoidance of solids are common in children with EoE [14]. Elemental formulas may be the sole source of nutrition or used as a supplement for those on a selective elimination diet. Unfortunately, elemental formulas have an unpleasant taste and may be poorly accepted by children, although infants usually do better. Taste fatigue can become an issue for those children who are willing to accept formula by mouth, especially when the use of formula is required for an extended period of time. Enteral tube feedings are often necessary as it can be very difficult for some children to drink the volume of elemental formula needed to meet nutritional requirements.

Enteral feeding methods include nasogastric (N/G) and gastrostomy tube (G Tube) feedings. Nasogastric tubes are typically used for short-term nutrition support. While there is no standardized definition of "short-term" use, if N/G tube feeds are needed for longer than 3–6 months, then gastrostomy tube feeds should be considered. While growth and development are of primary concern and may dictate the need for enteral feeding, the use of tube feedings presents both benefits and risks.

Infants and children learn how to eat as well as how not to eat. EoE and its symptoms can derail the development of oral feeding skills and alter the family dynamics at mealtime. In infants, learning to eat follows a predictable developmental sequence. The acquisition of feeding skills can be interrupted by illness, pain, environmental stressors, and tube feeds. Requirements for a liquid elemental diet or delayed introduction of solids and textures may impact feeding skill development. The use of N/G tube or G tube feeding may negatively impact feeding skill development by contributing to oral motor immaturity (such as poor jaw strength or tone) or oral sensory dysfunction. These problems may be a result of lack of experience or may be self-imposed as a result of symptoms or treatment. Oral sensory dysfunction manifests as food aversions, gagging with particular tastes or textures or specific refusals to bring food items to the mouth [14]. Lack of pleasant oral experiences leads to reduced motivation for eating and delayed oral skill development. In older children with EoE, the fear of foods getting "stuck" may contribute to altered patterns of eating.

In tube-fed children, there is a risk of altered feeding development and changes in mealtime dynamics. However, the use of tube feedings can significantly reduce parental anxiety over a child's inadequate oral intake. Tube feedings can reduce mealtime stress and lessen the tension between the child and the primary caregiver, thus paving the way for successful feeding therapy, if such therapy should be necessary.

Adverse events can occur during the administration of enteral feedings if proper care and monitoring are lacking. Previous studies have shown that between 20.9 and 43.5% of enteral tube placements are incorrect [15].

In the case of nasogastric tubes, there is a very real risk of incorrect tube placement, which is especially serious if the N/G tube is placed into the child's lungs. Inadvertent placement of an N/G tube into the esophagus significantly increases the risk of gastroesophageal reflux or aspiration into the lungs. There are several methods for measuring the placement length of the N/G tube as well as different types and sizes of N/G tubes. The nose-to-ear and then midway between xiphoid and umbilicus measurement is thought to be the most accurate means of measuring N/G tube length. The development of height-based formulas to predict esophageal length appear promising but are in need of more research [16]. Polyurethane nasogastric tubes are often used in children as these tubes may remain in place for up to 28 days before needing to be changed. The "gold standard" test for confirming correct placement of a nasogastric tube is by X-ray. This is not feasible for long-term use of N/G tubes or for patients who use N/G tubes at home. As there is no one nonradiologic method to confirm gastric placement of feeding tubes, a combination of some of the simpler and more accurate methods may be used and will help determine when an abdominal X-ray may be needed to confirm placement. Auscultation while injecting air into the feeding tube is not a reliable method for confirming N/G tube position as bowel or chest sounds may be misinterpreted as confirming gastric placement [17]. (Assessment of aspirate pH and color are the currently preferred method of confirming N/G tube placement). A pH of 5.5 or below is thought to indicate gastric placement. When gastric pH is greater than or equal to 6, using pH to predict tube location is of no benefit and the tube must be removed and replaced or a confirmatory abdominal X-ray obtained [17]. Gastric aspirates are cloudy, green, tan, off-white, bloody, or brown. Small bowel aspirates are typically yellow or bile colored. Pleural fluid is clear yellow and watery. Other less frequent complications associated with N/G tube use include perforation of the esophagus or stomach, obstruction of nasal breathing, and possibly increased incidence of sinusitis or ear infections [18].

Gastrostomy tubes allow for direct access into the stomach via an opening called a stoma and are used for long-term nutritional support. The obvious benefit to having a G Tube is the increased certainty that one is feeding into the child's stomach. Some children view the placement of N/G tubes as an invasive procedure and dislike the fact that having a visible N/G tube makes them appear different from other children. A gastrostomy tube reduces the impact of these issues. Gastrostomy tube feedings are tolerated well for the most part. However, they are not without complications. Infections, skin irritation, or breakdown from poor fitting tubes or leakage, and the development of painful or bleeding granulation tissue does occur with the use of gastrostomy tubes. There is no evidence that children with EoE experience more complications with gastrostomy tube use than do other children. As for any child with a gastrostomy tube, careful attention to care of the peristomal skin and periodic remeasuring for proper fit of the tube will help to reduce problems commonly associated with G Tube use.

Financial Considerations

Elemental formulas are quite expensive. The monthly cost of elemental formula for a patient needing 1,800 cal/day can easily exceed $1,000/month. Insurance coverage for these formulas varies, and intervention from the clinical team is almost always required to assist with preauthorization, letters of medical necessity, etc. Coverage is not always provided, despite aggressive efforts of the family and diligent advocacy of health-care providers. Some states have passed legislation-mandating coverage under specific conditions. A complete discussion of this issue is outside the scope of this chapter. But it should be noted that treatment with an elemental diet – even supplementation of solid food with elemental formula – may be cost-prohibitive for some families.

Food Reintroduction

An important part of nutritional management of EoE is the reintroduction of foods back into the diet. Once a normal biopsy has been achieved, on either an elemental diet or selective elimination diet (where more than one food was removed), foods can be added back into the patient's diet. Table 25.3 shows the general protocol used at the Children's Hospital of Philadelphia for reintroduction of foods after an elemental diet. Foods are classified into general families from group A (least allergic) to group D (most allergic).

Patients start with foods in column A and move to column B and so on. One new food is added per week, with a repeat endoscopy generally occurring 6–8 weeks after the last food is added. This process is repeated until a positive biopsy occurs. The foods that appear to cause abnormal biopsies are removed and others are tried. Most fruits and vegetables are considered low-risk foods for most patients with EoE. Therefore, they are typically the first to be reintroduced and more of them are added in-between endoscopies. The number of foods added between endoscopies decreases as the allergenicity of the food increases. Higher-risk foods such as grains,

Table 25.3 Food reintroduction following an elemental diet

A	B	C	D
Vegetables (non-legume):	*Tropical fruits*:	*"Allergic" fruit and vegetables*:	Most common foods
Carrots, squash, sweet potato, string beans, broccoli, lettuce	Banana, kiwi, pineapple, mango, papaya, guava, avocado	Apple, potato, peas	Corn
Fruit (non-citrus, nontropical):	*Melons*:	*Grains*:	Chicken
Pear, peaches, plum, apricot	Honeydew, cantaloupe watermelon	Rice, oat, barley, rye	Wheat
Citrus fruits:	*Berries*:	*Meat*[a]:	Beef
Orange, grapefruit, lemon, lime	Strawberry, blueberry, raspberry, cherry	Lamb, chicken, turkey, pork	Soy
	Legumes:	*Fish/shellfish*	Egg
	Lima beans, chickpeas, white/black/red beans	*Peanut and tree nuts*:	Milk
		Peanut, Almond, walnut, hazelnut, brazil nut, Pecan	

[a]Progress from well cooked to rarer

meats, eggs, soy and dairy often require individual trials, although specific methods of reintroduction will vary according to patient history and preference and clinical experience of the EoE team [3].

Nutritional Needs and Evaluation

Nutritional risks should decrease as foods are successfully reintroduced and dietary variety expands. Periodic reassessment of the diet via a 3-day food record can be helpful in adjusting micronutrient supplementation. Patients with preexisting feeding difficulties (food refusal, gagging/choking with foods, texture aversion) should have these behaviors reassessed throughout the course of treatment. If improvement is not observed once normal biopsies are achieved, a referral to a feeding specialist would be indicated to determine the need for behavioral therapy.

Patient Education

All caregivers and patients (once mature enough) should be educated on the need for allergen-avoidance to ensure the selection of safe products and food preparation. The RD should emphasize to all patients and caregivers the need to focus on what children can eat vs. what they cannot. All of the dietary treatments discussed here will impact the family's daily life, and this should be acknowledged. Families should be referred to appropriate resources for additional information and encouraged to investigate local support groups and/or online message boards. The American Partnership for Eosinophilic Disorders (http://www.apfed.org) is a valuable resource for many families and provides useful information which the families of newly diagnosed patients may find especially helpful.

Referrals for psychological counseling should be made if patients experience ongoing sadness or anger regarding their treatment plan.

Label Reading

Label-reading will become a crucial skill for all involved in food selection and preparation during an elimination diet. Legislation has been passed to assist patients and families with this task. The Food Allergen Labeling and Consumer Protection Act of 2004 (FALCPA) was implemented in January, 2006 [19]. An overview of the law follows here and complete details can be found on the Food Allergy and Anaphylaxis Network website at http://www.foodallergy.org. FALCPA mandates that any food product manufactured for sale in the Unites States must contain on the package label a clear listing of ingredients derived from commonly allergenic foods (milk, egg, soybean, wheat, peanut, tree nut, fish, crustacean shellfish). The law applies to conventional food products, dietary supplements, infant formulas, and medical foods; raw agricultural commodities are not affected. Manufacturers must also list the specific tree nut, fish, or crustacean shellfish used as an ingredient (mollusks are not considered major food allergens under FALCPA) [19].

Major food allergens must be listed on the product label in one of the following ways:

- In the ingredient list : "milk, egg, or soy"
- Parenthetically following the food protein derivative: "casein (milk)"
- Immediately below the ingredient list in a "contains" statement: "contains milk" [19]

Only one of these methods is required. Patients and families should be taught to avoid looking only for "contains" statements and continue to read ingredient lists as needed. Major food allergens must also be declared in spices, flavorings, colorings, or additives, or if used to aid in processing [19, 20]. These regulations apply only to ingredients derived from the eight foods listed above. Individuals who need to avoid ingredients not covered under FALCPA must contact the manufacturer to confirm product safety.

Some ingredients may be derived from an allergenic source but contain such insignificant amounts of the allergenic protein that they are usually well tolerated. Examples of this are lecithin (derived from soy) and kosher gelatin (derived from fish) [21, 22]. Highly refined vegetable oils derived from major food allergens are exempt from labeling requirements, as they contain very little protein and are not thought to pose a risk of allergic reaction [19–22].

Ingredients and manufacturing processes can change over time, and labels should be reviewed each time a food is purchased or consumed, even if the food has been used safely in the past. FAAN has available for purchase a Grocery Manufacturer's Directory and small pocket-sized laminated cards listing ingredients to avoid on specific allergen-free diets [23].

Patient/Family Education

Educational materials and instructions should be thorough, updated, and easily understood. Allergen-free sample menus can be used to help plan meals and snacks. Some families find it helpful for all family members to follow the prescribed diet restrictions, depending on the number of foods removed. This strategy can assist with dietary adherence in some cases, provided each family member's nutritional requirements are met. Lists of allergen-free foods should be provided along with information on where foods can be purchased. Food allergy cookbooks can also be useful. Patients and caregivers should be encouraged to try a variety of products, as able, and inquire about the safety of unfamiliar ingredients (Table 25.4).

The family should also receive guidance on how to manage diet restrictions when eating outside the home and/or on special occasions. Parents or caregivers should be

Table 25.4 Resources for eosinophilic disorders/food allergy

American partnership for eosinophilic disorders
http://www.apfed.org
CURED: Campaign urging research for eosinophilic disease
http://www.curedfoundation.org
Food allergy and anaphylaxis network
http://www.foodallergy.org
Kids with food allergies
http://www.kidswithfoodallergies.com
American academy of allergy, asthma and immunology
http://www.aaaai.org
American dietetic association
http://www.eatright.org

encouraged to contact their child's school to discuss the diet restrictions with not only the teacher but the school nurse, food service personnel, and school administration, if needed. It is usually best to contact restaurants ahead of time and visit during non-busy hours. Caregivers should ask questions about ingredients and food preparation or storage, so that the risk of cross-contamination can be considered.

The Food Allergy and Anaphylaxis Network (FAAN) has developed excellent educational materials for use in schools. Parents should be encouraged to familiarize themselves and their child's school with these materials. Additional resources for families are shown in Table 25.4.

Summary

Eosinophilic esophagitis can be successfully managed with careful dietary therapy, but diet restrictions present many challenges. The degree of food restriction can range from the elimination of just one food group to the elimination of all foods from a child's diet. An experienced registered dietitian is a crucial member of the multidisciplinary EoE team. Families must be educated appropriately to enhance success with adherence to specific diet plans. Children must be monitored closely to ensure nutritional needs are met and adequate growth occurs.

The impact of nutritional therapy on the patient's quality of life should be assessed on an ongoing basis.

References

1. Spergel JM, Andrews T, Brown-Whitehorn TF, Beausoleil JL, Liacouras CA. Treatment of eosinophilic esophagitis with specific food elimination diet directed by a combination of skin prick and patch tests. Ann Allergy Asthma Immunol. 2005;95(4):336–43.
2. Kagalwalla AF, Sentongo TA, Ritz S, et al. Effect of six-food elimination diet on clinical and histologic outcomes in eosinophilic esophagitis. Clin Gastroenterol Hepatol. 2006;4(9):1097–102.

3. Spergel J, Shuker M. Nutritional management of eosinophilic esophagitis. Gastrointestinal Endosc Clint N Am. 2008;18(1):179–94.
4. Kirby M, Danner E. Nutritional deficiencies in children on restricted diets. Pediatr Clin N Am. 2009;56:1085–103.
5. Christie L, Hine RJ, Parker JG, Burks W. Food allergies in children affect nutrient intake and growth. J Am Diet Assoc. 2002;102(11):1648–51.
6. Food and Nutrition Board Institute of Medicine. Dietary reference intakes – applications in dietary assessment. A report of the subcommittee on interpretation and uses of dietary reference intakes and the standing committee on the scientific evaluation of dietary reference intakes. Washington, DC: National Academy Press; 2000.
7. Food and Nutrition Board NRC. Recommended dietary allowances. 10th ed. Washington, DC: National Academy Press; 1989.
8. Mofidi S. Nutritional management of pediatric food hypersensitivity. Pediatrics. 2003;111 (6 Pt 3):1645–53.
9. Salman S, Christie L, Burks AW, McCabe-Sellers B. Dietary intakes of children with food allergies: comparison of the food guide pyramid and the recommended dietary allowances, 10th ed. J Allergy Clin Immunol. 2002;109:S214.
10. Crevel RW, Kerkhoff MA, Koning MM. Allergenicity of refined vegetable oils. Food Chem Toxicol. 2000;38(4):385–93.
11. Kelly K, Lazenby A, Rowe P, Yardley JH, Perman J, Sampson H. Eosinophilic esophagitis attributed to gastroesophageal reflux: improvement with an amino acid-based formula. Gastroenterology. 1995;109:1503–12.
12. Markowitz JE, Spergel JM, Ruchelli E, Liacouras CA. Elemental diet is an effective treatment for eosinophilic esophagitis in children and adolescents. Am J Gastroenterol. 2003;98(4):777–82.
13. Liacouras CA, Spergel JM, Ruchelli E, et al. Eosinophilic esophagitis: a 10-year experience in 381 children. Clin Gastroenterol Hepatol. 2005;3(12):1198–206.
14. Haas AM, Maune NC. Clinical presentation of feeding dysfunction in children with eosinophilic gastrointestinal disease. Immunol Allergy Clin N Am. 2009;29(1):65–75.
15. Ellett MLC, Croffie JMB, Cohen MD, Perkins SM. Gastric tube placement in young children. Clin Nurs Res. 2005;14(3):238–52.
16. Beckstrand J, Ellett MLC, McDaniel A. Predicting internal distance to the stomach for positioning nasogastric and orogastric feeding tubes in children. J Adv Nurs. 2007;59(3):274–89.
17. Metheny NA, Meert KL. Monitoring feeding tube placement. Nutr Clin Pract. 2004;19:487–95.
18. Metheny NA, Meert KL, Clouse RE. Complications related to feeding tube placement. Curr Opin Gastroenterol. 2007;23:178–82.
19. US Food and Drug Administration. Food Allergen Consumer Protection Act of 2004. 2004. http://www.cfsan.fda.gov. Accessed 9 June 2010.
20. US Food and Drug Administration. Questions and answers regarding food allergens including the food allergen consumer protection act of 2004. 4th ed. Oct 2006. http://www.cfsan.fda.gov. Accessed 9 June 2010.
21. Hefle SL, Taylor SL. How much food is too much? Threshold doses for allergenic foods. Curr Allergy Asthma Rep. 2002;2(1):63–6.
22. Taylor SL, Hefle SL. Food allergen labeling in the USA and Europe. Curr Opin Allergy Clin Immunol. 2006;6(3):186–90.
23. Munoz-Furlong A. Daily coping strategies for patients and their families. Pediatrics. 2003;111(6 Pt 3):1654–61.

Chapter 26
Oral Tolerance and Eosinophilic Esophagitis

Pooja Varshney and A. Wesley Burks

Keywords Eosinophilic esophagitis • Oral tolerance • Food allergy • Regulatory T cells • Oral immunotherapy

Introduction

Eosinophilic esophagitis (EoE) is an increasingly recognized disease process characterized by symptoms of vomiting, food refusal, and dysphagia associated with localized eosinophilic inflammation of the esophagus. Though the precise link is not completely understood, EoE has been shown to be highly associated with atopic disease. Sensitization to both food and environmental allergens has been seen in patients with EoE [1]. Studies have shown that a significant proportion of patients with EoE have evidence of allergic disease by history or skin testing [2]. In one series of 13 patients, 77% had a history of an allergic disorder (asthma, allergic rhinitis, urticaria, atopic dermatitis, food allergy, or drug allergy) and/or positive radioallergosorbent testing (RAST) or skin prick testing [3]. Another study of 21 children revealed that 68% of subjects had a positive result to foods on skin or RAST testing [4]. In patients with biopsy-proven EoE, elimination of positive foods identified by both skin prick testing and patch testing led to complete resolution of the clinical symptoms in 18 of 24 patients, suggesting a possible association [5].

The mucosal accumulation of eosinophils in the gastrointestinal tract suggests a Th2-mediated process [1]. Murine studies have shown impaired induction of esophageal

A.W. Burks (✉)
Department of Pediatrics, Division of Allergy and Immunology,
Duke University Medical Center, 2644, Durham, NC 27710, USA
e-mail: wesley.burks@duke.edu

C.A. Liacouras and J.E. Markowitz (eds.), *Eosinophilic Esophagitis*,
Clinical Gastroenterology, DOI 10.1007/978-1-60761-515-6_26,

eosinophilia in response to allergen in mice who are genetically deficient in signal transducer and activator of transcription 6 (STAT6), IL-13, IL-4, and IL-5, providing evidence that allergen-induced EoE is dependent on classic Th2 cytokine signaling [6]. Like other Th2-dependent disease processes, eosinophilic gastrointestinal diseases likely represent the interplay of extrinsic allergic triggers and intrinsic Th2 cytokines in genetically predisposed individuals [1].

The role of food allergy in EoE may be explained by a breakdown in oral tolerance or a failure in the induction of tolerance. Oral tolerance is the physiologic mechanism by which immune responses to an antigen are suppressed by prior administration of the antigen by the oral route [7, 8]. This normal process is crucial in allowing a wide array of dietary proteins access to the body without activating harmful immune responses.

Oral tolerance presumably evolved as an analog of self-tolerance to prevent potentially dangerous hypersensitivity reactions to harmless food proteins and commensal gut flora. The lumen of the gastrointestinal tract, the largest immunologic organ in the body, is continually exposed to numerous dietary proteins. Here, antigen-presenting cells encounter food proteins and subsequently activate regulatory T lymphocytes that reside in the loose connective tissue beneath the gastrointestinal epithelium [9]. These cells then suppress cellular and humoral immune responses to the protein. In nonallergic hosts, the majority of food proteins are absorbed without provoking injurious local or systemic immune responses [10]. The pathologic cellular and humoral immune responses that characterize food allergy likely result from either a failure in establishing tolerance or a breakdown in existing tolerance [9]. It is possible that similar mechanisms underlie the pathogenesis of EoE.

Mucosal Immunology and Fundamentals of Oral Tolerance

The surface area of the gastrointestinal mucosa exceeds that of the skin by several fold [10]. The gastrointestinal mucosa is also more permeable to antigens than intact skin and, therefore, represents the major site of contact with foreign antigenic materials. Approximately 130–190 g of food protein are absorbed daily in the gut [11]. Another source of natural antigenic stimulation is the resident gut microbiota, with approximately 10^{12} microorganisms per gram of stool [12]. The gut lodges the most abundant lymphoid tissue in the body, with 10^{12} lymphoid cells per meter of human small intestine; the population of immunoglobulin-secreting cells in the gut exceeds the total number found in all other lymphoid organs [13].

Foreign antigen exposure in the gut normally results in several major immunologic responses. The local production and release of noninflammatory secretory IgA antibody is the initial response occurring in the gastrointestinal mucosa. Antigens stimulate B lymphocytes in the organized mucosal lymphoid tissue. These cells migrate to distant mucosal and glandular sites and differentiate into

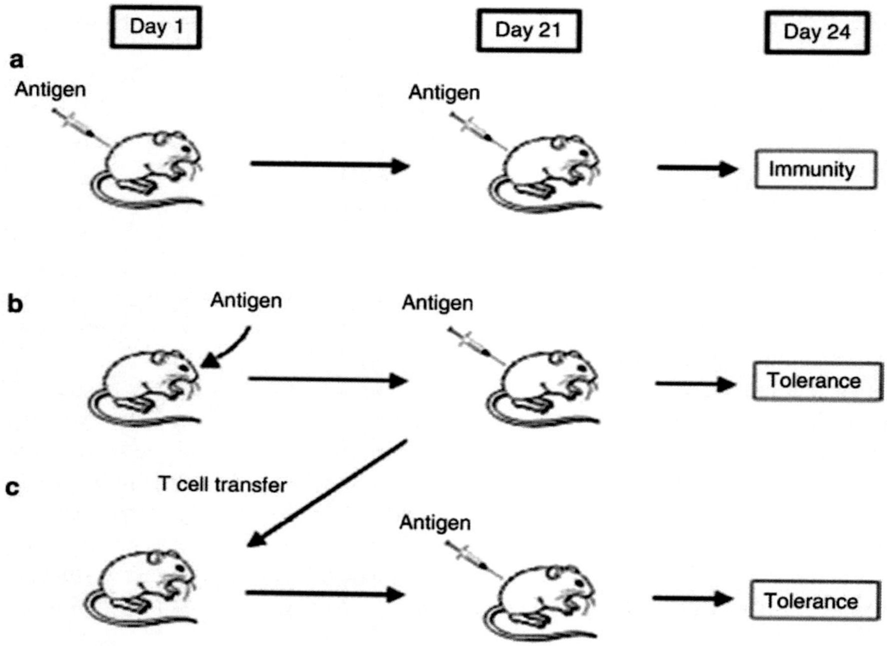

Fig. 26.1 Induction of oral tolerance. (**a**) Mice immunized subcutaneously and then boosted subcutaneously with an antigen show strong in vitro cell-mediated and antibody responses to the antigen. (**b**) When mice are first fed the antigen orally and then immunized subcutaneously, in vitro immune responses to the antigen are greatly reduced. (**c**) Transferring T cells from mice that were fed antigen to naive mice results in reduced in vitro immune responses to subsequent subcutaneous immunization. This shows that oral feeding of an antigen can induce a T cell-mediated active inhibitory immune response. Adapted from Chehade and Mayer. Oral tolerance and its relation to food hypersensitivities. J Allergy Clin Immunol. 2005;115(1):4, with permission

antigen-specific polymeric-IgA-producing plasma cells [14]. On subsequent exposure, polymeric IgA crosslinks luminal antigens and prevents their interaction with gut epithelial cells. Priming of the systemic immune system may also occur, activating humoral and cellular immunity to protect against the pathogen on future encounters [10].

In contrast to the activation of immunologic responses described above, exposure to dietary proteins and commensal bacteria in nonatopic hosts generally leads to a state of systemic and/or local immunologic tolerance, allowing these exogenous antigens access to the body [10]. In the mid-twentieth century, Chase and his colleagues established that oral feeding of an antigen induces T cell-mediated inhibition of subsequent immune responses, illustrating the concept of oral tolerance (Fig. 26.1) [7]. He contrasted the induction of oral tolerance from the generation of strong cell-mediated and humoral responses that follows subcutaneous immunization and booster administration of an antigen. Additional experiments demonstrated that the transfer of T cells from antigen-fed "tolerant" mice to naïve mice also resulted in reduced in vitro immune responses to subcutaneous immunization.

Exposure to food proteins and commensal gut flora exerts a stimulatory effect on the developing immune system [11]. Adult mice given a balanced diet consisting of amino acids but no intact food proteins have poorly developed gut-associated lymphoid tissue resembling that of suckling mice, with low levels of secretory IgA and fewer intraepithelial lymphocytes [15]. They also have a predominantly Th2 cytokine profile, with high concentrations of interleukin (IL)-10 and IL-4 and a low concentration of interferon-gamma (IFN-gamma). The presence of microbes in the murine gut also plays an important role in driving the expansion of B and T cells in Peyer's patches and mesenteric lymph nodes, illustrating the importance of commensal microbiota in the development of the mucosal immune system [16].

Antigen Processing in the Gastrointestinal Tract

The journey for a dietary protein involves multiple steps before tolerance or hypersensitivity is established. The digestion process itself, from salivary enzymes to gastric acid and luminal enzymes, promotes immunologic tolerance by degrading dietary proteins and destroying immunogenic epitopes [9]. The digestion of intact proteins to amino acid chains less than eight amino acids long renders them nonreactive with antigen recognition structures and thereby immunologically ignored [17]. Disruption of the enzymatic digestion process has been shown to impair tolerance in both animal and human models, leading to food hypersensitivity [18]. Peptic digests of bovine serum albumin (BSA) are tolerogenic when administered orally or directly injected into the mouse ileum [19]. Untreated BSA is immunogenic when administered to mice by ileal injection, yet tolerogenic when administered orally, likely due to degradation in the digestive tract. Clinical studies have also demonstrated the important role of enzymatic digestion in the induction of oral tolerance in humans. Pharmacologic suppression of gastric acid secretion by antiulcer medications has been associated with increased food-specific IgE production; impaired digestion of food proteins may render them potent sensitizers [20].

Proteins that are not degraded by gastrointestinal enzymes encounter the intestinal epithelium and the lymphoid tissue beneath it in several ways (see Fig. 26.2) [8]. Dendritic cells extend processes between epithelial cells to sample luminal antigens. M cells are specialized epithelial cells overlying Peyer's patches that take up particulate antigens and deliver them to subepithelial dendritic cells, which in turn present antigens to B cells in Peyer's patches. Soluble antigens, which are not efficiently taken up by M cells, cross the epithelium by transcellular or paracellular routes to the lamina propria, where they encounter T cells and macrophages. Intestinal epithelial cells act as nonprofessional antigen-presenting cells, endocytosing soluble antigens and presenting them to primed T cells.

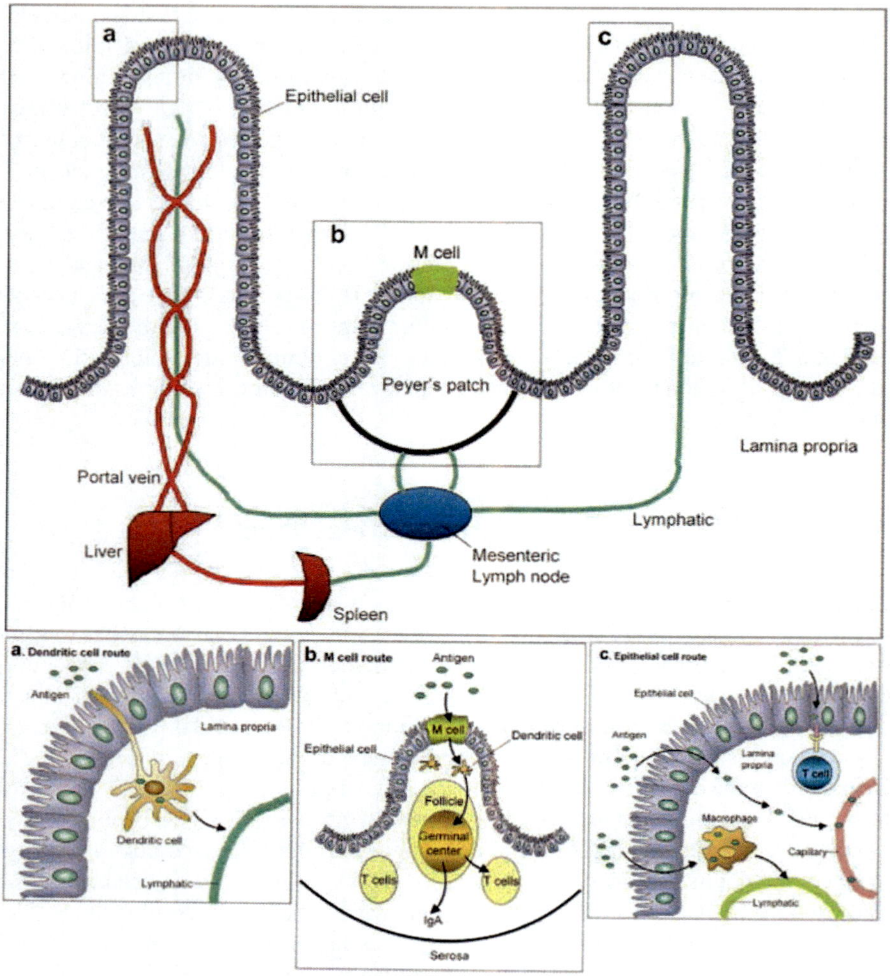

Fig. 26.2 Sites of antigen uptake in the gut. (**a**) Antigen can be sampled by dendritic cells that extend processes into the lumen. (**b**) M cells overlying Peyer's patches take up particulate antigens and then deliver them to dendritic cells in the subepithelial region and then to underlying B-cell follicles, where IgA commitment occurs. (**c**) Soluble antigens can cross the epithelium through transcellular or paracellular routes to then encounter T cells or macrophages in the lamina propria. Adapted from Chehade and Mayer. Oral tolerance and its relation to food hypersensitivities. J Allergy Clin Immunol. 2005;115(1):5, with permission

Mechanisms of Oral Tolerance

Oral tolerance is induced through two primary effector mechanisms – active suppression by regulatory T (Treg) cells and clonal anergy or deletion (see Fig. 26.3). The dose of the antigen is a key factor determining which will take place [21], although it is likely

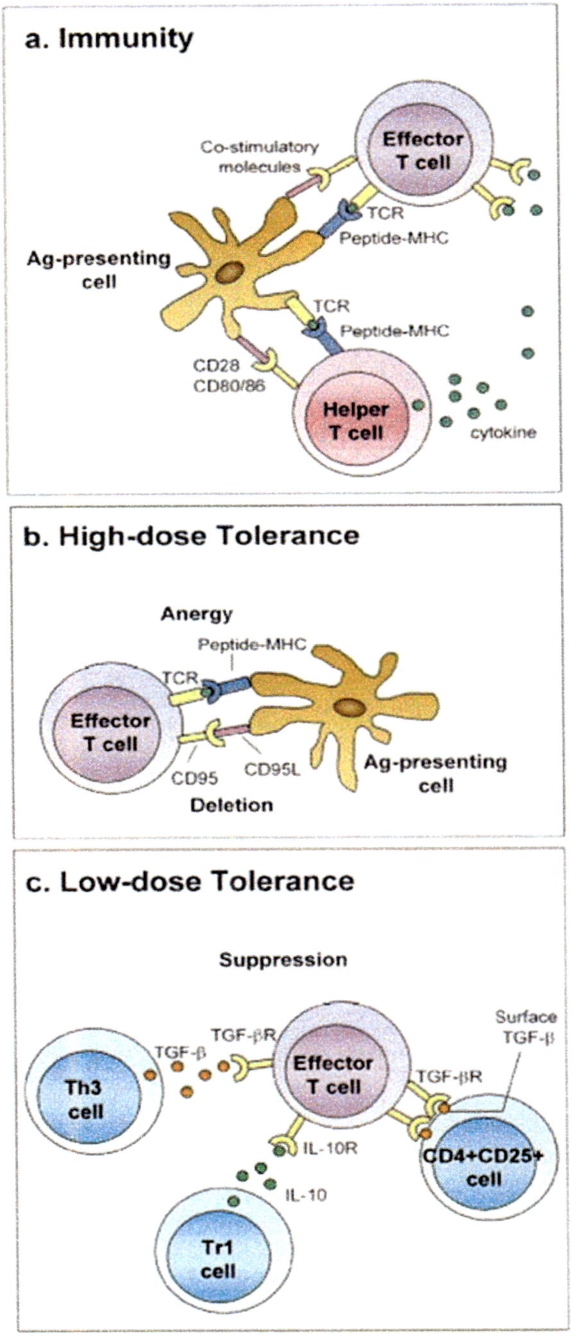

Fig. 26.3 Mechanisms of oral tolerance. (**a**) Generation of an immune response requires T-cell receptor ligation with peptide-MHC complexes in the presence of appropriate costimulatory molecules (CD80 and CD86) and cytokines. (**b**) High-dose tolerance is induced by T-cell receptor cross linking in the absence of costimulation or in the presence of inhibitory ligands (CD95 and CD95 ligand), leading to anergy or deletion, respectively. (**c**) Low doses of oral antigen lead to the activation of regulatory CD4+ CD25+ T cells, which suppress immune responses through soluble or cell surface-associated cytokines (IL-10 and TGF-β). *L* Ligand; *R* receptor. Adapted from Chehade and Mayer. Oral tolerance and its relation to food hypersensitivities. J Allergy Clin Immunol. 2005;115(1):7, with permission

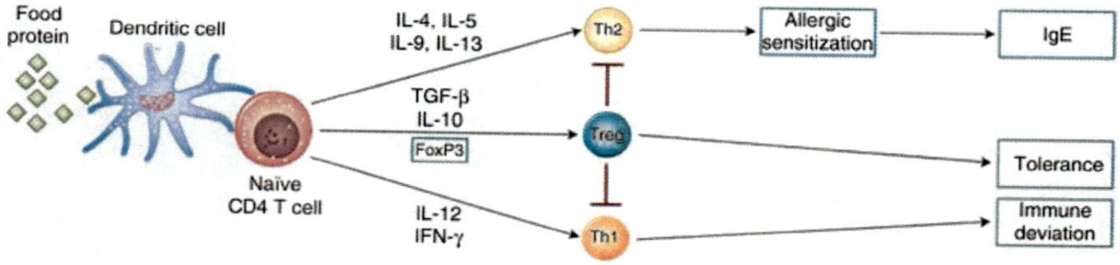

Fig. 26.4 Allergic sensitization vs. oral tolerance. Food antigen exposure in the gastrointestinal mucosal immune system can result in oral tolerance induction or allergic sensitization. FoxP3-forkhead box P3; IFN-interferon; IL-interleukin; TGF-transforming growth factor; Th-T-helper cell; Treg-T-regulatory cell. Adapted from Scurlock, Burks, and Jones. Oral immunotherapy for food allergy. Curr Allergy Asthma Rep. 2009;9(3):187, with permission

the two processes are not mutually exclusive. Low doses of antigen induce Treg cells that produce immunoregulatory cytokines such as transforming growth factor (TGF) beta and IL-10 and actively suppress reactive lymphocytes. Treg cells were initially characterized by their stable surface expression of the high-affinity component of the IL-2 receptor, CD25 [22]. More recently, studies have shown that subsets express the transcription factor forkhead box P3 (FOXP3), the key regulatory gene in the development of naturally occurring CD4+ Treg cells (see Fig. 26.4) [23]. Treg cells are functionally distinct from effector T cells by their ability to limit T cell proliferation and function [24]. CD4+ CD25+ Treg cells migrate to lymphoid organs and suppress effector cells through cell–cell interaction involving surface-bound TGF-beta [25], although their regulatory function can also occur independently of TGF-beta [26]. Treg cells also migrate to target organs, where they exert their immunosuppressive effects by releasing nonantigen-specific cytokines [10].

Defective Treg development has been shown to play a key role in the pathogenesis of autoimmune and allergic disease. Immune dysregulation, polyendocrinopathy, enteropathy, X-linked (IPEX) syndrome, which is caused by mutations in the gene encoding FOXP3, is characterized by autoaggressive lymphocyte clones due to a failure in Treg development [27]. An IPEX variant characterized by severe allergic as well as autoimmune manifestations has been described [28]. In this case, a mutation in a noncoding region of the FOXP3 gene results in a disorder characterized by severe food allergy, atopic dermatitis, elevated serum IgE, and eosinophilia in addition to enteropathy. Allergen-induced EoE pathogenesis is thought to be dependent on adaptive T cell immunity [29], and defects in Treg function may underlie the development of EoE. Recent work has demonstrated an imbalance in esophageal effector and Treg cells in a mouse model of EoE, suggesting that this may be a crucial factor in the promotion of pathogenic immunological responses in EoE [30].

Treg cells may also be important as a marker of tolerance in the setting of resolving food allergy. The appearance of circulating CD4+ CD25+ T cells has been associated with the development of tolerance in children with a history of non-IgE-medicated milk allergy [11]. Milk-tolerant children also had decreased in vitro proliferative responses to bovine beta-lactoglobulin in peripheral blood mononuclear cells compared with those who had persistent allergy. Similarly, the utility of Treg quantification is being investigated as a potential biomarker of tolerance in studies of oral immunotherapy (OIT) for food allergy. In ten subjects who received peanut OIT for as long as 36 months, the number of FoxP3 T cells increased approximately 1.5-fold in peanut-stimulated cells at 6 and 12 months and decreased thereafter, returning to baseline levels by 20 months [31].

Whereas low doses of antigen favor Treg-driven tolerance, high-dose tolerance is mediated by lymphocyte anergy or clonal deletion. Anergy can be induced through binding of a peptide antigen in the absence of costimulatory signals provided either by soluble cytokines (IL-2) or by interactions between receptors on T cells (CD28) and counterreceptors on antigen-presenting cells (CD80 and CD86) [32]. High doses of antigen induce deletion of reactive T cells by means of apoptosis. In mice transgenic for ovalbumin-specific T-cell receptor genes, oral antigen administration led to deletion of antigen-specific T cells in Peyer's patches [33]. The deletion was mediated by apoptosis of target cells. In the aforementioned study of open-label peanut OIT, genome-wide oligonucleotide microarray analyses compared transcription patterns in T cells obtained before and 6 months after OIT treatment and revealed downregulation of genes in several apoptosis pathways, although it is unclear at this time whether the observed changes included altered apoptosis of antigen-specific T cells [31]. To help isolate effects on antigen-specific T cells, studies using MHC class II/Ara h 2 peptide tetramers are currently underway.

It is likely that low- and high-dose tolerance mechanisms are not mutually exclusive and actually overlap in vivo. Cytotoxic T lymphocyte-associated antigen (CTLA-4) was first described in a pathway of anergy induction and has been shown to play a crucial role in the induction of high-dose tolerance [34]. However, CTLA-4-binding to T cells also leads to production of TGF-beta, an immunoregulatory cytokine that may counterbalance CD28-costimulation of T cell activation [35]. In addition, phagocytosis of apoptotic cells by macrophages results in induction of TGF-beta, further contributing to an immunosuppressive milieu favoring tolerance [36].

Factors Influencing Development of Tolerance

In addition to antigen dose, several other factors influence the development of tolerance, including antigen properties, route of exposure, age of the host, genetic factors, and gut flora (Fig. 26.4). Particulate antigens tend to be more allergenic than soluble antigens, although most food allergens are soluble proteins. Solubility can be altered by food preparation techniques and heat treatment. For example, roasting has been shown to progressively decrease the solubility of peanut proteins, rendering the protein more immunogenic and increasing the capacity of peanut-specific IgE to bind the protein when encountered in the gut [37]. Innate immunostimulatory properties of certain dietary proteins may also enhance their allergenicity and result in a Th2 response in genetically susceptible individuals. For example, the major glycoprotein peanut allergen, Ara h 1, was found to induce dendritic cells that prime Th2-skewed T cell responses [38].

The route of allergen exposure also plays an important role in the development of allergy or oral tolerance. As mentioned previously, oral administration of an antigen followed by subcutaneous immunization results in greatly reduced in vitro immune responses to the antigen, illustrating the concept of oral tolerance (Fig. 26.1) [7]. Food antigen exposure by other routes may result in sensitization and resultant allergy. In murine models, epicutaneous exposure to peanut protein induces a potent Th2 immune response, with high levels of IgE and IL-4 production, potentially preventing the induction of oral tolerance [39]. This principle may also be relevant to the pathogenesis of EoE, as epicutaneous allergen exposure in mice has been shown to prime for marked Th2-dependent esophageal eosinophilic inflammation with subsequent challenge [6]. Similarly, exposure to an inhaled respiratory allergen in mice was shown to promote eosinophilic esophagitis, suggesting common mechanisms regulating eosinophilic inflammation in the respiratory tract and esophagus [40]. In contrast, oral or intragastric allergen administration did not elicit eosinophilic inflammation in the esophagus.

As with other atopic conditions, host factors play a central role in the determination of food allergy or oral tolerance. An individual's genetic make-up plays an important role in whether exposure to a given protein results in sensitization or tolerance. Murine studies have demonstrated the strain-dependence of allergic responses. In a murine study of peanut allergen gene immunization, mice were immunized with plasmid DNA encoding Ara h 2, one of the major peanut allergens [41]. The response to subsequent peanut protein injection was strain-dependent; all of the C3H/HeSn mice but none of the AKR/J or BALB/c mice developed anaphylaxis. Similarly, EoE has been shown to have a strong familial association [2]. The sibling recurrence risk ratio λ_s for EoE has been estimated as approximately 80, with λ_s value of greater than 1 indicating increased risk of development of the disease among siblings of the proband compared with that of the general population [42]. Genome-wide expression analyses have identified *CCL26*, the gene encoding the eosinophil-specific chemoattractant eotaxin-3 as the most highly induced gene in EoE patients compared with its expression level in healthy individuals [43]. The disease-associated allele is only present in 14% of EoE cases, suggesting that additional risk variants exist. A recent genome-wide association study identified *TSLP* as an EoE susceptibility locus [44]. *TSLP* was found to be overexpressed in esophageal biopsies from individuals with EoE, similar to findings in lesional atopic dermatitis skin and the asthma-affected lung [45]. TSLP (thymic stromal lymphopoietin) has been implicated as a key initiator of allergic sensitization [46], which may prove to be a sentinel event in the pathogenesis of EoE.

The host's age is another factor influencing the development of oral tolerance. Immaturity of the immunologic and gastrointestinal systems predisposes infants to impaired tolerance and resultant food allergy [47]. Infants and young children have an immature gastrointestinal mucosal surface, with increased intestinal permeability, decreased gastric acidity, and decreased pancreatic enzyme production [48]. In addition, secretory IgA is absent in newborns. As a result, intact proteins are more likely to be systemically absorbed and may then stimulate the immune system and result in IgE production [47]. Furthermore, infants' immune systems are skewed toward Th2-skewed allergen-specific responses at birth [49]. These responses are rapidly suppressed during the first year of life in nonatopic children but persist in atopic children.

The resident flora of the gastrointestinal tract also plays a central role in the induction of oral tolerance. The maturation of gut-associated lymphoid tissue depends on the presence of commensal microorganisms [16]. After oral antigen administration, mice raised in germ-free environments maintained Th2-mediated immune responses characterized by production of IgE, IgG1, and IL-4 [50]. Reconstitution of the gastrointestinal tract with *Bifidobacterium infantis* restored the ability to induce oral tolerance, though only if performed in the neonatal period, thus demonstrating the shared roles of intestinal flora as well as age of exposure in the development of tolerance.

Conclusions

Oral tolerance is crucial in allowing a wide array of dietary proteins access to the body without activating harmful immune responses. A breakdown in oral tolerance mechanisms or a failure to establish tolerance can result in food allergy and may underlie the pathogenesis of EoE. Allergy has been implicated in the etiology of EoE based on patient characteristics, evidence of allergen sensitization, and in vivo and in vitro immunologic findings [51]. However, the precise role of food, cutaneous, or airborne allergen sensitization in the development of EoE has yet to be fully elucidated. Allergy may be a stimulus for the recruitment of eosinophils to the gastrointestinal tract or may lead to the failure of Treg cells leading to a disruption in low-dose oral tolerance [52]. A breakdown in mechanisms of high-dose oral tolerance, which include lymphocyte anergy or deletion, may also lead to the development of EoE as well as classic forms of food allergy. Further study to clarify the role of oral tolerance in the development of EoE can help identify potential prevention strategies and therapeutic targets.

References

1. Blanchard C, Rothenberg ME. Basic pathogenesis of eosinophilic esophagitis. Gastrointest Endosc Clin N Am. 2008;18(1):33–43. x.
2. Noel RJ, Putnam PE, Rothenberg ME. Eosinophilic esophagitis. N Engl J Med. 2004;351(9):940–1.
3. Vitellas KM et al. Idiopathic eosinophilic esophagitis. Radiology. 1993;186(3):789–93.
4. Orenstein SR et al. The spectrum of pediatric eosinophilic esophagitis beyond infancy: a clinical series of 30 children. Am J Gastroenterol. 2000;95(6):1422–30.
5. Spergel JM et al. The use of skin prick tests and patch tests to identify causative foods in eosinophilic esophagitis. J Allergy Clin Immunol. 2002;109(2):363–8.

6. Akei HS et al. Epicutaneous antigen exposure primes for experimental eosinophilic esophagitis in mice. Gastroenterology. 2005;129(3):985–94.
7. Chase M. Inhibition of experimental drug allergy by prior feeding of the sensitizing agent. Proc Soc Exp Biol. 1946;61:257–9.
8. Chehade M, Mayer L. Oral tolerance and its relation to food hypersensitivities. J Allergy Clin Immunol. 2005;115(1):3–12. quiz 13.
9. Burks AW, Laubach S, Jones SM. Oral tolerance, food allergy, and immunotherapy: implications for future treatment. J Allergy Clin Immunol. 2008;121(6):1344–50.
10. Faria AM, Weiner HL. Oral tolerance. Immunol Rev. 2005;206:232–59.
11. Karlsson MR, Rugtveit J, Brandtzaeg P. Allergen-responsive CD4+ CD25+ regulatory T cells in children who have outgrown cow's milk allergy. J Exp Med. 2004;199(12):1679–88.
12. Macfarlane GT, Macfarlane S. Human colonic microbiota: ecology, physiology and metabolic potential of intestinal bacteria. Scand J Gastroenterol Suppl. 1997;222:3–9.
13. Mestecky J, McGhee JR. Immunoglobulin A (IgA): molecular and cellular interactions involved in IgA biosynthesis and immune response. Adv Immunol. 1987;40:153–245.
14. Kraehenbuhl JP, Neutra MR. Transepithelial transport and mucosal defence II: secretion of IgA. Trends Cell Biol. 1992;2(6):170–4.
15. Menezes J, Da S, et al. Stimulation by food proteins plays a critical role in the maturation of the immune system. Int Immunol. 2003;15(3):447–55.
16. Hrncir T et al. Gut microbiota and lipopolysaccharide content of the diet influence development of regulatory T cells: studies in germ-free mice. BMC Immunol. 2008;9:65.
17. Aalberse RC. Structural biology of allergens. J Allergy Clin Immunol. 2000;106(2):228–38.
18. Untersmayr E, Jensen-Jarolim E. The role of protein digestibility and antacids on food allergy outcomes. J Allergy Clin Immunol. 2008;121(6):1301–8. quiz 1309–10.
19. Michael J. The role of digestive enzymes in orally induced immune tolerance. Immunol Invest. 1989;18:1049–54.
20. Untersmayr E et al. Anti-ulcer drugs promote IgE formation toward dietary antigens in adult patients. FASEB J. 2005;19(6):656–8.
21. Friedman A, Weiner HL. Induction of anergy or active suppression following oral tolerance is determined by antigen dosage. Proc Natl Acad Sci U S A. 1994;91(14):6688–92.
22. Sakaguchi S et al. Immunologic self-tolerance maintained by activated T cells expressing IL-2 receptor alpha-chains (CD25). Breakdown of a single mechanism of self-tolerance causes various autoimmune diseases. J Immunol. 1995;155(3):1151–64.
23. Hori S, Nomura T, Sakaguchi S. Control of regulatory T cell development by the transcription factor Foxp3. Science. 2003;299(5609):1057–61.
24. Ana I, Janine LC, Fiona P. Regulatory T cells suppress systemic and mucosal immune activation to control intestinal inflammation. Immunol Rev. 2006;212(1):256–71.
25. Nakamura K, Kitani A, Strober W. Cell contact-dependent immunosuppression by CD4(+) CD25(+) regulatory T cells is mediated by cell surface-bound transforming growth factor beta. J Exp Med. 2001;194(5):629–44.
26. Piccirillo CA et al. CD4(+)CD25(+) regulatory T cells can mediate suppressor function in the absence of transforming growth factor beta1 production and responsiveness. J Exp Med. 2002;196(2):237–46.
27. Ochs HD, Gambineri E, Torgerson TR. IPEX, FOXP3 and regulatory T-cells: a model for autoimmunity. Immunol Res. 2007;38(1–3):112–21.
28. Torgerson TR et al. Severe food allergy as a variant of IPEX syndrome caused by a deletion in a noncoding region of the FOXP3 gene. Gastroenterology. 2007;132(5):1705–17.
29. Mishra A et al. Critical role for adaptive T cell immunity in experimental eosinophilic esophagitis in mice. J Leukoc Biol. 2007;81(4):916–24.
30. Zhu X et al. An imbalance of esophageal effector and regulatory T cell subsets in experimental eosinophilic esophagitis in mice. Am J Physiol Gastrointest Liver Physiol. 2009;297(3):G550–8.
31. Jones SM et al. Clinical efficacy and immune regulation with peanut oral immunotherapy. J Allergy Clin Immunol. 2009;124(2):292–300. 300 e1–97.
32. Appleman LJ, Boussiotis VA. T cell anergy and costimulation. Immunol Rev. 2003;192:161–80.

33. Chen Y et al. Peripheral deletion of antigen-reactive T cells in oral tolerance. Nature. 1995;376(6536):177–80.
34. Samoilova EB et al. CTLA-4 is required for the induction of high dose oral tolerance. Int Immunol. 1998;10(4):491–8.
35. Chen W, Jin W, Wahl SM. Engagement of cytotoxic T lymphocyte-associated antigen 4 (CTLA-4) induces transforming growth factor beta (TGF-beta) production by murine CD4(+) T cells. J Exp Med. 1998;188(10):1849–57.
36. Freire-de-Lima CG et al. Uptake of apoptotic cells drives the growth of a pathogenic trypanosome in macrophages. Nature. 2000;403(6766):199–203.
37. Kopper RA et al. Peanut protein allergens: the effect of roasting on solubility and allergenicity. Int Arch Allergy Immunol. 2005;136(1):16–22.
38. Shreffler WG et al. The major glycoprotein allergen from *Arachis hypogaea*, Ara h 1, is a ligand of dendritic cell-specific ICAM-grabbing nonintegrin and acts as a Th2 adjuvant in vitro. J Immunol. 2006;177(6):3677–85.
39. Strid J et al. Epicutaneous exposure to peanut protein prevents oral tolerance and enhances allergic sensitization. Clin Exp Allergy. 2005;35(6):757–66.
40. Mishra A et al. An etiological role for aeroallergens and eosinophils in experimental esophagitis. J Clin Invest. 2001;107(1):83–90.
41. Li X et al. Strain-dependent induction of allergic sensitization caused by peanut allergen DNA immunization in mice. J Immunol. 1999;162(5):3045–52.
42. Blanchard C, Wang N, Rothenberg ME. Eosinophilic esophagitis: pathogenesis, genetics, and therapy. J Allergy Clin Immunol. 2006;118(5):1054–9.
43. Blanchard C et al. Eotaxin-3 and a uniquely conserved gene-expression profile in eosinophilic esophagitis. J Clin Invest. 2006;116(2):536–47.
44. Rothenberg ME et al. Common variants at 5q22 associate with pediatric eosinophilic esophagitis. Nat Genet. 2010;42(4):289–91.
45. Oyoshi MK et al. Cellular and molecular mechanisms in atopic dermatitis. Adv Immunol. 2009;102:135–226.
46. Liu YJ. TSLP in epithelial cell and dendritic cell cross talk. Adv Immunol. 2009;101:1–25.
47. Nowak-Wegrzyn A, Sampson HA. Adverse reactions to foods. Med Clin North Am. 2006;90(1):97–127.
48. Sampson HA. Food allergy. Part 1: immunopathogenesis and clinical disorders. J Allergy Clin Immunol. 1999;103(5 Pt 1):717–28.
49. Prescott SL et al. Development of allergen-specific T-cell memory in atopic and normal children. Lancet. 1999;353(9148):196–200.
50. Sudo N et al. The requirement of intestinal bacterial flora for the development of an IgE production system fully susceptible to oral tolerance induction. J Immunol. 1997;159(4):1739–45.
51. Furuta GT et al. Eosinophilic esophagitis in children and adults: a systematic review and consensus recommendations for diagnosis and treatment. Gastroenterology. 2007;133(4):1342–63.
52. Seibold F. Food-induced immune responses as origin of bowel disease? Digestion. 2005;71(4): 251–60.

Chapter 27
Treatment of Eosinophilic Esophagitis with Biological Agents

Kathryn A. Peterson, Molly O'Gorman, W. Daniel Jackson, and Gerald J. Gleich

Keywords Eosinophilic esophagitis • Dysphagia • Chest pain • Inflammation • Steroid administration

Introduction

Traditional therapies for eosinophilic esophagitis have focused on dietary modifications and/or anti-inflammatory treatments, primarily systemic or topical glucocorticoids. However, both such approaches are difficult to maintain for both patients and clinicians. Elemental diets, containing amino acids as a protein substitute plus simple carbohydrates and fatty acids, are effective in up to 98% of children [1–3], but due to poor palatability and cost, these diets often are not sustainable. A six-food elimination diet is effective in up to 78% of children and of adults [3, 4], but this diet is limited by significant noncompliance. Subsequently, clinicians have focused on the use of medications able to suppress inflammation for eosinophilic esophagitis (EoE). The first reports of the use of oral glucocorticoids [5] and swallowed aerosolized steroids for the topical treatment of EoE [6] were published in 1998. The results of the first randomized controlled trial of swallowed fluticasone in children with EoE in 2006 were disappointing, with only 50% of children achieving remission, compared to 9% of those receiving placebo [7]. The biopsies from the distal esophagus appeared more resistant to fluticasone administration arguing that perhaps the resistance to this therapy was related to the route of administration.

G.J. Gleich (✉)
Department of Dermatology, University of Utah Hospital,
30 North 1900 East, Salt Lake City, UT 84132, USA
e-mail: Gerald.gleich@hsc.utah.edu

C.A. Liacouras and J.E. Markowitz (eds.), *Eosinophilic Esophagitis*,
Clinical Gastroenterology, DOI 10.1007/978-1-60761-515-6_27,

Presently, the efficacy of suspension and viscous formulations of steroids are under investigation for EoE. Straumann recently reported success treating 18 adolescents and adults with EoE using 2 mg budesonide (0.25 mg/mL) suspension [8]. Two weeks of therapy with the suspension resulted in a drop of peak eosinophil counts from 148 to 18 eosinophils/high power field (HPF) with 13/18 patients achieving complete histological remission. A pilot trial of oral viscous budesonide demonstrated response (<7 eosinophils/HPF) in 80% of children [9]. In other studies of this issue, 15 children received 1–2 mg (dose dependent on height) oral viscous budesonide for 3 months with response (defined as less than 6 eosinophils/HPF) in 87% of children [9, 10]. Additionally, the children experienced substantial symptomatic relief.

However, although the side effects seen in the recent trials of swallowed topical budesonide suspensions have been minimal and systemic absorption of budesonide and fluticasone from the gastrointestinal tract also is minimal [11–13], concerns remain over possible candidal esophagitis and adrenal suppression associated with prolonged use of steroids. Additionally, a substantial number of children and adults are refractory to steroid administration and continue to suffer from ongoing dysphagia and chest pain.

Biological Agents

Neutralization of IgE by Omalizumab

EoE often develops in concert with atopy as suggested by the effectiveness of food avoidance in children. Food and aeroallergen sensitivities are found commonly, and asthma is relatively prevalent in such patients [14]. Indeed, there is abundant evidence implicating activation of mast cells and B cells within the esophagus. Vicario found evidence for in situ immunoglobulin production within the esophagus itself [15]. B cells and mast cells with bound IgE are increased in the esophagi of patients with EoE regardless of atopic status [15, 16]. Evidence of local immunoglobulin class switching has been detected via localization of germline transcripts, activation-induced cytidine deaminase, IgE heavy chain, and mature IgE mRNA within the esophageal tissue of EoE patients [17]. Additionally, >50% of EoE patients have elevated serum IgE levels and atopy [18], and the robust TH2 response may activate mast cells resident in the esophageal mucosa. Therefore, anti-IgE therapy may block the activation of such cells and reduce mediator release, including TNF-α and proteases release [19, 20].

Omalizumab is a humanized recombinant-derived IgG1 antibody which selectively binds to IgE. Currently omalizumab is approved for patients with moderate to severe asthma [21]. Omalizumab inhibits the binding of IgE to its high affinity receptor, FcεR1 (epsilon), by binding to the epitope on IgE that overlaps with the FceR1 binding site. In turn, IgE binding to mediator cells, such as mast cells and basophils, is inhibited thereby preventing release of mediators from these cells. Langerhans cells in the esophageal epithelium in eosinophilic esophagitis express FcεR1 in abundance, and the presence of FcεR1 is increased in EoE patients above that of controls, arguing that it plays a role in the immune response to allergens in the disease [22].

A trial evaluating the efficacy of omalizumab as compared to placebo in EoE was recently completed. Unfortunately, preliminary results do not show significant improvement in symptoms of dysphagia in 30 patients enrolled (Fang J, Gleich GJ, Peterson K. Omalizumab in the treatment of eosinophilic esophagitis. Unpublished, 2010). Additionally, omalizumab did not reduce the number of eosinophils within the esophagus of patients (peak proximal eosinophil counts before and after omalizumab therapy were 28 and 30/HPF, respectively). These preliminary results are surprising in view of the information discussed above suggesting the importance of IgE-mediated food allergy, and they argue that non-IgE-mediated mechanisms may be of greater importance in the pathogenesis of EoE than heretofore appreciated.

Treatment of EoE with TNF-α (Alpha) Antagonists

TNF-α (alpha) antagonists have been utilized in the treatment of gastrointestinal immune disorders for the last 10 years to downregulate the inflammatory pathway [23], and their use has benefitted patients, especially those with inflammatory bowel diseases, such as ulcerative colitis and Crohns' disease. In EoE, TNF-α (alpha) is elevated in the esophageal tissue of patients and is highly expressed by the esophageal epithelial cells [24, 25]. Additionally, evidence exists that eosinophils themselves produce TNF-α [26].

Infliximab is a chimeric (human–mouse) IgG1 monoclonal antibody against TNF-α (alpha) [27]. Straumann et al. tested the efficacy of inflixamab in three male patients with steroid-dependent EoE refractory to all other therapies [25]. All prior therapies were discontinued 4 weeks prior to the screening esophageal biopsies and eosinophil assessment. After the 4-week run-in period, patients were given two infusions of inflixamab at 0 and 2 weeks, and biopsies were obtained before and 4 weeks after the second dose. Eosinophil counts did not diminish although patients tolerated the infusions well. Tissue levels of TNF-α did not change significantly. Among other markers of inflammation, CD3+ cells decreased, but eotaxin-3 expression and tryptase-positive cells did not change. The authors comment that the value of the study is limited by its design as an open-label, nonrandomized pilot study with a small number of patients, and they emphasize that further studies with alternative dosing schedules are needed.

Treatment of EoE with Monoclonal Antibodies to IL-5

IL-5 is a primary TH2 cytokine involved in eosinophil inception, maturation, and release from the bone marrow [28, 29]. Additionally, it is involved directly in eosinophil longevity, activation, and survival. It has both systemic effects on eosinophils (including the trafficking of such cells) as well as local effects in the esophagi of EoE patients as a cytokine released directly from eosinophils themselves. IL-5 directly influences eosinophil responsiveness to local cytokines (such as eotaxin).

IL-5 has been implicated strongly as a pivotal cytokine involved in the development and perpetuation of esophageal eosinophilia [30]. Transgenic mice that overexpress IL-5 develop EoE [31, 32]. Antibodies against IL-5 prevent the development of EoE in these mice after the instillation of intranasal allergen. Further murine studies demonstrated that the EoE transcripts induced by intratracheal IL-13 were inhibited in the absence of IL-5 [33]. Yamazaki et al. demonstrated that the peripheral mononuclear cells of EoE patients as compared to controls develop increased levels of IL-5 when stimulated by allergens [34]. IL-5 mRNA levels were increased in the tissues of EoE patients as compared to normal controls [35].

Initial human trials investigating anti-IL-5 in the hypereosinophilic syndrome were promising [36] and a subsequent placebo-controlled multicenter trial showed the efficacy of anti-IL-5 treatment [37]. Subsequent investigations have explored the efficacy of anti-IL-5 in EoE. Mepolizumab is a fully humanized monoclonal IgG1 antibody specific for human IL-5 that blocks the ability of IL-5 to bind to the alpha chain of the IL-5 receptor on the eosinophil surface [38]. Mepolizumab reduces peripheral eosinophils by 90%. In a small pilot trial, mepolizumab reduced peripheral blood eosinophilia in four patients with hypereosinophilic syndrome, an effect that was sustained for 12 weeks after the last dose [36]. In this trial, one patient with esophageal tissue eosinophilia, presumably EoE, demonstrated a tenfold reduction of eosinophilic infiltration, suggesting that mepolizumab may be effective in the treatment of EoE.

A test of this concept was conducted in four EoE patients (mean esophageal eosinophilia of 37–66 eosinophils/HPF) with three infusions of mepolizumab, 10 mg/kg (maximum 750 mg), intravenously at monthly intervals [39]. Assessment with esophageal biopsies was performed 4 weeks after the last dose of mepolizumab. Eosinophil counts per HPF decreased from 66, 37, 43, 37 to 6, 3, 8, 8, respectively. All dysphagia symptoms improved and quality of life scores increased in all four patients.

Subsequently, Straumann et al. performed a double-blind, placebo-controlled study of mepolizumab at a dose of 10 mg/kg in 11 patients [24, 40]. In this trial, two intravenous infusions of mepolizumab or placebo were given at weeks 0 and 1. None of the patients achieved complete response (defined as less than 5 eosinophils/HPF) and continued on their allocated medications (mepolizumab at 1,500 mg or placebo) for two additional infusions at weeks 5 and 9 with repeat endoscopic assessments and biopsies at week 13. All responders entered into long-term follow-up off all medications, and final assessment was made at 43 weeks (34 weeks after the last infusion). Mepolizumab therapy resulted in reduction of esophageal eosinophilia of 54% (vs. 5% in the placebo group). There was no change in T cell (CD3+) or mast cells numbers in the esophagi of subjects. Eosinophil-derived neurotoxin (EDN) staining cells and extracellular EDN were reduced in the mepolizumab arm. Additionally, by week 13, there were significant reductions in remodeling factors (TGFβ1 (beta) and tenascin-c) in the mepolizumab arm compared to placebo. No changes in epithelial TNF-α or eotaxin-3 levels occurred. Symptoms were partially improved in the mepolizumab arm. However, by week 43, all patients in the mepolizumab arm reported significant worsening of their symptoms present at enrollment.

Reslizumab, a second humanized monoclonal antibody to IL-5 [41, 42], recently was tested for its efficacy in the treatment of EoE in a phase II/III randomized, double-blind, placebo-controlled multicenter clinical trial of pediatric patients (Spergel JM et al. Reslizumab in children and adolescents with eosinophilic esophagitis: results of a double-blind, randomized, placebo-controlled study. Unpublished, 2010). A total of 226 patients were enrolled with the following characteristics: 76% male, mean age 11.9 years, and 43% experienced dysphagia, 40% pain and 17% vomiting. Esophageal biopsies showed >24 eosinophils/HPF after treatment with a proton pump inhibitor for >4 weeks. Patients were randomized to placebo and treatment arms, and the treatment patients received doses of 1, 2, or 3 mg/kg. Reslizumab infusions were given at weeks 0, 4, 8, and 12. At the beginning of the study, the mean eosinophil count per high power field for the entire group was 106 eosinophils; at the end of the study, the median esophageal eosinophil counts per high power field were 93 for placebo and 37, 27, and 30 for the reslizumab doses 1, 2, and 3 mg/kg ($p<0.001$), respectively. All treatment groups, including placebo, reported improvement in the physician's EoE global assessment score, and the magnitude of the improvement did not differ between the placebo and the reslizumab groups. This surprising result showing no relief in the patient's symptoms could be interpreted as evidence that the presence or the numbers of the eosinophils is not related to the patient's disease severity, or alternatively, that the global assessment score may not be a correct tool to measure the response to the treatment.

Future Directions

A summary of prior tests of biological agents in EoE is presented in Table 27.1. New approaches for future treatment of EoE include further trials with antibodies to IL-5, introduction of eotaxin inhibitors, and use of IL-13 antagonists. The trials with reslizumab continue [42], although the initial results (see above) appear confusing. Eotaxin-3 is an obvious target, and antagonists are in the wings [43, 44]. Concerning IL-13, intratracheal instillation of IL-13 induced esophageal eosinophilia in a murine model, and the resulting eosinophilia was not produced in mice deficient in IL-5, eotaxin-1, and STAT6, suggesting that the IL-13-stimulated esophageal eosinophilia requires all of these molecules for its development. In the human esophagus, IL-13 induces the EoE transcriptome [17], and corticosteroid administration blunts this response, possibly identifying a mechanism by which steroids effect a benefit in EoE [45, 46]. CAT-354, a human monoclonal IgG4 antibody to IL-13, neutralizes IL-13 in human lung mast cells [47]. Phase I studies in asthma

Table 27.1 Biologic agents utilized for eosinophilic esophagitis

Medication	Mechanism of action	Trial	*N*	Design	Outcome
Omalizumab	Recombinant anti-IgE antibody	Fang et al. (Unpublished, 2010)	30	Randomized double-blind placebo controlled	No change in peak eosinophil count. No difference in symptoms as compared to placebo
Infliximab	Chimeric lgG1 anti-TNF antibody	Straumann et al. [26]	3	Prospective pilot use of only two infusions	One patient with improvement
Mepolizumab	Humanized monoclonal anti-IL-5 antibody	Stein et al. [39]	4	Prospective pilot trial with three infusions of 10 mg/kg	(1) Marked decrease in esophageal eosinophilia (2) Improved dysphagia + quality of life
Mepolizumab	Humanized monoclonal anti-IL-5 antibody	Straumann et al. [40]	11	Double blind placebo controlled of two infusions of 10 mg/kg weeks 0 and 1, then weeks 5 and 9	(1) Decreased esophageal eosinophilia (2) Decreased levels of esophageal TGFβ + tenascin
Reslizumab	Humanized monoclonal Ab to IL-5	Spergel (Unpublished, 2011)	226	Randomized double blind placebo control doses 1, 2, 3 mg/kg	Reduction of esophageal eosinophilia for all dose ranges

have shown it to be safe and tolerable to patients [48, 49]. Mice pretreated with intraperitoneal CAT-354 demonstrated blunted IL-13-induced esophageal eosinophilia production, arguing for a potential therapeutic role in EoE patients [50].

Current research has focused on the efficacy of anti-IL-5 treatment for EoE. Other possible targets for future study include TH2 cells and their cytokine production. Additionally, antibodies directed toward eosinophil recruitment and their interactions within the esophageal lumen may provide some therapeutic benefit to patients. Perhaps directly inhibiting eotaxin-3 expression in the esophageal epithelium may be the optimal target. Alternatively, the optimal treatment of EoE may be a combination of agents, such an administration of an antibody to IL-5 and another to eotaxin. Further development of biological agents may not only aid patients in overcoming their esophageal disease, but these agents may serve to provide insights into the pathogenesis and prognosis of EoE itself.

References

1. Liacouras CA et al. Eosinophilic esophagitis: a 10-year experience in 381 children. Clin Gastroenterol Hepatol. 2005;3(12):1198–206.
2. Spergel JM et al. Treatment of eosinophilic esophagitis with specific food elimination diet directed by a combination of skin prick and patch tests. Ann Allergy Asthma Immunol. 2005;95(4):336–43.
3. Kagalwalla AF et al. Effect of six-food elimination diet on clinical and histologic outcomes in eosinophilic esophagitis. Clin Gastroenterol Hepatol. 2006;4(9):1097–102.
4. Gonsalves N et al. A prospective clinical trial of six food elimination diet or elemental diet in the treatment of adults with eosinophilic esophagitis. Gastroentology. 2009;136(5 Suppl 1):A-126.
5. Liacouras CA et al. Primary eosinophilic esophagitis in children: successful treatment with oral corticosteroids. J Pediatr Gastroenterol Nutr. 1998;26(4):380–5.
6. Faubion Jr WA et al. Treatment of eosinophilic esophagitis with inhaled corticosteroids. J Pediatr Gastroenterol Nutr. 1998;27(1):90–3.
7. Konikoff MR et al. A randomized, double-blind, placebo-controlled trial of fluticasone propionate for pediatric eosinophilic esophagitis. Gastroenterology. 2006;131(5):1381–91.
8. Straumann A et al. Budesonide is effective in adolescent and adult patients with active eosinophilic esophagitis. Gastroenterology. 2010;139(5):1526–37. 1537 e1.
9. Aceves SS et al. Oral viscous budesonide: a potential new therapy for eosinophilic esophagitis in children. Am J Gastroenterol. 2007;102(10):2271–9.
10. Dohil R et al. Oral viscous budesonide is effective in children with eosinophilic esophagitis in a randomized, placebo-controlled trial. Gastroenterology. 2010;139(2):418–29.
11. Schaefer ET et al. Comparison of oral prednisone and topical fluticasone in the treatment of eosinophilic esophagitis: a randomized trial in children. Clin Gastroenterol Hepatol. 2008;6(2):165–73.
12. Noel RJ et al. Clinical and immunopathologic effects of swallowed fluticasone for eosinophilic esophagitis. Clin Gastroenterol Hepatol. 2004;2(7):568–75.
13. Remedios M et al. Eosinophilic esophagitis in adults: clinical, endoscopic, histologic findings, and response to treatment with fluticasone propionate. Gastrointest Endosc. 2006;63(1):3–12.
14. Roy-Ghanta S, Larosa DF, Katzka DA. Atopic characteristics of adult patients with eosinophilic esophagitis. Clin Gastroenterol Hepatol. 2008;6(5):531–5.
15. Vicario M et al. Local B cells and IgE production in the oesophageal mucosa in eosinophilic oesophagitis. Gut. 2009;59(01):12–20.
16. Abonia JP et al. Involvement of mast cells in eosinophilic esophagitis. J Allergy Clin Immunol. 2010;126(1):140–9.
17. Blanchard C et al. IL-13 involvement in eosinophilic esophagitis: transcriptome analysis and reversibility with glucocorticoids. J Allergy Clin Immunol. 2007;120(6):1292–300.
18. Furuta GT et al. Eosinophilic esophagitis in children and adults: a systematic review and consensus recommendations for diagnosis and treatment. Gastroenterology. 2007;133(4): 1342–63.
19. Rothenberg ME. Biology and treatment of eosinophilic esophagitis. Gastroenterology. 2009;137(4):1238–49.
20. Holgate S et al. The anti-inflammatory effects of omalizumab confirm the central role of IgE in allergic inflammation. J Allergy Clin Immunol. 2005;115(3):459–65.
21. Hendeles L, Sorkness CA. Anti-immunoglobulin E therapy with omalizumab for asthma. Ann Pharmacother. 2007;41(9):1397–410.
22. Yen EH et al. Comparative analysis of Fcεepsiv;RI expression patterns in patients with eosinophilic and reflux esophagitis. J Pediatr Gastroenterol Nutr. 2010;51(5):584–92.
23. Oussalah A, Danese S, Peyrin-Biroulet L. Efficacy of TNF antagonists beyond one year in adult and pediatric inflammatory bowel diseases: a systematic review. Curr Drug Targets. 2010;11(2):156–75.

24. Straumann A et al. Idiopathic eosinophilic esophagitis is associated with a T(H)2-type allergic inflammatory response. J Allergy Clin Immunol. 2001;108(6):954–61.
25. Straumann A et al. Anti-TNF-α (infliximab) therapy for severe adult eosinophilic esophagitis. J Allergy Clin Immunol. 2008;122(2):425–7.
26. Finotto S et al. TNF-alpha production by eosinophils in upper airways inflammation (nasal polyposis). J Immunol. 1994;153(5):2278–89.
27. Nam JL et al. Current evidence for the management of rheumatoid arthritis with biological disease-modifying antirheumatic drugs: a systematic literature review informing the EULAR recommendations for the management of RA. Ann Rheum Dis. 2010;69(6):976–86.
28. Matthaei KI, Foster P, Young IG. The role of interleukin-5 (IL-5) in vivo: studies with IL-5 deficient mice. Mem Inst Oswaldo Cruz. 1997;92 Suppl 2:63–8.
29. Sanderson CJ. The biological role of interleukin 5. Int J Cell Cloning. 1990;8 Suppl 1:147–53. discussion 153–4.
30. Stone KD, Prussin C. Immunomodulatory therapy of eosinophil-associated gastrointestinal diseases. Clin Exp Allergy. 2008;38(12):1858–65.
31. Mishra A. Mechanism of eosinophilic esophagitis. Immunol Allergy Clin North Am. 2009;29(1):29–40. viii.
32. Mishra A et al. An etiological role for aeroallergens and eosinophils in experimental esophagitis. J Clin Invest. 2001;107(1):83–90.
33. Mishra A, Rothenberg ME. Intratracheal IL-13 induces eosinophilic esophagitis by an IL-5, eotaxin-1, and STAT6-dependent mechanism. Gastroenterology. 2003;125(5):1419–27.
34. Yamazaki K et al. Allergen-specific in vitro cytokine production in adult patients with eosinophilic esophagitis. Dig Dis Sci. 2006;51(11):1934–41.
35. Tantibhaedhyangkul U et al. Increased esophageal regulatory T cells and eosinophil characteristics in children with eosinophilic esophagitis and gastroesophageal reflux disease. Ann Clin Lab Sci. 2009;39(2):99–107.
36. Garrett JK et al. Anti-interleukin-5 (mepolizumab) therapy for hypereosinophilic syndromes. J Allergy Clin Immunol. 2004;113(1):115–9.
37. Rothenberg ME et al. Treatment of patients with the hypereosinophilic syndrome with mepolizumab. N Engl J Med. 2008;358(12):1215–28.
38. Walsh GM. Mepolizumab and eosinophil-mediated disease. Curr Med Chem. 2009;16(36):4774–8.
39. Stein ML et al. Anti-IL-5 (mepolizumab) therapy for eosinophilic esophagitis. J Allergy Clin Immunol. 2006;118(6):1312–9.
40. Straumann A et al. Anti-interleukin-5 antibody treatment (mepolizumab) in active eosinophilic oesophagitis: a randomised, placebo-controlled, double-blind trial. Gut. 2009;59(01):21–30.
41. Reichert JM. Antibody-based therapeutics to watch in 2011. MAbs. 2011;3(1):76–99.
42. Walsh GM. Reslizumab for pediatric eosinophilic esophagitis. Immunotherapy. 2010;2(4):461–5.
43. Jin H et al. Expression and characterization of the chemokine receptor CCR2B from rhesus monkey. Biochem Pharmacol. 2003;66(2):321–30.
44. Zhang L et al. Functional expression and characterization of macaque C–C chemokine receptor 3 (CCR3) and generation of potent antagonistic anti-macaque CCR3 monoclonal antibodies. J Biol Chem. 2002;277(37):33799–810.
45. Zuo L et al. IL-13 induces esophageal remodeling and gene expression by an eosinophil-independent, IL-13R 2-inhibited pathway. J Immunol. 2010;185(1):660–9.
46. Neilsen CV, Bryce PJ. Interleukin-13 directly promotes oesophagus production of CCL11 and CCL24 and the migration of eosinophils. Clin Exp Allergy. 2010;40(3):427–34.
47. Kaur D et al. Mast cells express IL-13R alpha 1: IL-13 promotes human lung mast cell proliferation and Fc epsilon RI expression. Allergy. 2006;61(9):1047–53.
48. Singh D et al. A phase 1 study evaluating the pharmacokinetics, safety and tolerability of repeat dosing with a human IL-13 antibody (CAT-354) in subjects with asthma. BMC Pulm Med. 2010;10:3.

49. Oh CK et al. An open-label, single-dose bioavailability study of the pharmacokinetics of CAT-354 after subcutaneous and intravenous administration in healthy males. Br J Clin Pharmacol. 2010;69(6):645–55.
50. Blanchard C et al. Inhibition of human interleukin-13-induced respiratory and oesophageal inflammation by anti-human-interleukin-13 antibody (CAT-354). Clin Exp Allergy. 2005;35(8):1096–103.

Chapter 28
Feeding Disorders and Eosinophilic Esophagitis

Asim Maqbool and Colleen Lukens

Keywords Eosinophilic esophagitis • Feeding disorders • Feeding behaviors • Inflammation

Introduction

Feeding disorders from nonorganic etiologies are common in children. According to the Diagnostic and Statistical Manual of Mental Disorders (DSM-IV-TR), they occur in 25% of children under 6 years of age [1]. The incidence is thought to be greater in children with underlying medical conditions, as multiple aspects of a disease can adversely impact the development of normal feeding skills and contribute to maladaptive feeding behaviors. Eosinophilic esophagitis (EoE) is a chronic condition associated with inflammation in the esophagus as well as anatomical and functional digestive system impairments which pose a particular impediment to the development of normal feeding behavior and skills in children.

The objectives of this chapter are to review the medical aspects of EoE that impact feeding behavior, review the common clinical and behavioral presentations with which these patients may come to a clinician's attention, and provide an overview of a behavioral approach to the management of maladaptive feeding behaviors.

A. Maqbool (✉)
Pediatric Gastroenterology, Hepatology, and Nutrition, University of Pennsylvania School of Medicine, The Children's Hospital of Philadelphia, 34th and Civic Center Blvd, Philadelphia, PA 19104, USA
e-mail: maqbool@email.chop.edu

C.A. Liacouras and J.E. Markowitz (eds.), *Eosinophilic Esophagitis*, Clinical Gastroenterology, DOI 10.1007/978-1-60761-515-6_28,

Digestive Tract Factors

Esophagitis from any cause can be associated with feeding difficulty or reluctant swallowing. There are multiple causes of esophagitis in addition to EoE, including gastroesophageal reflux (GER), chemical ingestion (e.g., pill esophagitis, inflammation associated with caustic ingestions), infective esophagitis (e.g., candidal and viral), radiation esophagitis, and graft vs. host disease. Some of these conditions can co-exist, and there can be overlap in the symptoms observed, such as in the case of EoE and GERD. Esophagitis typically improves following treatment of the underlying condition(s); however, it can have lasting effects on a child's eating behavior.

Esophageal motor activity has been reported to be impaired in patients with esophagitis, particularly in patients with EoE [2]. Pediatric patients with GER – both with and without histological evidence of esophagitis – have impaired esophageal body motor abnormality as compared to patients without either condition [3]. A recent pediatric study compared healthy pediatric subjects without esophagitis to subjects with GER disease (GERD; when GER is considered pathological with adverse impact on health and behavior) and to subjects with EoE utilizing ph probe and esophageal manometry [2]. This study indicated the occurrence of GER in both the GERD and EoE groups, with the most GER noted predictably in the group of children diagnosed with GERD (by reflux index, longest duration of a reflux episode and total number of reflux episodes). Furthermore, abnormal peristalsis (>3 abnormal swallows) and abnormal stationary motility were noted in the EoE group only. These findings underline motility disturbances in two conditions that may coexist.

EoE can have a significant structural impact on the esophagus, with esophageal furrowing, rings, and strictures commonly described. These structural changes may pose anatomical impediments to normal swallowing function. For example, multiringed esophagus may be associated with an intermittent or more consistent dysphagia, and has been described as being more common in young males. While dysphagia has been demonstrated to improve with dilatation, repeated dilatations are often necessary [4], which may increase the risk for perforation. While thickening and furrowing are most commonly observed in younger children, esophageal trachealization and stricturing are thought to be more common in older children, adolescents, and adults. In addition to these findings existing in a continuum of possible presentations, they may represent the progression of untreated disease. Therefore, the onus is on care providers and health professionals to maintain an index of suspicion of this disorder and be cognizant of its typical presentations, to allow for early recognition, and early, aggressive management.

Clinical Presentations

The presenting signs and symptoms of EoE may vary with age, with failure to thrive and feeding difficulties common in infants, reflux symptoms and emesis in infants and young children, abdominal pain in pre-teens, and dysphagia and food impaction

Table 28.1 Common presenting symptoms of EoE in 562 pediatric subjects, by age

Symptom	Age, years (mean ± SD)	*n* (%)
Failure to thrive or feeding difficulties	2.8 ± 3.2	118 (21)
Gastroesophageal reflux or emesis	5.1 ± 4.1	158 (28)
Dysphagia or food impaction	11.1 ± 4.5	62 (11)

Modified from Spergel et al. J Pediatr Gastroenterol Nutr. 2009;48:30–6. Used with permission

in pre-teens, adolescents, and adults [5–7] (Table 28.1). Dysphagia has been reported by individuals of all ages, with dysphagia plus odynophagia and food impactions with or without strictures in older children and adults [8, 9]. A retrospective study of children presenting to a feeding disorders program identified food refusal, oral aversions, emesis, failure to gain weight, and eczema as the most common symptoms seen in children with an established diagnosis of EoE ($n=15$) [10].

Older children and adolescents with EoE can be misdiagnosed with eating disorders, particularly anorexia nervosa (AN). This is potentially counterproductive to management of EoE, particularly in terms of further development of feeding difficulty. These patients may not be referred for evaluation of EoE until they have demonstrated limited progress with treatment for AN. At that point in time, ongoing exposure to potentially allergenic foods can exacerbate disease as well as contribute to ongoing food refusal.

Growth and Nutritional Concerns

Failure to thrive may be a common presenting diagnosis for children with EoE and feeding disorders [10]. With restricted intake prediagnosis and as part of the management approach, these children may be susceptible to both macronutrient and micronutrient deficiencies. The severity of these deficiencies is based largely on the degree of self imposed or medically indicated restrictions on dietary repertoire in the food selective patient.

The first 2 years of life are nutritionally important from a neurocognitive perspective, and linear growth during the first 3 years of life predicts adult stature [11–13]. Given that EoE is most often diagnosed in children less than 6 years of age, and of that, the majority under 3 years of age [6], this chronic inflammatory disorder that limits oral intake can have a significant impact on growth and nutritional status. Christie et al. found that children with cow's milk protein allergy or children with two or more food allergies were shorter than children with only one allergy, based on height-for-age percentiles [14]. Furthermore, children who had cow's milk allergy or multiple food allergies consumed less dietary calcium than children who did not have cow's milk allergy and/or had only one food allergy. Animal protein is a rich source of bioavailable iron and zinc, and diets limited in these nutrients secondary to allergy concerns may place children at nutritional risk for deficiency states.

Table 28.2 The 10 most common foods identified to be associated with EoE in 562 pediatric subjects

Food	Occurrence (%)
Milk	17
Egg	11
Wheat	9.6
Soy	7.8
Corn	7.8
Beef	6.6
Chicken	6.1
Peanut	5.4
Potato	4.8
Rice	4.1

Modified from Spergel et al. J Pediatr Gastroenterol Nutr. 2009; 48:30–6. Used with permission

The types and numbers of foods to which patients may be allergic influence their clinical course and may impact feeding behavior. The most common foods to which patients with eosinophilic esophagitis may be allergic are commonplace and nearly ubiquitous in the diet [6] (Table 28.2). Complete food tolerance following a period of dietary elimination occurred in only 11 of 562 (2%) pediatric patients in a 14-year retrospective study. Thirty-three subjects (6%) had partial resolution of their food intolerance issues. Subjects who had complete resolution of food allergies were followed for an average of 5.2 years and the patients with partial resolution for 6.8 years, respectively. Therefore, it is safe to conclude that if management of EoE is based on restriction of food(s) to which patients may be allergic, this restriction is likely to be long term and may limit the dietary repertoire that patients are advised to eat.

Behavioral Presentation

Although there exists an increasing literature delineating the clinical presentation of EoE, there has been limited study of the behavioral manifestations of EoE. A 2007 task force comprising physicians participating in the First International Gastrointestinal Eosinophil Research Symposium (FIGERS) proposed consensus recommendations based on review of the available literature on the nature and treatment of EoE [15]. The committee described the presence of behavioral symptoms in young children with EoE including food refusal and failure to thrive as well as symptoms consistent with gastroesophageal reflux disease, including emesis and abdominal pain, while in older children, dysphagia and food impaction were observed. However, the final consensus statement indicated that it remains unclear whether EoE is characterized by a specific behavioral presentation.

Anecdotal reports suggest the presence of behavioral feeding problems consistent with those identified by the FIGERS task force. For example, Haas and colleagues described children with EoE as presenting with compromised nutritional status, food refusal, chronic discomfort associated with food and mealtimes, and delayed feeding skills [16]. The authors suggested that children with EoE may consume a limited variety and volume of food, demonstrate gagging and coughing during meals, and display learned feeding problems. Spergel et al. lend support to this suggested behavioral presentation, noting that the initial complaints of patients later diagnosed with EoE included feeding difficulty, gastroesophageal reflux disease, vomiting, abdominal pain, dysphagia, and food impaction [6]. Pentiuk, Miller, and Kaul documented the presence of specific behavioral feeding problems in a subset of children with EoE [10]. The authors examined a sample of children diagnosed with EoE who were referred to an interdisciplinary feeding program for evaluation and treatment of a feeding disorder. The children diagnosed with EoE presented with symptoms commonly associated with behavioral feeding disorders including food refusal, oral aversion, vomiting, and failure to gain weight. This data suggests that a subset of children with EoE may present with behavioral feeding problems but the true prevalence of behavioral feeding problems has not been clearly established.

The presence of behavioral feeding problems in children with EoE would not be surprising, given that gastrointestinal disorders (e.g., gastroesophageal reflux, food allergy or intolerance, constipation) are found to occur frequently in children presenting with pediatric feeding disorders. For example, Field, Garland, and Williams found that in a sample of children referred to a feeding clinic for evaluation of behavioral feeding problems, 50% presented with gastroesophageal reflux, 21% with food allergy and intolerance, and 15% with constipation [17]. Similarly, data collected from an interdisciplinary feeding intervention program indicated that 57% of children referred for intervention were diagnosed with gastroesophageal reflux, 17% presented with food allergy, and 24% presented with esophagitis or gastritis [18]. The occurrence of these gastrointestinal symptoms and associated discomfort can interrupt the progression of typical feeding behavior at any stage of feeding development, leading to the onset of maladaptive mealtime behaviors (Table 28.3).

Mealtime behavior problems are commonly demonstrated by young children as part of the course of typical feeding development [19, 20]. However, the mechanism by which these difficulties develop into feeding disorders is complex and their progression is influenced by multiple factors. Among them are the physical competence of the child, caregiver competency, appetite, ecological factors, parent–child interactions, child temperament, and medical conditions [20]. The reader is referred to other sources for an extensive discussion of the impact of these interacting factors (Table 28.4). For the purposes of this chapter, the development of behavioral feeding problems in children with EoE will be described using the two-factor model, which incorporates respondent (classical) and instrumental (operant) conditioning [21], focusing on the impact of medical conditions on typical feeding development.

Table 28.3 Adverse impact of EoE on typical feeding development

Age	Typical eating behavior [21, 34]	Symptoms of EoE	Resulting disruption in feeding development
0–3 months	Discomfort from hunger resolved by feeding on demand; dependent on breastmilk or formula	Frequent vomiting or other symptoms similar to GER	Can lead to weight loss necessitating more frequent feeding or supplemental nutrition
3–6 months	Introduction of complementary foods	Introduction of allergenic foods can lead to esophageal inflammation and discomfort	Discomfort can become associated with food and the feeding situation leading to food refusal
6–12 months	Finger feeding and reaching for utensil; introduction of solid food; introduction of cup	Discomfort associated with esophageal inflammation becomes associated with table food/chewable food	Can lead to difficulty advancing from pureed food to table food
		Treatment may necessitate dietary restriction	Can limit child's exposure to and experience with a wide variety of foods during a critical period in feeding development; may lead to overly selective diet
12–18 months	Can use utensils; self-feeding	Chronic discomfort leads to decreased interest in feeding experience	Child may demonstrate limited engagement in feeding process; may experience delayed development of self-feeding skills
12–24 months	Appetite decreases; food preferences increase; increased variability in volume and variety	Caregiver places increased demands at mealtime related to management of EoE (e.g., concern for weight loss, food restrictions)	Conflicts with increased autonomy seen at this age and may lead to negative caregiver–child interactions at mealtimes

Table 28.4 Resources regarding etiological factors related to the development of feeding disorders

Authors	Factors discussed
Fischer and Silverman [19]	Medical, anatomic/physiologic, developmental, interrelational, behavioral
Kedesdy and Budd [20]	Diet, physical competence, appetite, illness, interaction, child constitution, caregiver competence, systemic factors
Linscheid et al. [21]	Variability in appetite, social–emotional development of child, caregiver–child interaction, medical conditions, oral–motor competency, environmental experience

Conditioned Aversion

Many individuals report that they have experienced at least one conditioned food aversion in their lifetime. Conditioned food aversions are typically strong, such that they affect later food preferences, and they are easily generalized to other similar stimuli [22]. A conditioned food aversion is acquired when a negative or aversive stimulus becomes associated with food, subsequently leading to avoidance of either that particular food or the feeding experience entirely. It is hypothesized that a child who experiences discomfort while eating or in an eating-related situation may come to associate that discomfort with feeding-related stimuli.

Given the purported pain or discomfort experienced by individuals with EoE, it is suspected that a similar conditioning experience occurs [6, 15, 16]. It is hypothesized that high levels of eosinophils lead to inflammation and inflammation leads to clinical manifestations of vomiting and symptoms of gastroesophageal reflux [10]. If a child's daily feeding experience becomes associated with vomiting or pain related to inflammation in the gastrointestinal system, food refusal and other disruptive behaviors may develop as the child tries to avoid the feeding situation.

As well, components of the medical treatment of EoE may lead to conditioned aversion. For example, repeated endoscopic procedures as part of the course of intervention can produce anxiety associated with the feeding situation. Similarly, challenges with suspected allergenic foods may lead to physiologic reaction, further inflammation, and ongoing discomfort. As the child begins to associate food and the feeding situation with such discomfort, food refusal behaviors may develop in attempts to avoid the feeding situation and associated distress.

Finally, the course of treatment for EoE may require supplemental nutrition either orally or via tube feeding. Spergel and colleagues reported that of a sample of patients with EoE who required supplemental nutrition, 1/3 necessitated tube feeding [6]. Resumption of oral feeding following prolonged tube feeding is often a difficult process [23]. Children primarily dependent on tube feedings due to medical conditions receive a large portion of their estimated caloric needs via such supplementation. This caloric intake can lead to a decrease in appetitive motivation to consume food orally. As well, if children are repeatedly presented with food at times when they are not experiencing hunger, conditioned aversion can occur.

Environmental Contingencies

Food refusal behavior at mealtimes occurs commonly in young children [20, 21]. If challenging behaviors are managed effectively, they will decrease in frequency and severity. However, mealtime behavior problems may be maintained by environmental conditions, as what happens after the behavior alters the likelihood of the behavior occurring in the future. Factors in the environment can serve to inadvertently reinforce maladaptive eating behavior or punish appropriate eating behavior, leading to the development of a significant behavioral feeding problem.

For example, there exist environmental stimuli that reinforce food refusal behavior. It has been demonstrated that caregivers draw more attention to non-eating behavior than to adaptive eating behavior during a typical mealtime [24]. It is this attention that can inadvertently reinforce or maintain the problematic behavior, thereby increasing the frequency with which that behavior occurs at future mealtimes. If a child who experiences a conditioned aversion demonstrates food refusal behavior, a caregiver may provide attention to the food refusal, subsequently reinforcing that behavior. As well, a caregiver may allow the child to leave the feeding situation, reinforcing their escape from the mealtime situation.

In addition, there are environmental contingencies that punish adaptive eating behavior. For example, if consumed food leads to the production of eosinophils and subsequently inflammation in the gastrointestinal tract, it is possible that an individual can experience pain with further consumption of food. It is hypothesized that eating behavior can be punished by pain and discomfort, decreasing the likelihood that a child will continue to eat.

As described previously in this chapter, the management of EoE often involves an elimination diet. Limiting access to food or restriction of food as occurs with an elimination diet can lead to the development of food refusal and selectivity. For example, if a child requests food and it is repeatedly withdrawn or removed, the child's eating or requesting behavior may be extinguished via negative reinforcement. Such environmental contingencies decrease the probability that the child will request food again in the future.

Management

Feeding disorders require an integrated comprehensive approach, such as that afforded by multidisciplinary feeding teams (Fig. 28.1). Medical, nutritional, and behavioral aspects are important in addressing and managing feeding disorders in this setting [25]. These interventions are influenced by the medical management of EoE. They are dependent upon the reduction of inflammation and are affected by the nature and extent of food restriction and time course to reintroduction.

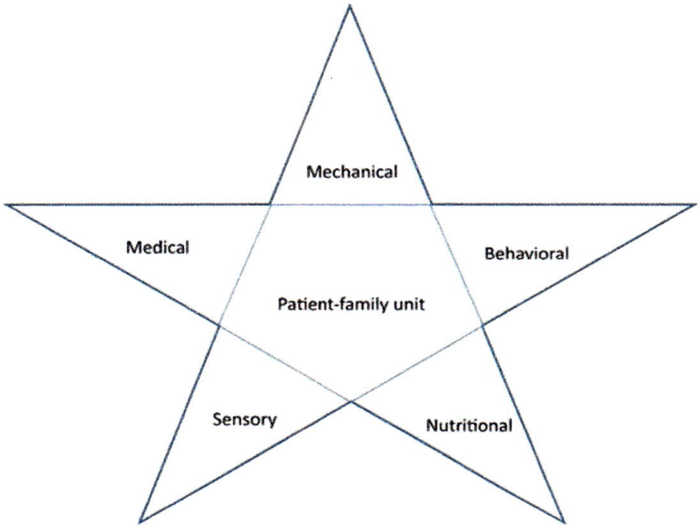

Fig. 28.1 An integrated approach to feeding disorders

Medical

The medical management of feeding problems associated with EoE primarily consists of diagnosis and management of EoE itself, by means of dietary restrictions, medications, or both. Repeat endoscopy following food eliminations or reintroduction is commonplace in the ongoing assessment and management of EoE. When treated aggressively and early, improvement and even resolution of feeding disorders is likely [10]. Additional interventions including use of medications and interventions for esophageal strictures are covered elsewhere in this book.

Nutrition

Children on restrictive diets may be at risk for macronutrient, caloric and micronutrient deficiencies, and subsequently, children with EoE may be at risk for malnutrition [26]. A large part of the medical management in pediatric EoE is based on restriction of dietary proteins. Specifically, the three most common dietary management approaches include removal of foods based on testing, removal of the most commonly responsible foods, or adoption of a semi-elemental or an elemental diet [27].

The adoption of the elemental diet may be a short-term or a long-term intervention. A small percentage of children completely outgrow all of their food allergies associated with EoE –2% in the 14-year experience of the Children's Hospital of Philadelphia [6]. However, resolution of these allergies, when they occur, can take several years [6].

Therefore, having a sound nutritional management plan to address nutrition and growth concerns is key. The use of a semi-elemental or an elemental diet as the sole source of nutrition is not only effective in the management of EoE, it may be required [27–29]. If voluntary oral intake is inadequate to meet caloric needs, supplemental enteral tube feeding may be required. The nutritional requirements for normal growth and development differ by age and by gender, and attention to meeting nutritional needs according to the Dietary Reference Intakes should be a cornerstone consideration in the medical management of these patients [30]. Elemental formula diets may not meet all micronutrient requirements, and supplemental micronutrient supplementation may be indicated.

Behavioral

There is some evidence that behavioral symptoms associated with EoE improve subsequent to the initiation of medical intervention (e.g., dietary manipulation, pharmacologic therapy) [31]. For example, in a sample of infants and toddlers diagnosed with EoE referred to a clinic for the treatment of pediatric feeding disorders, all children demonstrated normal endoscopic appearance as well as less than 5 eosinophils per HPF within a 3–12 month period subsequent to medical and nutritional intervention for EoE [10]. As well, 73% of the sample demonstrated improved oral intake and significant weight gain. However, these findings suggest that there is a small subset of children for whom disruptive mealtime behavior and food refusal behavior are maintained despite adequate medical management. It is this subset of children who may have developed a significant behavioral feeding problem warranting intervention.

There are multiple factors that contribute to the maintenance of feeding problems once medical management has been optimized, and these factors warrant different types of intervention. When environmental conditions contribute to the maintenance of feeding difficulties, behavioral intervention is warranted. Behavioral intervention entails the identification and manipulation of antecedent and consequential factors within the feeding environment with goals of altering mealtime behavior.

Behavioral intervention has been documented as an empirically validated treatment for the management of pediatric feeding problems [32]. Despite the documented effectiveness of behavioral intervention, such treatment is not recommended until medical management of EoE has been optimized in order to prevent further aversive conditioning. In a child with EoE, this would entail delaying the start of behavioral intervention until decreased esophageal inflammation is observed and the gradual reintroduction of foods has been recommended.

With regard to antecedent manipulation, precursors to the disruptive mealtime behavior can be altered to optimize the mealtime setting. For example, adequate management of discomfort (e.g., gastrointestinal difficulty) is crucial prior to conducting behavioral intervention. As well, appetite manipulation is imperative, particularly if supplemental nutrition has been introduced orally or via tube feeding. Maintaining a regular mealtime routine and schedule (e.g., meals at the table, appropriate seating, regular meal/snack schedule, limited distractions at mealtimes) despite tube feedings and supplemental nutrition optimizes appetite and increases the likelihood of successful behavioral intervention [33].

As well, contingency management is an important component of behavioral intervention [19]. By altering environmental conditions maintaining feeding difficulty, the interventionist attempts to change the likelihood of a particular behavior occurring at future mealtimes. For example, positive and negative reinforcement are utilized to strengthen adaptive mealtime behavior. Providing toys and attention to a child after they engage in behavior that supports eating may increase their positive eating behavior. As well, removal of a child from a presumably aversive feeding situation after they have demonstrated appropriate eating behavior is an example of negative reinforcement. Finally mild punishment can be implemented to decrease the occurrence of maladaptive mealtime behavior. For example, after a child engages in disruptive behavior or behavior incompatible with eating, a caregiver may remove attention and other potentially reinforcing stimuli from the feeding situation by turning away from the child.

Implications for Future Study

The behavioral presentation of EoE has not yet been clearly defined. However, given previous research on the behavioral expression of other gastrointestinal disorders it is likely that a subset of children with EoE present with behavioral feeding difficulties. Further research is necessary to better demarcate the nature and prevalence of these problems in children presenting specifically with EoE.

The behavioral manifestation of EoE may be important in determining treatment end points, as it is currently not clear if complete resolution of eosinophilia is crucial to prevent further complications or if reduction in symptoms (e.g., dysphagia, food impaction, vomiting, food refusal) is an adequate end point for treatment [15]. Further study of the behavioral manifestations of EoE as well as contributing risk factors could also inform preventive intervention. For example, early diagnosis and treatment from both a medical and behavioral standpoint is key, and may prevent the onset of more severe behavioral feeding problems. Families could be educated regarding appropriate feeding practices when dietary restrictions are imposed, when tube feeding is initiated, and when frequent endoscopy is prescribed. Finally, ongoing study of the effects of age on symptom resolution will be beneficial in recommending appropriate and effective intervention.

Summary

Eosinophilic esophagitis can adversely impact feeding development. Discomfort related to esophageal inflammation and vomiting can easily become associated with food and mealtimes, leading to maladaptive eating behavior. If this behavior persists following improvements in and resolution of the causative factors, a significant feeding disorder can develop. Early diagnosis and management of symptoms associated with EoE is vital in preventing the development of maladaptive feeding patterns. Early intervention is imperative to correct nutritional and behavioral abnormalities before they can adversely impact long-term nutritional and behavioral manifestations. Multidisciplinary feeding teams can be excellent and important resources in the integrative approach to the care of patients with EoE.

References

1. American Psychiatric Association. Task Force on DSM-IV. Diagnostic and statistical manual of mental disorders: DSM-IV-TR. 4th ed. Washington, DC: American Psychiatric Association; 2000.
2. Nurko S, Rosen R, Furuta GT. Esophageal dysmotility in children with eosinophilic esophagitis: a study using prolonged esophageal manometry. Am J Gastroenterol. 2009;104:3050–7.
3. Chitkara DK, Fortunato C, Nurko S. Esophageal motor activity in children with gastro-esophageal reflux disease and esophagitis. J Pediatr Gastroenterol Nutr. 2005;40:70–5.
4. Lee GS, Craig PI, Freiman JS, de Carle D, Cook IJ. Intermittent dysphagia for solids associated with a multiringed esophagus: clinical features and response to dilatation. Dysphagia. 2007;22:55–62.
5. Khan S, Orenstein SR, Di Lorenzo C, et al. Eosinophilic esophagitis: strictures, impactions, dysphagia. Dig Dis Sci. 2003;48:22–9.
6. Spergel JM, Brown-Whitehorn TF, Beausoleil JL, et al. 14 Years of eosinophilic esophagitis: clinical features and prognosis. J Pediatr Gastroenterol Nutr. 2009;48:30–6.
7. Orenstein SR, Shalaby TM, Di Lorenzo C, et al. The spectrum of pediatric eosinophilic esophagitis beyond infancy: a clinical series of 30 children. Am J Gastroenterol. 2000;95:1422–30.
8. Prasad GA, Talley NJ. Eosinophilic esophagitis in adults. Gastroenterol Clin North Am. 2008;37:349–68. v–vi.
9. Desai TK, Stecevic V, Chang CH, Goldstein NS, Badizadegan K, Furuta GT. Association of eosinophilic inflammation with esophageal food impaction in adults. Gastrointest Endosc. 2005;61:795–801.
10. Pentiuk SP, Miller CK, Kaul A. Eosinophilic esophagitis in infants and toddlers. Dysphagia. 2007;22:44–8.
11. Schroeder DG, Martorell R, Rivera JA, Ruel MT, Habicht JP. Age differences in the impact of nutritional supplementation on growth. J Nutr. 1995;125:1051S–9S.
12. Ruel MT, Rivera J, Habicht JP, Martorell R. Differential response to early nutrition supplementation: long-term effects on height at adolescence. Int J Epidemiol. 1995;24:404–12.
13. Pollitt E, Gorman KS, Engle PL, Rivera JA, Martorell R. Nutrition in early life and the fulfillment of intellectual potential. J Nutr. 1995;125:1111S–8S.
14. Christie L, Hine RJ, Parker JG, Burks W. Food allergies in children affect nutrient intake and growth. J Am Diet Assoc. 2002;102:1648–51.

15. Furuta GT, Liacouras CA, Collins MH, et al. Eosinophilic esophagitis in children and adults: a systematic review and consensus recommendations for diagnosis and treatment. Gastroenterology. 2007;133:1342–63.
16. Haas AM, Maune NC. Clinical presentation of feeding dysfunction in children with eosinophilic gastrointestinal disease. Immunol Allergy Clin North Am. 2009;29:65–75. ix.
17. Field D, Garland M, Williams K. Correlates of specific childhood feeding problems. J Paediatr Child Health. 2003;39:299–304.
18. Laud RB, Girolami PA, Boscoe JH, Gulotta CS. Treatment outcomes for severe feeding problems in children with autism spectrum disorder. Behav Modif. 2009;33:520–36.
19. Fischer E, Silverman A. Behavioral conceptualization, assessment, and treatment of pediatric feeding disorders. Semin Speech Lang. 2007;28:223–31.
20. Kedesdy JH, Budd KS. Childhood feeding disorders: biobehavioral assessment and intervention. Baltimore: Paul H. Brookes Publishing Co.; 1998.
21. Linscheid T, Budd KS, Rasnake LK. Pediatric feeding problems. In: Roberts M, editor. Handbook of pediatric psychology. New York: Guilford;2003:481–98.
22. Logue AW. Conditioned food aversion learning in humans. Ann N Y Acad Sci. 1985;443: 316–29.
23. Byars KC, Burklow KA, Ferguson K, O'Flaherty T, Santoro K, Kaul A. A multicomponent behavioral program for oral aversion in children dependent on gastrostomy feedings. J Pediatr Gastroenterol Nutr. 2003;37:473–80.
24. Stark LJ, Powers SW, Jelalian E, Rape RN, Miller DL. Modifying problematic mealtime interactions of children with cystic fibrosis and their parents via behavioral parent training. J Pediatr Psychol. 1994;19:751–68.
25. Aceves SS, Furuta GT, Spechler SJ. Integrated approach to treatment of children and adults with eosinophilic esophagitis. Gastrointest Endosc Clin N Am. 2008;18:195–217. xi.
26. Kirby M, Danner E. Nutritional deficiencies in children on restricted diets. Pediatr Clin North Am. 2009;56:1085–103.
27. Spergel JM, Shuker M. Nutritional management of eosinophilic esophagitis. Gastrointest Endosc Clin N Am. 2008;18:179–94. xi.
28. Markowitz JE, Spergel JM, Ruchelli E, Liacouras CA. Elemental diet is an effective treatment for eosinophilic esophagitis in children and adolescents. Am J Gastroenterol. 2003;98: 777–82.
29. Santangelo CM, McCloud E. Nutritional management of children who have food allergies and eosinophilic esophagitis. Immunol Allergy Clin North Am. 2009;29:77–84. Ix–x.
30. Otten JJ, Hellwig JP, Meyers LD. DRI, dietary reference intakes: the essential guide to nutrient requirements. Washington, DC: National Academies Press; 2006.
31. Liacouras CA, Spergel JM, Ruchelli E, et al. Eosinophilic esophagitis: a 10-year experience in 381 children. Clin Gastroenterol Hepatol. 2005;3:1198–206.
32. Kerwin ME. Empirically supported treatments in pediatric psychology: severe feeding problems. J Pediatr Psychol. 1999;24:193–214. discussion 5–6.
33. Linscheid TR. Behavioral treatments for pediatric feeding disorders. Behav Modif. 2006;30:6–23.
34. Schroeder CS, Gordon BN. Managing common problems: eating problems. In: Schroeder CS, Gordon BN, editors. Assessment and treatment of childhood problems: a clinician's guide. New York: Guilford; 2002. p. 81–114.

Chapter 29
Psychological Perspectives on Pediatric Eosinophilic Esophagitis

Mary Klinnert

Keywords Eosinophilic esophagitis • Psychosocial functions • Children • Adolescents • Chronic illness

Introduction

Eosinophilic esophagitis (EoE) is a recently described disorder marked clinically by symptoms of upper gastrointestinal distress and by histological evidence of increased eosinophils in the esophagus [1]. Although EoE has been reported in individuals across the lifespan, the disease has been most comprehensively described in children and adolescents [2]. In addition to further clarifications of EoE symptom presentation, current studies are investigating the pathophysiology of the disease as well as the effectiveness and outcome of treatments [3, 4]. Attention has now turned to the impact of the disease on the quality of life and psychosocial functioning of children and their families [5–7]. Since investigation of psychological aspects of EoE is in its infancy, little systematic information is available at this time. Nevertheless, with some information from recent and current studies as well as from clinical experience, it is possible to pose key questions about the impact of the symptoms and the treatments specific to EoE on quality of life for children and adolescents. Further, a great deal of information is available regarding psychosocial effects of various chronic illnesses on children, and extrapolations from previous

M. Klinnert (✉)
Department of Pediatrics, National Jewish Health,
1400 Jackson Street, Denver, CO, USA

Department of Psychiatry, School of Medicine, University of Colorado,
Aurora, CO, USA
e-mail: KlinnertM@NJHealth.org

C.A. Liacouras and J.E. Markowitz (eds.), *Eosinophilic Esophagitis*,
Clinical Gastroenterology, DOI 10.1007/978-1-60761-515-6_29,

studies are informative regarding likely effects on youth of all ages with EoE. This chapter reviews what is known about the impact of EoE on quality of life and psychosocial adjustment, discusses the bidirectional effects of pediatric chronic illness characteristics, psychosocial functioning, and quality of life, and examines the role of coping and adaptation in relation to psychosocial functioning and quality of life.

Demographics and Illness Characteristics of EoE in Children and Adolescents

To fully consider the quality of life impact and psychosocial aspects of EoE, it is important to understand the demographics of the disease, co-morbid conditions, diagnostic criteria, symptom patterns, and current treatments. Reports from numerous studies have indicated that children diagnosed with EoE are predominantly male with an approximate 3:1 ratio, and they range in age from 6 months to 21 years of age, with an average age of about 9 years [1, 8]. A recent report on 620 patients identified in the past 14 years found that 68% of the children were less than 6 years of age and 36% were younger than 3 years [8]. Families of patients were more likely to be Caucasian, affluent, highly educated, and to reside in suburban areas.

Increasingly, pediatric EoE is considered to be an allergic disease [9] and, like other allergic diseases, a chronic illness [3]. The majority of pediatric patients with EoE have co-morbid allergic disease such as eczema, allergic rhinitis, and asthma, as well as IgE-mediated food allergies [5]. Eosinophilic esophagitis may be seen as another manifestation of allergic disease in children, where the esophagus is the target organ responding to environmental antigens, in this case, food. Food allergies may be causative in more than 90% of patients, although IgE-mediated food allergies resulting in anaphylaxis have been documented for a smaller proportion of patients, ranging from 6 to 24% [9].

Although clinical symptoms of EoE are similar to those of gastroesophageal reflux disease (GERD), EoE is distinguished from GERD by the presence of eosinophils in the esophagus even after appropriate acid suppression. Endoscopy is thus required to document eosinophil levels. Recently established diagnostic criteria for EoE include the presence of 15 eosinophils per high power field, associated with characteristic clinical symptoms unresponsive to anti-reflux medication [1]. Presenting symptoms vary according to patient age [1, 2]. For infants and young children, typical presenting symptoms are reflux, gagging, choking, vomiting, and feeding aversion or refusal, resulting at times in failure to thrive [10, 11]. School-age children with EoE typically present with reflux, heartburn, regurgitation, vomiting, and abdominal pain. Dysphagia, or difficulty swallowing, and food impaction have been reported on occasion among school-age children [12], but become increasingly common in adolescence and are the primary presenting symptoms for adults.

Clinicians have consistently reported that presenting symptoms for EoE are nonspecific and highly variable among patients of all ages, and that there is often little relationship between symptom reports and histological findings. Several studies have shown that the association between symptoms and eosinophil counts is minimal [13–15]. Among a small number of pediatric patients, symptom reports were unrelated to eosinophil counts derived from endoscopies and, while endoscopy results showed evidence of remission through decreased eosinophil counts, no correlated changes were seen for symptom decreases or quality of life improvements [15]. In a larger study, symptom questionnaire and endoscopy results were evaluated for pediatric patients aged 3–18 who either had an EoE diagnosis but were not yet receiving treatment, or who were receiving follow-up assessments after treatment [14]. Children with untreated EoE had a higher symptom score than treated subjects, and for these untreated patients there was a modest correlation between symptom scores and the number of eosinophils found on biopsy. However, for the total sample there was no correlation between peak eosinophil counts and symptom scores. Importantly, among treated patients, 10% with persistent high eosinophil counts (i.e., with active EoE) reported no symptoms, while for 85% of patients, symptoms persisted despite histological resolution.

Some clarification of symptom patterns was provided in a study that used symptom scores to distinguish pediatric patients with EoE from a group with GERD and from control patients with and without allergies [13]. Symptom scores were higher for patients with EoE and GERD compared with the two control groups. Those with EoE and GERD complained of more nausea/vomiting, abdominal pain, heartburn/regurgitation, and nocturnal awakening than control groups. EoE patients were distinguished from GERD patients only by reports of dysphagia and anorexia/early satiety. Total symptom scores were uncorrelated with histological and endoscopic findings. However, the individual symptoms that distinguished EoE from GERD patients, dysphagia and dysphagia plus anorexia, were significantly correlated with severity ratings of histological and endoscopic findings. Dysphagia, typically reported by older children and adolescents, may have a different symptom status in comparison with the nonspecific symptoms reported for younger children.

The nonspecificity and high variability of EoE symptoms has many implications for the consideration of health-related quality of life and the relationship with psychosocial factors. For children and adolescents with EoE, the distinguishing diagnostic indicator is a high esophageal eosinophil count, while symptoms are highly variable. However, the psychological effects of EoE can be expected to be associated not with eosinophil counts, but with symptoms that are experienced or with treatments that are undergone. Given that children with EoE can have a wide variety of disease experiences, effects on quality of life or psychological adjustment can be expected to vary widely across individuals. Although decreases in symptoms may generally be associated with quality of life improvements, treatment may have clearer effects on some symptoms than on others, with associated improvements in quality of life or psychological adjustment more apparent for some children than for others. On the other hand, sometimes when symptoms fail to improve, psychological concerns may persist despite decreased eosinophil counts and histological disease remission. It may be important to provide behavioral treatment for certain nonspecific symptoms in their own right, albeit in parallel with the medical treatment. The complex interactions between symptoms and behavioral responses, such as those that occur with feeding disorders and persistent abdominal pain, impact quality of life and may lead to significant behavioral and emotional difficulties for children and adolescents with EoE.

The primary treatments that have been demonstrated to be effective for treating pediatric EoE are consistent with data indicating that food allergies underlie symptoms. Investigators have demonstrated that optimal treatments involve removal or avoidance of the offending foods or topical application of anti-inflammatory medications [16]. Removal of exposure to food is accomplished through partial or complete elimination diets, which involve restricting a selected set of foods from the diet or removing all foods from the diet and providing nutrition with elemental formulas either by oral ingestion or through feeding tubes. The dietary restrictions that are central to treatment of EoE may well constitute the most powerful factor impacting quality of life and psychosocial adjustment among children and adolescents with this disease.

With EoE, the treatment involving food restrictions at various levels is often a major cause of psychological distress. At times the distress due to the treatment far outweighs the distress related to symptoms, leading to a conundrum for patients and medical providers alike. With EoE, as with many other chronic illnesses, children often must continue to undergo treatments after symptoms have resolved in order to prevent further symptoms. For children in this situation, the disease experience primarily involves enduring treatments such as food restrictions, altered diets, and tube feeding for an indefinite period of time. In sum, emotional and behavioral responses to both symptoms and treatments for EoE have considerable potential for impacting quality of life and psychological adjustment for children and adolescents with this disease.

Impact of EoE on Quality of Life

The impact of disease on children and adolescents' health-related quality of life (HRQL) has been studied for a wide variety of illnesses that afflict pediatric patients. Studies of HRQL among children who have medical illnesses are concerned with the effects of the disease and associated medical treatments not only on the physical status, but also on the psychological and social aspects of children's lives [17]. HRQL instruments assess disease impact on academics, social interactions, extracurricular activities, and emotional functioning, as well as on health status. Generic instruments have been developed for the assessment of HRQL for children with health conditions and illnesses (e.g., Child Health Questionnaire-CHQ [18] and PedsQL™ [19]). Disease-specific instruments have also been developed for assessments of HRQL for a variety of pediatric diseases such as asthma, food allergies, and gastroesophageal reflux disease (GERD) [20–22].

In studies of HRQL, the primary focus is on the patient's subjective perceptions of their illness and its impact on their life. Thus, children and adolescents' self-report of their own experience provides the most valid HRQL information. Children of about age 8 years and older have been demonstrated as able to provide reliable reports of their subjective experience, although one self-report HRQL instrument has demonstrated reliability for children as young as 5 years of age [17, 19]. Proxy HRQL reports completed by parents, necessary for very young children, are often provided for older children and adolescents as well. However, there is evidence that quality of life ratings made by parents and physicians of chronically ill children may agree poorly with the children's own ratings, particularly for scales assessing subjective attributes such as emotions and pain [23]. Parents may overestimate quality of life effects on their children. Mothers of children with peanut allergy reported a greater impact on quality of life for their child in comparison with ratings made by siblings, fathers, or the peanut allergic children themselves [24]. In making proxy QOL ratings related to the impact of their children's asthma, parents' ratings were largely determined by their own psychological status rather than by objective measures of asthma care experienced by the children [25]. Similarly, when caregivers rated quality of life for their young children with otitis media, ratings of the children's quality of life was highly influenced by the caregivers' personal quality of life and functional health status [26]. Thus, while caregiver reports of children's HRQL are valuable and even necessary for young children, self-reports of the impact of the disease by children and adolescents with EoE on their quality of life are highly desirable.

At the present time, several studies of HRQL for pediatric patients with EoE are underway, but results are as of yet unavailable. However, one published study presents an initial view of qualitative information about HRQL for children and adolescents with EoE. Flood and colleagues [12] used an interview methodology to explore quality of life concerns among caregivers and pediatric patients with self-reported diagnoses of EoE. One-on-one interviews were conducted with parents of younger patients, age 2–7 years, and with older patients, age 8–17 years, about the effects that EoE had on the patients' everyday lives. Having EoE was reported to impact school attendance and school-related activities because of symptoms, and also academic performance because of difficulties with concentration. Both parents and older children reported that social interactions at school and outside of school were affected because of symptoms, as when feeling sick interfered with plans to play with friends, and also because dietary restrictions interfered with participating in activities such as school parties or eating with friends. Symptoms were reported to interfere with sports activities ranging from soccer to football.

There was a significant emotional impact reported as a result of having EoE [12]. Children of all ages experienced feelings of frustration and anger about not being able to eat the same foods as other children. They talked about having worries about eating the wrong food or having symptoms. Older children talked about feeling sad, depressed, unhappy, and tired of being sick. Parents reported that when their young children were having symptoms, they were often irritable and moody. Children and adolescents were unhappy about feeling different from others. For children of all ages, having EoE was reported to have a significant impact on their families. Older children were concerned about stress for the family or about the need for parents to adapt the family's eating patterns. Parents of younger children also talked about the effect of the EoE on family meals and restrictions on the family's ability to go out to eat or to participate in social events. Some parents noted a negative impact on the siblings of the child with EoE.

The concerns listed by the children and their parents illustrate how the symptoms of EoE and the treatments associated with it impact quality of life within all key domains of children's lives: physical, emotional, social, and school functioning [12]. For example, children reported that symptoms such as "feeling sick" led to restrictions on social activities. Notably, many of the concerns reported in this qualitative study stemmed from the effects of treatment, which for this sample of youngsters with EoE constituted dietary restrictions. The well-articulated emotional responses that occurred in response to both symptoms and treatment ranged across major categories of negative emotion, including anger/frustration, anxiety/worry, sadness/depression, and for younger children, irritability and moodiness.

While this initial qualitative study of QoL effects of EoE on children and adolescents was an important first step, future studies must attend carefully to the developmental status of the pediatric patients involved [7]. The changing impact of EoE across developmental stages of socioemotional development can hardly be overestimated. For each stage of development, pediatric patients have particular ways of communicating their symptom experiences and differing reactions to symptoms and to treatments. The disease impact occurs in social contexts that change with development and, perhaps most importantly, the contextual meaning of the disease experience for the child's emotional and social development changes dramatically with age.

For very young children, the social context in which EoE occurs is primarily confined to their immediate family, and for them the meaning of the disease is embedded in the quality of their interactions with their family members. For infants and toddlers, emotional responses to bodily sensations such as pain or nausea are expressed through behaviors such as food refusal, irritability and moodiness. Proxy reports of QOL for very young children are based on parents' observations and interpretations of the children's behavior. As noted above, parental reports of their young children's quality of life are influenced by their own psychological status and stress level [26]. But it is not just the reports that are influenced by parental variables; young children's behavior itself, while affected by multiple medical and developmental variables, is in part shaped by the parents' caregiving behavior and the nature of the parent–child interactions, including their emotional communications regarding the burden and meaning of the disease. Thus, quality of life and reports of quality of life for young children cannot really be separated from their parents' quality of life specific to the disease. Changes in disease status or treatment regimens, for better or worse, reflect the impact of the illness on both the child and the parent.

Preschool age children may not yet be able to complete questionnaires, but they are capable of verbally communicating their symptom experience and their feelings about the treatments they undergo. Proxy reports by parents of preschoolers' symptoms and quality of life, while still influenced by parents' emotional status and stress levels, can be based on verbal complaints of tummy pain or feeling sick. Preschoolers' emotional responses to their illness have to do not only with the physical discomfort they experience, but also with their observations of their own experience in relation to that of others. For example, preschoolers develop the ability to see that dietary restrictions apply to them and not to siblings or schoolmates. Nevertheless, their social context remains primarily centered within their family and they are amenable to parental influence such as being provided acceptable foods that are similar to those of their peers or being told that their food is "special." While children at the school entry age of 5–7 years of age undergo enormous shifts in cognitive and emotional development, they continue to be influenced primarily by the guidelines and support provided by their families.

An important developmental shift occurs when children are about 8 years of age, resulting in a qualitative change in their illness experience [20], and perhaps also in the factors affecting their quality of life. As noted, it is at this age that children are able to provide reliable reports of their physical and emotional state. Even while their family remains their primary social context, at this age children become increasingly peer-oriented. As they spend greater amounts of time away from home, dietary restrictions and limitations on social and academic activities can produce feelings of anger and frustration, as well as a heightened awareness of being different from others [12]. Thus, whereas they previously accepted their parents assurances and support, they no longer accept their disease status as being special, but instead begin to see their difference from peers in a negative light [20]. It is very important to assess quality of life for children in this age range independently from proxy reports made by their parents, as their views, attitudes, and feelings about their disease set the stage for their entry into adolescence. With adolescence, the social context involves even less parental supervision and more peer involvement, and is accompanied by the need to make independent decisions about handling social situations that involve eating. For teens, even more than in the younger years, disease-specific quality of life may be associated with overall psychological adjustment.

Just as the quality of life of chronically ill children is significantly impacted by the physical and emotional demands of the disease, so too is the quality of life of parents and siblings. Effects on parents of their children's chronic illness include time-consuming daily tasks, financial burdens, and effects on relationships within the family and social contacts outside the family [27]. Parents of chronically ill children aged 3–18 years from ten different types of pediatric chronic diseases had significantly lower health-related quality of life compared with parents of healthy school children. For the parents, the areas impacted included social activities, daily activities, vitality, and sleep. They reported fewer positive emotions and more depressive feelings than parents from the comparison group [28]. The areas of family life that are impacted by pediatric chronic illnesses are likely to be similar for families of children with EoE. Families of food-allergic children share with EoE several burdensome daily tasks, such as shopping for food the child is able to eat, adapting the family's diet to the needs of the food-allergic child, and explaining the condition to relatives, friends, and school personnel [29]. They also share with EoE the worries regarding nutritional sufficiency of acceptable food and the long-term impact on their child's growth and development [29].

Since the majority of children with EoE may be less than age 6 years [8], with symptoms often indistinguishable from GERD, the illness-related quality of life of caregivers of children with GERD are illustrative of parents' day-to-day concerns. Parents have described how routine care-giving activities for their children required extra work and care, such as special feeding techniques involving small portions, frequent feedings, and preparation of special meals or formulas [22]. The parents also talked about emotional concerns specific to their children's reflux and feeding problems, such as fearing that the child might choke on the their vomit when they put them to bed at night. Parents of children with food refusal and failure to thrive worried a great deal about their children's condition and prognosis. This is consistent with other studies that have documented high levels of parenting stress among parents of children with feeding disorders [30], a common condition among young children with EoE. Available information is mixed about effects of children's tube feeding on caregivers' emotional functioning and quality of life. Although feeding tubes can initially bring relief to parents concerned about their children's nutritional intake, one study showed that parents of children who had gastrostomy tubes had poorer quality of life in terms of social life, family life, sex life, and work [31]. However, another study showed no difference in rates of depression for caregivers of chronically ill children with a G-tube compared with those without [32].

Overall, available data indicate that both general concerns and burdens and EoE-specific issues have considerable impact on quality of life for the parents and siblings of children with EoE. However, like families of children with other diseases with comparable characteristics, families of children with EoE are likely to have varying emotional responses and coping strategies that result in a range of levels of adaptation.

Psychological Adjustment Among Children and Adolescents with Chronic Illness

To our knowledge, no systematic research has been published regarding psychological adaptation among pediatric EoE patients. However, there is consistent evidence that children with a variety of chronic illnesses have increased levels of emotional and behavioral difficulties in comparison with healthy children [33–35]. Most often, these studies show that the average level of increased problems, although statistically significant, is small [35], which suggests that there is a subset of children with considerable difficulty adapting to their illness although the remainder may be managing effectively. It is likely that a similar pattern will be found for children with EoE, such that most of the children will be found to be coping adequately, but a subset will be found to have adjustment problems that are concerning [7].

The physical symptoms experienced by chronically ill children, as well as the medical procedures and the treatments, can be thought of as a series of general and disease-specific stresses with which the child must find a way to cope. General stresses for chronically ill children include receiving a diagnosis for an illness that requires medical intervention, the possibility of long-term consequences on physical health, interference with developmentally normal experiences, feeling set apart from healthy children, and requirements for a variety and range of illness management strategies and behaviors. Other stresses associated with pediatric chronic illnesses are related to the unique characteristics of the disease and the treatments. Children have been shown to have more adjustment problems when their disease is visible, has an unpredictable course, is potentially fatal, or has a sensory or motor component [34]. In applying this to EoE, we might expect those children to have more difficulty adjusting to their disease who have visible symptoms such as vomiting at unpredictable times or food impactions in public settings. Children and adolescents who have food restrictions, who are on elimination diets, or who have gastrostomy tubes may experience these treatments as visible evidence that they are different from peers. Those with co-morbid, potentially anaphylactic food allergies may experience the anxiety that is associated with potentially life-threatening illness. While it is normal to have emotional responses to EoE-related stresses that include feelings of frustration, anxiety, or sadness, for some children these feelings are manageable, whereas for others the feelings can become overwhelming.

The manner in which children and adolescents cope with chronic illnesses has an important influence on their quality of life and psychological adjustment. Coping responses involve problem-solving behaviors or cognitive strategies that aid in managing negative emotional responses, and when children and adolescents with chronic illness are having difficulty coping, they often report both poor quality of life and negative mood [36]. Certain cognitive coping strategies have been associated with better adjustment and quality of life and fewer feelings of anxiety, depression, and stress. For 8- to 17-year-old youth with food allergies, more negative attitudes toward food allergy predicted more anxious and depressive symptoms as well as social stress [37]. For adolescents with inflammatory bowel disease, a coping strategy marked by a depressive cognitions (e.g., often worrying about things in the past, not being able to think of anything else but the problem) was related to poorer quality of life, while an optimistic coping style was related to better quality of life [38]. For adolescents with cystic fibrosis, the coping strategy of social comparison was related to higher quality of life, whereas depressive coping was negatively related to quality of life [39].

Disease severity might be expected to predict poor psychological adjustment, but studies of pediatric chronic illness have been mixed as to whether increased disease severity is related to more psychological problems [35, 40]. In fact, the differing results appear to be due to the measurement of disease severity. Objective measures of illness severity, such as those based on physiological data or clinician ratings, have tended to be unrelated to psychological problems, while it has been the patient or parent's perception of disease severity that has been correlated with psychological distress [39, 41]. Given that with EoE there is a minimal relationship between objective measures such as eosinophil counts and patients' symptoms, psychological adjustment problems can be expected to be associated primarily with symptoms. Patients with frequent vomiting or food impactions might be more affected socially and emotionally than patients with periodic reflux or those with no clinical symptoms, regardless of esophageal eosinophil counts.

Although EoE symptoms are generally nonspecific and variable, for pediatric patients with EoE and their families, several patterns of symptoms associated with characteristic child behaviors, family interactions, and psychological distress occur regularly. The age and developmental status of the patient is central to the nature of the adjustment difficulties that are encountered. Among infants and young children, the presenting symptoms of EoE are often feeding disorders, with organic and non-organic factors intertwined [42], accompanied by a great deal of emotional distress on the part of all family members. A different set of medical, behavioral, and emotional issues are raised for children who require tube feeding. Abdominal pain, often persistent regardless of histological remission, is yet another medical/psychological complex that can be problematic among school-age children with EoE. And concerns about peer status, stigma, and depression are yet another complex of areas of psychological distress that occur for older children and adolescents with persistent EoE disease. For each symptom pattern, there are complex relationships between EoE histology and symptoms, the child's emotional response to and coping with the disease, and interactions with the family and the family's coping responses. The complex interrelationships between disease symptoms, patient and family emotional and behavioral responses, and child adjustment are illustrated in several of the symptom patterns that occur with EoE.

Feeding Disorders

For infants and toddlers with EoE, the most common symptom presentation is food aversion or refusal, central components of feeding disorders among young children [1, 5, 10, 11]. Since more than a third of pediatric patients with EoE are less than 3 years of age [8], feeding disorders among patients with EoE are a common but significant problem. The nature of feeding dysfunction among children with eosinophilic gastrointestinal disease has been well described [43]. Feeding problems associated with eosinophilic gastrointestinal diseases include food refusal, gagging, coughing and vomiting, as well as delayed attainment of age-appropriate self-feeding skills and eating patterns [43]. These behaviors may lead to decreased variety and volume of oral intake, compromised nutritional status and may ultimately lead to failure to thrive [43].

The etiology of feeding problems among children with eosinophilic gastrointestinal diseases remains poorly understood. Although feeding disorders are known to occur in conjunction with a number of pediatric conditions, more than half of 700 young children with severe feeding problems had a gastrointestinal medical problem, and GERD was most frequently identified as the underlying medical condition [42]. Thus it is no surprise that feeding problems are common among children with EoE, since presenting symptoms for young children with EoE are the same as those for GERD. Among infants and toddlers with EoE who present with feeding problems, there appears to be an over-representation of neurodevelopmental disorders, with reports ranging from 12 to 67% of patients [10, 44]. This suggests that some children have oral motor or oral sensory deficits that have disrupted the normal process of learning to eat. For other children, the experience of pain with swallowing or reflux is believed to lead to a conditioned food aversion response. Thus, food aversion or intolerance is believed to stem from experiences of discomfort or pain with eating, leading to learned avoidance behavior in children too young to verbalize their pain. This causal pathway is supported by a study that showed that infants who have GERD during their first year of life were significantly more likely than healthy children to develop feeding problems within the following year [45], and it is likely that infants with EoE have a similar pattern. When children refuse food offered to them, parents often respond with altered feeding practices that reinforce ineffective eating behavior [43], setting in motion parent–child behavioral interaction patterns that can be extraordinarily resistant to change. Child behavioral patterns of food refusal are associated with significant stress for parents [30, 46, 47] and likely have a major impact on quality of life for siblings as well.

Research is needed to address various aspects of feeding disorders among children with EoE. There is a need for a description of the frequency of oral motor and oral sensory deficits among these children, as well as the role of behavioral issues in this group of children. It would be helpful to understand developmental predictors and correlates of feeding disorders as they relate to the development of EoE in infants and young children. For example, while the prevalence of feeding dysfunction is high among young children with EoE, as it is with the infants with GERD, not all children with EoE symptoms, such as reflux and vomiting, develop feeding problems. The question is, why is it that some infants who experience these unpleasant symptoms do not develop food aversion, while others develop frustrating and persistent problems that can become life threatening? What are the infant medical and temperamental characteristics, the parent physical and behavioral factors, and the environmental variables that constitute risk factors for the development of this difficult behavior pattern? There is also a need to assess the effectiveness of current interventions for these problem behaviors, and to understand what child and parent characteristics are associated with successful interventions. Ultimately, it will be important to understand the relationship between the course of EoE and the long-term nutritional and behavioral outcomes for children with onset of EoE in their first years of life. Future research must address these issues surrounding feeding dysfunction in children with EoE, where biological, behavioral, and relationship systems all play a role.

Tube Feeding

Another psychological adjustment necessary in children with EoE concerns tube feeding. Because allergic responses to food are the primary triggering factor for most pediatric patients with EoE, and removing foods from the diet is central to treatment, the provision of nutrition for these children can be extremely challenging. Treatment for some children involves placing nasogastric (NG) tubes for a limited period of time, in order to provide appropriate nutrition while allowing the esophagus to heal prior to re-introducing foods into the diet [48]. Some children continue to have high numbers of eosinophils in their esophagus and/or troublesome symptoms including the inability to ingest adequate nutrition and require gastrostomy tubes (G-tubes) [49]. The use of tube feeding in the treatment of EoE has clearly been associated with disease remission [48]. However, little information is available regarding the effect of either short- or long-term tube feeding on quality of life or behavioral and emotional functioning for children and adolescents with EoE, or on their families.

The use of feeding tubes in the treatment of EoE has the potential to seriously impact children in a number of ways, and the effect of tube feeding for any length of time on children with normal neurodevelopmental functioning is unknown. Although G-tube feedings ensure adequate nutrition, they may impede the development of oral feeding skills by decreasing children's hunger driven motivation to eat and by decreasing oral stimulation [50]. This may be a serious concern for infants and toddlers, who may miss oral stimulation and establishment of the connection between hunger and eating during critical periods for the development of eating behavior [43]. For older children with independent eating skills, eliminating the connection between hunger and eating may compound eating problems, making difficult the reinstatement of eating [50]. No information is available about how school-age children with NG or G-tubes feel about their bodies or about being different from others. Equally important for older children are the emotional effects of removing food from the diet and the resulting impact on social activities and peer relationships. Thus, research is needed to investigate multiple aspects of this common treatment, both concurrently with tube placement, but also over time, in order to discover the short- and long-term effects on eating behavior, quality of life, and psychological adjustment.

Abdominal Pain

Abdominal pain, frequently a primary presenting symptom for EoE, represents another area in which medical and psychological factors are often inextricably intertwined. Although clinical symptoms of EoE are notoriously nonspecific, which is why the diagnosis depends on histological findings [14], some symptoms are more nonspecific than others. Dysphagia and anorexia/early satiety may be the most specific of reported symptoms, since they distinguished EoE patients from GERD patients [13], whereas abdominal pain may be the most nonspecific. In the study by Aceves, abdominal pain was present for both EoE and GERD patients, although it was among the symptoms distinguishing those two groups from normal controls [13]. In a group of 49 pediatric patients age 3–18 with diagnosed EoE, 69% reported experiencing abdominal pain; this was the most commonly reported symptom from this sample [14]. Among treated EoE patients who achieved histological remission, 88% continued to report symptoms. Given its frequency, abdominal pain is likely one of the symptoms that persisted after remission. Although explanations for the persistence of abdominal pain are being conceptualized and investigated [14], it seems that many patients with EoE who by objective measures have been successfully treated continue to have complaints of abdominal pain.

The frequent persistence of abdominal pain in patients with EoE, regardless of treatment status or histological resolution, suggests that behavioral treatment specific to managing or alleviating the pain may be indicated. Assuming that pharmacological and nutritional interventions are already in place, behavioral treatment could follow the model of treatments for recurrent or functional abdominal pain, which have been shown to be moderately effective [51]. These cognitive behavioral treatments include cognitive coping, progressive muscle relaxation and/or diaphragmatic breathing, and contingency management training for parents. The cognitive aspect involves addressing the appraisal of pain as a serious threat with responses of fear and avoidance of activities, a style of coping that interferes with children's ability to engage in developmentally appropriate activities [52]. Contingency management examines and addresses the manner in which parents, teachers, and health care providers respond to the child's pain behavior. Protective and anxious responses can promote the child's focus on the pain, increased anxiety, and withdrawal from school and other activities. In contrast, an active approach to pain management and maintenance of daily activities helps a child to stay fully functional and less anxious, and leads to better quality of life.

Research is needed to investigate the relationship between abdominal pain and physiological aspects of EoE, such as eosinophil counts and levels of stomach acid. In addition, the reciprocal relationship between abdominal pain and psychological factors merits investigation. Family stress levels and child or adolescent psychological functioning in relation to abdominal pain, both prior to and following evaluation and treatment for EoE might be explored. In a study of youth ages 8–17 with abdominal pain but no known gastrointestinal or chronic illness, family stress and psychological functioning was assessed prior to diagnostic esophagogastroduodenoscopy [53]. For girls, depression predicted positive biopsy findings (including high levels of eosinophils for some children), while for boys, positive biopsies were predicted by family stress. These results are suggestive regarding relationships between stress, physiological processes, and symptoms. Also in need of investigation is the effectiveness of behavioral approaches for pain management with children with EoE who have persistent abdominal pain.

Social Stigma and Adherence

As previously noted, children from about 8 years of age onward often struggle with feelings of self-consciousness and being different. For youngsters with EoE, these feelings may occur related to symptoms, as when a 12-year-old with dysphagia chokes on food in the school cafeteria. However, with EoE the dietary restrictions appear to be even more salient than the symptoms, as they impact all domains of children's and teens' lives [12]. The array of feelings related to being different from others has been commonly noted among older children and adolescents across a range of chronic illnesses. Adolescents with celiac disease vividly described how adherence to their prescribed diet complicated their social relationships by drawing attention to themselves and making visible their otherwise invisible medical condition [54].

For youth with EoE, dietary adherence might be compromised. as a result of difficult social interactions resulting from limited diets. Dealing with similar concerns, older children and adolescents with food allergy were concerned about the lack of understanding on the part of others and the social embarrassment they experienced when attempting to avoid certain foods; as a result they sometimes felt that "just chancing it would be okay." [55] In a study of risk-taking behavior among adolescents with food allergy, a substantial number of the teens reported eating foods that "may contain" the foods to which they were allergic [56]. It seems likely that adolescents with EoE would have very similar experiences with their dietary restrictions as those reported by the adolescents with celiac disease and food allergies. If teens at risk for anaphylaxis take chances with possible exposure to foods, it seems very likely that the same behavior occurs for teens with EoE, where there is a less clear connection between ingesting restricted food and experiencing symptoms or developing increased eosinophils in the esophagus.

Little is known about dietary adherence among children and adolescents with EoE. It is unclear how completely parents manage their children's diets, and to what extent they do it independently of or in concert with diets of other family members. It is also unknown how well older children and adolescents comply with their dietary restrictions when they are on their own, or when they are at home in the family context. Drawing from research regarding adherence with other chronic illnesses, it is hypothesized that dietary adherence is predicted by understanding the illness, by the quality of parent–child relationships, and by the child's psychological and social adjustment. Teens with food allergy who had better peer relationships and who had disclosed their illness to their friends took fewer risks with food [56]. Research is needed to determine how youngsters and their families manage and adhere with their dietary restrictions, about the burden involved, and also about factors that facilitate or impede adherence. Only by knowing to what extent families and children follow their diets will it be possible to evaluate the effectiveness of dietary restrictions in treating EoE. Further, only by systematically evaluating the perceived burden of dietary restrictions on children and families will it be possible to make treatment decisions that optimize effectiveness while minimizing burden.

Coping in Families of Children and Adolescents with EoE

There are many demands on families of a child with EoE, from the onset of symptoms and requirements for medical appointments and diagnostic procedures, to the acceptance of a diagnosis and collaborative decision-making on a treatment plan. Not only are there medical issues to comprehend; parents also are responsible for integrating treatment plans into the family structure. They must determine how food restrictions will be accomplished and how special diets will be instituted, they must develop an understanding of the nutritional adequacy of recommended diets, and they may need to learn how to manage tube feeding. There are logistical issues of medical appointments, insurance concerns, and financial burdens. Besides these practical matters, parents have the task of helping the child with EoE to understand and cope with the illness and the related treatment plans and lifestyle changes that ensue. Further, they assume the responsibility of doing this in a developmentally appropriate, sensitive, and emotionally attuned manner. Finally, most parents attempt to stretch their attention and emotional and material resources to meet the needs of the other children in the family, and to create a family environment of mutual support and cohesiveness.

No wonder that parents of children with EoE, like parents of other chronically ill children, often feel extremely stressed, and sometimes experience anxiety and depression. A large epidemiological study showed that mothers of chronically ill children reported more negative affect than those of healthy children, and mothers and fathers were 2–3 times more likely to seek mental health treatment [57]. Across different pediatric chronic disorders, mothers' adjustment problems were found to be one standard deviation above the mean for the general population [58]. Although families can experience considerable stress and distress as they learn to cope with their children's chronic illness, overall their responses to children's illnesses vary along a continuum, with many families coping extraordinarily well while a subset of families experience considerable difficulty. In this way parents and family coping responses parallel those of the children, with the majority managing well. Recent research regarding families of children and adolescents with health problems has supported the overall competence of families in adapting to and managing their children's illnesses [41], and emphasizes the importance of focusing on families' competence and the adaptive processes they employ.

As research is initiated regarding psychosocial aspects of EoE for children and adolescents, it is also important to investigate how the illness affects the child's family. Consideration must be given to effects of the illness on parents and children's quality of life, on their psychological adjustment, and their overall adaptation. While appreciating the burdens and demands of the disease and the impact of the disease on pediatric patients and their families, it is important to maintain focus on families' competence. The overall goal is to understand the adaptive and coping processes, by developing an understanding of families' experiences and how they deal with the demands they encounter. By gaining a thorough understanding of these complex processes, it will be possible to better support families as they learn to cope with and achieve optimal adaptation for the child with EoE and for the entire family.

Implications for Psychological Care of Children and Adolescents with EoE

Clearly, there are many ways in which EoE impacts the quality of life and psychological adjustment of children and their families. For physicians and health care providers of these children and families, concerns about impact on quality of life have risen to the forefront, along with medical discoveries and treatment innovations. Attention by clinicians to both children and parents' emotional responses and their coping effectiveness is critical if one is to have a child and family-centered approach to caring for EoE. The problems that children present in response to inquiries about their quality of life point to the issues that are particularly salient for them, and their attitude toward their illness provides a window into their coping strategies. Similarly, the questions that parents raise indicate which of the multiple facets of their child's care is foremost among their concerns.

Although attention by the clinician to the child and parents' concerns is a crucial first step in facilitating families' coping, a routine assessment by a psychosocial clinician that focuses on emotional concerns, quality of life issues, and coping strategies is an extremely helpful second step. The content of this quality of life assessment depends on each individual child's developmental status as well as disease phase, whether it be in the stage of diagnostic testing, treatment planning and institution, or follow-up evaluation. Families may be dealing with symptom management, with implementation of food restrictions, or with introducing food back into the diet. Each family has unique concerns about how to manage these issues and tasks. The quality of life assessment necessarily includes brief interventions such as anticipating with families the stages and components of evaluation and treatment of EoE, educating them regarding illness demands and coping challenges experienced by other families, and clarifying the family's specific questions, concerns, and coping style. Finally, the quality of life assessment allows a review of the patient and family's emotional functioning and overall adaptation, with an opportunity to evaluate for risk factors of significant co-morbid psychological conditions such as depression and anxiety.

The third level at which psychosocial issues can be addressed for pediatric patients with EoE and their families involves behavioral counseling or psychotherapy. The physician can make referrals based on clinical observations, or the need for treatment may become apparent during the quality of life assessment. Behavioral counseling may be required for patients having difficulties with EoE-specific issues such as self-image, peer relationships, or treatment adherence. Children with abdominal pain may benefit from pain management treatment. Anxiety and depression occur for a subset of children and adolescents with chronic illness, and these patients require treatment from mental health professionals. Children with asthma have been shown to benefit from group art therapy [59], and it is likely that children with EoE would benefit similarly from the opportunity to express their feelings about their disease and share their experiences with others who have similar problems. Parent counseling to address young children's emotional, behavioral, or sleep regulation can be a useful adjunct to medical and feeding therapy. Finally, family therapy can be extremely helpful for parents and children struggling with the emotional burden of EoE, since family cohesion and open expression of feelings are associated with better child adjustment to chronic illness [60].

Summary

For pediatric patients with EoE, symptoms, the nonspecific and variable symptoms and treatment involving dietary restrictions often have a major impact on the quality of life of the children and adolescents and on that of their families. Psychological adjustment among children and adolescents with EoE may be impacted to a lesser degree, but a subset of children will likely develop concerning psychological difficulties that require treatment. Several patterns of symptoms and behavioral responses that are specific to EoE, including feeding dysfunction, tube feeding, and abdominal pain, can lead to considerable psychological difficulty, and older children and adolescents may be affected by problems often associated with chronic illness, including stigma, adherence challenges, and depression. Families of children with EoE experience a variety of burdens and challenges, and it is important to provide appropriate levels of intervention while supporting families' competence.

References

1. Furuta GT, Liacouras CA, Collins MH, et al. Eosinophilic esophagitis in children and adults: a systematic review and consensus recommendations for diagnosis and treatment. Gastroenterology. 2007;133(4):1342–63.
2. Liacouras CA, Spergel JM, Ruchelli E, et al. Eosinophilic esophagitis: a 10-year experience in 381 children. Clin Gastroenterol Hepatol. 2005;3:1198–206.
3. Aceves SS, Bastian JF, Newbury RO, Dohil R. Oral viscous budesonide: a potential new therapy of eosinophilic esophagitis in children. Am J Gastroenterol. 2007;102(10):2271–9.
4. Konikoff MR, Noel RJ, Blanchard C, et al. A randomized, double blind, placebo-controlled trial of fluticasone propionate for pediatric eosinophilic esophagitis. Gastroenterology. 2006;131(5):1381–91.
5. Atkins D, Kramer R, Capocelli K, Lovell M, Furuta GT. Eosinophilic esophagitis: the newest esophageal inflammatory disease. Nat Rev Gastroenterol Hepatol. 2009;6:267–78.
6. Franciosi JP, Liacouras CA. Eosinophilic esophagitis. In: Furuta GT, Atkins D, Alam R (eds). Immunology and Allergy Clinics of North America: Eosinophilic Gastrointestinal Diseases. Volume 29(1). Philadelphia: W.B. Saunders Company, 2009.
7. Klinnert MD. Psychological impact of eosinophilic esophagitis on children and families. In: Furuta GT, Atkins D, Alam R (eds). Immunology and Allergy Clinics of North America: Eosinophilic Gastrointestinal Diseases. Volume 29(1). Philadelphia: W. B. Saunders Company, 2009.
8. Spergel JM, Brown-Whitehorn TF, Beausoleil JL, et al. 14 years of eosinophilic esophagitis: clinical features and prognosis. J Pediatr Gastroenterol Nutr. 2009;48:30–6.
9. Jyonouchi S, Brown-Whitehorn TA, Spergel JM. Association of eosinophilic gastrointestinal disorders with other atopic disorders. In: Furuta GT, Atkins D, Alam R (eds). Immunology and Allergy Clinics of North America: Eosinophilic Gastrointestinal Diseases. Volume 29(1). Philadelphia: W. B. Saunders Company, 2009.
10. Pentiuk SP, Miller CK, Kaul A. Eosinophilic esophagitis in infants and toddlers. Dysphagia. 2007;22:44–8.
11. Putnam PE. Evaluation of the child who has eosinophilic esophagitis. In: Furuta GT, Atkins D, Alam R (eds). Immunology and Allergy Clinics of North America: Eosinophilic Gastrointestinal Diseases. Volume 29(1). Philadelphia: W. B. Saunders Company, 2009.

12. Flood EM, Beusterien KM, Amonkar MM, et al. Patient and caregiver perspective on pediatric eosinophilic esophagitis and newly developed symptom questionnaires. Curr Med Res Opin. 2008;24(12):3369–81.
13. Aceves SS, Newbury RO, Dohil MA, Bastian JF, Dohil R. A symptom scoring tool for identifying pediatric patients with eosinophilic esophagitis and correlating symptoms with inflammation. Ann Allergy Asthma Immunol. 2009;103:401–6.
14. Pentiuk S, Putnam PE, Collins MH, Rothenberg ME. Dissociation between symptoms and histological severity in pediatric eosinophilic esophagitis. J Pediatr Gastroenterol Nutr. 2009;48:152–60.
15. Stoltenberg AM, Melin-Aldana H, Li B, Kagalwalla AF, Sentongo TA, Nelson SP. Gastroesophageal reflux symptoms and quality of life do not correlate with esophageal histopathology in children with eosinophilic esophagitis. J Pediatr Gastroenterol Nutr. 2004;39:S243–4.
16. Aceves SS, Furuta GT, Spechler SJ. Integrated approach to treatment of children and adults with eosinophilic esophagitis. In: Furuta GT, Lightdale CJ (eds). Gastrointestinal Endoscopy Clinics of North America: Eosinophilic Esophagitis. Volume 18(1). Philadelphia: W.B. Saunders Company, 2008.
17. Maity S, Thomas AG. Quality of life in paediatric gastrointestinal and liver disease: a systematic review. J Pediatr Gastroenterol Nutr. 2007;44(5):540–54.
18. Landgraf JM, Abetz L, Ware JE. Child health questionnaire (CHQ): a user's manual. Boston, MA: The Health Institute, New England Medical Center; 1996.
19. Varni JW, Limbers CA, Burwinkle TM. Impaired health-related quality of life in children and adolescents with chronic conditions: a comparative analysis of 10 disease clusters and 33 disease categories/severities utilizing the PedsQL 4.0 Generic Core Scales. Health Qual Life Outcomes. 2007;5:43.
20. DunnGalvin A, de BlokFlokstra BMJ, Burks AW, Dubois AEJ, Hourihane JOB. Food allergy QoL questionnaire for children aged 0–12 years: content, construct, and cross-cultural validity. Clin Exp Allergy. 2008;38:977–86.
21. Juniper EF, Guyatt GH, Epstein RS, Ferrie PJ, Jaeschke R, Hiller TK. Evaluation of impairment of health related quality of life in asthma: development of a questionnaire for use in clinical trials. Thorax. 1992;47:76–83.
22. Kim J, Keininger DL, Becker S, Crawley JA. Simultaneous development of the pediatric GERD caregiver impact questionnaire (PGCIQ) in American English and American Spanish. Health Qual Life Outcomes. 2005;3:5.
23. Janse AJ, Sinnema G, Uiterwall CS, Kimpen JL, Gemke RJ. Quality of life in chronic illness: children, parents and paediatricians have different, but stable perceptions. Acta Paediatr. 2008;97(8):1118–24.
24. King R, Knibb R, Hourihane JB. Impact of peanut allergy on quality of life, stress and anxiety in the family. Allergy. 2009;64:461–8.
25. Price M, Bratton D, Klinnert M. Determinants of caregiver report of asthma quality of life. Ann Allergy Asthma Immunol. 2002;89:572–7.
26. Boruk M, Lee P, Faynzilbert Y, Rosenfeld R. Caregiver well-being and child quality of life. Otolaryngol Head Neck Surg. 2007;136:159–68.
27. Stein R, Riessman C. The development of an impact-on-family scale: preliminary findings. Med Care. 1980;18:465–72.
28. Hatzmann J, Heymans H, Ferrer-i-Carbonell A, van Praag B, Grootenhuis M. Hidden consequences of success in pediatrics: parental health-related quality of life-results from the care project. Pediatrics. 2008;122:e1030–8.
29. Cohen B, Noone S, Munoz-Furlong A, Sicherer S. Development of a questionnaire to measure quality of life in families with a child with food allergy. J Allergy Clin Immunol. 2004; 114(6):1159–63.
30. Greer A, Gulotta C, Masler E, Laud R. Caregiver stress and outcomes of children with pediatric feeding disorders treated in an intensive interdisciplinary program. J Pediatr Psychol. 2008;33(6):612–20.

31. Wong C, Akobeng A, Miller V. Quality of life of parents of children on home parenteral nutrition. Gut. 2000;46:294–5.
32. Heyman M, Harmatz P, Acree M, et al. Economic and psychologic costs for maternal caregivers of gastrostomy-dependent children. J Pediatr. 2004;145:511–6.
33. Hysing M, Elgen I, Gillberg C, Lundervold AJ. Emotional and behavioural problems in subgroups of children with chronic illness: results from a large-scale population study. Child Care Health Dev. 2009;35(4):527–33.
34. Lavigne JV, Faier-Routman J. Psychological adjustment to pediatric physical disorders: a meta-analytic review. J Pediatr Psychol. 1992;17(2):133–57.
35. McQuaid EL, Kopel SJ, Nassau JH. Behavioral adjustment in children with asthma: a meta-analysis. J Dev Behav Pediatr. 2001;22(6):430–9.
36. Reinfjell T, Hjemdal O, Aune T, Vikan A, Diseth T. The pediatric quality of life inventory (PedsQL) 4.0 as an assessment measure for depressive symptoms: a correlational study with young adolescents. Nord J Psychiatry. 2008;62(4):279–86.
37. LeBovidge JS, Strauch H, Kalish LA, Schneider LC. Assessment of psychological distress among children and adolescents with food allergy. J Allergy Clin Immunol. 2009;124:1282–8.
38. Van der Zaag-Loonen HJ, Grootenhuis MA, Last BF, Derkx HHF. Coping strategies and quality of life of adolescents with inflammatory bowel disease. Qual Life Res. 2004;13:1011–9.
39. Staab D, Wenninger K, Gebert N, et al. Quality of life in patients with cystic fibrosis and their parents: what is important besides disease severity? Thorax. 1998;53:727–31.
40. Klinnert MD, McQuaid EL, McCormick D, Adinoff AD, Bryant NE. A multimethod assessment of behavioral and emotional adjustment in children with asthma. J Pediatr Psychol. 2000;25:35–46.
41. Kazak AE, Rourke MT, Navsaria N. Families and other systems in pediatric psychology. In: Roberts MC, Steele RG, editors. Handbook of pediatric psychology. 4th ed. New York: Guilford; 2009. p. 656–71.
42. Rommel N, De Meyer A, Feenstra L, Veereman-Wauters G. The complexity of feeding problems in 700 infants and young children presenting to a tertiary care institution. J Pediatr Gastroenterol Nutr. 2003;37:75–84.
43. Haas AM, Maune NC. Clinical presentation of feeding dysfunction in children with eosinophilic gastrointestinal disease. In: Furuta GT, Atkins D, Alam R (eds). Immunology and Allergy Clinics of North America: Eosinophilic Gastrointestinal Diseases. Volume 29(1). Philadelphia: W. B. Saunders Company, 2009.
44. Assa'ad AH, Putnam PE, Collins MH, et al. Pediatric patients with eosinophilic esophagitis: an 8-year follow-up. J Allergy Clin Immunol. 2007;119(3):731–8.
45. Nelson S, Chen E, Synair G, et al. One-year follow-up of symptoms of gastroesophageal reflux during infancy. Pediatrics. 1998;106(6):1–4.
46. Powers S, Byars K, Mitchell M, Patton S, Standiford D, Dolan L. Parent report of mealtime behavior and parenting stress in young children with type 1 diabetes and in healthy control subjects. Diabetes Care. 2002;25(2):313–8.
47. Silverman A, Tarbell S. Feeding and vomiting problems in pediatric populations. In: Roberts MC, Steele RG, editors. Handbook of pediatric psychology. 4th ed. New York: Guilford; 2009. p. 429–45.
48. Markowitz JE, Spergel JM, Ruchelli E, Liacouras CA. Elemental diet is an effective treatment for eosinophilic esophagitis in children and adolescents. Am J Gastroenterol. 2003;98(4):777–82.
49. Goldberg E, Kaye R, Yaworski J, Liacouras C. Gastrostomy tubes: facts, fallacies, fistulas, and false tracts. Gastroenterol Nurs. 2005;28(6):485–94.
50. Byars K, Burklow K, Gerguson K, et al. A multicomponent behavioral program for oral aversion in children dependent on gastrostomy feedings. J Pediatr Gastroenterol Nutr. 2003;34:473–80.
51. Huertas-Ceballos A, Logan S, Bennet C, Macarthur C. Psychosocial Interventions for recurrent abdominal pain (RAP) and irritable bowel syndrome (IBS) in childhood. Cochrane Database Syst Rev. 2008.

52. Walker L, Jones D. Psychosocial factors: impact on symptom severity and outcomes of pediatric functional gastrointestinal disorders. J Pediatr Gastroenterol Nutr. 2005;41:S51–2.
53. Puzanovova M, Rudzinski E, Shirkey K, Cherry R, Acra S, Walker L. Sex, psychosocial factors, and reported symptoms influence referral for esophagogastroduodenoscopy and biopsy results in children with chronic abdominal pain. J Pediatr Gastroenterol Nutr. 2008;47:54–60.
54. Olsson C, Lyon P, Hornell A, Ivarsson A, Sydner YM. Food that makes you different: the stigma experienced by adolescents with celiac disease. Qual Health Res. 2009;19(7):976–84.
55. DunnGalvin A, Gaffney A, Hourihane JB. Developmental pathways in food allergy: a new theoretical framework. Allergy. 2009;64(4):560–8.
56. Sampson MA, Munoz-Furlong A, Sicherer SH. Risk-taking and coping strategies of adolescents and young adults with food allergy. J Allergy Clin Immunol. 2006;117(6):1440–5.
57. Cadman D, Rosenbaum P, Boyle M, Offord D. Children with chronic illness: family and parent demographic characteristics and psychosocial adjustment. Pediatrics. 1991;87:884–9.
58. Wallander J. Special section editorial: current research on pediatric chronic illness. J Pediatr Psychol. 1993;18:7–10.
59. Beebe A, Gelfand E, Bender B. A randomized trial to test the effectiveness of art therapy for children with asthma. J Allergy Clin Immunol. 2010;126(2):263–6.
60. Wallander J, Varni J. Effects of pediatric chronic physical disorders on child and family adjustment. J Child Psychol Psychiatry. 1998;39(1):29–46.

Chapter 30
Eosinophilic Esophagitis: Treatment Approach in Adults

Ikuo Hirano

Keywords Eosinophilic esophagitis • Gastroesophageal reflux disease • Dysphagia • Endoscopy

Introduction

Since its recognition as a distinct clinical entity in the mid 1990s, eosinophilic esophagitis (EoE) has emerged as one of the common and readily treatable causes of dysphagia in adults. Over the past 15 years, studies have identified a number of medical, dietary, and endoscopic therapies that are highly effective at remedying the symptoms, signs, and histopathology of EoE in both children and adults. This chapter will focus on the management of EoE in adults based primarily upon the adult literature with reference to key pediatric studies.

Goals of Therapy

The overall goals of therapy of EoE include not only alleviation of presenting symptoms and signs but also prevention of disease recurrence, improvement in quality of life, and preclusion of complications. Substantial dietary limitation, alteration in eating habits, food impaction, and esophageal perforation may result from

I. Hirano (✉)
Division of Gastroenterology, Northwestern University Feinberg School of Medicine, Chicago, IL, USA
e-mail: i-hirano@northwestern.edu

C.A. Liacouras and J.E. Markowitz (eds.), *Eosinophilic Esophagitis*, Clinical Gastroenterology, DOI 10.1007/978-1-60761-515-6_30,

the submucosal fibrosis, esophageal stricture formation, and narrow caliber esophagus that characterize EoE in adults. Understanding the natural history of EoE is of central importance. If EoE is a self-limited condition, short-term therapy or observation would be reasonable. On the other hand, a chronic and progressive course would favor early intervention and maintenance therapy. Unfortunately, little is known regarding the natural history, creating a challenge in patient management, particularly in those with minimal or no symptoms. In the longest follow-up study to date, Straumann et al. followed 30 adult patients for an average of 7.2 years in the absence of medical or dietary therapy [1]. All patients survived the study period in good health in a stable nutritional state, but 97% continued to experience dysphagia. Dysphagia increased in 23%, was stable in 37%, and improved in 37%. Esophageal eosinophilia persisted but demonstrated an overall decline in most patients. That one third of the cohort received esophageal dilation likely affected the reported symptom outcome but not the histologic sequellae as supported by a recent study of dilation in EoE [2]. A recent preliminary study found a significant correlation between the duration and severity of symptoms in a cohort of 125 adult EoE patients [3]. When examined over a 30-year time frame, patients with longer duration of dysphagia presented at the time of EoE diagnosis with a greater frequency of dysphagia and severity of food impaction. While several chronic esophageal disorders including gastroesophageal reflux disease, tylosis, and radiation esophagitis have been associated with an increased risk of esophageal squamous and adenocarcinoma, no cases of esophageal neoplasia related to EoE have been reported. Barrett's metaplasia has been reported in patients with EoE but it is unclear as to whether this is a causal relationship or just chance co-existence of two conditions. Spontaneous remission of EoE has been reported, but this occurs quite infrequently based on natural history data and placebo response rates in controlled trials.

Uncertainty exists regarding the most pertinent endpoints of treatment of EoE. Symptoms are a commonly tracked outcome by clinicians. Caution is needed, however, in the interpretation of symptom improvement as many patients modify their diets to minimize ingestion of foods that are difficult to swallow whereas others have very sporadic symptoms that may not manifest during a short follow-up period. Additional patients alter their eating habits to allow for more meticulous mastication and prolonged meal times. While such alterations may result in a patient reporting minimal dysphagia, a substantial reduction in quality of life may result from adverse effects on social interaction and meal enjoyment [4]. More objective treatment outcomes include endoscopic esophageal mucosal changes, radiographic presence of esophageal strictures, alterations in esophageal mural distensibility, and histopathology [5]. Detection of these consequences of EoE may be important measures and need further validation in prospective studies. In many existing studies, response is determined by a reduction in tissue eosinophilia. However, the appropriate degree of reduction is uncertain and different target endpoints have been used including <15, <10, or <5 eosinophils per high power field (eos/hpf). Other markers of tissue injury such as markers of eosinophil activation, basal cell hyperplasia, or subepithelial fibrosis may be as important as the actual number of eosinophils [6].

Furthermore, histologic resolution of inflammation on esophageal mucosal biopsies could be misleading. The inflammatory process within the esophagus is patchy and limited biopsy sampling could introduce error in interpretation [7]. Furthermore, studies have demonstrated that esophageal eosinophilia can extend to involve the submucosa as well as muscularis layers, regions that are not routinely sampled by esophageal mucosal biopsies [8, 9].

The majority of the published therapeutic studies to date have focused on therapeutic outcomes of symptoms and esophageal eosinophilia. When comparing existing treatment studies, differences in patient selection, definition of therapeutic response, and duration of treatment are important parameters that may explain heterogeneity in results. More recently, investigations have included additional parameters of histologic tissue injury such as submucosal fibrosis as well as anatomic and physiologic consequences of EoE determined by use of high frequency endoluminal ultrasonography and esophageal mural compliance [5, 9]. Development of an EoE activity index is underway that combines clinical with endoscopic and histologic parameters and will offer a validated assessment of patient response to therapy.

Evaluation Prior to Initiation of Therapy

The management of EoE in adults begins with recognition of the disease. EoE is considered in adults with dysphagia and food impactions, regardless of the presence or absence of heartburn. Endoscopic evidence of esophageal signs of EoE include rings, longitudinal furrows, white exudates, or edema. Biopsies should be obtained even when these features are absent since up to 9% of adults may have a normal appearance to the esophagus on EGD [10]. The practice of empiric, large caliber esophageal dilation in patients with unexplained dysphagia should generally be avoided given reported complications of dilation in EoE. Instead, biopsies of the esophagus for unexplained dysphagia can identify patients with EoE who would benefit from medical or dietary therapy and a conservative approach to esophageal dilation. Other less common presentations of EoE in adults include atypical chest pain or heartburn that does not respond to empiric PPI therapy. In such cases, the utility and cost-effectiveness of esophageal biopsies to rule out EoE is uncertain. Prospective studies have shown that the diagnostic yield of this approach is low in the absence of symptoms of dysphagia. On the other hand, several case reports have described patients suspected of having reflux refractory to medical or surgical fundoplication who were subsequently diagnosed with EoE [11, 12]. Improvement in the patients was subsequently achieved after treatment of EoE [11].

In patients with suspected EoE, multiple mucosal biopsies should be obtained since the inflammatory changes are often not uniform but patchy. Both a pediatric and adult study of histologic variability in EoE demonstrated that the yield for detection of esophageal eosinophilia defined by greater than 15 eos/hpf was maximized by acquisition of six esophageal biopsies [7, 13]. The number of biopsies necessary increases if a higher threshold number of eos/hpf is used to define the disease. In terms of location of biopsies, the practice of obtaining separate biopsies from the proximal or mid esophagus rather than distal esophagus is based on the notion that reflux is associated with distal inflammation that may include eosinophils. The accuracy of this protocol is unproven. Selective biopsies from only the proximal esophagus may improve the specificity of the diagnosis of EoE at the expense of sensitivity. There is also variability in the location of biopsies with some centers obtaining proximal and others mid esophageal biopsies. While the optimal location of biopsies remains uncertain, multiple biopsies from different regions of the esophagus are recommended to maximize detection of esophageal eosinophilia.

Once the presence of increased esophageal eosinophilia has been established in symptomatic patients, secondary causes of esophageal eosinophilia need to be considered. Most secondary etiologies including inflammatory bowel disease, drug hypersensitivity reactions, and parasitic disease should be apparent from a review of the patient's past medical history. Concomitant eosinophilic gastroenteritis (EoG) is an association that may necessitate additional biopsies of the gastric and small bowel mucosa at the time of endoscopy. However, EoG is uncommon and the majority of EoG patients present with symptoms as well as endoscopically evident mucosal features that would prompt biopsy acquisition.

Gastroesophageal reflux disease (GERD) has become increasingly difficult to differentiate from EoE [14]. Studies from the eighties equated esophageal eosinophilia with the diagnosis of GERD. In the early 1990s, reports described EoE as a entity distinct from GERD based either on lack of response to proton pump inhibitor (PPI) therapy or absence of distal esophageal acid exposure on ambulatory pH testing. Over the past decade, it has become evident that EoE and GERD not only frequently coexist but moreover that treatment of acid reflux is effective in a significant proportion of patients with symptoms, endoscopic features, and histopathology that are consistent with EoE. A symptom profile of dysphagia and food impaction in an atopic individual combined with characteristic features on EGD is highly predictive of esophageal eosinophilia but does not predict responsiveness to PPI therapy. Several pediatric and adult series demonstrated normalization of symptoms and tissue eosinophilia after PPI therapy [15–18]. On the other hand, the presence of GERD defined by an abnormal pH study does not preclude the presence of EoE. Increased acid exposure exists in patients whose esophageal eosinophilia persists in spite of PPI therapy [15, 19]. Whether patients with significant tissue eosinophilia responsive to PPI therapy should be diagnosed with GERD or a PPI responsive form of EoE is uncertain. GERD may be involved in the pathogenesis of EoE by reducing tissue integrity that allows exposure of esophageal antigen presenting cells to dietary allergens. Furthermore, acid exposure increases eosinophil viability and the release of mediators involved in eosinophil recruitment. Owing to the ease and safety profile of PPI therapy, a trial of PPI therapy is reasonable in patients with suspected EoE. Available data, although limited, does not support the routine use of pH monitoring in the evaluation of EoE if the intent is the identification of patients who will benefit from PPI therapy.

Initial Therapy for EoE: Drugs, Diet, or Dilation?

If symptoms and eosinophilia persist despite a trial of acid-suppression, primary treatment options for EoE are discussed with the patient. Over the past 15 years, a number of medical, dietary, and endoscopic approaches have emerged (Table 30.1) [20]. Medical and dietary therapies are effective at reducing symptoms as well as tissue eosinophilia. The degree to which the structural alterations are reversible with medical or dietary therapy is uncertain. For adults, topical steroids are the most commonly used treatment given the ease of administration and published data supporting their efficacy and safety. Several prospective, uncontrolled studies and five, randomized controlled trials have evaluated the effectiveness and efficacy of steroids, respectively [21–27]. With the exception of one study, the adult trials with topical steroids have consistently demonstrated marked, significant clinical and histologic improvement after therapy administered from 15 days to 3 months. Histologic response rates defined by less than 6 eos/hpf were achieved in recent studies in over 70% of patients. Endoscopic signs of rings, furrows, and strictures visibly improve but may not completely resolve [27] (Fig. 30.1). Significant variability in the degree of response to topical steroids has been observed. Interestingly, in pediatric studies, allergic individuals identified by reactivity on skin testing and taller subjects demonstrated lower response rates [21, 22]. The data suggest that the efficacy of topical steroids may be affected by the dose of steroid as well as degree of underlying atopy. The mode of administration via swallowed aerosolized particles or viscous liquid preparations may affect the delivery and contact time of the steroid with the esophageal mucosal surface. Based on pediatric data, the efficacy of topical and systemic steroids appears comparable [25]. Adherence compliance with prolonged therapy has been a concern as the symptomatic benefits are not immediate and tend to last for prolonged periods after cessation.

Limitations of topical steroids include disease recurrence in 90% following cessation and uncertainty regarding long-term safety [28]. A proportion of patients have limited responsiveness to topical steroids perhaps owing to drug delivery, intrinsic steroid resistance, or an underlying strong allergic predisposition. Whether such patients would respond to higher doses of topical steroids, therapy directed at allergic environmental triggers, or systemic steroids has yet to be determined. The primary side effect of topical steroids has been oropharyngeal or esophageal candidiasis. A prospective study in children administered fluticasone at doses of 220–440 μg QID found esophageal candidiasis in 15% of patients, although the patients did not report symptoms attributable to the infection [25]. Potential concerns for steroid side effects such as adrenal insufficiency or osteoporosis have not been reported. Pharyngeal irritation is more commonly reported with aerosolized steroid and may be related to contact irritation by the propellant.

Available data support the effectiveness of dietary therapy in adults with EoE although the majority of studies have been from pediatric centers. The three dietary approaches used in children include (1) elemental diet, (2) allergy testing directed elimination diet, and (3) empiric elimination diet [28–30]. Although pediatric series

Table 30.1 Treatment options for eosinophilic esophagitis

Treatment	Advantages	Disadvantages
Medications		
Topical steroids (Fluticasone, Budesonide)	Ease of administration	Esophageal Candidiasis
	Consistent effectiveness in uncontrolled studies	Recurrent disease after cessation
	High degree of efficacy in randomized controlled trials	
Systemic steroids	High degree of efficacy in randomized, controlled trials	Toxicities of systemic steroid
	Ease of administration	Recurrent disease after cessation
Antihistamines	Ease of administration	Limited data to support effectiveness
Proton pump inhibitor	Moderate effectiveness	Unclear whether response is specific for GERD or a PPI reponsive form of EoE
	Safety profile	
Leukotriene antagonist	Symptom improvement in uncontrolled studies	High doses may be needed for effect
		No change in esophageal eosinophilia
		Side effects of nausea and myalgias
Immunomodulator	Steroid sparing agent	Immunosuppression
		Side effect profile
		Limited data (three patients) to support effectiveness
Anti-TNF therapy	Rationale based on increased	No clinical improvement in a small, uncontrolled trial
	Tissue expression of TNF	
Anti-IL-5 therapy	Rationale based on role of IL-5 in systemic eosinophilic disorders	Limited data to support efficacy
Cromolyn sodium	Rationale based on asthma model	Limited pediatric data does not support effectiveness
Diet		
Elemental	High degree of effectiveness	Poor palatability
		Requires prolonged period of food reintroduction
	Avoidance of long-term use of medications	Need for repeated EGD and biopsies to identify allergen
Directed elimination	High degree of effectiveness	Skin prick test with poor predictive value
	Theoretical advantage of more selective diet	Atopy patch testing not standardized or widely available
	Avoidance of long-term use of medications	Need for repeated EGD and biopsies to identify allergen
Empiric elimination	High degree of effectiveness	Need for repeated EGD and biopsy to identify allergen
	Avoidance of long-term use of medications	High degree of vigilance to avoid contamination
Dilation		
	High degree of effectiveness	Reports of esophageal laceration causing significant pain and infrequent hospitalization
	Prolonged symptom response without medications	Infrequent reports of esophageal perforation

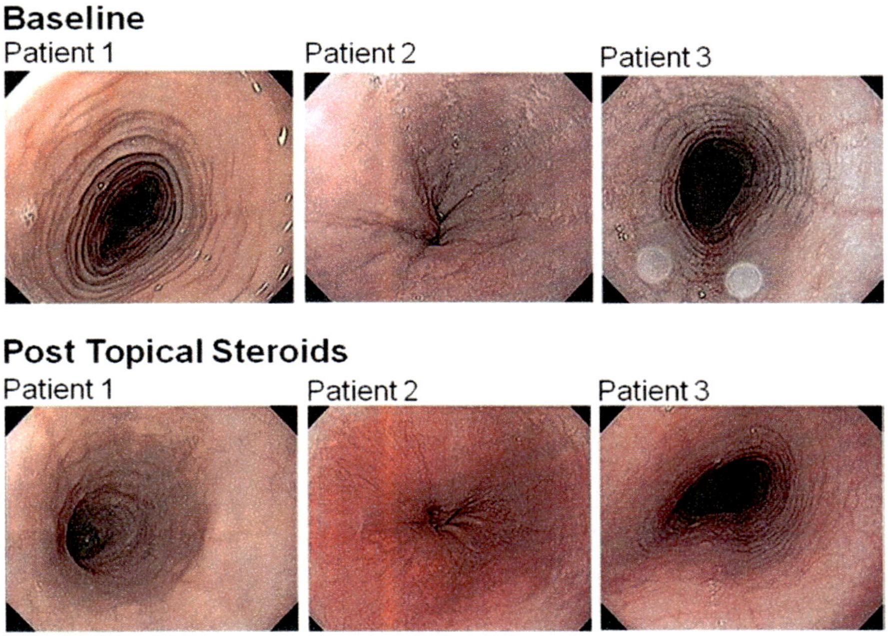

Fig. 30.1 Endoscopic features of eosinophilic esophagitis before and after topical steroid administration in three adult patients with eosinophilic esophagitis. Patient 1 has esophageal rings and furrows, patient 2 has longitudinal furrows and exudates, and patient 3 has rings, furrows, and exudates (*upper panel*). All three patients show improvement in the endoscopic signs after 6 weeks of topical fluticasone (*lower panel*)

describe hundreds of EoE patients treated effectively with diet, none of the series have been randomized controlled trials. It is important to emphasize that the goal of dietary therapy is not only achieving symptomatic and histologic disease remission but moreover the identification of specific food allergens. Patients view the dietary approach as a non pharmacologic intervention that seeks to remove environmental triggers to their disease. The dietary approach requires a highly motivated patient willing to avoid several common foods for a defined period of time with vigilance regarding dietary contamination. The success is optimized by close supervision by a dietician with experience in food allergy. A recently completed prospective study of 50 adults at Northwestern applied the empiric elimination of common food allergens (wheat, milk protein, soy, egg, nuts, and seafood) for 6 weeks followed by systematic food reintroduction [31]. Histologic response rates defined by less than 10 eos/hpf was achieved in 70%. Symptom improvement in dysphagia occurred in almost every patient with demonstrable improvement in endoscopic abnormalities (Fig. 30.2). Milk and wheat were the most common food triggers identified. Based on the response to food reintroduction testing among responders, skin prick testing for food allergens led to both false negative and false positive results in the majority of patients.

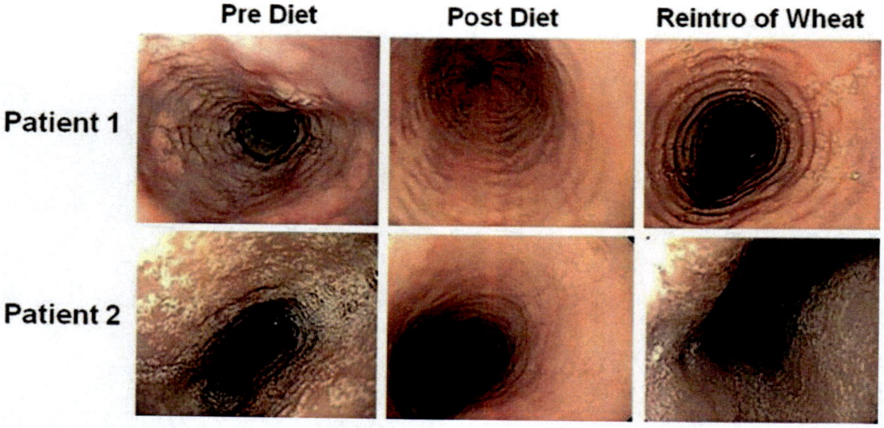

Fig. 30.2 Endoscopic features of eosinophilic esophagitis before and after six-food elimination diet (SFED) in two adult patients with eosinophilic esophagitis. Patient 1 has esophageal exudates and furrows while patient 2 has longitudinal furrows and exudates (*left panel*). Both patients show improvement in the endoscopic signs after 6 weeks of dietary elimination (*middle panel*). During reintroduction, both patients had recurrent symptoms, endoscopic signs, and esophageal eosinophilia following reintroduction of wheat (*right panel*)

Disadvantages of elimination diet therapies include the potential impact on patient quality of life during the initial elimination phase of the diet as well as long-term selective elimination of specific food(s). The reintroduction phase generally incorporates not only symptom assessment but also periodic endoscopic surveillance for recurrent esophageal eosinophilia. The performance of multiple EGD with biopsies is associated with both time and expense for patients. The accuracy of following only symptom rather than symptom and histologic recurrence upon food reintroduction has not been determined. Two factors limit the use of pure symptom data in the identification of food triggers. First, the inflammatory response to ingested allergens follows a delayed rather than immediate hypersensitivity reaction making it challenging for patients to temporally link food ingestion with recurrent symptoms. Second, tracking dysphagia as a primary determinant of response is problematic as the symptoms are intermittent. A noninvasive biomarker of disease activity would greatly improve the acceptance of the dietary therapy of EoE. Moreover, an allergy assay which accurately predicts causative food allergens would clearly be ideal. The long-term effectiveness of dietary elimination and eventual ability to reintroduce identified food triggers are the subject of ongoing investigations. The role of treatment of aeroallergies as primary or adjunctive therapy in EoE remains speculative.

Esophageal dilation was one of the first therapies used for adult patients with EoE. Early reports of complications related to esophageal dilation in EoE included not only chest pain but also perforation generated trepidation among gastroenterologists. Of the 84 adult patients reported prior to 2008 who underwent dilation,

5% experienced an esophageal perforation and 7% were hospitalized for chest pain [32]. Further compounding this concern were early reports of esophageal tears and perforations from food impactions and diagnostic endoscopies, suggesting a particular susceptibility for esophageal mural fragility in EoE [33]. Such findings led to a consensus statement publication that recommended that medical or dietary therapy for EoE be attempted prior to the performance of esophageal dilation [34].

Two recent retrospective studies from adult centers reported complication rates for sequellae of perforation or pain requiring hospitalization that were considerably lower than that of initial reports [2, 35]. No perforations were reported among 243 patients undergoing esophageal dilation. Incorporating this new data, the perforation rate for dilation is 1.5%, with chest pain in 7% and chest pain requiring hospitalization in 2%. An important factor that may have influenced the higher complication rates in earlier reports has to do with disease awareness. Many of the initial reports of esophageal perforation occurred in patients in whom EoE was not initially recognized and prior to publications describing the dangers of esophageal dilation. As such, the greater safety reported in the studies by more recent series may reflect the adoption of a more conservative approach by gastroenterologists aware of the potential hazards of dilation in EoE.

In spite of the greater safety margin reported in these recent studies of esophageal dilation, the role of dilation as a primary therapy of EoE is still controversial and should be individualized until more data is available. In adults, EoE generally affects otherwise healthy, young to middle-aged patients who, if given the option, might prefer periodic dilation to regular use of a medication or an elimination diet. Dilation can provide immediate and long-lasting relief of dysphagia in patients with high-grade esophageal strictures [2]. On the other hand, monotherapy with dilation does not improve the underlying inflammatory process. One would not recommend dilation without PPI therapy for a peptic stricture, so should EoE, also a reversible chronic inflammatory condition, be any different? If medical or dietary therapy is selected as initial therapy, it seems reasonable to determine the clinical response prior to dilation. The rapid and potentially long-lasting benefits of dilation should be weighed against the substantial consequences of esophageal perforation, albeit rare.

At this time, there is no prospective data to guide the decision for selecting the optimal initial therapy for patients with eosinophilic esophagitis. The available data supports the use of topical steroids, diet, or dilation as effective means of managing the dysphagia that dominates the clinical presentation in adults. The only randomized, controlled trials performed to date establish the efficacy of topical steroids. A stepwise approach using monotherapy is suggested whereby patients are initially placed on a trial of PPI therapy (Fig. 30.3). Unresponsive patients meeting the current consensus statement definition of primary EoE are offered therapy with either diet or steroids, with selected patients undergoing esophageal dilation. Patients who are unresponsive to initial therapy can be switched to an alternative therapy. The role for initial combination therapy, other than dilation with topical steroids, has not been evaluated.

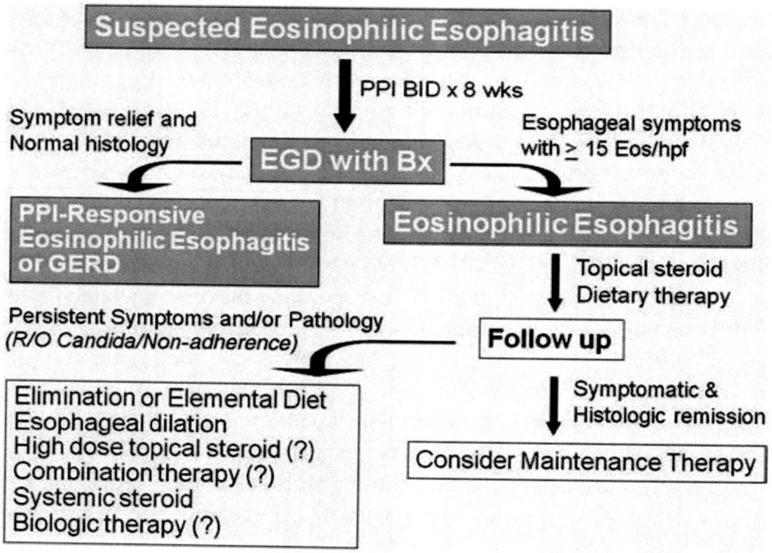

Fig. 30.3 Suggested management algorithm for eosinophilic esophagitis in adults. Patients presenting with esophageal symptoms, typically dominated by dysphagia and food impaction, in the setting of history of atopy are suspected of having eosinophilic esophagitis. Highly sensitive endoscopic signs with esophageal eosinophilia are supportive findings in patients having undergone upper endoscopy. A treatment trial of double-dose proton pump inhibition is followed by an upper endoscopy with esophageal biopsies. Patients with persistent symptoms combined with histologic evidence of esophageal eosinophilia meet the current consensus statement definition of eosinophilic esophagitis. Primary therapy with either topical steroids or dietary elimination is discussed. Use of esophageal dilation is considered in selected patients. A follow-up endoscopy with biopsy provides information regarding the endoscopic and pathologic response to initial therapy but may not be necessary for all patients. Patients who do not respond to initial therapy are then candidates for secondary therapies

Patients Refractory to Therapy

Patients demonstrating limited response to initial therapy include those with persistent symptoms, those with persistent esophageal inflammation and those with both. When both symptoms and inflammation persist, the initial therapy needs to be reevaluated. Patients not responding to topical steroids should be questioned as to compliance and appropriate method of administration. Dose escalation with topical steroids is a consideration as higher response rates were noted in studies using fluticasone at 880 μg BID compared with those using 440 μg BID. However, this comparison is made between different studies that enrolled different EoE populations. While systemic steroids were shown to have similar efficacy to topical steroids in a pediatric, controlled trial, the histologic improvement was more complete with systemic steroids supporting a potential role for systemic steroids in patients unresponsive to topical steroids [25]. Anecdotal reports have noted patients who failed to respond to swallowed fluticasone by inhaler administration who responded to liquid budesonide. Dietary therapy is an option for patients unresponsive to topical steroids although there is no data regarding the effectiveness of this approach. Uncontrolled data point to a greater response to elemental compared to empiric elimination diet therapy. Alternate medical therapies including montelukast, cromolyn sodium, or antihistamines have shown limited benefits in a few, small uncontrolled studies [36]. Combination therapies with steroids and montelukast or steroids with antihistamines have not been reported. Esophageal dilation is a useful adjunctive therapy that has been used in combination with medical therapy [2]. Safety concerns that support a conservative dilation strategy were discussed in the preceding section.

Patients with resolution of eosinophilia but continued dysphagia may have developed esophageal strictures amenable to esophageal dilation. It should be noted that the reversal of esophageal submucosal fibrosis and remodeling in EoE may require prolonged therapy over months whereas the tissue inflammatory response may reverse within days of topical corticosteroid administration. A prospective adult study detected significant improvement in endoscopic detection of esophageal strictures following 3 months of fluticasone [27].

Novel biologic therapies have emerged for the treatment of EoE. Anti-IgE, anti-IL-5, anti-TNF therapies have all been reported in very small series as discussed in a prior chapter. The controlled study of anti-IL-5 therapy in a group of 11 adults with steroid dependent or unresponsive disease showed significant reductions in both tissue and peripheral eosinophilia but did not achieve its primary endpoint of achieving <5 eos/hpf and did not demonstrate significant symptom benefit [37]. Trials examining anti-IL-13 are ongoing at this time. Analogous to their use in inflammatory bowel disease, biologic therapy offers the potential therapy as disease modifying agents. More data on their use as monotherapy or in combination with existing therapies are needed.

Treatment of Asymptomatic Patients

From the American Gastroenterological Association consensus statement, patients with significant esophageal eosinophilia on esophageal biopsy but without symptoms would not meet the definition of EoE [34]. However, as noted above, patients may have significant esophageal structural alterations and strictures but not report dysphagia due to careful mastication, prolonged meal times, and/or food avoidance. The same situation is encountered in patients initially diagnosed with EoE but achieving symptom but not histologic remission following medical or dietary therapy. Currently, there is little information to support additional treatment of such individuals. A more proactive approach might be considered in patients with higher degrees of esophageal stenosis. Given the uncertainties regarding the natural history of EoE, it seems prudent to advise clinical follow-up for patients with esophageal eosinophilia even in the absence of symptoms.

Maintenance Therapy

Maintenance therapy is an important consideration for EoE patients since the majority develop recurrent symptoms and histopathology upon cessation of therapy with either topical or systemic steroids. Maintenance therapy is not discussed after elimination diet therapy as it assumed that patients continue to abstain from identified trigger foods. As there is limited data to suggest that EoE is a progressive disorder that leads to increased esophageal structuring over time, long-term therapeutic strategies should be individualized. For patients with mild and intermittent dysphagia without significant strictures or food impaction, intermittent on-demand topical steroids may be appropriate assuming that the patient is reliable and has clinical follow-up. For patients with severe dysphagia, repeated food impaction and high-grade esophageal strictures at presentation and who respond to initial medical therapy, maintenance therapy seems reasonable. Lowering the dosage of topical steroids below that used to induce clinical remission is a consideration but a recent study that attempted this strategy noted a significant reduction in treatment efficacy. Maintenance with nonsteroid medications such as antihistamines, immunomodulators, or leukotriene antagonists has been reported in very small retrospective case series. Finally, the prolonged relief of dysphagia reported after esophageal dilation needs to be considered given the inconvenience and potential side effects of long-term medical or dietary therapy.

References

1. Straumann A, Spichtin HP, Grize L, Bucher KA, Beglinger C, Simon HU. Natural history of primary eosinophilic esophagitis: a follow-up of 30 adult patients for up to 11.5 years. Gastroenterology. 2003;125(6):1660–9.
2. Schoepfer AM, Gonsalves N, Bussmann C, et al. Esophageal dilation in eosinophilic esophagitis: effectiveness, safety, and impact on the underlying inflammation. Am J Gastroenterol. 2010;105(5):1062–70.
3. Toto E, Kern E, Moy N, Kwasny M, Gonsalves N, Hirano I. Duration of dysphagia is associated with increased frequency of dysphagia and food impaction in adults with eosinophilic esophagitis. Gastroenterology. 2010;138(5):S-176.
4. Kern E, Taft T, Moy N, Kwasny M, Gonsalves N, Keefer L, et al. Patient reported outcomes in adults with eosinophilic esophagitis. Gastroenterology. 2010;138(5):S-175.
5. Kwiatek MA, Hirano I, Kahrilas PJ, Rothe J, Luger D, Pandolfino JE. Mechanical properties of the esophagus in eosinophilic esophagitis. Gastroenterology. 2011;140:82–90.
6. Aceves SS, Newbury RO, Dohil R, Bastian JF, Broide DH. Esophageal remodeling in pediatric eosinophilic esophagitis. J Allergy Clin Immunol. 2007;119(1):206–12.
7. Gonsalves N, Policarpio-Nicolas M, Zhang Q, Rao MS, Hirano I. Histopathologic variability and endoscopic correlates in adults with eosinophilic esophagitis. Gastrointest Endosc. 2006;64(3):313–9.
8. Stevoff C, Rao S, Parsons W, Kahrilas PJ, Hirano I. EUS and histopathologic correlates in eosinophilic esophagitis. Gastrointest Endosc. 2001;54(3):373–7.
9. Fox VL, Nurko S, Teitelbaum JE, Badizadegan K, Furuta GT. High-resolution EUS in children with eosinophilic "allergic" esophagitis. Gastrointest Endosc. 2003;57(1):30–6.

10. Sgouros SN, Bergele C, Mantides A. Eosinophilic esophagitis in adults: what is the clinical significance? Endoscopy. 2006;38(5):515–20.
11. Kelly KJ, Lazenby AJ, Rowe PC, Yardley JH, Perman JA, Sampson HA. Eosinophilic esophagitis attributed to gastroesophageal reflux: improvement with an amino acid-based formula. Gastroenterology. 1995;109(5):1503–12.
12. Dellon ES, Farrell TM, Bozymski EM, Shaheen NJ. Diagnosis of eosinophilic esophagitis after fundoplication for 'refractory reflux': implications for preoperative evaluation. Dis Esophagus. 2010;23(3):191–5.
13. Shah A, Kagalwalla AF, Gonsalves N, Melin-Aldana H, Li BU, Hirano I. Histopathologic variability in children with eosinophilic esophagitis. Am J Gastroenterol. 2009;104(3):716–21.
14. Spechler SJ, Genta RM, Souza RF. Thoughts on the complex relationship between gastroesophageal reflux disease and eosinophilic esophagitis. Am J Gastroenterol. 2007;102(6):1301–6.
15. Molina-Infante J, Ferrando-Lamana L, Gallardo BP, et al. Systemic clinicopathologic follow up on high dose acid suppression is mandatory to avoid eosinophilic esophagitis overestimation in adults. Gastroenterology. 2010;138(5):S1073.
16. Morrow JB, Vargo JJ, Goldblum JR, Richter JE. The ringed esophagus: histological features of GERD. Am J Gastroenterol. 2001;96(4):984–9.
17. Dranove JE, Horn DS, Davis MA, Kernek KM, Gupta SK. Predictors of response to proton pump inhibitor therapy among children with significant esophageal eosinophilia. J Pediatr. 2009;154(1):96–100.
18. Ngo P, Furuta GT, Antonioli DA, Fox VL. Eosinophils in the esophagus–peptic or allergic eosinophilic esophagitis? Case series of three patients with esophageal eosinophilia. Am J Gastroenterol. 2006;101(7):1666–70.
19. Shah A, Kagalwalla AF, Gonsalves N, Melin-Aldana H, Li BU, Hirano I. Histopathologic variability in children with eosinophilic esophagitis. Am J Gastroenterol. 2009;104(3):716–21.
20. Garrean C, Hirano I. Eosinophilic esophagitis: pathophysiology and optimal management. Curr Gastroenterol Rep. 2009;11(3):175–81.
21. Dohil R, Newbury R, Fox L, Bastian J, Aceves S. Oral viscous budesonide is effective in children with eosinophilic esophagitis in a randomized, placebo-controlled trial. Gastroenterology. 2010;139(2):418–29.
22. Konikoff MR, Noel RJ, Blanchard C, et al. A randomized, double-blind, placebo-controlled trial of fluticasone propionate for pediatric eosinophilic esophagitis. Gastroenterology. 2006;131(5):1381–91.
23. Straumann A, Conus S, Degen L, et al. Budesonide is effective in adolescent and adult patients with active eosinophilic esophagitis. Gastroenterology. 2010;139(5):1526–37.
24. Peterson KA, Thomas KL, Hilden K, Emerson LL, Wills JC, Fang JC. Comparison of esomeprazole to aerosolized, swallowed fluticasone for eosinophilic esophagitis. Dig Dis Sci. 2010;55(5):1313–9.
25. Schaefer ET, Fitzgerald JF, Molleston JP, et al. Comparison of oral prednisone and topical fluticasone in the treatment of eosinophilic esophagitis: a randomized trial in children. Clin Gastroenterol Hepatol. 2008;6(2):165–73.
26. Remedios M, Campbell C, Jones DM, Kerlin P. Eosinophilic esophagitis in adults: clinical, endoscopic, histologic findings, and response to treatment with fluticasone propionate. Gastrointest Endosc. 2006;63(1):3–12.
27. Lucendo AJ, Pascual-Turrion JM, Navarro M, et al. Endoscopic, bioptic, and manometric findings in eosinophilic esophagitis before and after steroid therapy: a case series. Endoscopy. 2007;39(9):765–71.
28. Liacouras CA, Spergel JM, Ruchelli E, et al. Eosinophilic esophagitis: a 10-year experience in 381 children. Clin Gastroenterol Hepatol. 2005;3(12):1198–206.
29. Spergel JM, Andrews T, Brown-Whitehorn TF, Beausoleil JL, Liacouras CA. Treatment of eosinophilic esophagitis with specific food elimination diet directed by a combination of skin prick and patch tests. Ann Allergy Asthma Immunol. 2005;95(4):336–43.
30. Kagalwalla AF, Sentongo TA, Ritz S, et al. Effect of six-food elimination diet on clinical and histologic outcomes in eosinophilic esophagitis. Clin Gastroenterol Hepatol. 2006;4(9):1097–102.

31. Gonsalves N, Yang G, Doerfler B, Ritz S, Ditto A, Hirano I. Prospective clinical trial of allergy testing and food elimination diet and food reintroduction in adults with eosinophilic esophagitis. Gastroenterology. 2008;134(4):A104.
32. Hirano I. Dilation in eosinophilic esophagitis: to do or not to do? Gastrointest Endosc. 2010;71(4):713–4.
33. Straumann A, Rossi L, Simon HU, Heer P, Spichtin HP, Beglinger C. Fragility of the esophageal mucosa: a pathognomonic endoscopic sign of primary eosinophilic esophagitis? Gastrointest Endosc. 2003;57(3):407–12.
34. Furuta GT, Liacouras CA, Collins MH, et al. Eosinophilic esophagitis in children and adults: a systematic review and consensus recommendations for diagnosis and treatment. Gastroenterology. 2007;133(4):1342–63.
35. Dellon ES, Gibbs WB, Rubinas TC, et al. Esophageal dilation in eosinophilic esophagitis: safety and predictors of clinical response and complications. Gastrointest Endosc. 2010;71(4):706–12.
36. Attwood SE, Lewis CJ, Bronder CS, Morris CD, Armstrong GR, Whittam J. Eosinophilic oesophagitis: a novel treatment using Montelukast. Gut. 2003;52(2):181–5.
37. Straumann A, Conus S, Grzonka P, et al. Anti-interleukin-5 antibody treatment (mepolizumab) in active eosinophilic oesophagitis: a randomized, placebo-controlled, double-blind trial. Gut. 2010;59(1):21–30.

Chapter 31
Eosinophilic Esophagitis: Treatment Approach in Children

Jonathan E. Markowitz and Chris A. Liacouras

Keywords Eosinophilic esophagitis • Gastroesophageal reflux • Dysphagia • Food intolerance

Introduction

Over the past 20 years, eosinophilic esophagitis (EoE) has become one of the most discussed diseases among pediatric gastroenterologists and allergists in the United States. According to a consensus statement drafted by a multidisciplinary working group, EoE is a clinicopathological disease characterized by symptoms such as gastroesophageal reflux, dysphagia, or feeding intolerance (although not limited to these) in the presence of at least 15 eosinophils seen per microscopic high powered field in at least one biopsy specimen taken from the esophagus, without another identifiable etiology [1]. Likely owing to a combination of increased awareness among physicians and an increasing incidence among the population, EoE is now one of the most important chronic gastrointestinal diseases to affect children. Yet, despite the increased attention paid to this problem, there remains considerable debate as to the optimal way to diagnose and treat the disorder. This chapter will discuss the various potential approaches to diagnosing and treating EoE with regard to the latest information on the subject.

J.E. Markowitz (✉)
Department of Pediatrics, Pediatric Gastroenterology and Nutrition,
Greenville Hospital System University Medical Center,
200 Patewood Drive, Suite A-140, Greenville, SC 29615, USA
e-mail: JMarkowitz@ghs.org

C.A. Liacouras and J.E. Markowitz (eds.), *Eosinophilic Esophagitis*,
Clinical Gastroenterology, DOI 10.1007/978-1-60761-515-6_31,

Diagnosis

Although it may seem self-evident, the single most important aspect in devising a treatment strategy for EoE is ensuring that the diagnosis is correct. In many circumstances, diagnosing EoE in a pediatric patient is relatively straightforward. However, there exist some important, but subtle guidelines to confirming the diagnosis that when not followed may leave the diagnosis in doubt.

The gold standard for the diagnosis of EoE is endoscopy with biopsy. Without the demonstration of increased numbers of esophageal eosinophils, the diagnosis cannot be confirmed. However, as mentioned previously, EoE is a clinicopathologic diagnosis; the absence of appropriate clinical and histopathologic findings should immediately raise concern over alternative diagnoses. In the pediatric patient, the clinical findings tend to be more variable than those currently reported in adults. While adult patients with EoE most commonly present with dysphagia, esophageal narrowing, and food impaction [2], children with EoE may present with a wide array of complaints [3]. The youngest patients with EoE may manifest only nonspecific symptoms such as irritability, feeding refusal, or regurgitation. As the age at presentation increases, symptoms tend to include complaints of abdominal pain, gastroesophageal reflux, vomiting, and dysphagia. Food impaction is less common in children than adults, and when seen is typically present in teenagers. It should be noted that all of these symptoms are also commonly seen in children with uncontrolled acid reflux.

Early studies of EoE tended to differentiate gastroesophageal reflux disease (GERD) from EoE by measures such as pH-metry [4]. Early dogma was that the presence of a significant amount of reflux on a pH study was inconsistent with a diagnosis of EoE. Today, the co-existence of EoE and GERD remains a point of contention among experts. Historically, the presence of eosinophils in the esophagus was felt to be an indicator of GERD, although the reports that first suggested this association usually detailed relatively low eosinophilic density in the esophagus compared to the typical EoE patient [5]. Later, retrospective analysis demonstrated that density of eosinophils in the esophagus predicted response to acid suppression [6]. Patients with low levels of eosinophils in the esophagus were most likely to respond and those with the highest levels unlikely. Patients with moderate eosinophil levels tended to respond but relapse.

However, clinical experience reveals that separation of EoE and GERD is not so clearcut. Case reports have detailed patients with extremely high density of esophageal eosinophils that have had resolution of symptoms and eosinophilia on acid suppression alone [7, 8]. Today, some suggest there are two forms of EoE – those patients who respond to acid suppression and those who are nonresponsive. This dichotomy is problematic from a diagnostic standpoint as it could be argued that EoE responsive to acid suppression would better be characterized as eosinophilic GERD, or reflux esophagitis with a predominance of eosinophils. The importance of this characterization derives from choosing the appropriate treatment for the disorder. And, although one cannot necessarily define a disease by its response to therapy, the exclusion of another identifiable cause of esophageal eosinophilia remains an important aspect in making the diagnosis. As such, if acid suppression results in improvement in the eosinophilia without other intervention, one could argue the correct diagnosis is truly acid reflux and not EoE. Aside from reflux, other causes of esophageal eosinophilia include hypereosinophilic syndrome, eosinophilic gastroenteritis, inflammatory bowel disease, and parasitic infection. The presence of any of these diagnoses would also exclude EoE.

With this particular conflict in mind, it is optimal to treat a child with suspected EoE with acid suppression prior to the definitive diagnostic test of endoscopy with esophageal biopsy. It is potentially problematic that there is no definitive guideline for the type of acid suppression, dose, or duration that should be employed prior to endoscopy. Intuitively, aggressive acid suppression with a proton-pump inhibitor would provide the most definitive evidence of response or lack of it. Several PPIs are FDA-approved for children aged 1 and above with dosing guidelines based on weight, allowing for a reasonable standardization of dosing. Subsequently, the presence of a high density of esophageal eosinophils (15 or more per microscopic high powered field), after a reasonable treatment course of acid suppression, coupled with ongoing clinical symptoms, is necessary to make the diagnosis of EoE. Endoscopic findings of EoE such as mucosal furrowing, rings, or white plaques increase the suspicion of EoE, but none of these are entirely specific to the disorder [3]. In rare cases, circumstances exist where endoscopy may not be able to be delayed long enough to allow for a course of acid suppression. In particular, patients with food impaction, severe dysphagia or significant weight loss and a narrowed esophagus may warrant emergent or urgent endoscopy. In those circumstances, while a presumptive diagnosis of EoE can be made, a definitive diagnosis should be reserved until GERD can be reasonably excluded as a potential etiology. This can be facilitated with pH-metry and/or impedance analysis, which allows for earlier assessment of the presence of acid reflux; however, reflux and eosinophilic esophagitis can co-exist in some patients. Longitudinal follow-up of these patients remains the best way to determine the actual etiology of their findings.

Initial Management

The initial management of the patient with EoE depends on a number of factors including the severity of symptoms, medical resources available to the patient and providers, the experience and preference of the treating physician, and the motivation and financial resources of the patient and their family. Among the most commonly utilized treatments are steroids (both systemic and topical), dietary elimination (empiric or directed based on allergy testing), and elemental diet. In addition, PPI therapy, while not a primary therapy for EoE, is often utilized as a concomitant therapy because of secondary reflux symptoms due to an abnormally functioning esophagus. Each treatment choice has potential benefits and can be justified based on the available published experience. Likewise, each has its liabilities.

Corticosteroids

Systemic corticosteroids have been previously shown to be effective in treating several allergic disorders associated with increased eosinophils, including asthma, eczema, and eosinophilic gastroenteritis [9–11]. In patients with EoE, several reports have demonstrated a rapid and complete improvement in symptoms and histology when they are treated with oral steroids such as prednisone and methylprednisolone [3, 12]. The advantages of systemic steroids include ease of administration, rapid onset of response, and very high response rate. However, the toxicities relating to prolonged steroid use are well documented, and the high relapse rate of EoE after this treatment is discontinued limit the utility of oral steroids as a maintenance therapy. Presently, systemic steroids should be reserved for isolated cases such as patients who have esophageal strictures or small caliber esophagus causing significant dysphagia, food impaction, weight loss, or severe swallowing problems that require a rapid treatment response prior to other treatments being instituted.

Topical corticosteroids were first suggested as a potential treatment for EoE a few years after systemic steroids were demonstrated to be effective [13]. The first trials of topical steroids utilized aerosolized forms of steroids originally developed for inhalation as a treatment for asthma. These aerosolized preparations were swallowed rather than inhaled, in an effort to coat the surface of the esophagus and limit their systemic exposure. Utilization of budesonide in some preparations further reduced the likelihood of systemic side effects, owing to rapid first-pass hepatic metabolism [14, 15]. The use of topical steroids proved to be successful in reducing symptoms as well as eosinophilic inflammation. However, as seen with systemic steroid therapy, the effect of topical steroids has been shown to be limited as symptoms and esophageal eosinophilia almost always recur when the medication is weaned or discontinued. Although significant side effects of topical steroids have yet to be reported, esophageal candidiasis has been seen in a proportion of patients who receive this therapy [16]. In addition, some have raised concerns about growth, changes in the hypothalamic–pituitary–adrenal axis and bone density, but these abnormalities have yet to be demonstrated. Because of the currently reported minimal risk of systemic side effects, many advocate ongoing treatment with topical steroids, while others suggest intermittent treatment. To date, there is no maintenance method that has been proven to be most effective. It also remains to be seen whether this therapeutic approach reduces esophageal inflammation enough to prevent long-term complications such as fibrotic changes in the esophagus.

An alternative approach to aerosolized topical steroids, budesonide, such as would be used in a nebulizer, has been made into a viscous solution for ingestion [17]. Viscous budesonide exhibits an effect similar to that seen with the swallowed aerosolized steroid. The side effects are similar and the risk of systemic effects should also be comparable. A recent trial of this preparation in children with EoE has been ongoing and has had encouraging results [18]. At this point, it appears that effectiveness of both forms of topical steroid therapy are similar and that selection should depend on a discussion between the physician, the patient, and his or her family.

Dietary Therapy

From the time that EoE was first recognized, it was strongly suggested that it was an allergic disease. The original case series that demonstrated improvement in esophagitis on an elemental diet laid the groundwork for using restriction of food antigens as a treatment for EoE [19]. In that series, patients not only responded to an elemental diet, but they also developed a recurrence of symptoms when they were re-exposed to the offending foods. Subsequent studies have confirmed that restriction of food antigens can result in both a significant symptomatic and histologic improvement of EoE. While there is little debate on these points, the difficulty lies in how best to determine which and how many food antigens are causing the clinical symptoms and esophageal eosinophilia.

Elemental Diet

Among all of the methods for restricting foods from the diet, the administration of an elemental diet utilizing a strict amino acid-based formula has shown the highest response rate both clinically and histologically. Multiple reports have demonstrated that greater than 95% of patients respond both clinically and histologically to the introduction of an elemental diet [3, 20]. Reports suggest that symptom resolution may occur as quickly as within the first week of starting the diet. Follow up biopsies, 1 month after starting treatment, show essentially complete resolution of eosinophilia in many cases. Of the commonly accepted treatments for EoE, treatment with elemental diet can be considered the most efficacious. However, the effectiveness of the diet, meaning the utility in real-world situations rather than controlled trials, may be limited because of several logistical issues associated with this treatment.

The greatest limitation to the use of an elemental diet is palatability. In general, the more elemental the protein source in a formula, the more unpalatable it tends to be. Further adding to the poor taste is the presence of a high proportion of MCT oil and lack of sweet-tasting sugars. When introduced early in life, children commonly adjust to the taste of elemental formulas; however, the initiation of these formulas in a child or adolescent who is already used to a more normal diet is often a difficult proposition. At 30 kcal/oz, the elemental formulas designed for use in children over 1 year of age require relatively large volumes over the course of a day to provide adequate nutrition. A minimum of 1 L of formula is commonly administered in the smallest of children, while older children and adolescents may need 2 or more liters of formula per day. In many cases, children are unable to drink this volume of formula, necessitating enteral tube feeding via nasogastric tubes or a surgically or endoscopically placed gastrostomy tube.

Another problem is that the cost of elemental formulas tends to be higher than intact protein formulas or hydrolyzed protein formulas. The cost takes on more importance because it is common for medical insurers to exclude formula from their basic coverage, thus, leading to significant out-of-pocket expenditure for the family. Emotional costs also exist because of quality-of-life issues. Using a strict elemental diet not only removes individuals from the social aspects of eating but also impacts the rest of the family who may be asked to alter their diet in support of the patient.

It is important that those who attempt to use an elemental diet receive close observation to ensure that their nutritional needs are being met. This includes total calories as well as macro- and micronutrients. Nutritional deficiencies have been recognized in children on exclusive elemental diets for prolonged periods [21]. It is advisable that a pediatric dietitian or nutritionist or a physician with expertise in nutritional management oversee the administration of elemental diet in order to minimize the risks of this form of treatment. These patients may also need the support of social work, case management, psychology, and feeding specialists.

Dietary Restriction

Despite the high success rate of elemental diets in patients with EoE, there are numerous advantages to being able to eat an intact protein diet. Choosing which foods to restrict from the diet can be difficult, yet choosing correctly is vital to the success of this approach. The decision on how to restrict the diet also depends on the resources available to the patient. The two most common approaches to dietary restriction are an empiric diet (based on the removal of the most common problematic food antigens) and a directed diet (based on the results of allergy testing).

Empiric food elimination of the most common causative foods has been shown to be an effective approach in children. In 2006, Kagalwalla compared the clinical and histological response of a six-food elimination diet (SFED) that restricted cow's milk, soy protein, peanut, wheat, egg, and shellfish to another cohort of EoE patients who received an elemental diet [22]. Seventy-four percent of the SFED group showed a histologic response after a minimum of 6 weeks of treatment, with peak eosinophil count dropping from about 80 eosinophils per high power field to 13. While these results were favorable, those who received an elemental diet over that time period showed a more complete histologic response.

Meanwhile, directed dietary therapy has also been shown to be successful. As mentioned in previous chapters, while the exact type of allergic response in patients with EoE is unknown, allergy testing may still be beneficial. Often patients with EoE have reactions to multiple foods. Spergel demonstrated that many patients with EoE manifest evidence of both immediate-type (IgE-mediated) and delayed-type (T-cell mediated) allergy [23]. Traditional skin prick testing provides evidence of IgE-mediated food allergy while atopy patch testing may provide supplemental data on delayed-type hypersensitivity reactions to foods. When utilized together, the sensitivity of these forms of testing tend to be high, but the specificity is variable. These tests increase the likelihood that specific dietary elimination will be successful, however, false positives and false negatives frequently occur. When utilized, the elimination of foods identified by testing is usually employed for a minimum of

4–6 weeks, followed by EGD to confirm a histologic response. While clinical improvement may take place within the first few weeks of food elimination, it remains critical to re-evaluate the mucosal response with biopsy in both clinical responders and nonresponders. It is not uncommon for symptoms to wax and wane even when inflammatory activity remains constant. Further, because many symptoms of EoE are not specific to this disorder, it is important to confirm that ongoing symptoms are truly due to ongoing eosinophilic inflammation and not another cause such as acid reflux.

As with elemental diet, it is highly advisable to have a dietitian available to the family that undertakes any dietary therapy, whether directed by allergy testing or empiric therapy. Just like the use of elemental formulas, restrictive diets put patients at risk for macro- and micro-nutrient deficiencies [24, 25]. Additionally, the ubiquitous nature of certain types of food antigens such as wheat, soy, and cow's milk make complete elimination extremely difficult. A skilled dietitian who has experience counseling patients and their families on recognizing food antigens in ingredient lists can greatly help to prevent inadequate response due to inadvertent exposure to foods. Further support for patients can be provided through organizations such as the Food Allergy and Anaphylaxis Network (FAAN) and the American Partnership for Eosinophilic Disorders (APFED).

Suggested Approach to the Pediatric Patient with Eosinophilic Esophagitis

Despite the growing experience with EoE over the past 15 or more years, there remains debate as to the best approach to the newly diagnosed patient. In some chronic disorders such as inflammatory bowel disease, the treatment approach is based on a "pyramid" where initial treatment is given to most patients and subsequent treatments are given to those with persistent disease activity [25]. In this model, initial treatment usually is considered the safest, while each subsequent treatment offers the prospect for improved effectiveness but also may include increased risk of side effects. In EoE, the approach to treatment is more varied, following more of a "hopscotch" game where there is no definitive starting point and patients may "skip" over certain treatments in lieu of others. The lack of a consistent and sequential treatment strategy stems not only from a lack of head to head trials of treatments but also relates to differences in the resources available in different areas of the country. With this in mind, we suggest a treatment guideline similar to that suggested in Fig. 30.3.

EGD with biopsy is the only standard with which the diagnosis of EoE can be made. Wherever possible, EGD should be delayed until an adequate trial of acid suppression can be given. A minimum of 4 weeks of therapy with a PPI given at high dose is optimal. In children, many experts in EoE suggest using twice daily dosing of a PPI, at a dose up to 1 mg/kg/dose, to a maximal adult dose. Ongoing clinical symptoms coupled with significant isolated esophageal eosinophilia of greater than 15 or more eosinophils per microscopic high powered field (400×)

without significant eosinophilia in other areas of the GI tract is sufficient for the diagnosis of EoE. In circumstances where the EGD is performed prior to an adequate trial of acid blockade above, it would be advisable to evaluate for significant acid reflux as a potential cause of the esophageal eosinophilia. This can be accomplished by pH-metry with or without impedance analysis, or by subsequent trial of acid blockade and re-evaluation of the esophageal mucosa.

Following a diagnosis of EoE, either dietary restriction/elimination or the use of topical steroids should be instituted. In certain circumstances, such as a significant small caliber esophagus or multiple food impactions a more aggressive initial treatment approach, such as systemic steroids or esophageal dilatation may be needed. Often, the therapeutic choice is made depending on the resources of the physician and after a discussion with the patient and family. When considering the use of diet restriction/elimination, in cases where allergy testing does not reveal any potential foods for removal, or where the dietary restrictions prove too difficult for the family to maintain, topical steroid therapy should be considered. Alternatively, in patients who are unable to comply with using topical steroids, dietary restrictions should be considered. During any therapy, a repeat EGD is recommended (minimum 4–6 weeks later) to document resolution of inflammation. As mentioned previously, close follow-up is required regardless of treatment choice. When using dietary restrictions, one must make sure that adequate nutrition is supplied and that growth is maintained. When using steroids, medication side effects and growth also require monitoring. After the initiation of therapy, we advise that acid suppression be maintained throughout the treatment process until a final course of therapy has been chosen.

With regard to topical steroid therapy, initial dosing is usually twice daily. The duration of treatment with topical steroids remains unclear, but it is widely believed that disease almost always relapses upon discontinuation of treatment. Most EoE experts advocate decreasing the dosing schedule once symptoms are controlled and inflammation improves. Topical steroid therapy should be maintained as long as is necessary to maintain a symptomatic remission. Some will choose to discontinue therapy periodically, with a plan to restart treatment once symptoms re-emerge. A repeat EGD is recommended after medication changes (minimum 4–6 weeks) to document resolution of inflammation. Presently, it remains unclear what degree of eosinophilia presents a risk for long-term complications such as esophageal fibrosis and stricture formation but generally it is felt that lower numbers of eosinophils are better.

With regard to dietary elimination, once remission is achieved with dietary therapy, food challenges with restricted foods can be started. Symptom relapse following introduction of a previously restricted food is adequate to define failure on reintroduction, but lack of symptoms does not ensure that disease has not relapsed. After the introduction of one or a small group of foods, an endoscopy should be performed to confirm that there has not been a subclinical relapse. The number of foods to be introduced before endoscopy is a matter of choice. Endoscopy between each food introduction is the most definitive way to evaluate each food, but is costly and results in cumulatively more risk, albeit small. However, the more foods introduced between each endoscopy introduce less certainty as to which food or foods are responsible if a relapse is found. As a guideline, it is reasonable to introduce a few lower-risk foods at a time between endoscopy, while performing endoscopy between single food introductions of higher-risk or foods that are more of a staple of the typical diet, such as egg, milk, and wheat.

Summary

Eosinophilic esophagitis presents challenges to the patient, family, and treating physician. While there are several effective treatments available, each is accompanied by particular drawbacks. In choosing a treatment, one must consider the severity of symptoms, the resources available to the treatment team, and the quality-of life-impact that treatment will have on the patient and the family. In the future, head-to-head evaluations of the treatments may provide better information as to the best approach. For now, it is advisable for the treating physician to be familiar and comfortable with all of the available treatments and tailor therapy to the individual patient.

References

1. Furuta GT, Liacouras CA, Collins MH, Gupta SK, Justinich C, Putnam PE, et al. Eosinophilic esophagitis in children and adults: a systematic review and consensus recommendations for diagnosis and treatment. Gastroenterology. 2007;133:1342–63.
2. Prasad GA, Alexander JA, Schleck CD, Zinsmeister AR, Smyrk TC, Elias RM, et al. Epidemiology of eosinophilic esophagitis over three decades in Olmsted County, Minnesota. Clin Gastroenterol Hepatol. 2009;7:1055–61.
3. Liacouras CA, Spergel JM, Ruchelli E, Verma R, Mascarenhas M, Semeao E, et al. Eosinophilic esophagitis: a 10-year experience in 381 children. Clin Gastroenterol Hepatol. 2005;3:1198–206.
4. Liacouras CA. Eosinophilic esophagitis in children and adults. J Pediatr Gastroenterol Nutr. 2003;37 Suppl 1:S23–8.
5. Winter HS, Madara JL, Stafford RJ, Grand RJ, Quinlan JE, Goldman H. Intraepithelial eosinophils: a new diagnostic criterion for reflux esophagitis. Gastroenterology. 1982;83:818–23.
6. Ruchelli E, Wenner W, Voytek T, Brown K, Liacouras C. Severity of esophageal eosinophilia predicts response to conventional gastroesophageal reflux therapy. Pediatr Dev Pathol. 1999;2:15–8.
7. Molina-Infante J, Ferrando-Lamana L, Ripoll C, Hernandez-Alonso M, Mateos JM, Fernandez-Bermejo M, et al. Esophageal eosinophilic infiltration responds to proton pump inhibition in most adults. Clin Gastroenterol Hepatol. 2011;9(2):110–7.
8. Ngo P, Furuta GT, Antonioli DA, Fox VL. Eosinophils in the esophagus–peptic or allergic eosinophilic esophagitis? Case series of three patients with esophageal eosinophilia. Am J Gastroenterol. 2006;101:1666–70.
9. Markowitz JE, Russo P, Liacouras CA. Solitary duodenal ulcer: a new presentation of eosinophilic gastroenteritis. Gastrointest Endosc. 2000;52:673–6.
10. Park HS, Kim HS, Jang HJ. Eosinophilic gastroenteritis associated with food allergy and bronchial asthma. J Korean Med Sci. 1995;10:216–9.

11. Redondo-Cerezo E, Cabello MJ, Gonzalez Y, Gomez M, Garcia-Montero M, de Teresa J. Eosinophilic gastroenteritis: our recent experience: one-year experience of atypical onset of an uncommon disease. Scand J Gastroenterol. 2001;36:1358–60.
12. Liacouras CA, Wenner WJ, Brown K, Ruchelli E. Primary eosinophilic esophagitis in children: successful treatment with oral corticosteroids. J Pediatr Gastroenterol Nutr. 1998;26:380–5.
13. Faubion Jr WA, Perrault J, Burgart LJ, Zein NN, Clawson M, Freese DK. Treatment of eosinophilic esophagitis with inhaled corticosteroids. J Pediatr Gastroenterol Nutr. 1998;27:90–3.
14. Aceves SS, Bastian JF, Newbury RO, Dohil R. Oral viscous budesonide: a potential new therapy for eosinophilic esophagitis in children. Am J Gastroenterol. 2007;102:2271–9. quiz 80.
15. Aceves SS, Dohil R, Newbury RO, Bastian JF. Topical viscous budesonide suspension for treatment of eosinophilic esophagitis. J Allergy Clin Immunol. 2005;116:705–6.
16. Teitelbaum JE, Fox VL, Twarog FJ, Nurko S, Antonioli D, Gleich G, et al. Eosinophilic esophagitis in children: immunopathological analysis and response to fluticasone propionate. Gastroenterology. 2002;122:1216–25.
17. Aceves SS, Newbury RO, Chen D, Mueller J, Dohil R, Hoffman H, et al. Resolution of remodeling in eosinophilic esophagitis correlates with epithelial response to topical corticosteroids. Allergy. 2010;65:109–16.
18. Dohil R, Newbury R, Fox L, Bastian J, Aceves S. Oral viscous budesonide is effective in children with eosinophilic esophagitis in a randomized, placebo-controlled trial. Gastroenterology. 2010;139:418–29.
19. Kelly KJ, Lazenby AJ, Rowe PC, Yardley JH, Perman JA, Sampson HA. Eosinophilic esophagitis attributed to gastroesophageal reflux: improvement with an amino acid-based formula. Gastroenterology. 1995;109:1503–12.
20. Markowitz JE, Spergel JM, Ruchelli E, Liacouras CA. Elemental diet is an effective treatment for eosinophilic esophagitis in children and adolescents. Am J Gastroenterol. 2003;98:777–82.
21. Jones M, Campbell KA, Duggan C, Young G, Bousvaros A, Higgins L, et al. Multiple micronutrient deficiencies in a child fed an elemental formula. J Pediatr Gastroenterol Nutr. 2001;33:602–5.
22. Kagalwalla AF, Sentongo TA, Ritz S, Hess T, Nelson SP, Emerick KM, et al. Effect of six-food elimination diet on clinical and histologic outcomes in eosinophilic esophagitis. Clin Gastroenterol Hepatol. 2006;4:1097–102.
23. Spergel JM, Beausoleil JL, Mascarenhas M, Liacouras CA. The use of skin prick tests and patch tests to identify causative foods in eosinophilic esophagitis. J Allergy Clin Immunol. 2002;109:363–8.
24. Noimark L, Cox HE. Nutritional problems related to food allergy in childhood. Pediatr Allergy Immunol. 2008;19:188–95.
25. Hanauer SB. Clinical perspectives in Crohn's disease. Turning traditional treatment strategies on their heads: current evidence for "step-up" versus "top-down". Rev Gastroenterol Disord. 2007;7 Suppl 2:S17–22.

Index

C.A. Liacouras and J.E. Markowitz (eds.), *Eosinophilic Esophagitis*, Clinical Gastroenterology, DOI 10.1007/978-1-60761-515-6,

D

E